Genetic Improvement of Farmed Animals

Genetic Improvement of Farmed Animals

Geoff Simm

University of Edinburgh, UK

Geoff Pollott

Royal Veterinary College, London, UK

Raphael Mrode

Scotland's Rural College, Edinburgh, UK

and

International Livestock Research Institute, Nairobi, Kenya

Ross Houston

The Roslin Institute, University of Edinburgh, UK

Karen Marshall

International Livestock Research Institute, Nairobi, Kenya

CABI

CABI is a trading name of CAB International

CABI
Nosworthy Way
Wallingford
Oxfordshire OX10 8DE
UK

Tel: +44 (0)1491 832111
Fax: +44 (0)1491 833508
E-mail: info@cabi.org
Website: www.cabi.org

CABI
745 Atlantic Avenue
8th Floor
Boston, MA 02111
USA

Tel: +1 (617)682-9015
E-mail: cabi-nao@cabi.org

References to Internet websites (URLs) were accurate at the time of writing.

A catalogue record for this book is available from the British Library, London, UK.

Library of Congress Cataloging-in-Publication Data

Names: Simm, Geoff, 1959- author. | Pollott, Geoffrey, author. | Mrode, R. A., author. | Houston, Ross, author. | Marshall, Karen, author.
Title: Genetic improvement of farmed animals / Geoff Simm, Global Academy of Agriculture and Food Security, University of Edinburgh, UK, Geoff Pollott, Royal Veterinary College, London, UK, Raphael Mrode, Scotland's Rural College, Edinburgh, UK, and International Livestock Research Institute, Nairobi, Kenya, Ross Houston, The Roslin Institute, University of Edinburgh, UK, Karen Marshall, International Livestock Research Institute, Nairobi, Kenya.
Description: Wallingford, Oxfordshire, UK ; Boston, MA : CABI, [2020] | Includes bibliographical references and index. | Summary: "Comprehensive, yet concise and approachable, Genetic Improvement of Farmed Animals provides a thorough grounding in the basic sciences underpinning current farmed animal breeding practice. The text relates science to practical application in all the major farmed animal species: cattle, sheep, goats, poultry, pigs and fish"--Provided by publisher.
Identifiers: LCCN 2019054983 (print) | LCCN 2019054984 (ebook) | ISBN 9781789241723 (hardback) | ISBN 9781789241716 (paperback) | ISBN 9781789241730 (ebook) | ISBN 9781789241747 (epub)
Subjects: LCSH: Livestock--Genetic engineering. | Livestock improvement.
Classification: LCC SF756.5 .S56 2020 (print) | LCC SF756.5 (ebook) | DDC 636.08/21--dc23
LC record available at https://lccn.loc.gov/2019054983
LC ebook record available at https://lccn.loc.gov/2019054984

ISBN-13: 9781789241723 (hardback)
9781789241716 (paperback)
9781789241730 (ePDF)
9781789241747 (ePub)

Commissioning Editor: Alexandra Lainsbury
Editorial Assistant: Lauren Davies
Production Editor: Tim Kapp

Typeset by SPi, Pondicherry, India

Contents

The online resources referred to in the text can be found at: www.cabi.org/openresources/41723

Foreword

Animal breeding has a long history, probably as long as domestication itself. Well before the current knowledge of genetics, people understood the importance of choosing the best animals to become parents and of avoiding unhealthy and aggressive animals. Darwin was fully aware of the achievements of animal breeders and used breeding of fancy pigeons as an analogy of natural selection. He even started breeding and crossing pigeons himself in his garden. It is also clear that breeding, moving hand-in-hand with major changes in both feeding and management, especially in the past half century or so, has had an enormous impact on animal production, leading to higher production efficiency and lower prices for the consumer.

Although the principles of breeding are easy to grasp, modern animal breeding methodology is anything but. For most important traits, there is continuous variation among animals and they generally do not fall into a few easily separated classes. Even if they do, for example, healthy and sick animals, the underlying reason is normally not a single malfunctioning gene. It is increasingly clear that most traits are affected by many genes and also by environmental factors. The task is no longer selecting the best animals to become parents, based on their own performance, but selecting as parents those animals that give the best progeny.

To resolve this, we need to collect large amounts of data on phenotypes and sometimes genotypes of farmed animal populations. To utilize these data sets we require sophisticated statistical methods, combined with well-designed software and substantial computing power. This makes learning animal breeding difficult for students, and also difficult for teachers, I might add. Although the underlying theory and methods are the same for all species, the structure of the industry and the animal populations, economic conditions, biological constraints and actual applications differ markedly between farmed animal species. Learning the theory without connecting it to real-life situations is not a recipe for success, especially not within agricultural sciences.

Therefore, it is with great pleasure I welcome the book on *Genetic Improvement of Farmed Animals*, by Geoff Simm, Geoff Pollott, Raphael Mrode, Ross Houston and Karen Marshall. This is an extensively updated and expanded edition of the previous book by Simm, which focused on cattle and sheep. Now there are completely new sections on poultry, pig, aquaculture and goat breeding. There is also new information on estimation of genetic variation and methods for phenotype recording, and chapters have been updated with the latest knowledge related to genomic evaluations. The book ends with an interesting discussion of the sustainability dimension of livestock production. So, in short, I am convinced that this book will make the lives of teachers and their students much easier!

Erling Strandberg
Professor of Animal Breeding and Genetics
Swedish University of Agricultural Sciences, Uppsala

Preface

For over 10,000 years the fortunes of the human race have been closely intertwined with the husbandry of livestock. For much of this time, whether knowingly or unknowingly, livestock have been changed genetically by subjective means. Some of the scientific foundations for more objective genetic improvement methods were laid over 120 years ago, and others followed from the 1900s to the 1930s. However, it is only over the past 70 years or so that these have been applied to any great extent in livestock improvement. These objective methods are based on measurement of performance in economically important traits. To date they have been used most widely in pig, poultry and dairy cattle breeding, and to a lesser extent in beef cattle, sheep, goat and fish breeding. They have been used widely in industrialized countries, and much less so in lower-income countries.

In those parts of the world where it has been used effectively, genetic improvement of farmed animals has contributed to increasing the availability and affordability of highly nutritious food, and so to food security, and it has improved resource-use efficiency per unit of product. However, some applications have had a negative impact on animal health and welfare, and others have led to erosion of genetic resources. Also, the availability of relatively cheap livestock products, partly as a result of genetic improvement, is a major driver of the so-called 'livestock revolution' – the rapid growth in global demand for livestock products, which exacerbates the environmental impact of our food systems. The wider use of existing scientific methods in animal breeding, and the development of new and more sustainable ones, could help to meet the challenge of feeding well the dramatically increased human population over the next few generations. We hope that the book will help to equip and inspire future generations of students, researchers and practitioners to rise to these massive challenges, and develop even more sustainable livestock breeding practices in future.

The book is based on *Genetic Improvement of Cattle and Sheep* by Geoff Simm, first published in 1998 by Farming Press, and the 2000 reprint with amendments, subsequently published by CABI. There have been many developments in animal genetics since then, which we describe here. We have also expanded the species coverage of the book and included applications in both developed and developing countries.

The first chapter in the book sets the scene for modern livestock breeding, by looking at the origins and rôles of today's livestock breeds. The next four chapters deal with the scientific principles of livestock improvement. Chapter 2 outlines some of the basic principles in genetics and attempts to illustrate the link between genes and the performance of individual farm animals, or populations of them. In Chapter 3 the main strategies for genetic improvement are discussed. The factors which affect responses to within-breed selection, and some of the tools and technologies used, especially for more effective within-breed selection, are discussed in Chapters 4 and 5. Chapter 6 explores in more depth how we analyse variation in farm animals. Chapter 7 discusses approaches to predicting breeding values. Chapters 8 to 13 deal with the application of these principles in practical breeding programmes in dairy cattle, beef cattle, sheep and goats, poultry, pigs and aquaculture. Finally, Chapter 14 discusses some of the key societal, technical and ethical challenges facing farm animal production in general, and animal breeding and genetics in particular. It discusses how livestock breeders, scientists and others might respond to ensure wide societal and animal benefits from future breeding schemes. There is a glossary of technical terms at the end of the book. These terms are given in italics in the text when first mentioned.

The fairly wide use of statistics in modern methods of animal breeding is often off-putting to both students and practitioners. We have tried to keep the use of statistics to a minimum, but a little understanding of some of the basics goes a long way. So, some statistical methods are described, but little or no prior knowledge is assumed. New techniques from molecular biology are having a major impact in animal breeding. But, here too, there is a risk that the technology and language could widen the gulf between developer and user. We have tried to outline the current and potential applications and value of these techniques without going into too much detail on the molecular methods themselves. If parts of some chapters are too detailed, the summaries at the end of each chapter should provide enough information to allow readers to move on to the next chapter.

We have tried to illustrate as many of the principles of animal breeding as possible by the use of practical examples. For reasons of convenience and familiarity, many of these examples are from work done by us and our colleagues, but there are many other examples in the scientific literature which are just as relevant. To keep the book as readable as possible, we have kept direct references to published work to a minimum. The full list of sources appears at the end of each chapter. Where possible we have tried to use recent reviews of a subject area, rather than individual papers. If you want to know more about a subject, these reviews are a good place to start. Also, we have listed examples of recommended reading at the end of the chapters.

Happy reading!

Acknowledgements

The book is based on *Genetic Improvement of Cattle and Sheep* by Geoff Simm, first published in 1998 by Farming Press, and the 2000 reprint with amendments, subsequently published by CABI. We repeat our heartfelt thanks here to the very many colleagues that contributed to the earlier text, and who are acknowledged individually there.

We thank Professor Erling Strandberg of SLU, Sweden for generously providing the Foreword to this book.

We are very grateful to Dr Santiago Avendaño of Aviagen Group and Prof Dr Rudolf Preisinger, Chief Technical Officer – Layers, of the EW GROUP GmbH for their advice on Chapter 11. Likewise, we thank Dr Grant Walling and Stephen Waite of JSR Genetics and Dr Pieter Knap of Genus PLC for their advice on Chapter 12.

We also thank the following colleagues for allowing us to use their excellent photos in the book: Professor Peter Amer (Abacus Bio, NZ); Professor Alan Archibald, Norman Russell, Dr Christine Tait-Burkard and Professor Ian Wilmut (all Roslin Institute, UK); Dr Sandra Eady (CSIRO, Armidale, Australia); Carey Coombs; Richard Fuller; Dr Kreg Leymaster (formerly United States Department of Agriculture (USDA) Meat Animal Research Center, Clay Center, Nebraska); Professor John Robinson (formerly Scotland's Rural College; SRUC); Royal Agricultural Society of England; Dr Gary Snowder (formerly USDA, Idaho); Professor Dave Thomas (formerly of University of Wisconsin, Madison, USA); Dr Grant Walling (JSR Genetics); Dr Alison Van Eenennaam (University of California, Davis, USA); Tim White and Dr Mark Young. Marianne Farish (SRUC), Dr Alastair Hamilton (Hendrix Genetics), and the International Livestock Research Institute very kindly provided cover photos.

We thank the many colleagues who kindly gave us access to their unpublished data, or helped by producing data, figures, etc. for examples – they are credited in the tables and figures concerned. We also thank the many authors and publishers who kindly gave their permission to reproduce direct or amended versions of their material, or to reproduce material for which they are copyright holders. These original sources are noted in the table or figure captions concerned, and full details are given in the reference list at the end of each chapter.

Table 2.6 is reproduced with permission from Wiley, ©Malcolm B Willis 1991. We thank the US Congress, Office of Technology Assessment and US Department of Energy for the use of Figs 2.5 and 2.6, and USDA for multiple tables and figures. We thank the Biotechnology and Biological Sciences Research Council, Swindon, UK for permission to use their material in Fig. 2.7. Extracts from Veterinary Genetics by F. W. Nicholas (1996) in Chapters 2 to 4 are reproduced with permission of Oxford Publishing through PLSclear. Material from Animal Production and BSAS Occassional Publications is reproduced in Chapters 3 and 8 with the permission of the British Society of Animal Science. Table 5.2 is reproduced with the permission of the British Cattle Breeders Club. Fig. 5.11 is reproduced from Trends in Genetics Science with permission from the Licensor via PLSclear. We are grateful to Sam Boon (Agriculture and Horticulture Development Board; AHDB) for providing material for figures in Chapters 9 and 10, and to AHDB and Signet Breeding Services for their permission to reproduce this. Table 10.16 is reproduced from the Journal of Dairy Science with permission from the Licensor via PLSclear. Figure 10.22 is reproduced from Livestock Production Science with permission from the Licensor via PLSclear. We thank Dr Susanne Hermesch on behalf of the President of the Internatiuonal Committee of the World Congress on Genetics Applied to Livestock Production for permission to reproduce material in Table 10.2. The extracts from the Banner Committee Report in Chapter 14 are Crown copyright; Crown copyright is reproduced with the permission of the Controller of Her Majesty's Stationery Office.

Special thanks to Professor Mike Coffey, Abbygail Wells, Karolina Kaseja and colleagues at Edinburgh Genetic Evaluation Services (EGENES), SRUC, who assisted in generating data from the UK national dairy and Langhill databases used in many figures. In addition, valuable contributions from Marco Winters of AHDB on dairy cattle genetics in the UK are appreciated. Thanks to Toine Roozen and Valentina Palucci of the Interbull Centre, Upsalla, Sweden, for permission to reproduce material shown in Chapter 8 and providing information for Table 8.10. In addition, we wish to express our gratitude to colleagues at the various national genetic evaluation centers, especially for permission to use their data in Fig. 8.21.

We thank SRUC for their permission to reproduce many diagrams and excerpts from tables, as indicated in the text.

We also thank our employers for their support in this venture and Lyndsey Hayes and Karen Paterson for their admin support. We also thank the funders of our research and the many breeders and breeding organizations who have worked with us, for their interest and support in getting research into practice.

We are very grateful to Caroline Makepeace, Alex Lainsbury, Lauren Davies and Tim Kapp at CABI for their support in writing this book, for their patience in waiting for it, and for their editorial input.

Finally, we are all very grateful to friends and members of our families who provided support in many ways during this lengthy project.

1 The Origins and Rôles of Today's Livestock Breeds

Natural Selection and Evolution

Animals come in an incredible variety of sizes, shapes and colours. Just why this is so has occupied many great minds over the centuries. Most biologists today believe that the species which we farm, keep as pets, observe in the wild or see on our screens, and those now extinct, evolved by the process of *natural selection*. Although several 19th century naturalists and philosophers contributed ideas, Charles Darwin is usually credited with putting together a cohesive theory of natural selection in 1838. He later explained this in his book *On the Origin of Species* – or *On the Origin of Species by Means of Natural Selection, or the Preservation of Favoured Races in the Struggle for Life,* to give it its full title – first published in 1859.

The main principles of Darwin's theory of natural selection are that species can change over time, and that their survival or 'success' depends on how well they 'fit' their environment – what one of Darwin's supporters, Thomas Huxley, described as 'the survival of the fittest'. The key to this process is variation between individuals, in particular variation which is (at least partly) inherited from one generation to the next. Darwin recognized the 'many slight differences which appear in the offspring from the same parents' – it is these differences which natural selection, or breeders of domestic livestock, can act upon. Those individuals which have favourable attributes stand a higher chance of surviving and reproducing than those that do not.

This theory provides an explanation of how the huge variety of animal species, and other species, has arisen from the earliest primitive forms of life. Chance variations in the size or shape or functioning of animals, over the course of millions of years, has allowed them to adapt to particular environments, or niches. Some species have been able to adapt to and profit from major changes in the environment while others, such as the dinosaurs, have not and have become extinct. Many new species have emerged, usually as a result of physical isolation of part of a population – for example, when continents drifted apart – or due to isolation of other kinds, such as increasing dependence on a particular type of food. One of the most famous examples of natural selection comes from Darwin's visit to the Galapagos Islands. There, he noticed the wide variety in the size and shape of the beaks of different species of finches, which was related to the way in which each species obtained its food. Although Darwin's work is usually linked to evolution and natural selection of wild animals, he was well aware of, and greatly influenced by, the changes in domestic animals brought about by *artificial selection* in these species by early livestock breeders, as shown in his 1868 work *The Variation of Animals and Plants Under Domestication* (Darwin, 1868).

Darwin's theory was highly controversial at the time, but there is now overwhelming evidence, from many branches of science, that it is substantially correct. For more details of the background to Darwin's work, and developments from it, see Leakey (1986), Clutton-Brock (1987), Futuyma and Kirkpatrick (2017) and Walsh and Lynch (2018).

Domestication

Over the last 250,000 years, the human population has increased from an estimated 3 million to over 7.7 billion (Clutton-Brock, 1987; UN, 2019). During this time, the life expectancy of humans has also increased substantially. The increase in population size has occurred in four main surges. The first was stimulated when our early ancestors learned to use tools and make fire – attributes which allowed them to spread from the tropical regions in which they first evolved to inhabit colder, northern areas. The second surge (the first 'agricultural revolution') occurred about 12,000 to 10,000 years ago, when humans began to cultivate plants and domesticate

Genetic Improvement of Farmed Animals (G. Simm *et al.*)
DOI: 10.1079/9781789241723.0001

animals after the end of the last ice age. The third surge in population size began with increased industrialization. For example, in Britain the population increased from about 5.5 million to about 10.75 million in the 18th century, with a particularly rapid rise in the second half of the century (Hall and Clutton-Brock, 1989). The fourth surge in population size followed the so-called 'green revolution' in the mid-1900s, which saw the introduction of new crop varieties, chemical fertilizers and pest controls. The world's population is expected to approach 11.0 billion by the end of this century (UN, 2019). Feeding this growing population well, while protecting the natural systems on which we all depend, is one of the greatest challenges facing humanity – a topic we touch on throughout the book and return to in more detail in Chapter 14.

When humans first spread northwards, they were primarily hunters who adapted their own lifestyle to that of their prey (Clutton-Brock, 1987). Some groups, such as the Indigenous Peoples of North America following herds of bison, or Sámi people following reindeer, continued this lifestyle. Others learned to modify the behaviour of some of their prey species, and so began the process of domestication.

Of the very large number of animal species, very few have been successfully domesticated. Francis Galton (Darwin's cousin) wrote an essay on domestication in 1865, and he suggested that the process of domestication happened by trial and error. He reasoned that '..a vast number of half-unconscious attempts have been made throughout the course of ages, and that ultimately, by slow degrees, after many relapses, and continued selection, our several domestic breeds became firmly established'. Galton also identified six conditions for successful domestication of a species of animals, including their ability to breed in captivity, to cope with earlier weaning than normal, to adapt to artificial feeding and husbandry, to be reasonably placid and amenable to being herded and closely confined, and to have products valuable to our ancestors (Clutton-Brock, 1987).

Sheep and goats were probably the first of our current farm livestock species to be domesticated, about 10,000 years ago, though domestication of the dog began about 2000 years earlier. They were followed by cattle and pigs, and later still by horses. The process continues today with domestication of new species used in aquaculture. Domestication has led to many differences from the wild ancestors – either as a direct result of domestication itself, by chance, by natural selection or, directly or indirectly, as a result of artificial selection. Usually, there is a much greater diversity in appearance of the domestic strains of livestock than in their wild counterparts. In many cases the domestic strains of terrestrial livestock differ from the *wild type* in physical appearance, including a shortening of the facial region of the skull and the jaws, longer ears, longer or curling tails, differences in the size or shape of horns, differences in coat or feather colour, and a wide range in the thickness of the coat, depending on the local climate (Clutton-Brock, 1987). Most domestic species have a higher concentration of fat in their carcass than their wild ancestors (Fig. 1.1). Also, most *breeds* of domestic sheep have lost the characteristic of completely shedding wool in the summer. (In some countries where the costs of shearing are high in relation to the value of the wool, there is renewed interest in this ability to shed wool naturally. See Chapter 10 for more details.)

Modern livestock breeders are sometimes accused of producing maladapted breeds or individuals (see Chapters 8 to 13), but it is interesting to note that as long ago as 450 BC there were strains of fat-tailed sheep in Arabia with tails so long and fat that shepherds crafted small wooden trailers, harnessed to the sheep, to prevent their tails from dragging on the ground (Clutton-Brock, 1987).

The domestication of livestock species continues to be a well-researched topic with the inevitable appearance of conflicting theories. We do not intend to explore these in detail in this book, but there are several authoritative treatments of the subject. In the initial pages of their survey of the state of the world's animal genetic resources the Food and Agriculture Organization (FAO) of the United Nations (UN) (2015a, pp. 5–23) outline much of the recent work on domestication of livestock species. Needless to say, the advent of molecular genomic methods has contributed to this debate and the paper by Magee *et al.* (2014) in a whole edition of *Animal Frontiers* devoted to domestication issues is a useful source of information. Also, Bruford *et al.* (2003) and Weiner and Wilkinson (2011) put domestication into a modern genetic context. The paper by Mignon-Grasteau *et al.* (2005) approaches domestication from a resource allocation perspective, whereas Driscoll *et al.* (2009) provide an evolutionary viewpoint of domestication.

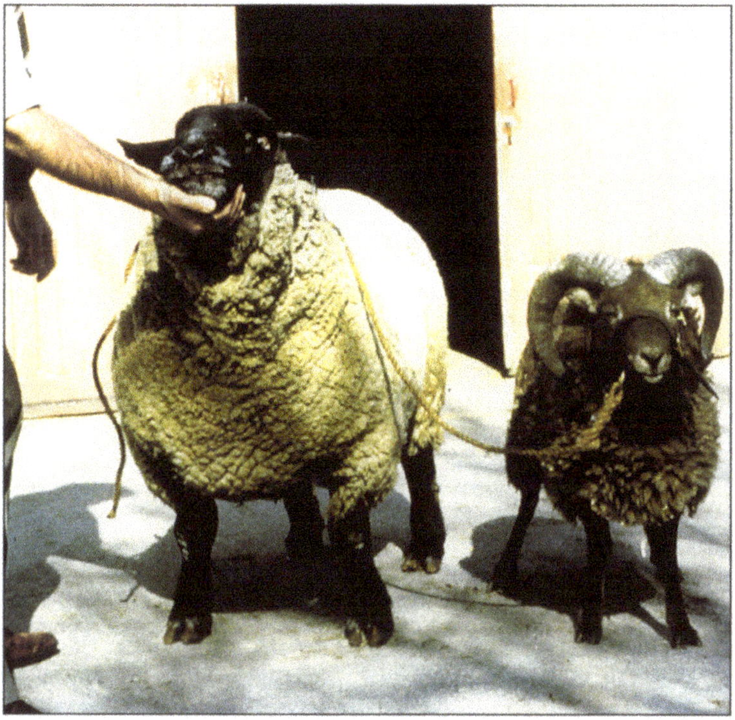

Fig. 1.1. Domestication has brought about many changes in animals, including changes in size and fatness. This figure shows a Suffolk ram, a breed that has undergone many generations of selection for growth and meat production, compared to a Soay ram, a breed that has undergone very little artificial selection and retains many of the characteristics of its wild predecessors, including a leaner carcass than many 'improved' breeds. (Courtesy of Professor John Robinson.)

Livestock Breeds and Their Origins

A breed of livestock is basically a recognized interbreeding group of animals of a given species. In most cases, animals which belong to the same breed are of fairly uniform appearance. This appearance is inherited, and usually distinguishes the breed concerned from other breeds. However, in other cases animals are considered to belong to the same breed by virtue of their geographical location, and there is quite wide variation in their appearance. Breeds have been created by 'reproductive isolation' – that is, the formation of separate groups of animals, where mating occurs within the groups but not usually between them. This is analogous to the way in which new species or sub-species of wild animals evolve, except that the reproductive isolation of wild animals often occurs due to geographical dispersion, whereas reproductive isolation of domestic breeds is usually imposed by humans.

The UK Farm Animal Genetic Resources Committee define a breed as: '...an interbreeding population of husbanded or formerly husbanded domesticated animals of consistent genotype and phenotype with a recognized history and administrative framework' (Defra, 2012).

The FAO (2007) define a breed as:

> Either a subspecific group of domestic livestock with definable and identifiable external characteristics that enable it to be separated by visual appraisal from other similarly defined groups within the same species or a group for which geographical and/or cultural separation from phenotypically similar groups has led to acceptance of its separate identity.

See FAO (2007, pp. 339–340) for further discussion on the concept of breeds, including these cultural and geographical distinctions.

Within many breeds there is further subdivision into strains or lines. These share a common ancestry, but have become reproductively isolated, to varying extents, as a result of physical separation or pursuit of different breeding objectives. For example, many of the strains of black and white Friesian or Holstein dairy cattle around the world originate from importations of Dutch Black Pied animals, mostly in the 19th century. In many countries these local strains have been crossed, over the last few decades, to North American Holstein strains to increase yield. (See FAO (2015a) for more information on the classification and recent status of livestock breeds.)

Distinct breeds of dogs, cattle and sheep had been developed by Ancient Egyptian civilizations by about 4000 years ago (Clutton-Brock, 1987). In Northern Europe, there is little evidence of the presence of distinct breeds until the Roman period (about 2000 years ago). The Romans are thought to have made positive efforts to improve their stock, possibly by selective breeding of favoured animals.

There was probably a slow evolution of livestock breeds, with strong regional ties, until a couple of centuries ago. In Britain, the impetus for more rapid livestock improvement came in the second half of the 18th century with the dramatic increase in the size of the human population and the need for greater food production. By the earlier part of that century there were already some notable changes in agriculture which increased production, including the enclosure of land into fields, drainage of land, felling of woodland, improvement of roads, the use of root crops as winter feed for livestock, and the start of mechanization (Hall and Clutton-Brock, 1989).

Robert Bakewell (1725–1795) is usually regarded as the pioneer of livestock improvement as we know it (Fig. 1.2). He and his followers employed *linebreeding* – the mating of closely related animals – which had been practised quite effectively in racehorses already. He also appears to have made widespread use of comparisons of growth and feed intake to help his selection decisions, and to have used both measurements and preserved specimens to allow him to chart his progress. Bakewell was particularly associated with the improvement of the Leicester breed of sheep and the Longhorn

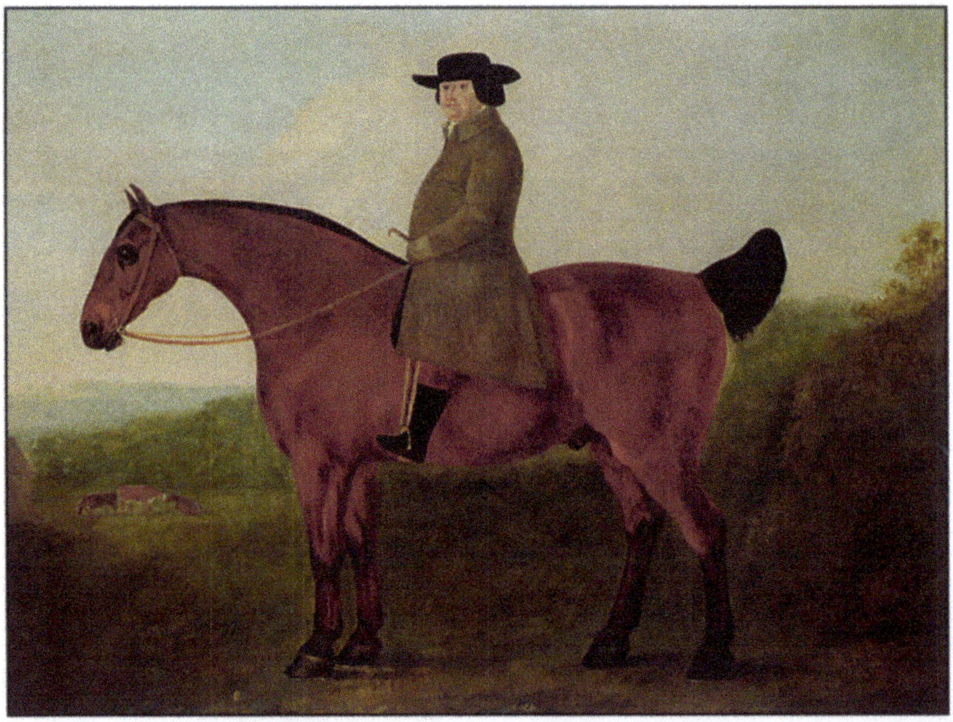

Fig. 1.2. 'Robert Bakewell at Dishley Grange' by John Boultbee. (Courtesy of the Royal Agricultural Society of England.)

breed of cattle. His Dishley or New Leicester breed of sheep (Fig. 1.3) was created from other sheep breeds in Leicestershire and Lincolnshire and was of uniform appearance by 1770. He selected for improved mutton production and, as a result, sheep of his own breed were claimed to reach market a year sooner than the usual 3 or 4 years of age (Hall and Clutton-Brock, 1989). Incidentally, much of this early selection in meat breeds, together with husbandry methods of the time, produced extremely fat animals. Fat was in great demand at that time, at least in the high proportion of the human population which was engaged in physically demanding work. Over the last few decades, with a more sedentary lifestyle and consumer preferences for leaner meat, reversing the propensity of animals to fatten has been a major preoccupation of livestock breeders and scientists.

Bakewell began letting out rams for hire for the mating season from about 1760. He is reputed to have ridden on horseback around his customers' fields, comparing the progeny of different rams, and

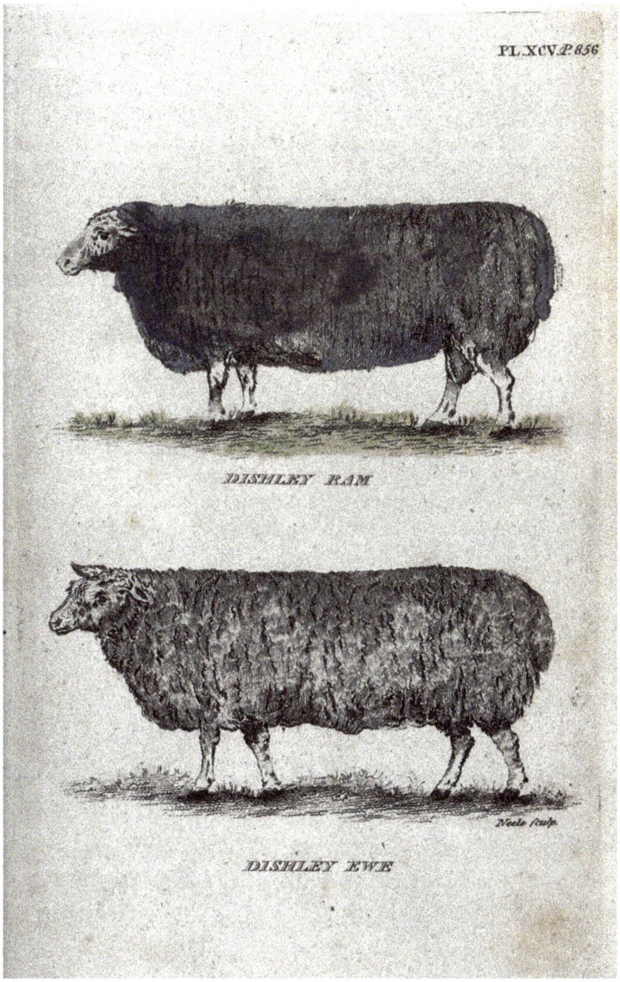

Fig. 1.3. 'A Dishley ram and a Dishley ewe', coloured stipple engraving by James Joshua Neele. (Source: Wellcome Collection gallery (2018-03-21), available at https://wellcomecollection.org/works/htzkhx5u CC-BY-4.0 (accessed 7 December 2019).)

using the best of these rams at home – an early, informal example of *progeny testing* (see Chapter 4). Bakewell established the Dishley Society which laid down the rules for ram letting for Leicester breeders, and was, in many respects, a forerunner for today's *pedigree* breed societies. Anyone who is shocked by the spiralling price records in some of today's pedigree sheep sales will be interested to know that in 1789 Bakewell made 1200 guineas from letting a single ram for one season (Hall and Clutton-Brock, 1989). This is equivalent to about £150,000 at today's prices, and it must have caused a few raised eyebrows at the time! Many British sheep breeds are thought to have some New Leicester ancestry, but the Border Leicester and Leicester Longwool are comparatively pure descendants (Hall and Clutton-Brock, 1989).

Bakewell had less success in improving the meat qualities of the Longhorn breed of cattle, but his followers did achieve success with the Shorthorn breed (see Fig. 1.4). The *Coates Herd Book* for this breed was founded in 1822 (some 31 years after the first stud book for thoroughbred horses), and herd or flock books for many other breeds of cattle, pigs and sheep around the globe followed (Hall and Clutton-Brock, 1989).

For many decades afterwards, in many breeds, the new profession of pedigree breeding in Britain enjoyed an enviable reputation for producing quality *purebred* livestock. The evidence for that is still visible today in the wide geographical distribution of British breeds and, less obviously, in the contribution they made to the formation of many other breeds around the globe. However, there are few of these British breeds which still enjoy this reputation today. To some extent this is a result of the pre-eminence of a small number of breeds in today's more specialized agricultural industries. Those breeds which have been selected for current market needs (e.g. efficient production of eggs, lean meat, milk solids or wool of specific fibre diameter) have expanded at the expense of those which have not. This process has been stimulated by vast improvements in international communication and transport and accelerated by techniques like *artificial insemination* and *embryo transfer*. Many people believe that we now depend too heavily on a small number of very specialized breeds, and that we need to do more to protect those which are declining in numbers. The subject of conservation of genetic resources is very topical, and some of the issues involved are discussed in more detail in Chapter 4.

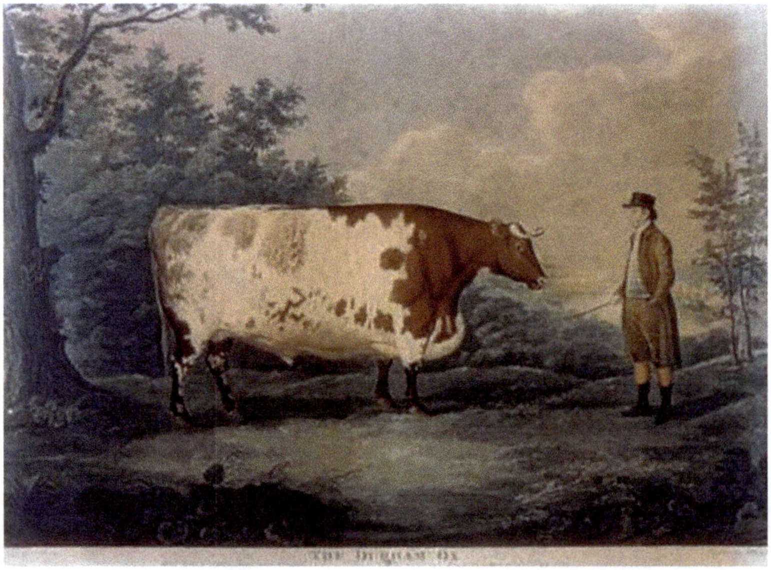

Fig. 1.4. 'The Durham Ox' by John Boultbee. The animal was bred by pioneering Shorthorn breeder Charles Colling in 1796. (Source: Family collection, Public Domain, available at: https://commons.wikimedia.org/wiki/File:Durham_Ox.jpg (accessed 7 December 2019).)

The Rôles of Livestock

The rôles that livestock play today are varied and diverse, particularly so in low- and middle-income countries (Herrero *et al.*, 2013; Smith *et al.*, 2013; Hoffman *et al.*, 2014; ILRI, 2019). These rôles include supporting livelihoods and economies, food and nutritional security, human health and environmental health (ILRI, 2019), as discussed further below. Other rôles that livestock may play in low- and middle-income countries are illustrated in Table 1.1.

The majority of farmed animals globally are found in Africa and Asia (see Fig. 1.5). Many of the examples of genetic improvement programmes we give later in the book are from Europe, North America and Oceania, as this is where they have been applied longest and most widely. However, the principles usually apply generally, and we hope that these examples assist those promoting the wider use of sustainable livestock breeding globally.

The livestock sector supports the livelihoods of more than 1 billion people globally and contributes 40% of the global value of agricultural output (ILRI, 2019). It is estimated that there are around 770 million poor livestock keepers, living on less than US$2 per day (2010 data from Robinson *et al.*, 2011), the majority of these in Sub-Saharan Africa (30%), South Asia (43%) and East Asia and the Pacific (22%). The world's high-value agricultural commodities are, in decreasing order of average annual values for 2007 to 2016: rice, pig meat, cow milk, cattle meat, maize, chicken meat, wheat, potatoes, eggs and sugar cane. Thus, livestock-derived foods constitute five of the world's ten highest-value agricultural commodities (ILRI, 2019).

On food and nutritional security, eggs, dairy and meat provide the world with 40% of its protein and 18% of its calories (ILRI, 2019). In addition, livestock-derived foods provide essential micronutrients that are absent or at low concentrations, or not readily bioavailable, in plant-based diets. The consumption of livestock-derived foods in the first 1000 days of life (from conception to 2 years old) has been shown to lead to clear nutritional benefits, particularly in Africa and South Asia where undernutrition is highest (Grace *et al.*, 2018). Human health benefits also derive from the livelihood benefits of livestock keeping, which allow people to make better choices on diet and healthy foods (ILRI, 2019).

Livestock can also enhance environmental health by helping to make optimal use of plant biomass. The majority (86%) of livestock feed at a global level comprises materials that are not edible by humans, including grass and fibrous vegetation, crop residues (stalks and leaves) after grain harvest, and other food waste (ILRI, 2019). Livestock are able to covert these to readily available nutrients for human use (FAO, 2016). Livestock also provide other ecosystem services, for example, livestock grazing (when managed correctly) can increase land cover and biodiversity as well as help control weeds and invasive species, and roaming livestock distribute nutrients across landscapes via manure and urine (FAO, 2016). Likewise, expansion of aquaculture can ease pressures on populations of wild marine animals, albeit often with considerable environmental impacts on coastal ecosystems (Ahmed and Thompson, 2019).

Table 1.1. Examples of rôles of livestock to their keepers in developing and emerging economies. (Adapted from Marshall, 2014.)

Rôle	Examples
Income	Sale of livestock and/or their products
Food security	Provision of animal-source foods such as meat, milk, blood and eggs
Vulnerability reduction	Diversifying livelihood options, such as in mixed crop-livestock systems
Inputs into crop production	Draught power/animal traction, manure for soil fertilization
Savings and insurance	Disposal (sale or exchange) in times of need
Transportation	Transportation
Shelter, bedding, clothing, footwear	Shelter, bedding, clothing, footwear made from fibres, hides and skins
Benefit from common property resources	Means for households to benefit from common property resources – such as communal grazing areas
Energy/fuel	Use of manure as a fuel for cooking or heating; use of manure for biogas production
Ecosystem services	Weed eradication, seed dispersal, and bush encroachment control
Socio-cultural	Used in festivals/dowry, as a source of pride

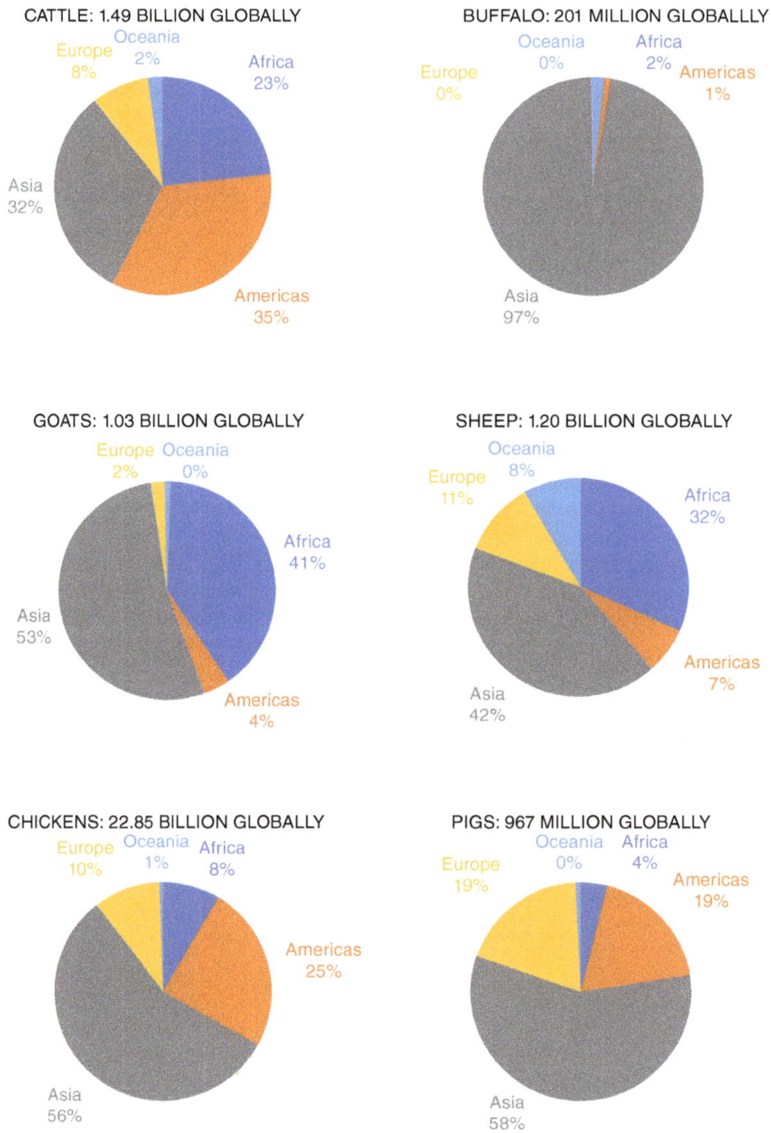

Fig. 1.5. Global population numbers and locations of major terrestrial farmed animal species. (From FAO, 2015b).

Livestock can also have negative consequences, including: overconsumption of livestock-derived foods by wealthier sectors of society, contributing to obesity; zoonotic diseases (diseases transmitted between animals and humans); illness caused by the consumption of contaminated food; increased antimicrobial resistant pathogens due to imprudent use of antimicrobial drugs; and environmental harms, such as the production of greenhouse gases, contribution to land degradation and biodiversity reduction (FAO, 2006; ILRI, 2019). Care needs to be taken to understand and balance the negative and positive impacts of livestock keeping (Herrero *et al.*, 2009) – topics we explore further in the final chapter.

Summary

- The huge variety of animal and other species that we see today, together with those now extinct, evolved by the process of natural selection.
- The key to natural selection, and to the artificial selection practised by breeders, is the inherited variation in many characteristics that exists between individual animals.
- Domestication of animals began 12,000 to 10,000 years ago. Whether or not it has been done knowingly, artificial selection, as well as natural selection, has been practised among domestic animals ever since then.
- Although distinct breeds or strains of cattle and sheep existed long before then, the practices of pedigree recording and selection of related animals with the aim of breed improvement date from the mid-1700s. The formation of herd books began early in the following century.
- Livestock continue to have a wide range of important rôles globally, with a range of positive and negative societal and environmental impacts, which need to be managed and balanced.

References

Ahmed, N. and Thompson, S. (2019) The blue dimensions of aquaculture: A global synthesis. *Science of the Total Environment* 652, 851–861.

Bruford, M.W., Bradley, D.G. and Luikart, G. (2003) DNA markers reveal the complexity of livestock domestication. *Nature Reviews Genetics* 4, 900-910. Available at: https://www.nature.com/articles/nrg1203 (accessed 29 August 2020).

Clutton-Brock, J. (1987) *A Natural History of Domesticated Mammals*. British Museum (Natural History), London.

Darwin, C. (1859) *On the Origin of Species by Means of Natural Selection, or the Preservation of Favoured Races in the Struggle for Life*. John Murray, London.

Darwin, C. (1868) *The Variation of Animals and Plants Under Domestication*. Vols. I and II. John Murray, London.

Defra (2012) UK Country Report on Farm Animal Genetic Resources 2012. Available at: https://assets.publishing.service.gov.uk/government/uploads/system/uploads/attachment_data/file/191781/pb13938-fangr-country-report-2012.pdf (accessed 20 September 2019).

Driscoll, C.A., Macdonald, D.W. and O'Brien, S.J. (2009) From wild animals to domestic pets, an evolutionary view of domestication. *Proceedings of the National Academy of Science* 106(Suppl 1), 9971–9978. DOI: 10.1073/pnas.0901586106.

FAO (2006) *Livestock's Long Shadow. Environmental Issues and Options*. Livestock Environment and Development/Food and Agriculture Organization of the United Nations, Rome. Available at: http://www.fao.org/3/a-a0701e.pdf (accessed 30 June 2019).

FAO (2007) *The State of the World's Animal Genetic Resources for Food and Agriculture*. Rischkowsky, B. and Pilling, D. (eds). FAO, Rome. Available at: http://www.fao.org/docrep/010/a1250e/a1250e00.htm (accessed 22 November 2019).

FAO (2015a) *The Second Report on the State of the World's Animal Genetic Resources for Food and Agriculture*. Commission on Genetic Resources for Food and Agriculture, Food and Agriculture Organization of the United Nations, Rome. Available at: http://www.fao.org/3/a-i4787e.pdf (accessed 14 May 2019).

FAO (2015b) FAOSTAT. Available at: http://www.fao.org/faostat/en/#data/QL (accessed 5 May 2019).

FAO (2016) *The Contributions of Livestock Species and Breeds to Ecosystem Services*. Food and Agricultural Organisation of the United Nations, Rome. Available at: http://www.fao.org/3/a-i6482e.pdf (accessed 14 May 2019).

Futuyma, D.J. and Kirkpatrick, M. (2017) *Evolution,* 4th edn. Oxford University Press, Oxford.

Grace, D., Dominguez-Salas, P., Alonso, S., Lannerstad, M., Muunda, E. *et al* (2018) *The Influence of Livestock-derived Foods on Nutrition During the First 1,000 Days of Life*. ILRI Research Report 44. Nairobi. Available at: https://hdl.handle.net/10568/92907 (accessed 5 May 2019).

Hall, S.J. and Clutton-Brock, J. (1989) *Two Hundred Years of British Farm Livestock*. British Museum (Natural History), London.

Herrero, M., Thornton, P.K., Gerber, P. and Reid, R.S. (2009) Livestock, livelihoods and the environment: understanding the trade-offs. *Current Opinion in Environmental Sustainability* 1, 111–120. DOI: 10.1016/j.cosust.2009.10.003.

Herrero, M., Grace, D., Njuki, J., Johnson, N., Enahoro, D. *et al*. (2013) The roles of livestock in developing countries. *Animal* 7, 3–18. DOI: 10.1017/S1751731112001954.

Hoffman, I., From, T. and Boerma, D. (2014) *Ecosystem Services Provided by Livestock Species and Breeds, with Special Consideration to the Contributions of Small-scale Livestock Keepers and Pastoralists*. Background Study Paper No. 66 Rev.1. FAO Commission on Genetic Resources for Food and Agriculture. Available at: http://www.fao.org/3/a-at598e.pdf (accessed 14 May 2019).

ILRI (2019) *Options for the Livestock Sector in Developing and Emerging Economies to 2030 and Beyond. Meat: The Future Series. World Economic Forum, Geneva, Switzerland*. Available at: https://www.weforum.org/whitepapers/meat-the-future-series-options-for-the-livestock-sector-in-developing-and-emerging-

economies-to-2030-and-beyond (accessed 14 May 2019).
Leakey, R.E. (1986) *The Illustrated Origin of Species by Charles Darwin*, abridged and introduced by Richard E. Leakey. Faber and Faber, London.
Magee, D.A., MacHugh, D.E. and Edwards, C.J. (2014) Interrogation of modern and ancient genomes reveals the complex domestic history of cattle. *Animal Frontiers* 4, 7–22. DOI: 10.2527/af.2014-0017.
Marshall, K. (2014) Optimizing the use of breed types in developing country livestock production systems: a neglected research area. *Journal of Animal Breeding and Genetics* 131, 329–340. DOI: 10.1111/jbg.12080.
Mignon-Grasteau, S., Boissy, A., Bouix, J., Faurea, J-M., Fisherd, A.D. *et al*, (2005) Genetics of adaptation and domestication in livestock. *Livestock Production Science* 93, 3–14. DOI: 10.1016/j.livprodsci.2004.11.001.
Robinson, T.P., Thornton, P.K., Franceschini, G., Kruska, R.L., Chiozza, F. *et al.* (2011) Global Livestock Production Systems. FAO and ILRI. Available at: http://www.fao.org/3/i2414e/i2414e00.htm (accessed 14 May 2019).
Smith, J., Sones, K., Grace, D., MacMillan, S., Tarawali, S. and Herrero, M. (2013) Beyond milk, meat, and eggs: Role of livestock in food and nutrition security. *Animal Frontiers* 3, 6–13. DOI: 10.2527/af.2013-0002.
UN (2019) World Population Prospects 2019. United Nations Population Division, New York. Available at: https://population.un.org/wpp/ (accessed 18 June 2019).
Walsh, B. and Lynch, M. (2018) *Evolution and Selection of Quantitative Traits*. Oxford University Press, Oxford.
Weiner, P. and Wilkinson, S. (2011) Deciphering the genetic basis of animal domestication. *Proceedings of the Royal Society B* 278, 3161–3170. DOI: 10.1098/rspb.2011.1376.

Recommended Reading

Animal Frontiers (2014) The human–animal bond and domestication: Through the ages ... animals in our lives. *Animal Frontiers*, 4, Issue 3. https://academic.oup.com/af/issue/4/3.
Clutton-Brock, J. (1987) *A Natural History of Domesticated Mammals*. British Museum (Natural History), London.
FAO (2015) *The Second Report on the State of the World's Animal Genetic Resources for Food and Agriculture*. Commission on Genetic Resources for Food and Agriculture, Food and Agriculture Organization of the United Nations, Rome. Available at: http://www.fao.org/3/a-i4787e.pdf (accessed 14 May 2019).
Futuyma, D.J. and Kirkpatrick, M. (2017) *Evolution,* 4th edn. Oxford University Press, Oxford.
Hall, S.J. and Clutton-Brock, J. (1989). *Two Hundred Years of British Farm Livestock*. British Museum (Natural History), London.
Leakey, R.E. (1986) *The Illustrated Origin of Species by Charles Darwin*, abridged and introduced by Richard E. Leakey. Faber and Faber, London.
Mason, I.L. (1996) *A World Dictionary of Livestock Breeds, Types and Varieties,* 4th edn. CAB International, Wallingford, UK.
Ryder, M.L. (1983) *Sheep and Man*. Duckworth, London.
Stanley, P. (1995) *Robert Bakewell and the Longhorn Breed of Cattle*. Farming Press, Ipswich, UK.

2 Genes, Genetic Codes and Genetic Variation

Introduction

The previous chapter outlined the long history of livestock improvement by subjective means. Some of the scientific foundations for more objective genetic improvement of livestock were laid towards the end of the 1800s, and others followed from the 1900s to the 1930s. However, it is only over the past 70 years or so that these methods of selection (i.e. based on measurements of performance) have become fairly widely used in pig, poultry and dairy cattle breeding and, to a lesser extent, in beef cattle, sheep, goat and aquaculture breeding. Where they have been applied, these scientific methods have helped to increase the output and resource use efficiency, reduce production costs, decrease the price and improve the quality of food and other animal products. The wider use of existing scientific methods in animal breeding, and the development of new ones, could help to meet the challenge of feeding a dramatically increased human population sustainably over the next few generations and contribute towards reducing greenhouse gas emissions per unit of product.

There have been contributions to objective methods of livestock improvement from several branches of science, and many of these are explained in later chapters. However, it is from the science of genetics that some of the most important contributions have come. School lessons on Mendel and his experiments with peas, or laboratory practical classes studying the genetics of fruit flies or mice, can seem distant from the business of breeding better farm animals. However, most of the principles of genetics established in these model species, which most of us have encountered at some time, apply equally to farm livestock in the modern era. A little understanding of these principles goes a long way towards understanding modern approaches to livestock improvement, which are described later in the book. Hence, the purpose of this chapter is to introduce some of these principles, and to begin to explain the link between basic genetics and the genetic improvement of traits of economic or other importance in farmed animals. The first part of the chapter deals with *chromosomes* and *genes* – the means by which animal characteristics are 'passed on', or *inherited*, from one generation to the next. The next section deals with the structure and function of genes in a little more detail. Then the influence of genes on animal performance, and some of the different types of gene action, are discussed. Finally, the genetic basis of traits of economic importance in farm livestock is examined.

With any specialist subject, one of the most off-putting things for a newcomer is the language used by 'insiders'. The main function of technical terms is to provide a sort of shorthand means of communication. Many of the technical terms in widespread use in genetics and livestock improvement are introduced in this chapter, but remember there is nothing mystical about these terms, they are meant to aid communication, not make it harder! There is a glossary at the end of the book if you need a reminder of the meaning of some of these technical terms.

Chromosomes and Genes

What was not clear in Bakewell's or Darwin's time, was just how characteristics were passed on, or inherited, from one generation to the next. Although knowledge will continue to evolve in genetics, major advances have been made during the 20th and 21st centuries. Ironically, it was during Darwin's lifetime that the first seeds were sown (no pun intended!) by the monk and naturalist, Gregor Mendel, though the significance of Mendel's work was not appreciated widely until much later. Mendel worked in a monastery in what is now Brno, in Czechia. Much of his work was with peas and, in 1865, he reported that some characteristics such as flower colour, height of plants, seed shape and texture,

Genetic Improvement of Farmed Animals (G. Simm *et al.*)
DOI: 10.1079/9781789241723.0002

followed particular patterns of inheritance (Mendel, 1865). This he attributed to 'elements', which were inherited from each parent. We now call these elements genes.

By the early 1900s a great deal of effort had gone into studying the process of cell division using the microscope. These studies revealed structures, which were named chromosomes, present in the *nucleus* of all cells, and which these early biologists suspected were involved in the process of inheritance (see Fig. 2.1). We now know that these suspicions were true and that genes occur in sequences, often likened to a string of beads, on the chromosomes. In eukaryotes (organisms with cell nuclei enclosed within membranes) there are typically hundreds or a few thousand genes on each chromosome.

The chromosomes can be seen clearly with the aid of a microscope only at certain stages of cell division; at other times they are difficult to distinguish. (The complete set of chromosomes is known as a *karyotype*; see Fig. 2.2.) In all cells except the *gametes* – that is, the sperm and eggs – the chromosomes occur in pairs, with the number of pairs being a characteristic of the species. For example, humans have 23 pairs of chromosomes in each of the body cells, pigs have 19 pairs, sheep have 27 pairs, cattle have 30 pairs, chickens have 39 pairs, and most farmed Atlantic salmon have 29 pairs (the *diploid* number of chromosomes is the total number of chromosomes that a species has, i.e. 30 × 2 = 60 for cattle). When sperm and eggs are created in the reproductive organs (testes and ovaries), each sperm and

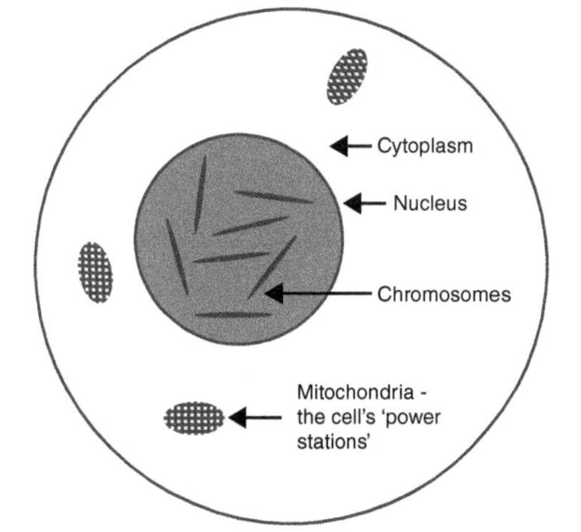

Fig. 2.1. Diagram of a cell illustrating chromosomes in the nucleus (not all chromosomes are shown).

each egg receives only a single set of chromosomes. In other words, the sperm or eggs of humans, pigs, sheep, cattle, chickens and Atlantic salmon carry 23, 19, 27, 30, 39 and 29 single chromosomes, respectively (this is known as the *haploid* number of chromosomes). When a sperm fertilizes an egg, the resulting embryo carries the original number of paired chromosomes. While the majority of livestock species are diploid (i.e. have two sets of chromosomes), there are several groups of fish species that exhibit *polyploidy* (i.e. they have four or more sets of chromosomes). This is particularly true in species-rich orders such as *Perciformes* or *Cypriniformes* (Comber and Smith, 2004). Several of the most commonly farmed fish (e.g. common carp and Atlantic salmon), are recent tetraploids that are thought to be in the process of reverting back to the diploid state.

In some species, particular pairs of chromosomes can be distinguished from one another, when viewed under a microscope, by differences in their size or shape, and by visible differences in the patterns of banding after staining (see Figs 2.3 and 2.4). These patterns of banding are nature's equivalent of the bar codes on most items we buy. Differences in the size, shape and banding patterns have allowed identification and numbering of each pair of chromosomes in some species, but in others, such as cattle and sheep, this is difficult because some pairs are very similar in appearance. Although different pairs of chromosomes may differ in size, the two members of each pair of chromosomes are the same size, with the exception of one pair, the sex chromosomes. The convention is to number the chromosomes in order of size from largest (chromosome 1) to smallest (species haploid number minus one) with the sex chromosomes numbered last.

In the body cells of female mammals there are two sex chromosomes of similar size, termed X chromosomes. In the body cells of male mammals, there is one X chromosome, and a smaller Y chromosome (see Fig. 2.2). Hence, in mammals it is the sperm which determines the sex of the resulting embryo. This is because all eggs carry an X chromosome, but sperm carry either an X or a Y sex chromosome. Eggs fertilized by sperm carrying an X chromosome develop into females, while eggs fertilized by sperm carrying a Y chromosome develop into males. (A single gene on the Y chromosome causes the development of males, from what would otherwise become females.) The reverse is true in birds: sperm carry the same sex chromosomes, but eggs carry either male or female sex chromosomes. All chromosomes,

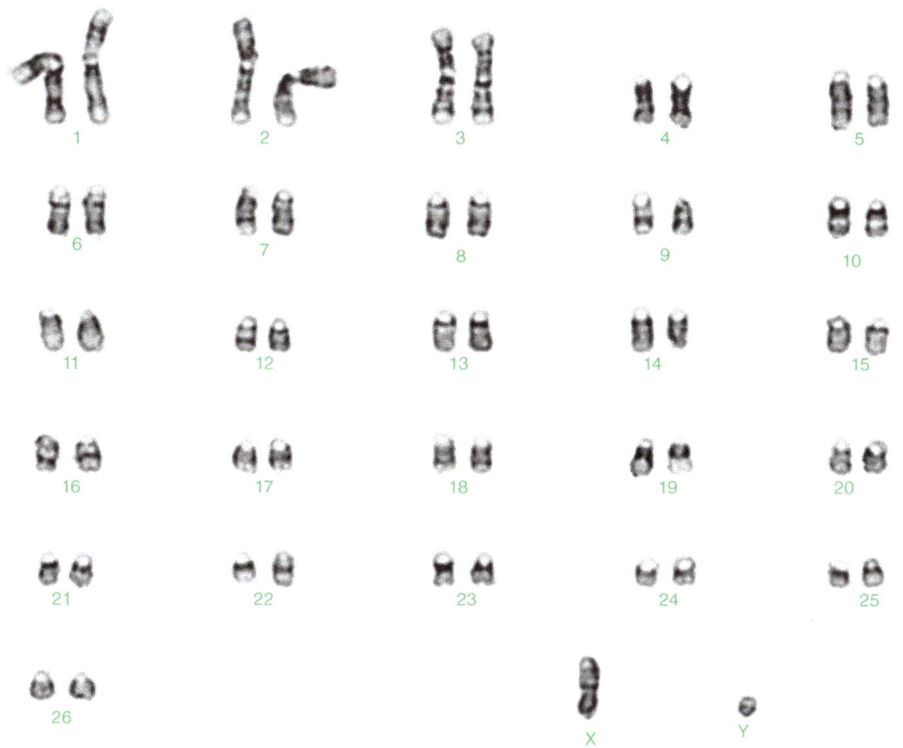

Fig. 2.2. Karyotype of the sheep – a photograph of the chromosomes at a particular stage of cell division, which has been cut up and rearranged to show all pairs of chromosomes in order. (Available at: https://commons.wikimedia.org/wiki/File:Karyotype_of_sheep_(Ovis_aries).png from Singh *et al.*, 2011; CC-BY-3.0; accessed 7 December 2019.)

apart from the sex chromosomes, are called *autosomes*, and the genes on these chromosomes are said to be *autosomal*. Genes on the sex chromosomes are said to be *sex linked*. (For more details on chromosomes see Nicholas (1987, 2010). Sex determination is more varied and complex in fish, often being multifactorial, and dimorphism (difference in size) between the male and female sex chromosomes is atypical (Martínez *et al.*, 2014).

The Structure and Function of Genes

DNA and genetic codes

One of the most significant scientific events of the 20th century was the discovery of the chemical structure of the material of which chromosomes and genes are made: *deoxyribonucleic acid* or *DNA* for short. This discovery was published by James Watson and Francis Crick and others in 1953 (see the Online Mendelian Inheritance in Animals (OMIA, 2019) website for this and other landmark papers in genetics). Although the detail of the structure of DNA is outside the scope of this book, there are a few points about it that help to explain how genes function, and how genetic variation arises among farmed animals, or any other form of life. DNA molecules are made up of two strands, or backbones, a bit like the sides of a very long ladder, with cross linkages between these strands, equivalent to the rungs on the ladder (see Fig. 2.5). The cross linkages are made up of pairs of different chemical substances called *bases*. There are four different bases which make up the cross linkages: adenine (abbreviated to A), thymine (T), guanine (G) and cytosine (C), which form pairs in a particular way. Thymine always pairs with adenine, and guanine always pairs with cytosine. This means that if the sequence of bases on one strand of the DNA molecule is known, then the sequence on the complementary

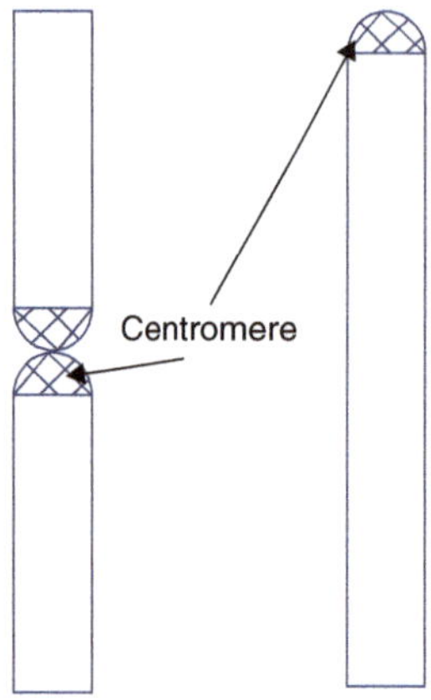

Fig. 2.3. Chromosomes have different shapes – some chromosomes have a constricted area called the *centromere* at or near the middle; others have the centromere at one end. Most sheep chromosomes and all cattle chromosomes, apart from the sex chromosomes, are of the second type. Pig and fish chromosomes are a mixture of the two types, while chicken chromosomes are mostly of the latter type.

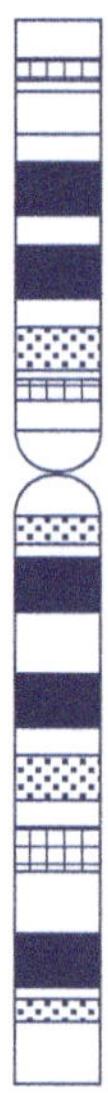

Fig. 2.4. The patterns of banding on sheep chromosome number 3, after a particular method of staining. Darker bands in the diagram represent greater intensity of staining. The patterns are used to distinguish pairs of chromosomes from one another. The bands on each chromosome of a species have been given internationally agreed numbers, for ease of reference. (After Ansari *et al.*, 1993; redrawn from a map produced from the SheepBase World Wide Web site using Anubis mapping software (Simm, 1998).)

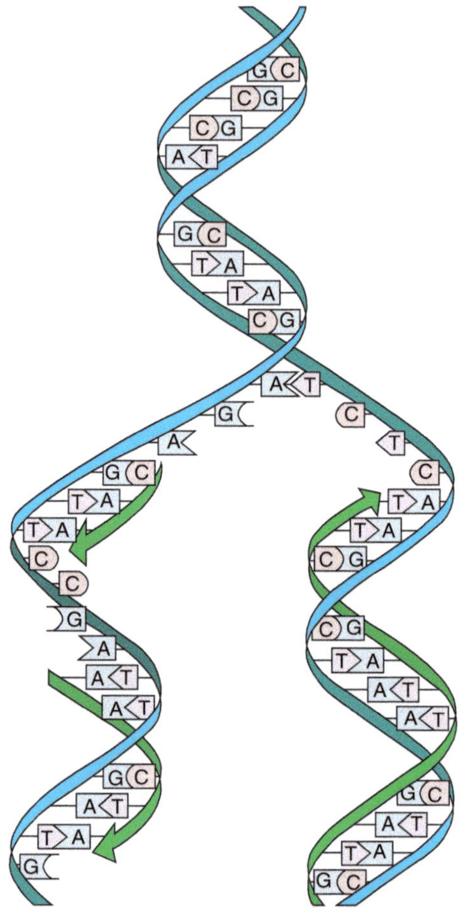

Fig. 2.5. The structure of DNA, especially the pairing of the bases adenine (A) with thymine (T) and guanine (G) with cytosine (C). The diagram also shows how the DNA molecule unwinds during replication, with each single strand acting as a template for the synthesis of a new complementary strand. (Available at: https://commons.wikimedia.org/wiki/File:DNA_replication_split.svg; accessed 7 December 2019; CC-BY-SA 3.0; by Madeleine Price Ball.)

strand can be worked out. The whole molecule of DNA (the long ladder) is twisted into a corkscrew shape, which gives rise to the commonly used description of a 'double helix'. Genes are effectively segments of the ladder, made up of long *sequences* of these base pairs. The DNA is intertwined with proteins called histones, which together are packaged into the nucleus of cells as a substance called *chromatin*.

Genes are both the design plans and the instruction manuals for all living creatures. They provide the instructions for a newly fertilized egg to grow into an adult, and for the body to go about its business at all times. Also, genes are the means by which these instructions are passed from one generation to the next. Each of these functions rests heavily on the structure of DNA, and the fact that (errors aside) the bases which make up DNA always pair in the same way.

Genes are made up of sequences of bases at particular locations in DNA molecules, but they account for less than 3% of the total DNA in chromosomes (the entire *genome*). Genes function by providing the basis for the production of proteins, a process called *coding*. Many of these proteins are themselves 'signals' which control biochemical processes elsewhere in the body (e.g. the enzymes involved in controlling digestion, or the hormones controlling growth, reproduction and lactation), aided by non-protein-coding variation which determines their *transcription* and *translation* (see next few paragraphs). Others are 'structural' proteins which are used directly in the growth or repair of body tissues such as muscle, internal organs, skin or hair, or they are secreted in milk and eggs.

Wherever a gene occurs in a DNA molecule, the sequences of bases on one side of the strand forms a template for the production of a series of amino acids. Amino acids are the building blocks from which proteins are made. Sets of three bases together in DNA are called a *triplet*, and each triplet either forms the code for producing a particular amino acid, or it signals where a gene stops or starts. Since there are 64 possible combinations of the four bases into triplets, but only 20 amino acids, it follows that several triplets code for the same amino acid or there is some redundancy in the set of possible triplets. For example, the triplets TTT and TTC both code for the amino acid phenylalanine, and the triplets TCT, TCC, TCA and TCG all code for the amino acid serine. (See Nicholas (2010) for the full set.)

Genes are long sequences of these triplets. Typical sizes of various units of genetic information in cattle are shown in Table 2.1. The sequence of triplets makes up a code, or template, for the production of particular proteins. In order for the template to be 'read', the double strand of DNA unwinds and the base pairs become separated temporarily (equivalent to unzipping a zip fastener) to leave a sequence of unpaired bases. A single-strand sequence of complementary bases is then formed from this template by a substance closely related to DNA, called *messenger ribonucleic acid* (*mRNA*). This process is called transcription. Groups of three bases in

Table 2.1. The relative size of different 'units of genetic information' in cattle. (From Zimin *et al.*, 2009; Nicholas, 2010).

Unit of genetic information	Relative size (number of bases or base pairs)
A triplet/codon	3 bases
A gene (informative part)	Range from ~1,000 bases to ~40 kb
A chromosome (for species like cattle with 30 pairs)	Range from 40 to 160 Mb
The entire genome (all of the genetic information contained on a single member of each pair of mammalian chromosomes)	About 3,000,000,000 base pairs

mRNA, which code for the production of an amino acid, are known as *codons*. Messenger RNA strands leave the nucleus and move to the *ribosomes*, the cell's 'protein factories', where the appropriate protein is synthesized (translation; see Figs 2.6 and 2.7 for more details).

Although all body cells in the same animal carry the same genetic code, different cells have very different functions. Specialized cell types express only the subset of genes present in their genome that is relevant to their particular function. The same triplets appear to code for the same amino acids in all animals, and virtually the same genes are present in all animals. It is simply the presence or absence of a few triplets, or different combinations of these triplets, arranged over a different number of chromosomes, and variation in the number of copies of genes, which distinguish different species.

The traditional explanation of a gene and its function given in the preceding paragraphs allow a basic understanding of how genetics works. However, we now know that in reality, things are more complicated than this. Although we tend to concentrate on the protein-coding part of the genome, i.e. the genes, there are in fact many other DNA features on a typical eukaryotic chromosome. Genes themselves comprise several components including *introns* (non-protein-coding regions), *exons* (protein-coding regions) and several regions controlling and regulating gene expression. The so-called 'non-coding parts' of the genome outside of the genes comprise many different types of DNA features, including promoters, enhancers, insulators, cytosine methylation, scaffold/matrix attachment region sequences, pseudogenes and genes of non-coding RNAs, as well as transposons and

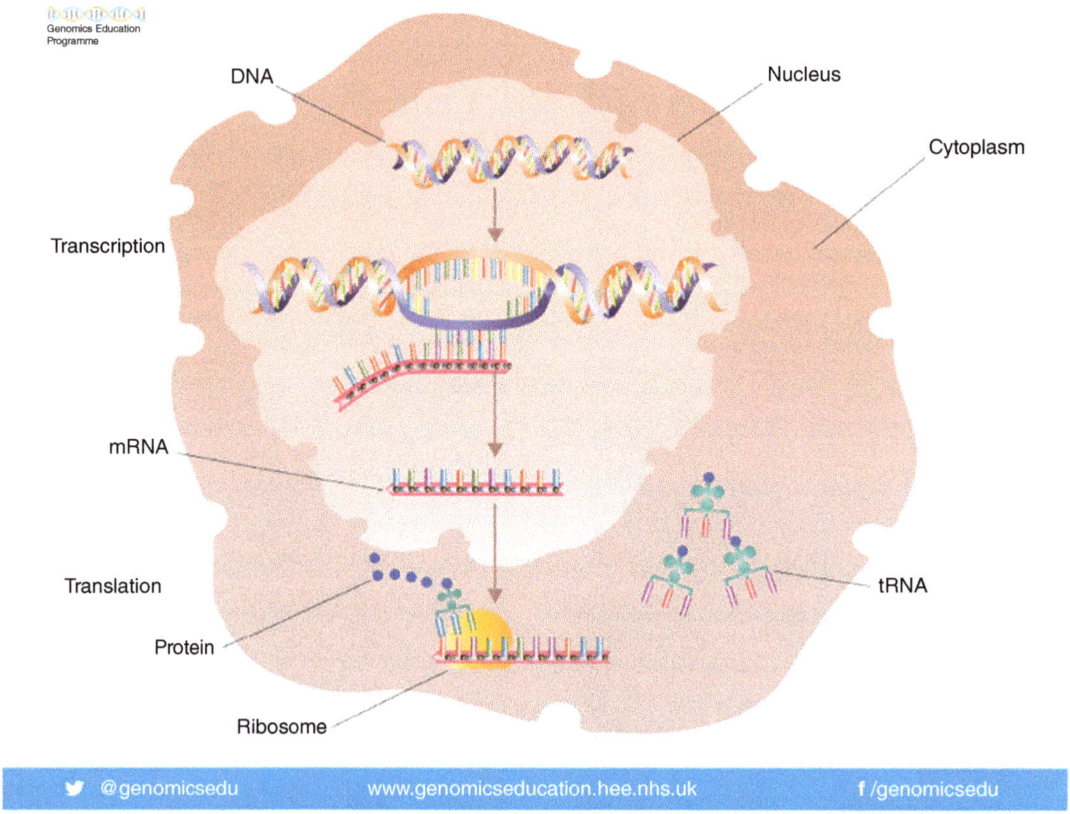

Fig. 2.6. How genes function. Genes form templates for the production of a series of amino acids which make up a protein. In order for the template to be 'read', the double strand of DNA unwinds and the base pairs become separated temporarily to leave a sequence of unpaired bases. A single-strand sequence of bases is then formed from this template by *messenger RNA* (*mRNA*) – which is very similar to DNA (this process is called transcription). This messenger RNA leaves the nucleus and moves to a ribosome in the cytoplasm of the cell. These ribosomes are the cell's protein factories. Another type of RNA (transfer RNA or tRNA) is involved in transporting free amino acids in the cell to the ribosomes for assembling proteins, a process called translation. (From https://www.flickr.com/photos/genomicseducation/13083355814, accessed 7 December 2019; CC-BY 2.0; NHS HEE Genomics Education Programme www.genomicseducation.hee.nhs.uk.)

simple repeats of centromeric and telomeric regions of chromosomes. Many of these features contribute to the regulation of the expression of genes, while others may exist in the genome without any discernible function to the animal, or so we may think at present. A full explanation of all these DNA features is outside the scope of this book but a review by Patrushev and Kovalenko (2014) provides a good introduction to the topic.

It is pertinent to ask what proportion of the genome is functioning to control the traits we are interested in. Not surprisingly, the answer is controversial. As Patrushev and Kovalenko (2014) outline, there is a division of opinion in the scientific world between those who

> believe that most of non-coding sequences are not functional and reflect evolutionary accumulation of shatters of genes no longer needed or represent selfishly multiplying DNA. Another group of researchers supposes that most of the non-coding sequences should be functional.

You can read the various arguments in their paper. However, one of the striking facts about human, and by implication other mammalian, genomes is

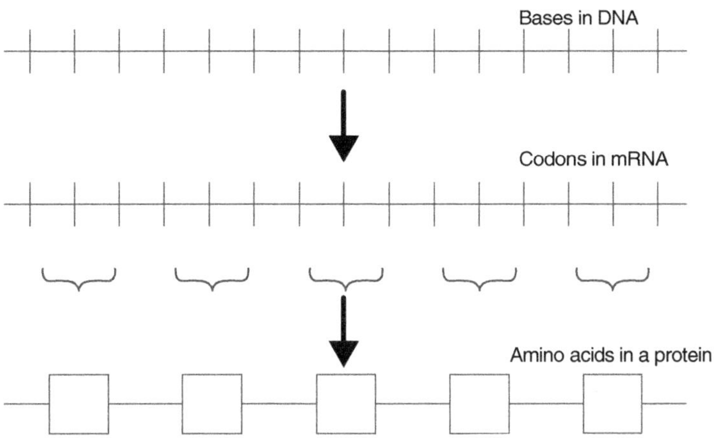

Fig. 2.7. The relationship between the sequence of bases in DNA, codons in mRNA and amino acids in a protein. (From Biotechnology and Biological Sciences Research Council, 1996.)

that only ~3% of the genome comprises the exons in genes and only 1.2% of base positions code for amino acids. There is evidence that a large amount of DNA in the non-coding part of the genome (~97%) has a function, since it is transcribed into various molecules, and it also appears to be conserved relatively unchanged between generations, and even between species. The traits we are interested in are also affected by these non-coding regions of DNA and any changes in some of these features will also change the way the protein-coding parts of the genome are regulated and controlled, and hence how animals differ.

By now you may be confused about what a gene is. You are not alone. Technically, it is better to use the correct descriptive terms for the parts of the genome that we are talking about. However, for simplicity, we will continue to use the term gene to mean the protein-coding part of the genome, but be aware that other features close to, or more distant from, the protein-coding parts of the genome may give rise to variation in traits of interest in livestock. In livestock genetics a related term, *quantitative trait locus* (QTL), which is discussed in detail later, refers to any part of the genome which affects the traits of interest in our breeding programmes. QTL may lie within protein-coding regions or non-coding regions, or both.

So, to recap, genetic variation in traits of interest in livestock may arise from variation in the coding regions of genes (traditionally viewed as the basis of all genetic variation), variation in regions of the genome affecting gene transcription or translation, or variation in other regions whose function we do not yet fully understand but may well be described in the near future.

Loci and alleles

As described above, the chromosomes occur in pairs in the body cells of all animals, with one member of each pair coming from the father via the sperm and one from the mother via the egg. Genes occur in a particular sequence along the chromosome. So, for instance, as a result of the *gene mapping* activities that are outlined in Chapter 5, the gene affecting the presence or absence of horns in many *Bos taurus* cattle breeds is now known to be on chromosome 1. (Animals that have horns and those that are naturally hornless are called horned and polled, respectively.) This gene will be located at the same position on each member of the pair for chromosome 1 – the one from the father and the other from the mother – and the gene will be in this location for all animals of the breed or species. This location, or the site of a gene on a chromosome is called a *locus* (the plural is *loci*; see Fig. 2.8). Each locus is generally in the same position on the chromosome for all animals of a species. However, at that locus the two members of a pair of chromosomes may have either identical or slightly different segments of DNA present. Often segments of DNA at a single locus differ only by the substitution of one base pair for another. In a population of animals there may be

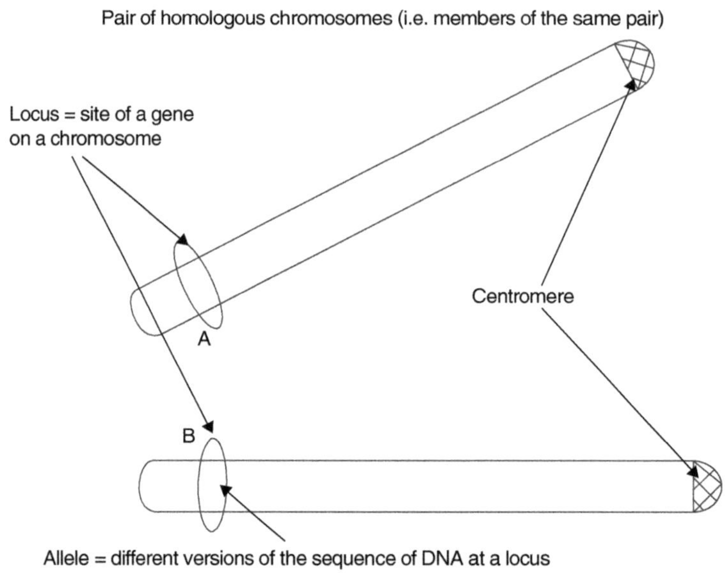

Fig. 2.8. A locus is the site where a particular gene is located on the chromosome; alternative forms of DNA sequence at any locus are termed alleles. In this example the two members of a pair of chromosomes are carrying different alleles, one abbreviated to A and the other to B. In a given breed, or in the population as a whole, there may be many other alleles possible at this locus (e.g. C, D, E), but individual animals can only carry either two copies of the same allele, or one copy of two different alleles. Often alleles differ only because of the substitution of a single base pair by another alternative pair of bases in their DNA sequence.

several alternative segments of DNA present at a given locus, but an individual diploid animal can carry a maximum of two different versions – one on each of a pair of chromosomes. It is the particular form of the segment of DNA on a chromosome which is called a gene or, more properly, an *allele*. (As we have seen, the word gene gets used interchangeably to mean the site, or locus, and the actual form of DNA present, or allele). As an analogy, think of the two members of any pair of chromosomes as being streets of the same length, each with the same number of houses, but with houses of various designs. The locus on a chromosome is equivalent to the house number or address, while the allele describes the type of house that is built there.

Transfer of genetic codes during cell division

Cell division is a vital part of both the growth and development of animals from a single cell to an adult containing millions of cells, and the production of the sex cells or gametes (sperm and eggs). There are different types of cell division involved in growth and reproduction. These are called *mitosis* and *meiosis* respectively, and they are outlined below.

Mitosis

During growth and development, the purpose of normal cell division is to create more cells which carry identical genetic information. This type of cell division is called mitosis or *multiplication division*. It creates two 'daughter cells' from one original cell, with the nucleus of each daughter cell containing a copy of the complete original set of chromosomes. There are several steps involved in producing copies of each of the chromosomes; the most important ones for our purpose are illustrated in Fig. 2.9. The first step involves duplication of each chromosome. This is achieved by the DNA molecule unwinding from its tightly coiled shape. Then the two strands of DNA separate, i.e. the ladder is pulled apart down the middle of each rung. Next, new bases, which are present in the nucleus, move in to join up with each strand of DNA in the usual formation – thymine pairing with adenine and guanine with cytosine (as shown already in Fig. 2.5).

When this process is complete for each of the original strands, there are two identical molecules of DNA (two ladders). At this stage, the two copies of each original chromosome, called *chromatids*, are still joined at the centromere. They then line up in the centre of the cell and separate, so that one copy ends up in the nucleus of each 'daughter' cell.

Meiosis

Sperm and eggs are produced by specialized cells in the reproductive organs. The type of cell division involved here is called meiosis or *reduction division*. It is illustrated in Fig. 2.10. In the early stages of sperm and egg production the process of cell division in the reproductive organs is similar to that which occurs during the growth of an animal. However, there are some very important differences in the later stages.

The first of these is a phenomenon known as *recombination* or *crossing over*, which occurs just before the division of cells during the production of sperm and eggs. Once the chromosomes have been copied, but while the two chromatids are still attached to each other, segments of one of the paternally-derived chromatids may swap with a corresponding segment on a maternally-derived chromatid. This is illustrated further in Fig. 2.11. The segments of chromosome which cross over correspond exactly in location, so there is no change in the size of chromosomes after crossing over. Recombination simply leads, as the name suggests, to new combi-

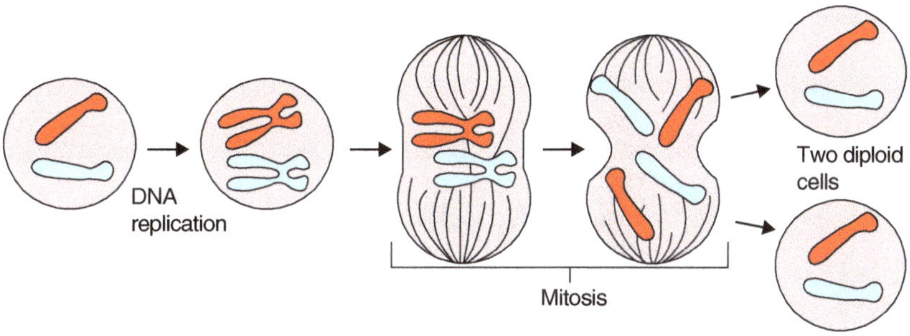

Fig. 2.9. Mitosis. Mitosis creates identical copies of chromosomes during the multiplication of cells that accompanies normal growth, development and tissue repair. (From https://commons.wikimedia.org/wiki/File:Major_events_in_mitosis.svg after Mysid, US National Center for Biotechnology Information (Public domain).)

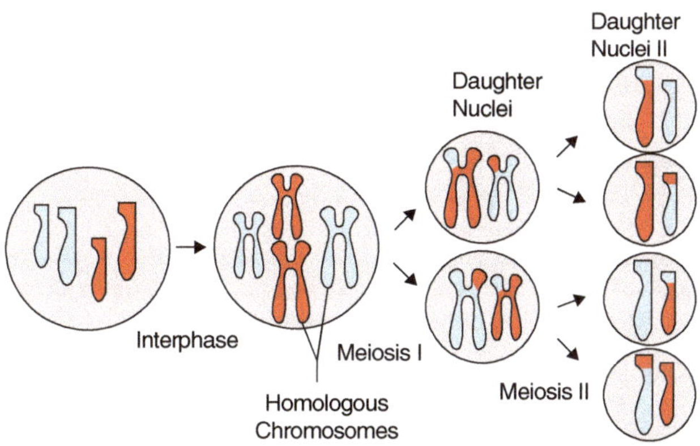

Fig. 2.10. Meiosis. This is the type of cell division involved in the production of the sex cells or gametes. The resulting cells get only a single set, rather than a pair of chromosomes. The normal complement of pairs of chromosomes is restored at fertilization. (From https://commons.wikimedia.org/wiki/File:Meiosis_Overview_new.svg#filelinks; CC-BY-SA-4.0; by Rdbickel.)

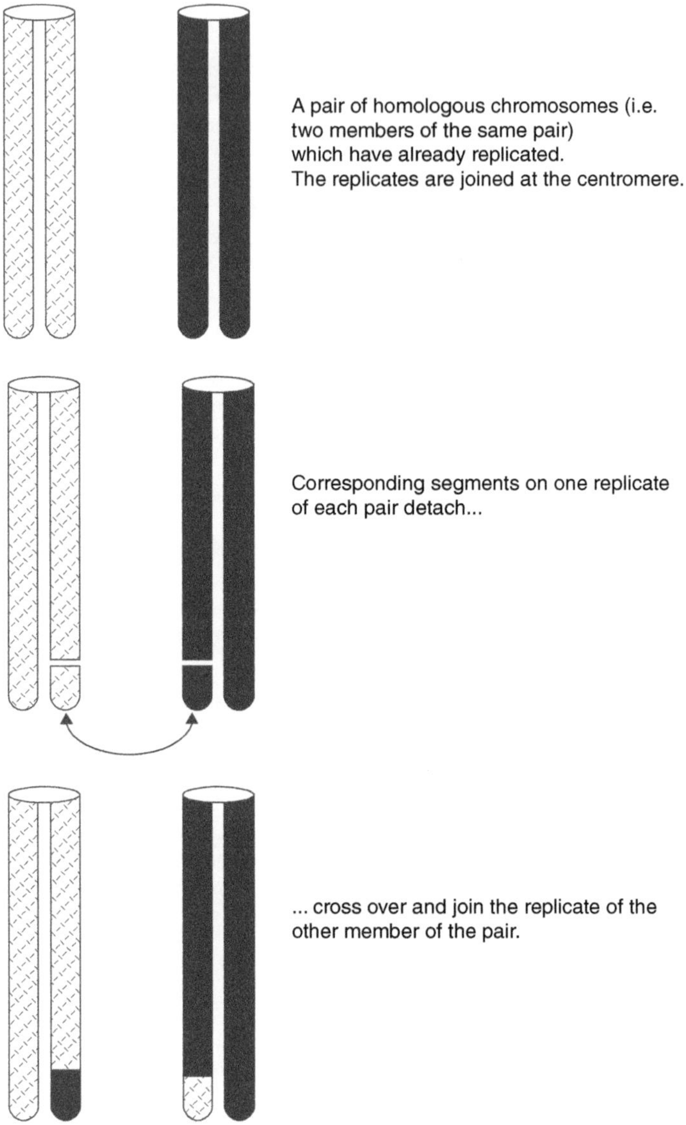

Fig. 2.11. The process of recombination or crossing over. This involves segments on the maternally-derived and paternally-derived members of a pair of chromosomes swapping over during meiosis, prior to formation of sperm and eggs. Characteristics that are controlled by genes close together on the same chromosome tend to be inherited together. These genes are said to be linked. Characteristics controlled by genes further apart on the same chromosome will be inherited together less often, as a result of recombination.

nations of genes on each of the two chromosomes involved – some of these came from the animal's father, and others from its mother. (Recombination also occurs between the two identical chromatids, but since the two segments which swap over are identical, there is no effect on the genetic make-up of the resulting chromosomes.) Typically, there are two or three recombination events per chromosome during the formation of sperm and eggs. This means that chromosomes in sperm or eggs are made up of a 'patchwork' of segments originating from the father and mother of the animal producing the sperm or egg. Because segments of the chromosome are involved in crossing over, genes which are closer together on the same chromosome will tend to cross over together more often than genes which are far apart on the same chromosome. This is known as *linkage*, and it is one reason why some characteristics appear to be inherited together. Linkage of genes has enabled the creation of genome maps, and linkage-based QTL mapping studies, which have underpinned many recent advances in livestock breeding, as explained in Chapter 5.

Meiosis also differs from mitosis in that the cells which become sperm or eggs receive only a single set of chromosomes. For example, the sperm or eggs of cattle carry 30 individual chromosomes, rather than the 30 pairs found in other cells. Whether a sperm or egg receives a copy of the maternally- or the paternally-derived member of a particular pair of chromosomes is an entirely chance event. On average, each sperm and each egg will carry half paternally-derived and half maternally-derived chromosomes, but there will be quite wide variation in this, purely by chance. This variation is termed *Mendelian sampling*. As explained above, recombination causes a further mixing of maternally- and paternally-derived genes. As a result of the chance sampling of chromosomes, and of recombination, sperm and eggs contain a largely independent assortment of the genes of the animals producing them. Exceptions occur in the case of genes which happen to be located close together on the same chromosome and so tend to be inherited together. It is worth noting that this re-sorting of genes by crossing over is an important process for producing new combinations of alleles within species and, together with new *mutations* (see next section), it provides us with a continuing source of variation in the traits that we breed for.

Mutation

Another event associated with cell division which has important consequences for genetic variation in animals is mutation. There are two main types of mutation. The first, called *chromosomal mutation*, involves changes in the number or structure of chromosomes. This often has a profound effect and is believed to be a major source of embryonic mortality (see Nicholas (2010) for other examples of the effects of this type of mutation). The second type of mutation is termed a *gene* or *point mutation*. Whether cell division is occurring during growth or in the production of sperm and eggs, the copying of DNA is usually correct, so that each new strand is identical to the original strand from which it was copied. However, occasionally mistakes are made and the sequence of bases in the new copy of the DNA strand is slightly different from that in the original strand. Some of these gene mutations are corrected by special repair enzymes within the cell. If uncorrected mutations occur in any part of the body other than the reproductive organs, they may interfere with the functions of that organ in the animal, but they will not affect the genetic make-up of offspring. If, on the other hand, gene mutations occur in cells responsible for producing sperm or eggs in the reproductive organs, they lead to a change in the genetic code of offspring. Studies on the *whole genome sequence* of humans has revealed that there is one mutation in every 30 million base positions on average, and single gene studies put the mutation rate at about 2×10^{-5}, i.e. 1 in 50,000 (Xue *et al.*, 2009).

Variation among alleles at any locus is a direct result of gene mutations at some time in the past. The name mutation conjures up images of freaks of nature. In fact, the majority of gene mutations which occur have little or no effect on an animal. But some do have an effect, and that effect can be negative. For example, there are quite a few genetic disorders of farm animals which have arisen because of a mutation in a sequence of bases coding for important enzymes (see Nicholas (2010) and OMIA (2019) for more details). Other gene mutations may have a positive effect. For example, the variation in colour, shape or function of wild animals which allows them to exploit new habitats or sources of food is partly a result of mutations. Similarly, much of the variation among farm animals which is exploited by selection is a result of mutations of positive effect occurring over many generations both before and after domestication.

Tracking genes across generations

Tracking the contribution of chromosomes and genes across generations is quite confusing, but it is important in order to understand the degree of similarity between relatives (we will return to this in Chapters 6 and 7). It is easiest to follow if we consider three generations of animals. In this example, the oldest generation are the grandparents. The middle generation of animals, the ones producing the sperm or the eggs in this example, are the parents. The animals resulting from the sperm and eggs produced by the parents are the offspring. Each of the parents received half of their genes from their father and half from their mother (the grandparent generation). *On average*, the sperm and eggs produced by the parent generation will carry equal numbers of genes from each grandparent. However, any particular gene carried by the sperm or egg must come from only one of the two possible grandparents. So, by chance, an individual sperm or egg may have more or less than 50% of its genes from a particular grandparent. This happens because of the separation and chance sampling or *segregation* of paternally- and maternally-derived genes during meiosis in the production of a sperm or egg. So, all offspring get *exactly* half of their genes from each parent, but individuals may get more or less than a quarter of their genes from each grandparent (though across the offspring generation as a whole, animals will get an *average* of one-quarter of their genes from each grandparent). It is worth emphasizing that this *potential* inequality of genetic contributions is from the grandparents, and not the parents of the offspring which results from the sperm or egg concerned. Figure 2.12 illustrates this process.

Genes, Genotypes and Phenotypes

It will be easier to understand more about the way that genes or alleles affect the appearance or performance of animals by considering the inheritance of coat colour as an example. In some livestock breeds there are several different versions of a gene affecting colour that can occur at a single site or locus. However, individual animals will have a maximum of two of these versions present at a locus – one on each chromosome. (In some breeds,

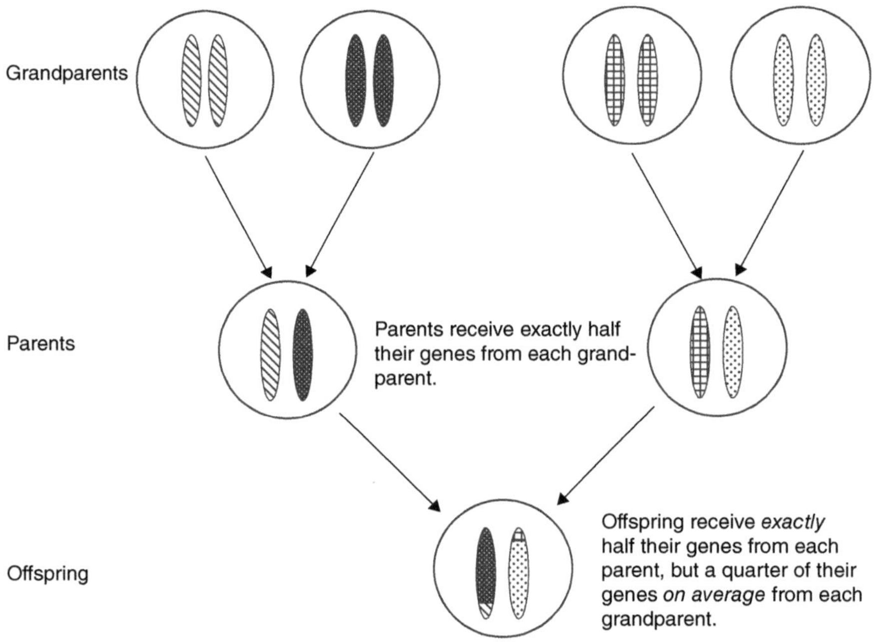

Fig. 2.12. The transmission of genes from grandparents to grand-offspring. This illustrates that, although offspring get exactly half of their genes from each parent, the contributions from grandparents can vary. On average one-quarter of an animal's genes will come from each grandparent, but by chance individual animals may receive greater or smaller contributions from particular grandparents. In this example, only a single pair of chromosomes is shown in each generation. These are equivalent pairs in each animal, but they are shown in different patterns to make it easier to follow their transmission. For any particular pair of chromosomes, offspring could potentially inherit one chromosome each from a single grandparent - so only two of the four grandparents' genes would be represented. However, in practice, recombination mixes the contributions of grandparents to particular chromosomes in offspring. Also, when *all* chromosomes are considered, the contribution of each grandparent is likely to be more equal (i.e. closer to 25%).

there is more than one locus involved in determining colour, but for simplicity only a single locus is considered here.) The effect of different genes can be seen clearly in the coat colour of the Shorthorn breed of cattle. In this breed there are three main colours observed – red, white and roan. Combinations of these colours can appear also – for example, some animals have patches of both solid red and solid white – but for simplicity only the three single colours are considered here. What we observe when we look at animals, or measure them in some way, is referred to as the *phenotype*, so in Shorthorn cattle there are three main phenotypes for coat colour – red, white and roan (see Fig. 2.13). These coat colours are determined at a single locus with two versions of the gene, or two alleles, involved. One of these alleles codes for red coat colour (abbreviated R here) and the other one codes for white (abbreviated W here). All Shorthorn calves get a copy of one of these coat colour genes from their father and one from their mother. So, there are three possible combinations of these genes in the calves. These are: two copies of the red gene (RR – these calves are red), two copies of the white gene (WW – these calves are white), or one copy of each of the genes (RW – these calves are roan). The particular combination of genes or alleles which an animal inherits is called its *genotype*. In this case there are three possible genotypes for coat colour - RR, WW and RW, although there are only two genes or alleles involved, R and W. Except in the case of a few, rare genes, it does not matter which parent contributes which allele to the offspring, the effect is the same. That is, a calf which receives an R gene from its sire and a W gene from its dam will be the same colour as one which gets the R gene from its dam and the W gene from its sire. In both of these cases, the genotype is abbreviated in the same way (RW). In breeds where there are three genes or alleles at a single locus for coat colour, six different combinations of these are possible. That is, six different genotypes are possible. If there are four genes involved at a single locus, then there are ten different genotypes, and so on.

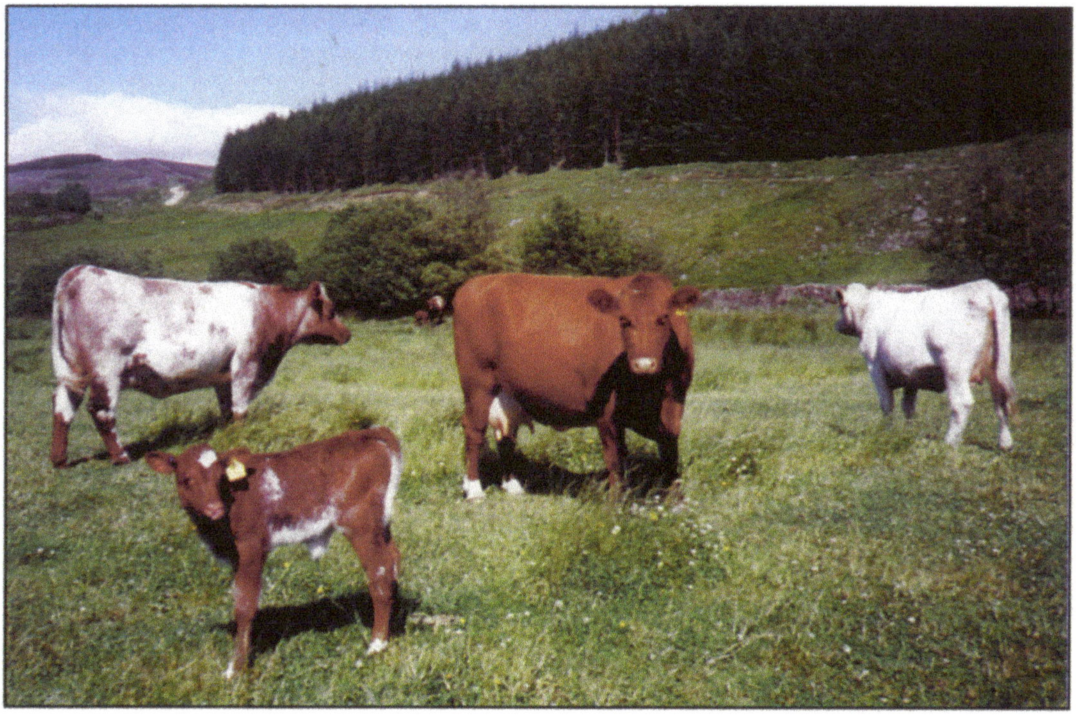

Fig. 2.13. Red, white and roan Shorthorn cattle. (Courtesy of Carey Coombs.)

Animals that carry two copies of the same gene or allele, for example the RR or WW Shorthorn cattle, are said to be *homozygous* for that particular gene or allele. Those animals which carry different copies of a gene, such as the RW Shorthorns, are said to be *heterozygous*. (The corresponding nouns are *homozygote* and *heterozygote*.)

Predicting the outcome of matings among different genotypes

Obviously, breeders of farm livestock would like to be able to predict the outcome of matings between different pairs of parents so that they can make the best mating decisions. Unfortunately, the coat colour example used above is one of the few cases where we can actually tell the genotype of the animal by looking at it. Most of the traits of economic importance in farm animals are controlled by genes at many different loci and have many 'shades' of performance, rather than discrete categories like coat colour. Despite this, understanding what happens at a single locus with visible effects is an important step towards understanding the more complex situation when many genes are affecting a trait.

Although genes or alleles are present in pairs in the nucleus of body cells – one on each member of a pair of chromosomes – this pairing of alleles is broken during the production of sperm or eggs. That is, the alleles which were paired in parents pass to the next generation singly. This 'un-pairing' and mixing of alleles or genes is termed segregation, as mentioned earlier. Mendel was the first to demonstrate this process, and to link it to visible effects such as seed type and flower colour in plants. The study of single genes and their effects is often termed *Mendelian genetics* in recognition of this. The ratios of different offspring genotypes expected from matings between particular genotypes of parents are often called the *Mendelian segregation ratios*.

For more details on Mendel's work, see the list of recommended reading at the end of the chapter. For the latest information on the molecular characterization of Mendelian traits, and some of the early landmark publication in genetics, see the OMIA (2019) website. Many examples of Mendelian traits have been described for livestock and domestic animals and are curated in the OMIA database. This database is a very useful starting point to investigate the genetic basis of any particular condition or trait, either new or established. Each 'Mendelian' gene has a reference in this database which we shall use throughout this book when they are first mentioned. So, the Shorthorn coat-colour example has the reference OMIA 001216-9913. If you use a search engine with this reference, or use the numerical part in the OMIA database itself, you will be directed to a page containing a summary of what is known about the *variants* of the gene causing different coat colours in Shorthorns plus the references describing its discovery. This is a very useful resource for about 3500 such Mendelian traits in livestock and domesticated animals. Incidentally, there is an equivalent resource for human genetics called the Online Mendelian Inheritance in Man (OMIM) database.

Table 2.2 shows how the outcome of matings between particular genotypes can be predicted for a single locus of interest. The main principles are that at any locus an individual animal has two alleles present, one derived from each parent. If the animal is a homozygote these two alleles will be of the same type. If the animal is a heterozygote the two alleles will be different. Normally, when animals produce sperm or eggs, the two alleles at any locus will be represented equally, i.e. half of the sperm or eggs will carry copies of one of the alleles, and half will carry copies of the other. For example, half of the sperm from an RW Shorthorn bull will carry the R allele, and half will carry the W allele. So, the first step in predicting the outcome of a mating is to 'split' the genotype of each parent down into the two individual alleles or genes which their sperm or eggs will carry at the locus of interest. Which particular egg a female sheds, and which particular sperm fertilizes that egg, are entirely random or chance events. So, we have to calculate the probability or expected frequency of all possible offspring genotypes which could result from a given mating.

To do this it is easiest to write down the two types of sperm and eggs on adjacent sides of a grid (or *Punnett square*, named after its originator) consisting of four cells. This grid is the shaded part of Table 2.2. Next, all four combinations of alleles from the sperm and eggs are entered into the appropriate part of the grid. On average, one-quarter of the offspring from a particular type of mating are expected to have the genotype in each of the four grid squares. Some of the grid squares contain the same offspring genotype, so the frequencies of these are simply added together. For example, as shown in Table 2.2, matings between RW Shorthorn bulls and RW Shorthorn cows are expected to result in ¼ RR, ½ RW and ¼ WW calves; a segregation ratio of 1:2:1. On average, half of the RW calves get their R gene from their father, and half get their R gene from their mother.

Table 2.2. Calculating the expected offspring genotype frequencies at a single locus, such as that determining coat colour in Shorthorn cattle, following matings between parents of different genotype.

(a) Mating between RW bull and RW cow

		Type of sperm from RW bull	
		½ R	½ W
		Expected offspring genotypes and their frequencies	
Type of egg from RW cow	½ R	¼ RR	¼ RW
	½ W	¼ RW	¼ WW

Expected *genotype frequency* of offspring: ¼ RR, ½ RW, ¼ WW

(b) Mating between RW bull and RR cow

		Type of sperm from RW bull	
		½ R	½ W
		Expected offspring genotypes and their frequencies	
Type of egg from RR cow	½ R	¼ RR	¼ RW
	½ R	¼ RR	¼ RW

Expected genotype frequency of offspring: ½ RR, ½ RW. The same outcome is expected from matings between RR bulls and RW cows.

(c) Mating between RR bull and WW cow

		Type of sperm from RR bull	
		½ R	½ R
		Expected offspring genotypes and their frequencies	
Type of egg from WW cow	½ W	¼ RW	¼ RW
	½ W	¼ RW	¼ RW

Expected genotype frequency of offspring: all RW

(d) Mating between RR bull and RR cow

		Type of sperm from RR bull	
		½ R	½ R
		Expected offspring genotypes and their frequencies	
Type of egg from RR cow	½ R	¼ RR	¼ RR
	½ R	¼ RR	¼ RR

Expected genotype frequency of offspring: all RR. Similarly, all of the offspring from matings between WW bulls and WW cows will be WW.

It is worth stressing that these are *expected* genotype frequencies, and that the *actual* frequencies observed can depart quite widely from these expectations, especially when the outcomes of only a few matings are considered. For example, a single Shorthorn calf born from a mating between an RW bull and an RW cow must fall into only one of the three genotypes expected, and so the expected ratio of colours cannot be reached. In fact, if we look at any less than four calves born from matings between RW Shorthorn bulls and cows we cannot possibly reach the expected ratio of genotypes. Even with four calves from this type of mating, there is less than a 20% chance of getting the expected frequency of genotypes. In practice, we would need many more observations to get close to the expected ratio of genotypes. It is easy to demonstrate this by putting a ball marked R and a ball marked W in a box. These represent the alleles produced by one parent. Then two balls, representing the alleles produced by the other parent, are put in a second box. The boxes are shaken to mix up the balls, and then one ball is drawn from each box, representing the chance combination of alleles from the two parents at fertilization. The combination of the two letters corresponds to the new animal's genotype. The balls are then replaced and the whole exercise is repeated a number of times, to simulate repeated matings.

So, it is worth remembering that expected genotype frequencies tell us what to expect on average. Actual observations can depart quite widely from these expectations, especially when the number of observations is small. (See Van Vleck *et al.* (1987) for more details of how to calculate the probability of getting particular genotypes from different numbers of matings.)

Genotype and gene (or allele) frequencies

The method described above for predicting the outcome of matings is useful if there is only a small number of animals involved. However, it can be extended to larger numbers of animals, as long as we know how many animals there are of each genotype in the herd or flock, or in the whole breed. The proportion of animals of each genotype is called the *genotype frequency*. It is simple to calculate if the different genotypes can be distinguished – it is just the number of animals of each genotype present, expressed as a fraction or percentage of the total (i.e. the total genotype frequency must add up to 1 or 100%). For example, if we had a herd of 100 Shorthorn cows comprising 30 red, 50 roan and 20 white cows, the genotype frequency in the herd would be 30% RR, 50% RW and 20% WW (or 0.3, 0.5 and 0.2, respectively). These genotype frequencies can be used to calculate the expected outcome of matings to bulls of a particular genotype. If only a single bull is used, the genotype frequencies can be calculated in three steps.

1. Calculating the expected outcome of matings between this bull genotype and each of the cow genotypes, as shown in Table 2.2. For example, if a red bull was used the expected outcome of the matings to these three cow genotypes is:

		Offspring		
Bull	Cows	RR	RW	WW
RR	RR	1 (100%) RR	–	–
RR	RW	0.5 (50%) RR	0.5 (50%) RW	–
RR	WW	–	1 (100%) RW	–

2. 'Weighting' the results according to the genotype frequencies of cows in the herd. In this case there are 30% RR cows, 50% RW cows and 20% WW cows, so the weighted proportions of expected offspring genotypes as a result of mating each cow genotype to an RR bull is:

Cow genotype	Proportion of herd of this genotype	Weighted proportion of offspring of each genotype following mating to an RR bull (column 2 in this table multiplied by the proportion of each offspring genotype expected, taken from the table above)		
		RR	RW	WW
RR	0.3 (or 30%)	0.3 × 1 = 0.3 (30%) RR	–	–
RW	0.5 (or 50%)	0.5 × 0.5 = 0.25 (25%) RR	0.5 × 0.5 = 0.25 (25%) RW	–
WW	0.2 (or 20%)	–	0.2 × 1 = 0.2 (20%) RW	–

3. Totalling the expected proportion of calves of each genotype. In this case the overall proportion of different calf genotypes is 0.55 (or 55%) RR plus 0.45 (or 45%) RW.

If more than one genotype of bull is involved, then this process has to be repeated for each genotype, and the results weighted according to the genotype frequency of bulls. This approach soon gets laborious when there are several genotypes of each sex involved. Although it is useful to know the genotype frequency in an initial group of animals, once the numbers are large, and we consider the results of several generations of matings, it is often more convenient to think of *gene (or allele) frequency*. As the name suggests, gene (or allele) frequency is based on a count of the genes (or alleles) present in a specific population, rather than the genotypes. This is also more logical as it is individual genes or alleles, not genotypes, that get passed from parent to offspring.

To calculate the *gene frequency* we have to split each different genotype down into its two constituent alleles, and then weight these according to the proportion of the herd or flock carrying these alleles. For example, RR Shorthorn cattle carry only R genes; WW animals carry only W genes; RW animals carry half R genes and half W genes. Hence, the frequency of the R gene can be calculated as:

(1 × RR genotype frequency) + (0.5 × RW genotype frequency)

So, in our herd of 100 cows made up of 30% RR, 50% RW and 20% WW animals, the frequency of the R gene is:

(1 × 0.3) + (0.5 × 0.5) = 0.55

Similarly, the frequency of the W gene can be calculated as:

(1 × WW genotype frequency) + (0.5 × RW genotype frequency)

= (1 × 0.2) + (0.5 × 0.5)

= 0.45

Or more conveniently, since only two genes are involved, the frequency of the W gene is simply:

1 – frequency of R gene

= 1 – 0.55

= 0.45

If there is no selection for or against particular alleles at a locus, no mutation and no movement of animals into or out of a large random-mating population of animals, then the gene and genotype frequencies in that population tend to stay the same from one generation to the next. This is called the *Hardy-Weinberg equilibrium*, after the mathematician and the physician who demonstrated it independently in the early 1900s. (This is described mathematically as: $p^2 + 2pq + q^2 = 1$ where p and q are the allele frequencies of two alleles at a locus and the three terms in the model relate to the genotype frequencies of a homozygous, heterozygous and the alternate homozygous genotype, respectively.) So, without forces such as selection operating, the variation in a population is maintained rather than disappearing over time. In farm animal breeding the conditions for the Hardy-Weinberg equilibrium are rarely met, and so we can expect gene and genotype frequencies to change. For a start, the populations are usually relatively small (e.g. individual herds or flocks, or even all herds or flocks which inter-breed in a particular country), and so changes may occur by chance alone. These chance changes in gene frequency are called *genetic drift*. Also, there are often imports or exports of breeding stock to or from a particular breeding population. Finally, most breeding programmes are geared towards widespread use of parents with favourable characteristics, and away from random mating. So, selection in farm animals usually changes gene and genotype frequencies, but this is not usually obvious, unless selection is for something as visible as coat colour. For example, if the herd of cows mentioned above was bred entirely to WW (white) bulls, then the frequency of the W allele would be higher in the calves than it was in the original herd of cows. If female calves from this new generation were in turn bred to a white bull, then the frequency of the W allele would increase further in their offspring. If matings were always made to WW bulls, the R gene would eventually disappear altogether from the herd. In this case the frequency of the W allele would be 1, and that of the R allele would be 0. The W allele is then said to be *fixed* in this population, and the R allele *lost* from it.

If we know the frequency of a particular allele of interest, we can estimate how many generations of selection it would take to increase or decrease the frequency by a certain amount. This is useful in planning eradication of genetic diseases controlled by single genes, or increasing the frequency of a favourable single gene in a breed; for example, a single gene affecting the cheese-making properties of cows' milk, or one affecting fertility in sheep. It is generally easier to alter the frequency of a gene which is already at an intermediate frequency, than to alter the frequency of a gene which is already at either a very high or very low frequency. (For more details on these calculations, and their application, see Nicholas (1987) and Falconer and Mackay (1996).)

Sources of genetic variation between animals

Genetic improvement depends on genetic variation. If there is no genetic variation between animals in traits of interest, there can be no improvement. To put it another way, if there are no animals genetically better than the rest, there is no way of picking better parents to breed from, regardless of the animals' phenotypes. The most important sources of genetic variation between individuals or groups of animals have been mentioned in the preceding sections, but genetic variation is so central to genetic improvement that it is worth discussing them in more detail here. These sources of variation are:

- differences in gene (allele) frequencies;
- segregation of genes (alleles);
- recombination; and
- mutation.

Differences in gene (allele) frequencies are a major source of variation between groups of animals of a particular species. If we look far enough back into history, then all animals of the same species have common ancestors. Offspring get half of their genes from each parent, and this continues down the generations. So, at first sight, we might expect distant ancestors and current animals to have copies of the same genes. However, as mentioned earlier, there is an element of chance as to which half of each parent's alleles the offspring receive. This means that some alleles carried by parents may never appear in offspring, while others may appear often. If you toss a coin often enough you expect it to land on 'heads' 50% of the time, and on 'tails' 50% of the time, but with a short sequence of tosses you often get several heads in a row, or several tails in a row. So it is with the transfer of alleles from one generation to the next. A parent which is heterozygous at any locus is expected to produce half of its sperm or eggs carrying each of the two alleles. However, because only a few offspring are produced, by chance these may all carry copies of the same allele. This can lead to changes in gene frequency. In the case of domestic livestock species, the populations have expanded enormously, and have become subdivided. So, there may be differences between sub-populations by chance alone. Also, these species have been subject to many generations of natural and artificial selection. As a result, particular alleles present in the original population may have been lost altogether or, at the other extreme, all of the animals may carry two copies of the same allele at a particular locus, i.e. they have become fixed. Between these two extremes, different breeds or groups of animals may have different allele frequencies.

Perhaps it is easiest to visualize this by considering genes for coat colour again. In some breeds of cattle or sheep all of the animals are the same colour, whereas in others there are several different colours. Coat colour in all mammals appears to be controlled by a series of at least six loci, with several alleles possible at each locus (Nicholas, 1987, 2010; OMIA, 2019). The reason why some breeds have little or no variation in colour, while others show wide variation, is that some of the alleles at some loci have been lost in the less variable breeds, either by chance or deliberate selection. In the Icelandic breeds of cattle, sheep and horses, and a few other breeds, there has been little or no systematic selection for or against particular colours, and so there is a huge range in coat colour (see Fig. 2.14). In contrast, in many other cattle breeds coat colour is effectively determined at a single locus. This may be because there is only variation at a single locus (i.e. there are two identical alleles at each of the other loci), or because any variation at other loci is masked by the alleles present at a single locus. So, in breeds where all the animals are the same colour, it is likely that the allele for this colour has become fixed, while those which produced other colours in ancestors have been lost, or that the effect of any remaining alleles for other colours is 'masked'. (This process of masking is discussed in the next section.)

Within a population of animals, genetic variation also occurs because of segregation. As explained earlier, this is a consequence of parents carrying two copies of each gene, one on each member of the pair of chromosomes concerned, but sperm and eggs carrying only a single copy of each gene at any locus. When animals reproduce, the sperm or eggs they produce carry half of their genes, but the particular sample of genes which any sperm or any egg carry is down to chance. Chance is also involved in which particular egg is shed by a female, and which particular sperm successfully fertilizes this egg. Similarly, recombination helps to 'mix' the genes present in a breed, herd or flock, and to create new combinations of genes on a particular chromosome, which contributes to genetic variation.

The different genes present at any locus have arisen because of mutations at some time in the past. Until relatively recently, new gene mutations were considered to be a minor source of genetic variation, and usually to have negative effects. However, it is now recognized that they make an important contribution to genetic variation, and that their effects are sometimes beneficial. New gene mutations are

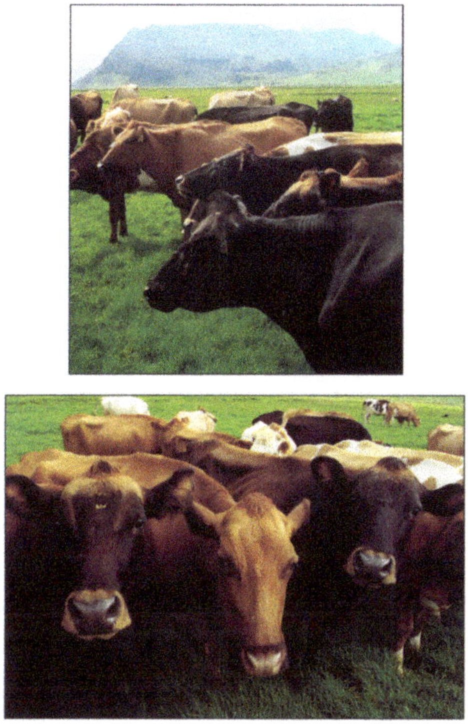

Fig. 2.14. Icelandic cattle showing some of the many coat colours still present in this breed. (Photos by Geoff Simm.)

a particularly important source of variation in populations which have been under selection for a long time. They are largely responsible for most selected populations continuing to change, even after many generations of selection. Without mutation as a source of new variation very highly selected populations would reach a plateau or limit in the character under selection (see Simm *et al.*, 2004).

To use a card-playing analogy, the first three sources of genetic variation mentioned above – differences in gene frequency, segregation and recombination – all cause variation by shuffling and splitting the existing pack. However, mutation can create completely new cards.

Types of Gene Action

Additive and non-additive gene action

So far, we have considered only the simplest type of gene action where the heterozygous animals show characteristics of both of the homozygous types. In the Shorthorn coat-colour example discussed earlier, for instance, the heterozygous animals had both red and white hairs, whereas the homozygous types had either red or white hairs. In this case there is said to be *co-dominance*, or no *dominance*. The equivalent type of gene action when performance is measured on some scale occurs when heterozygotes are exactly intermediate to the two homozygous types. In these cases the type of gene action is described as *additive*. However, there are several other types of gene action, collectively called *non-additive* types of gene action. These are *complete dominance*, *partial* (or *incomplete*) *dominance* and *overdominance*. The distinctions between these types of gene action, and some practical examples, are discussed below. These types of gene action are also illustrated in Fig. 2.15.

Co-dominance, no dominance or additive gene action

The inheritance of red, white and roan coat colour in Shorthorn cattle, described above, is a good

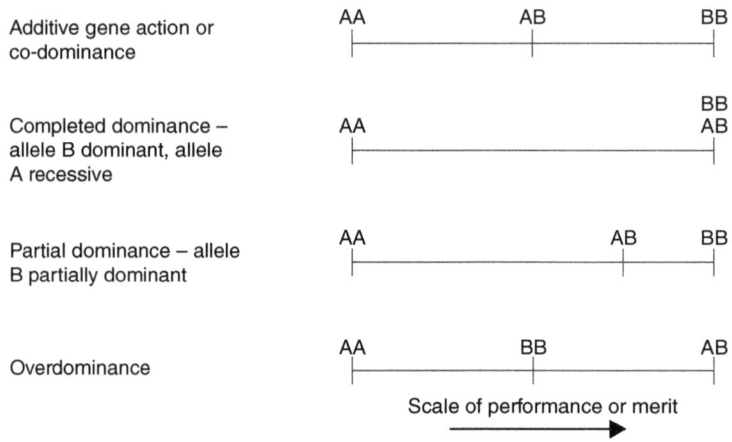

Fig. 2.15. Four different types of gene action. The horizontal scale shows some visible or measurable 'performance' characteristic in animals. This could be a trait like colour or blood group with few alternatives, or a trait like milk yield or live weight measured on a continuous scale. Co-dominant gene action gives heterozygotes which show characteristics of both homozygous types, e.g. they have both red and white hairs in the case of Shorthorn coat colour, or they have two blood haemoglobin types, whereas homozygotes have only one. The equivalent type of gene action when performance is measured is called additive gene action. Additive gene action gives heterozygotes with performance midway between the two homozygotes. With complete dominance, heterozygotes have the same level of performance as one of the homozygotes. The performance of heterozygotes is less extreme with partial dominance (see the text), but still closer to that of one of the homozygotes. Overdominance leads to heterozygotes which are more extreme in performance than either homozygote. (After Falconer and Mackay, 1996.)

example of co-dominance. (As mentioned before, as well as occurring singly, these colours can occur in combination, but for simplicity this is ignored here.) In this breed, the segment of DNA which we call the gene R, leads to the production of red pigment in the coat hairs. In animals which have two copies of this gene, all of the hairs will be red. The gene W leads to no pigment production, and the hairs appear white. Animals with two copies of this gene appear all white. Heterozygous animals get one copy of each gene, and so have some pigmented hairs and some unpigmented hairs, and they appear roan. Similarly, this type of gene action is often seen when the products of a gene – such as enzymes or blood types – can be detected directly. Advances in molecular biology allow direct analysis of the sequence of bases seen in alternative alleles at many loci in farm animals. Sequences of DNA used as '*markers*' – potential indicators of improved performance – are often co-dominant. That is, the two alternative sequences seen in homozygotes can both be detected in heterozygotes (see Chapter 5).

The Booroola gene (denoted FecB; OMIA 000383-9940) in sheep provides a good example of the equivalent form of gene action – additive gene action – in characteristics which are counted or measured, rather than showing obvious visible differences like colour. The Booroola gene was discovered in the late 1970s in Merino sheep in Australia, but it has been introduced since then to a number of other breeds and countries. (It is now believed that the gene was introduced to Australian Merino sheep via importations of Garole sheep from India in the late 1700s; see review by Fogarty (2009).) The Merino breed normally has a relatively low number of lambs, but animals carrying the Booroola gene were noticed because of their high fecundity. Closer examination of the results of matings between fecund and normal animals showed that a single gene was involved, which had an approximately additive effect on ovulation rate. In other words, the performance of heterozygous animals is close to the average of that of the homozygous normal animals (often referred to as the wild type) and those homozygous for the Booroola gene. The genotype of normal animals is denoted ++, the genotype of those carrying one copy of the Booroola gene is denoted B+, and the genotype of those carrying two copies of the Booroola gene is denoted BB. In one well-documented experiment the ++, B+ and BB Merino ewes had ovulation rates of about 1.40, 2.82 and 4.38 ova, respectively, so each copy of the B gene added an extra 1.4 to 1.6 ova (Piper *et al.*, 1985). Figure 2.16 shows the results of a more recent review of crossing experiments involving Booroola Merinos, which show a similar effect on ovulation rate (Fogarty, 2009). The term additive refers to the fact that there is a linear association, or smooth progression, between the number of copies of a gene and some characteristic of the animal - in this case ovulation rate.

Complete dominance

Unfortunately, with non-additive gene action it is not always this easy to tell what the genotype of an animal is from its phenotype. To illustrate this, let us look at another coat-colour example (OMIA 001199-9913). Most Aberdeen Angus cattle are black, but there is also a red gene in the breed. Animals which carry two copies of the black gene appear black (this genotype is abbreviated to BB here), and those that carry two copies of the red gene appear red (this genotype is abbreviated bb here; the rationale for these abbreviations follows shortly). However, when these two types of animals are mated to each other, all of the resulting calves are black (they have the genotype Bb). So, in this case, there are still two genes and three genotypes involved, but only two phenotypes – black or red. It is not possible to tell from looking at the black animals whether or not they carry the red gene (i.e. whether they are BB or Bb). This type of gene action is called complete dominance, usually referred to simply as *dominance*. It occurs when the effect of one allele is completely masked, or overridden, by the presence of another. In this case, a single copy of the red gene is completely masked by the presence of a single copy of the black gene. The black gene is called a *dominant gene*, while the red gene is called a *recessive gene*. The expected genotype frequencies of offspring from different matings, the segregation ratios, can be calculated as shown in Table 2.2. The results for all possible matings between BB, Bb and bb animals are summarized in Table 2.3. (The black or red coat colour seen in Holstein Friesians and several other breeds is inherited in the same way as that described here for the Angus breed.)

If a gene acts co-dominantly, and it also has a readily visible effect, then the heterozygotes can be distinguished by their appearance or phenotype, as in the case of roan Shorthorn cattle. If there is complete dominance, as in the case of coat colour in the Aberdeen Angus or Holstein Friesian breeds, then the heterozygotes cannot be distinguished by their appearance. These heterozygotes are also called *carriers* of a recessive gene. In some cases it is possible to detect carriers from a blood test (e.g. when carriers of a genetic disease produce different levels of a particular enzyme from homozygous normal animals), but there are often still animals whose genotype remains uncertain. In other cases, until

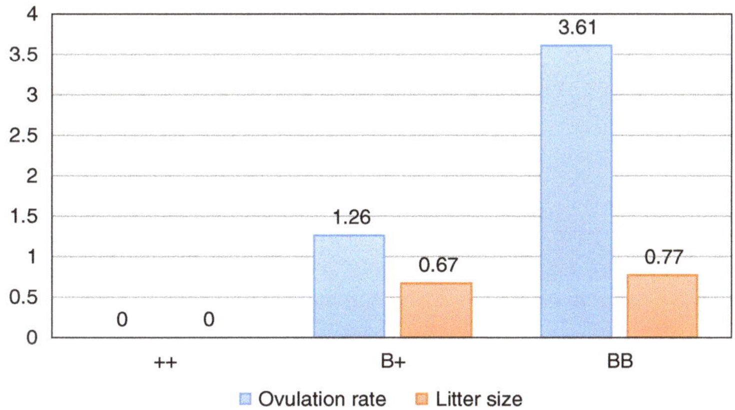

Fig. 2.16. The effect of different genotypes, with respect to the Booroola gene (FecB), on ovulation rate and litter size of sheep. The chart shows the mean ovulation rates and litter sizes of B+ and BB ewes compared to those of ++ animals. There appears to be additive gene action on ovulation rate. The effects on mean litter size appear to be partially dominant, probably as a result of higher prenatal mortality in larger litters. (Data from Fogarty, 2009.)

the development of DNA-based tests which have revolutionized the management of recessive genes in general and inherited disorders in particular, the only way of detecting heterozygotes or carrier animals when a recessive gene is involved was to do test matings. This involves mating animals of unknown genotype to those of known genotype, and making an inference about the unknown genotype based on the frequency of offspring of different types. For example, if a black Angus bull is mated to red Angus cows we would expect to get no red calves at all if the bull is a homozygote (BB). But, if he is a heterozygote or carrier (Bb), we would expect to get 50% red calves, on average.

There are many genetic diseases in farm animals which are under the control of single recessive genes (see OMIA, 2019) and where test matings of this type have been used to prevent carriers being used inadvertently. For example, there is a condition called tibial hemimelia syndrome (OMIA 001009-9913) which occurs in the Galloway cattle breed. Homozygous recessive calves have severely shortened and twisted hind limbs and a large abdominal hernia. Affected calves are usually born alive but die soon after birth. In the mid-1970s, a screening programme was operated by the Galloway Cattle Society and the then East of Scotland College of Agriculture, to check that Galloway bulls were not carriers of the gene concerned, before they were used for artificial insemination (AI). Since the condition is lethal, and so no homozygous recessive cows were available, a herd of known carrier cows was established, and test matings were made to these cows.

Table 2.4 shows the number of offspring from test matings of this type required to achieve different probabilities of detecting carriers of a recessive gene. The table also shows the numbers of offspring required from matings to recessive homozygous animals, when these are available, and for matings to offspring of the parent under test. Test matings for recessive genes should be made with these minimum numbers of offspring in mind. For example, to have a 95% chance of detecting a bull carrying a copy of the gene causing a defect like the tibial hemimelia syndrome, the bull under test would need to be mated to enough known carrier cows to produce 11 progeny. To have a 99% chance of detecting a carrier bull, 16 progeny would be needed. Of course, whenever a single affected offspring is produced the test is complete, and the animal under test is known to be a carrier.

One of the spin-offs from the developments in molecular genetics (see Chapter 5 for more details)

Table 2.3. Expected offspring genotype frequencies, or segregation ratios, and corresponding phenotypes following matings between parents of different genotype for coat colour in the Aberdeen Angus cattle breed. (After Nicholas, 1987.)

	Expected genotype frequency (segregation ratio) among offspring			Corresponding phenotypes	
Type of mating	BB	Bb	bb	Black	Red
BB × BB	1	0	0	1	0
BB × Bb	½	½	0	1	0
BB × bb	0	1	0	1	0
Bb × Bb	¼	½	¼	¾	¼
Bb × bb	0	½	½	½	½
bb × bb	0	0	1	0	1

Table 2.4. Number of offspring required from different types of test mating to achieve probabilities of 95%, 99% or 99.9% of detecting a carrier of a recessive gene. (After Nicholas, 1987.)

	Number of offspring required to reach this probability of detecting carriers		
Animal under test mated to:	95%	99%	99.9%
Homozygous recessive (i.e. affected) animals	5	7	10
Known heterozygotes (carriers)	11	16	24
Its own offspring	23	35	52

is that DNA-based tests for carriers of recessive genes affecting colour, polledness, genetic diseases, and many other characteristics of interest, are becoming available (see OMIA, 2019).

When the exact location of the gene of interest is known, then these tests can detect carriers with 100% certainty. However, if the exact location of the gene of interest is unknown, but the location of a closely linked gene is known, this can be used as a marker. Because the gene of interest and the marker occur close together on the same chromosome, they will usually be inherited together. Recombination may separate them occasionally, but this will occur less frequently the closer together the loci for the marker gene and the gene of interest are. So, a test for a particular marker genotype may indicate the presence of the favoured genotype for the trait of interest. As mentioned above, a useful feature of many DNA markers is that, even if the gene acts non-additively at the level of the trait of interest (e.g. colour or polledness), markers at the DNA level are co-dominant and so heterozygotes are readily detectable.

Whether the location of the gene of interest is known, or whether it is the location of a marker which is known, DNA tests on blood or other tissue can be used to detect carriers, with lower welfare and financial costs than test mating programmes such as that described above. Many such DNA tests are already in use for a range of genetic disorders in dairy cattle. For example, BLAD (bovine leucocyte adhesion deficiency; OMIA 000595-9913) and DUMPS (deficiency of uridine monophosphate synthase; OMIA 000262-9913) are both genetic diseases of cattle that are controlled by single genes. To prevent the inadvertent widespread use of carriers through AI, and hence the risk of producing homozygous affected animals in later generations, most young dairy bulls of affected breeds are screened using DNA-based tests prior to entering progeny tests, and homozygous affected or carrier animals are excluded. DNA-based tests are also available now for cattle which are carriers of the horned gene and for a range of coat-colour alleles in several species. See Innovate UK (2019) for valuable guidance on managing or removing inherited diseases using molecular genetic techniques and Pollott (2018) for a discussion of how to detect new recessive genetic diseases.

Partial dominance

Partial dominance occurs when the effect of one allele is partially, but not completely, masked by the presence of another allele. In other words, the 'performance' of heterozygotes is closer to one type of homozygote than the other. Although the effect of the Booroola gene (OMIA 000383-9940) is additive with respect to ovulation rate, the gene appears to show partial dominance with respect to litter size. In this case the B+ genotype is much closer to the BB genotype in litter size than to the ++ genotype (i.e. the B gene appears to be partially dominant; see Fig. 2.16).

In some cattle breeds there is a single gene present which causes extreme muscularity or *double muscling* (muscular hypertrophy; OMIA 000683-9913). This is particularly common in the Belgian Blue and Piedmontese breeds. Although the results are somewhat inconsistent, from some studies it has been suggested that the double muscling gene (myostatin, or *GDF8,* its abbreviated gene identifier) is partially dominant to the gene for normal muscularity. In other words, heterozygotes are closer to homozygous double-muscled animals in appearance and performance than to the homozygous normal animals (see Aiello *et al.* (2018) for a comprehensive review).

Overdominance

Overdominance occurs when heterozygotes show more extreme performance than either homozygote. This type of gene action is probably quite rare, at least for traits of economic importance. The Inverdale gene (OMIA 000386-9940), which affects fertility in sheep, provides a good example of overdominance. The gene was discovered in Romney sheep which had been screened, on the basis of high fertility, into a research flock at the Invermay Agricultural Centre in New Zealand. Romney ewes carrying a single copy of the Inverdale gene have litter sizes about 0.58 lambs higher than normal Romney ewes. (Because of higher neonatal lamb mortality, this is reduced to about 0.17 extra live lambs at 1 day of age.) However, ewes carrying two copies of the Inverdale gene are completely infertile, as they have undeveloped ovaries (Davis, 2004).

Other types of gene action and inheritance

Sex-linked genes

As mentioned earlier, genes are either located on the autosomes (i.e. on any of the chromosomes except the sex chromosomes), or they are located on the sex chromosomes, in which case they are said to be sex linked. Since there is only one pair of sex chromosomes in each cell, and many more pairs of autosomes, it follows that the majority of genes are autosomal. However, there are a few important or interesting examples of sex-linked genes in farm livestock. These include the Inverdale fertility gene (OMIA 000386-9940) in sheep which was mentioned above. The Inverdale gene is located on the X chromosome, so females can carry 0, 1 or 2 copies of the gene (abbreviated ++, I+ and II, respectively), while males, which have only one copy of the X chromosome, carry either 0 or 1 copy of the gene (abbreviated + and I). Hence, calculating segregation ratios for sex-linked genes is a bit more complicated than it is for autosomal genes. The key is to calculate genotype frequencies separately for male and female offspring. This is illustrated for a hypothetical X-linked gene in Table 2.5 (few genes have been identified on Y chromosomes). An added complication in the case of the Inverdale gene is that females homozygous for the Inverdale gene (II) are infertile, so not all types of matings listed produce offspring.

Sex-limited gene action

Sex linkage is not the only route for the sex of an animal to affect gene expression. Sex-linked genes occur on the sex chromosomes. But, autosomal genes may be *sex limited*, even though two copies of the genes are carried by both sexes, if the trait they affect is only shown by one sex, e.g. milk production or ovulation rate are only observed in females.

Sex-influenced gene action

The expression of genes may be *sex influenced*, without being sex linked or sex limited. For example, in some sheep breeds, including the Merino and the Welsh Mountain, the males are usually horned and the females usually polled even though they have the same genotype (OMIA 000483-9940). The polled locus is not on one of the sex chromosomes, so it is not sex linked. Similarly, there is no basic biological reason for horn growth to be sex limited – the fact that both the males and females of many other sheep breeds are horned proves the point. So, there must be another mechanism, such as the level of circulating sex hormones, which alters the expression of the horned gene in some breeds, depending on the sex of the animal. The coat colour of some cattle breeds, such as the Jersey and Guernsey, is darker in males than females, probably for similar reasons.

Genomic imprinting

In most cases, it does not appear to matter which sex of parent an animal inherits an allele from – the effects are the same. For instance, in the Shorthorn coat-colour example mentioned earlier, it does not matter whether roan calves get their R allele from their sire or their dam, they still turn out to be roan. However, there are a few known cases (and probably many more unknown ones) where this rule does not hold, and the effects of a particular genotype on the appearance or function of an animal depend on which parent contributed each allele (Surani and Allen, 1990). This phenomenon is called *genomic imprinting*. Most of the known

Table 2.5. Expected offspring genotype frequencies for a hypothetical sex-linked gene S, on the X chromosome, following matings between parents of different genotype. (The Inverdale fertility gene in sheep follows this pattern of inheritance, except that females homozygous for the Inverdale gene (II) - equivalent to the SS genotype in this example - are infertile, so not all types of matings listed here produce offspring.)

Type of mating		Expected genotype frequencies in offspring				
		Female offspring			Male offspring	
Sire	Dam	SS	S+	++	S	+
S	SS	1	0	0	1	0
S	S+	½	½	0	½	½
S	++	0	1	0	0	1
+	SS	0	1	0	1	0
+	S+	0	½	½	½	½
+	++	0	0	1	0	1

examples of this type of gene action are in laboratory animals or humans, but there is a suspected case of this in sheep. This is the so-called *callipyge* gene (OMIA 001354-9940), which causes extreme muscularity in sheep (Cockett *et al.*, 1996; see Figs 2.17 and 2.18). Initially this was thought to act like an autosomal dominant gene, but studies on the pattern of inheritance suggest that lambs that inherit the callipyge gene from their dam do not show extreme muscularity. This type of inheritance was termed 'polar overdominance' and the callipyge gene is an example of an imprinted gene. Imprinting is an example of an *epigenetic* process, in which the inheritance of changes in phenotypes are not the result of changes in DNA sequence (Nicholas, 2010).

Pleiotropy

Often an allele at a single locus has an influence on more than one animal characteristic. This is known as *pleiotropy*, and a gene which affects several characteristics is said to have a *pleiotropic* effect. For instance, as mentioned above, the single gene, myostatin, is believed to be responsible for double muscling in several cattle breeds, and this condition is often associated with reduced fertility, lower calf survival and sometimes with increased stress susceptibility (OMIA 000683-9913; Aiello *et al.*, 2018). The homozygous polled condition in goats leads to the development of intersex animals, rather than females (OMIA 000483-9925; Boulanger *et al.*, 2014). Also, there are associations between the Merle coat-colour gene (OMIA 000211-9615) and eye and other defects in dogs, and between the Overo coat-colour gene (OMIA 000214-9796) and lethal intestinal obstructions in horses (Nicholas, 2010). There are many other less dramatic and less obvious cases of pleiotropy in traits of economic importance in cattle and sheep.

Epistasis

We have already seen that the effect of one allele at a single locus can be influenced by the presence of another allele at that locus on the other member of a pair of chromosomes – this is termed dominance. When the presence of an allele at one locus masks the effect of an allele *at a different locus*, this is termed *epistasis*. While it is likely that epistasis affects many traits of economic importance in farm

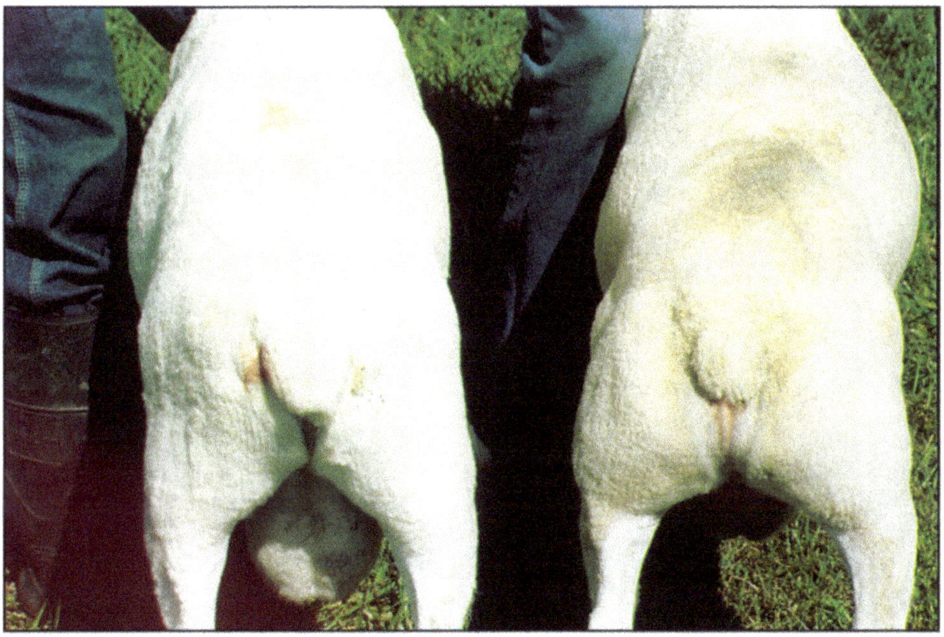

Fig. 2.17. Dorset-Romanov F_1 lambs – the lamb on the left is not carrying a callipyge gene, the lamb on the right is heterozygous for the callipyge gene. (Courtesy of Dr K.A. Leymaster.)

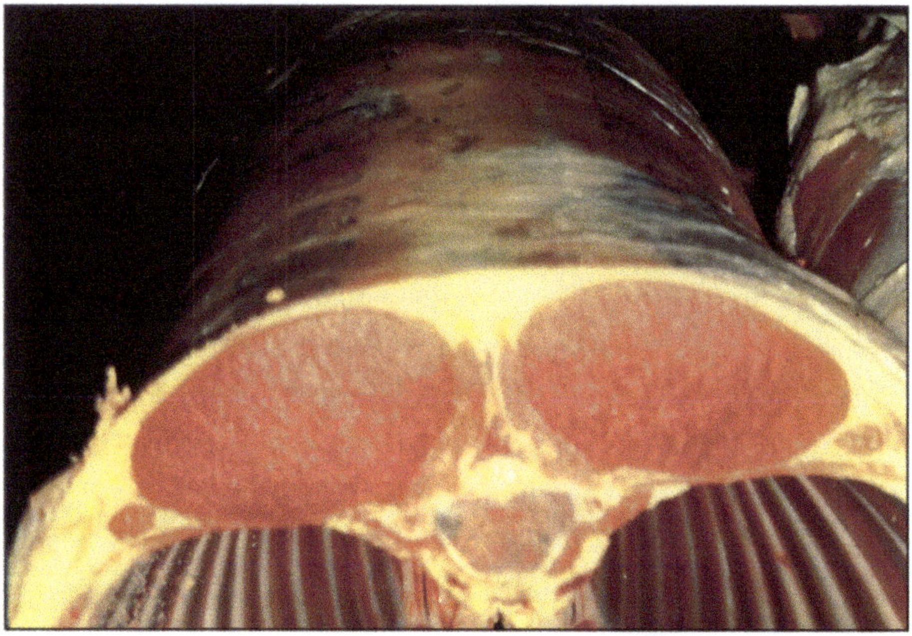

Fig. 2.18. Cross section of a carcass from a lamb carrying the callipyge gene. (Courtesy of Dr G.D. Snowder.)

animals, once again it is easiest to visualize the effects of epistasis from a coat-colour example. The example that is probably familiar to most people is that of coat colour in Labrador Retriever dogs. Colour is controlled by two alleles at each of two loci, called the B (OMIA 001249-9615) and E (OMIA 001199-9615) series. In the presence of the dominant E allele (either one or two copies), one or two copies of the dominant allele B leads to black animals (i.e. BB and Bb are both black), while homozygous recessive animals (bb) are chocolate coloured. All animals which are homozygous for the recessive e allele are yellow, regardless of their genotype at the B locus (though their noses are different colours!). These combinations of genotypes, and their effect on colour, are summarized in Table 2.6. A similar example occurs in some cattle breeds, such as the Simmental (OMIA 001545-9913; OMIA 001199-9913). In Europe, most Simmentals are either deep red, or a lighter yellow colour, in each case with a white face and markings. In fact, both types carry two copies of the red allele, but the expression of these is influenced by the presence or absence of an allele at a different locus which causes dilution of coat colour. Without the dilution allele, the cattle appear red, but with either one or two copies of the dilution allele, they appear yellow (Gutiérrez-Gil *et al.*, 2007).

Table 2.6. The epistatic effect of coat-colour genes in Labrador Retrievers (Willis, 1991)

Genotypes				Phenotype
BBEE	BbEE	BBEe	BbEe	Black
bbEE	bbEe			Chocolate
BBee	Bbee			Yellow (black nose)
bbee				Yellow (liver nose)

Incomplete penetrance and variable expressivity

There are some genetic disorders in animals which are known to be the result of a single recessive gene, but not all homozygous recessive animals show the disease. This is termed *incomplete penetrance*. (It may be a result of epigenetic or environmental influences, or different mutations occurring within the same gene.) A good example of incomplete penetrance occurs in the malignant hyperthermia syndrome in pigs (OMIA 000621-9823). Animals affected by this disorder show increased body temperature, muscle rigidity and respiratory complications, leading to death, when they are exposed to mild stress. Fortunately, a test has existed for many years which allows pig breeders to check whether prospective breeding animals are susceptible. The original test (now superseded by a DNA-based test) involved allowing pigs to breathe halothane vapour, an anaesthetic. Those which reacted by showing a stiffening of the muscles were classified as susceptible (the majority showed a complete recovery from the test). However, a proportion of animals were misclassified as reactors or non-reactors. Although the frequency of misclassifications was reduced with increasing experience of the person conducting the test, there was still less than 100% detection of affected animals.

A similar situation arises with a few other genetic disorders caused by a single gene. In these cases, all animals of the affected genotype show the disease, as expected, but they show it to varying extents. A good example is the condition known as 'mulefoot' which occurs in cattle (OMIA 000963-9913) and pigs (OMIA 000963-9823). It is believed to be caused by a single gene which is recessive in cattle but dominant in pigs. Affected animals have solid hooves, rather than the usual cloven hooves. However, animals with the mulefoot genotype can have from one to four feet affected. This is known as *variable expressivity* (Van Vleck *et al.*, 1987).

There are many situations in animal breeding where the inheritance of particular phenotypes cannot be explained in terms of the animal's genotype at a single locus. In a few cases, such as those outlined above, this may be due to incomplete penetrance or variable expressivity. However, in the vast majority of cases, it is much more likely that the phenotypes observed are the result of the action of genes at more than one locus, or that the phenotype is affected by non-genetic factors (e.g. feeding and management) as well as by genes at one or more loci (so-called *polygenic traits*). These situations are discussed in later sections in this chapter.

Cytoplasmic or mitochondrial inheritance

For generations, livestock breeders have claimed that particular maternal lineages have special attributes. Dairy cattle breeders in particular stress the importance of 'cow families'. Until recently, these claims were often dismissed by scientists as being chance effects, or wishful thinking. However, there is now some evidence of a real effect of cow families, albeit small. So far, the discussion of the transmission of genetic material has focused solely on DNA in the nucleus of cells. While the majority of the DNA is in the nucleus, there are small amounts outside the nucleus, in the cytoplasm. In particular, there is DNA in the *mitochondria* (see Fig. 2.1). These are small structures in the cytoplasm of cells which are responsible for energy generation – the cell's 'power stations'. Because it is only eggs, and not sperm, which contain mitochondria, it is possible that mitochondrial DNA, which gets passed from mother to daughter in vertebrate species, is responsible for the apparent superiority of some cow families. Proving or disproving this from records of performance is incredibly difficult. For example, mothers and daughters usually occur in the same herd, and it is difficult to distinguish between preferential treatment of favoured families and true *mitochondrial inheritance*. Nonetheless, several studies indicate that up to 5% of the total variation in performance could be due to cytoplasmic effects (Gibson *et al.*, 1997; Maniatis and Pollott, 2002).

Names and abbreviations of genes

At this point, it is worth mentioning the way genes are named and abbreviated in Mendelian genetics, because this is often based on their type of gene action. Dominant, co-dominant or additive genes are sometimes abbreviated by using an upper case letter (e.g. R and W in the Shorthorn examples above, and B for the black gene in the Angus breed) while recessive genes are abbreviated by using the lower case version of the letter used to abbreviate the dominant gene. For example, b was the name used for the red gene in the Angus example above; the gene was called b rather than r, to denote that red is recessive to the black gene.

In other cases, one or more letters are used to denote the name of the locus. These are often taken from the character affected by the locus, the name of the person who discovered it, or the place of discovery. Superscripts may be used to denote the alleles that are found there. This is particularly useful if there are more than two alleles at a locus. For example N^d, N^t, and n are the names of three alleles affecting medullation, or hairiness, of the fleece in Romney sheep (OMIA 000443-9940); the n comes from Nielson, the name of the owner of the property on which a ram with an exceptionally hairy fleece was first found. (The N^d and N^t alleles – and a third allele, N^j, discovered in a part Border

Leicester part Romney flock – increase medullation compared to the normal type. This increases the value of the fleece for carpet manufacture and has led to the formation of three new breeds, the Drysdale, the Tukidale and the Carpetmaster based on these three alleles respectively; see Nicholas (1987) for more details.) In cases where an allele is a rare or unusual version of a normal type, the symbol + is sometimes used to denote the normal allele (the wild-type allele), and a letter is used to denote the unusual version (as with the Booroola gene). For sex-linked genes, the genotype is often presented as a superscript on the letter X or Y, depending on which chromosome the gene is located. For example, the full description of the genotype of a ewe heterozygous for the Inverdale gene is Fec X^{I+}. In this case Fec is an abbreviation of fecundity.

The consistent naming of genes has become very important as the molecular genetic revolution has unfolded. Clearly, the scientific community needs to standardize the names of the 25,000 or so genes in the species being studied. International committees oversee the naming of newly discovered genes in an attempt to maintain consistent methods and unique names and to improve communication (see Hu *et al.*, 2014). However, for genes whose effect has been known for a long time, such as those affecting coat colour, there are often many alternative names in use for the locus and its alleles. Also, similar loci and alleles occur across species, and they may have different names in each. Gene names are commonly abbreviated with upper case italicized letters and their equivalent proteins are named similarly but in unitalicized lettering.

The Nature of Traits of Interest in Farmed Animals

Qualitative and quantitative traits

So far, most of the examples of types of gene action in farm animals that we have discussed have concerned coat colour. Characteristics like coat colour and polledness, where the animals can be divided into discrete types with no intermediates, are called *qualitative characteristics*. It was this type of characteristic in plants, such as flower colour and seed coat type, that Mendel studied. Many of these characteristics are controlled by single genes. Also, these traits are often entirely controlled by genes and are unaffected by non-genetic influences. For example, except in rare cases of nutrient deficiency, the coat colour of animals is usually controlled entirely by genes and is unaffected by the type of feed offered.

However, most traits of economic importance in livestock are either expressed in units which can be counted (e.g. numbers of lambs born or weaned, number of services per conception) or, more often, measured on a continuous scale (e.g. kilogram of live weight, litres of milk, millimetres of fat) rather than falling into discrete categories. These are called *quantitative* characteristics. Most of these quantitative traits (also called *metric traits*) are affected by many genes, rather than single genes. Additionally, most of these traits are affected, to a greater or lesser extent, by non-genetic influences. These non-genetic influences are collectively called the *environment*. This includes factors such as the standard of feeding and management of the animal, geographic or climatic influences on performance, together with a host of other chance influences, such as exposure to disease agents. For example, there is an important genetic component to the milk yield of dairy cows, but the actual yield achieved by cows depends not only on their *genetic merit* (the sum of the total effects of genes on milk yield), but also on how well they are fed and managed.

The bridge between Mendel's work on qualitative characters and the genetic basis of measured or quantitative traits was made in the first couple of decades of the 1900s by R. A. Fisher in Britain and Sewall Wright in the USA. The application of these ideas in animal breeding was pioneered by J. L. Lush in the USA in the 1930s. (See OMIA (2019) for landmark papers on genetics by these and other authors.)

Genetic and environmental influences

An important concept in animal breeding is that the genotype of an animal confers on it a particular value for a given trait. Across the whole population of animals, the average performance of animals will be a reflection of their average genetic merit. However, the performance of individual animals may appear better or worse than their true genetic merit, depending on whether they receive a favourable or unfavourable environment. For instance, the milk yield of a cow of very high genetic merit may be quite low if she happens to be in a herd in which she is fed poorly.

Conversely, a cow of lower genetic merit may produce much higher yields than the cow mentioned previously, as a result of being kept in a herd which is well fed.

To summarize, for most quantitative traits, the phenotype (P), or observed performance of an animal depends on the genotype (G) it inherits and the environment (E) it 'receives'. This is often abbreviated to the simple mathematical *model* (after Falconer and Mackay, 1996):

Phenotype (P) = Genotype (G) + Environment (E)

The genotype of an animal can be split further into additive genetic effects (i.e. the combined effects of all genes which act additively on the trait of interest; abbreviated to A), plus non-additive genetic effects, due to dominance and epistasis, abbreviated to NA, so:

Genotype (G) = Additive genetic (A) + Non-additive genetic (NA)

and

Phenotype (P) = Additive genetic (A) + Non-additive genetic (NA) + Environment (E)

For most quantitative characteristics it is the additive genetic part of the animal's genotype which we try to measure and alter by selection – this part is also termed its *breeding value*. There are good methods available for predicting the breeding value, or additive genetic merit of individual animals, and for predicting changes in the additive genetic merit of a herd or flock from one generation to the next. The former is discussed in Chapter 7 and the latter in Chapter 4. However, it is very difficult to assess the effects of dominance and epistasis on quantitative traits. They are treated largely as 'noise' in within-breed genetic improvement programmes, though they are important in *crossbreeding*. It is simplest to think of the non-additive effects acting alongside the additive part of the animal's genotype, either to enhance or diminish the performance of the animal, in a way which is difficult to predict. For example, live weight in cattle is probably affected by genes at tens or hundreds of loci, some with additive gene action, and some with non-additive gene action (i.e. there is dominance or epistasis or both). Selection on *predicted breeding values* (i.e. additive genetic merit) is expected to give a fairly smooth increase in the average weight of animals in the herd, year by year. But in practice, non-additive gene action can create irregularities in response. For instance, one of the many loci affecting live weight might have two alternative alleles (H and h), one (H) showing partial dominance over the other (h). Let us assume that, on average, the HH animals are 10 kg heavier than the hh animals and the Hh animals are 8 kg heavier than the hh animals. If we select for higher live weight, we will tend to get more HH animals and fewer hh animals; we are increasing the frequency of the H allele and decreasing the frequency of the h allele. However, the increments in performance are not equal as we substitute h alleles by H alleles; there is a bigger increment in response from replacing an hh animal by an Hh animal (8 kg on average) than from replacing an Hh by an HH (2 kg on average). So, non-additive gene action such as this contributes to unevenness in *response to selection* (see Chapter 3).

The fact that there are so many grades or levels of performance in quantitative traits, as a result of many genes and the environment acting together, means that it is usually impossible to observe the Mendelian segregation ratios seen in qualitative characteristics. However, this segregation is still happening and the principles of inheritance of quantitative traits are exactly the same as those already described for traits like coat colour – it is simply harder to see what is happening. Most of the following chapters are about the methods that are used to surmount the problem of not being able to detect different genotypes easily, in order to make genetic improvement in quantitative traits.

Traits affected by single genes

There are many examples of traits of importance where a single gene is known or thought to be involved. In farm animals these include:

- coat and feather colour (OMIA 001216-9913, OMIA 001249-9615, OMIA 001199-9615; although several loci are involved, in many breeds there is no variation at some of these loci, or this is masked by variation at other loci, so control of colour is often effectively at a single locus);
- polledness in cattle (OMIA 001736-9913, OMIA 000483-9913; absence of horns; the polled gene P is dominant to the horned gene p in *Bos taurus* cattle breeds), sheep (OMIA 000483-9940) and goats (OMIA 000483-9925; inheritance is more complex and breed dependent);
- muscular hypertrophy, or double muscling, in cattle (OMIA 000683-9913);

- muscularity in some sectors of the Poll Dorset sheep breed in the United States, and now other breeds which have been mated to Poll Dorset animals carrying the gene concerned (OMIA 001354-9940; the callipyge gene);
- milk protein types (κ-casein (OMIA 002033-9913) and β-lactoglobulin (OMIA 001437-9913)) affecting cheese-making properties and protein yield of cows' milk;
- a number of genetic diseases and disorders, including tibial hemimelia (OMIA 001009-9913), 'amputated lethal' or 'bulldog calf' syndrome (OMIA 001926-9913), BLAD (OMIA 000595-9913) and DUMPS (OMIA 000262-9913) in cattle; 'spider syndrome' (OMIA 001703-9940 – chondrodysplasia) in sheep; porcine stress syndrome (OMIA 000621-9823);
- susceptibility to scrapie in sheep (OMIA 000944), and infectious pancreatic necrosis in salmon (Houston *et al.*, 2010);
- wool fibre diameter in Romney sheep, and breeds derived from it (OMIA 000443-9940); and
- fecundity in Merino sheep and other breeds that have been crossed to the Merino (OMIA 000383-9940 – the Booroola gene), and in Romney sheep (OMIA 000386-9940 – the Inverdale gene).

Many of the traits listed above are qualitative (i.e. they have discrete phenotypes) but, as discussed earlier, the Booroola gene provides a good example of a single gene that influences a quantitative characteristic. (See Georges *et al.* (2019) for more examples.)

Traits affected by many genes

Usually it is impossible to equate the appearance or performance of an animal with its genotype at a single locus, in the way we have done already for coat colour and the Booroola gene. This is because several or many genes, as well as non-genetic factors, are influencing the phenotype, or measured performance of the animals. These traits are said to be under polygenic control. Even so, what we see when we measure the performance of animals is the net result of Mendelian segregation at many different loci.

Figure 2.19 illustrates this. If we consider a hypothetical (but quite feasible) example of a single locus affecting milk yield additively, with only two alleles possible at that locus, A and B, then there are three possible genotypes: AA, AB and BB. If the A allele has no effect on average lactation yield, but each copy of the B allele adds 50 kg milk to the average yield, then there will be three discrete levels of performance due to variation at this locus. AA

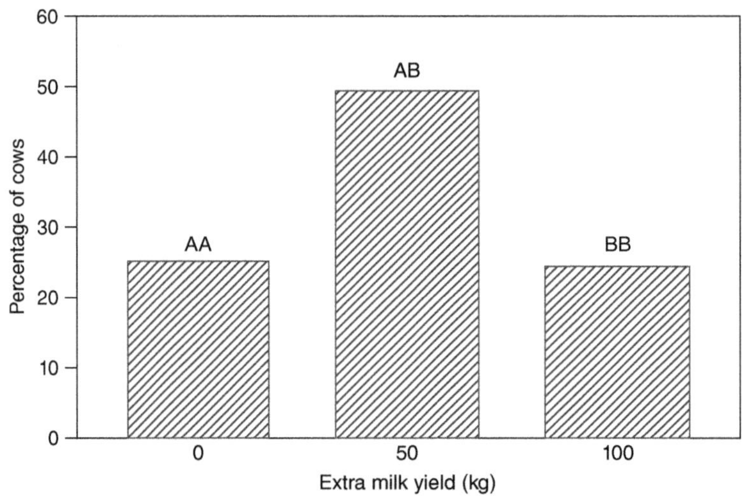

Fig. 2.19. Histogram showing the proportion of cows with different yield levels as a result of variation in genotype at a single locus. The horizontal scale shows the yield level, increasing from left to right. In this example there are three yield levels: 0 kg extra for the AA cows, 50 kg extra for the AB cows and 100 kg extra for the BB cows. The vertical scale shows the proportion of cows that fall into each yield level. In this example, the gene frequency is 0.5, so there are 25% AA cows, 50% AB cows and 25% BB cows. (After Nicholas, 1987; Falconer and Mackay, 1996.)

cows will produce no extra milk, AB cows will have 50 kg higher average yield (i.e. + 50 kg from the single copy of the B allele), and BB cows will produce an extra 100 kg of milk (two copies of the B allele, each worth 50 kg). If the frequency of the A and B allele is the same (0.5), then 25% of the cows will be AA, 50% will be AB, and 25% will be BB. This leads to the distribution shown in the figure.

If we consider a second locus affecting yield, also with two alleles acting additively (J and K) and independently from the first locus (i.e. they are not linked), then there are nine genotypes possible for the two loci considered together. These are shown in Table 2.7. If the J allele has no effect on yield, but each copy of the K allele adds 100 kg, then the three genotypes at this locus will produce 0 kg (JJ), 100 kg (JK) and 200 kg (KK) extra milk. Although there are nine different genotypes, several of these have the same 'value', so only seven different levels of performance are observed. Figure 2.20 shows the expected distribution of yield deviations assuming gene frequencies of 0.5 at each locus, and thus genotype frequencies of 25% AA, 50% AB and 25% BB, and 25% JJ, 50% JK and 25% KK.

Comparing Figs 2.19 and 2.20 shows that as the number of loci affecting performance increases, so too does the number of 'levels' of performance. As the number of loci increases, eventually these levels merge together and the distribution of performance in a population of animals follows a smooth bell-shaped distribution. The performance of most animals falls near the middle of this distribution, and relatively few animals have performance at either extreme. The fact that feeding, management and other non-genetic factors influence performance, also helps to produce a smooth curve. This curve is termed the *normal distribution*, it has a bell shape and is characteristic of many traits of importance in farm animals which are influenced by many genes. Figures 2.21 and 2.22(a) show distributions of the actual live weights of Suffolk ram lambs from a single flock and the milk yields of Holstein Friesian dairy cows from several herds. These distributions are already fairly smooth, but if we repeated this exercise with data from many more animals, the distributions would become even smoother. (As explained later, the distributions also get smoother when some of the known environmental influences on performance are accounted for.)

The distributions such as those shown in Figs 2.21 and 2.22(a) are quite useful in animal breeding, but there are several additional steps which can increase their value further. The shape of a distribution can be influenced by the number of 'bands' of performance which are used to group animals. For instance, if we chose to count the number of cows with total lactation milk yields in only three bands, say between 0–4000, 4001–8000 and 8001–12,000 kg, we would get a rather narrow, spiky distribution. If we went to the other extreme, and chose 120

Table 2.7. The proportion of cows with different yield levels as a result of variation in genotype at two independent loci. The grid shows all possible combinations of genotypes at the two loci, the expected frequency of these combined genotypes given gene frequencies of 0.5 at each locus (this is obtained by multiplying together the genotype frequencies at the first and second loci – for example, if the frequency of the AA genotype is 0.25 and the frequency of the JJ genotype is 0.25, the expected frequency of the AAJJ genotype is 0.25 × 0.25 = 0.0625 or 6.25%), and the expected extra yield as a result of the B allele at the first locus increasing yield by 50 kg per copy, and the K allele at the second locus increasing yield by 100 kg per copy.

	Genotype at first locus, genotype frequency and effect on yield		
Genotype at second locus, genotype frequency and effect on yield	AA 25% 0 kg	AB 50% +50 kg	BB 25% +100 kg
JJ 25% 0 kg	AAJJ 6.25% 0 kg	ABJJ 12.5% +50 kg	BBJJ 6.25% +100 kg
JK 50% +100 kg	AAJK 12.5% +100 kg	ABJK 25% +150 kg	BBJK 12.5% +200 kg
KK 25% +200 kg	AAKK 6.25% +200 kg	ABKK 12.5% +250 kg	BBKK 6.25% +300 kg

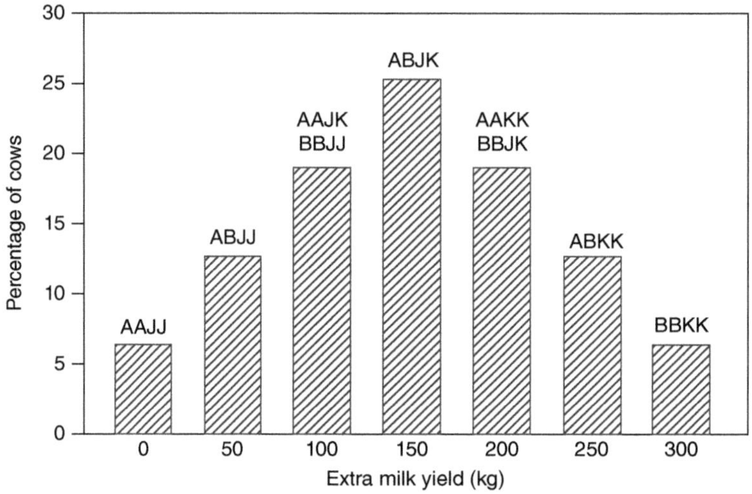

Fig. 2.20. Histogram showing the proportion of cows with different yield levels, expressed as deviations from the average for the herd, as a result of variation in genotype at the two independent loci described in the text and Table 2.7. The horizontal scale shows the yield level, increasing from left to right. In this example there are seven yield levels. The vertical scale shows the proportion of cows which fall into each yield level. The genotype frequencies are 25% AA, 50% AB and 25% BB, and 25% JJ, 50% JK and 25% KK. (After Nicholas, 1987; Falconer and Mackay, 1996.)

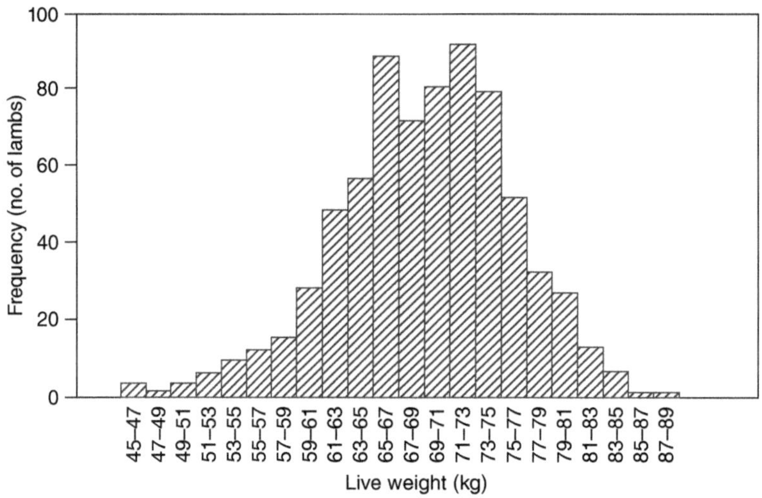

Fig. 2.21. Distribution of the 21-week live weight of over 700 ram lambs, recorded over 9 years, in the SAC Suffolk flock.

bands, in increments of 100 kg, then we would end up with a fairly flat distribution. However, if the number of bands is chosen carefully, comparing the shapes of distributions can be highly informative. For instance, Fig. 2.22(b) shows the distribution of milk protein percentages for the animals whose yields were shown in Fig. 2.22(a). In both cases, performance has been grouped in increments of about 5–6% of the mean performance (300 kg milk and 0.2% protein). The graphs show that there is a narrower distribution, or less variation, in milk protein percentage than in milk yield. Although the

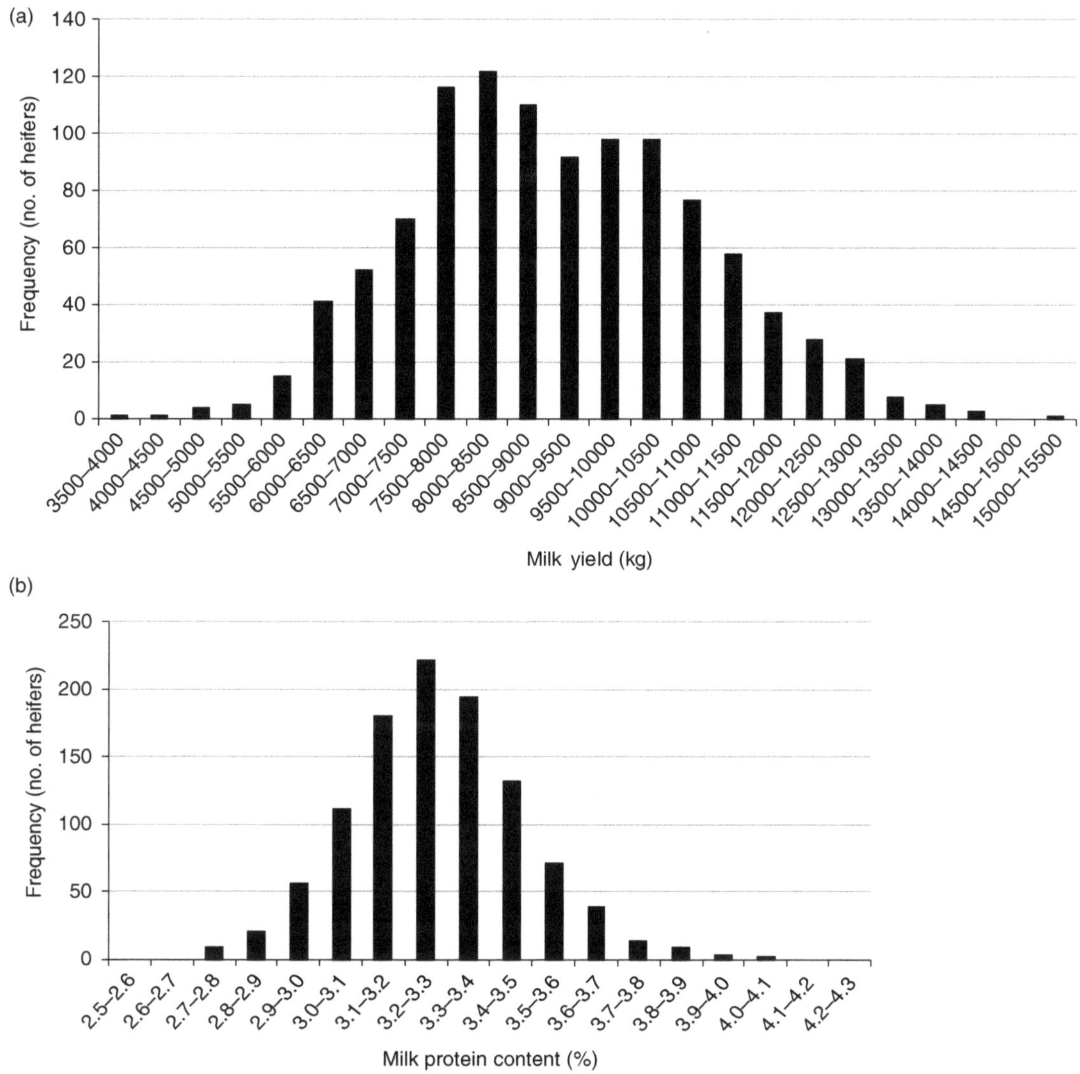

Fig. 2.22. (a) Distribution of the 305-day lactation yields of about 1000 Holstein Friesian heifers that calved in 2018 from a sample of UK herds. (b) Distribution of milk protein contents for the same animals. In both cases performance has been grouped in increments of about 5–6% of the mean performance (500 kg milk and 0.2% protein). (EGENES, Scotland's Rural College.)

amount of variation in a trait can be influenced by management, such as the quantity and quality of feed offered, it is also a biological characteristic of the trait concerned. Measuring the total amount of variation and apportioning this to genetic and non-genetic effects is central to livestock improvement. Later in this chapter, and in Chapter 6, we discuss how this variation is measured; how the measurements are used in improvement programmes is described in Chapters 4 and 7.

At this point, it is worth mentioning another group of traits of interest in animal breeding. The animals' phenotypes for these traits fall into only two, or a small number, of categories. However, they are not inherited in a simple Mendelian way like coat colour, etc., but are influenced by many genes and the environment, just like the normally-distributed traits described above. Ovulation rate and litter size in most sheep breeds (excluding those with the Booroola gene, which has a big impact on litter size), survival and multifactorial diseases such as mastitis are good examples.

Although there are many genes and environmental factors influencing ovulation rate and litter size, most ewes have either 0, 1, 2 or 3 lambs. Similarly, cows or ewes are either unaffected or affected by mastitis (often coded 0 and 1, respectively). In these cases, it is still useful to think of an underlying normal distribution of the causal effect, but the distribution now has one or more *thresholds* which determine the phenotype. For example, within breeds of sheep, ovulation rate, and hence litter size, is partly influenced by an underlying distribution of body condition. Below a certain threshold body condition, a ewe may shed only a single egg, while above it she may shed two. Above an even higher threshold body condition she may shed three eggs, and so on. It may be easier to understand the concept of thresholds from an analogy – that of hen eggs sold on the basis of weight. The weight of eggs follows a normal distribution, but in many countries, eggs are sold according to a small number of bands (e.g. small, medium, large, extra large). The weight of an egg in relation to a series of thresholds determines which band it falls into.

In the case of multifactorial diseases, it is common to think of an underlying normal distribution of *liability* to be affected by the disease. At one end of this distribution there are animals which have a favourable genotype and a favourable environment, and they have a low liability of being affected by the disease. At the other end of the distribution, there are animals who have the worst possible combination of genes and environment, and they are much more liable to be affected by the disease. Dealing with this sort of trait is more complex than dealing with traits like milk yield, and special statistical methods have been developed for the purpose (see Falconer and Mackay (1996) for more details).

Measuring Variation in Performance

Earlier in this chapter we saw that, even when distributions are drawn on a comparable scale, there can be differences in the spread of the distributions, which are characteristics of the traits concerned. For example, there was a wider spread in the distribution of cows' milk yields than in the distribution of their milk protein concentrations. Distributions for the same trait may vary also, depending on the range of genotypes, and the range of environments present. For example, we would expect a wider distribution of yields in a herd using bulls of both very good and average genetic merit for yield than in a herd which only used good bulls. Similarly, we would expect a wider distribution of yields in a herd which fed cows *ad libitum* than in a herd where all the cows received a fixed quantity of feed per day. This is because under *ad libitum* feeding, there is likely to be a wider range of feed intakes than under restricted feeding, and feed intake affects yield.

So far, we have only described the shape of these distributions or amounts of variation in words, but it is important to actually measure the spread of distributions of performance. This is achieved using a statistic called the *variance* (defined as the mean-squared deviation from the mean) or its square root which is called the *standard deviation*.

Variances can only be calculated for a group, or population as it is often called, of animals. The first step in doing so is to prepare a list of performance records for that group of animals, such as live weights, milk yields or egg weights. The best way to do this is to transfer a file of records from a farm database into a spreadsheet using rows as a record for each animal and a column for each of the measured traits that you want to analyse. Simple statistics of your data such as the mean (or average), the variance and standard deviation (the square root of the variance) can then be calculated quite easily using the functions available in the spreadsheet. Table 2.8 gives a simple illustration of calculating the mean (average), variance and standard deviation of the 20-week weights of ten lambs.

Variances are measured in 'squared units', e.g. kg squared (kg^2) or litres squared (l^2), and these are difficult to interpret. Hence the popularity of standard deviations which are expressed in the same units that the records were measured in, for example kg or l, just like the mean (or average) of the trait.

Spreadsheet 2.1 in the online resources repeats the data in Table 2.8 so that you can try these calculations using the spreadsheet's mean (average), variance and standard deviation calculation functions. Try it and see if you get the same answers as shown in Table 2.8.

Now have a go at analysing the data in Spreadsheet 2.2 (see online resources). Here we have four traits

Table 2.8. Calculation of the variance and standard deviation of lamb weights. The unshaded cells show the records, the calculations are shown in the shaded areas.

Animal identity	20-week weight (kg)	Deviation from mean (kg)	Squared deviation (kg^2)
1	70	+5	+25
2	73	+8	+64
3	61	−4	+16
4	58	−7	+49
5	63	−2	+4
6	67	+2	+4
7	60	−5	+25
8	68	+3	+9
9	69	+4	+16
10	61	−4	+16
Total	650	0	228 kg^2
Mean	65 kg	**Variance** (total from column 4, divided by 9 [n = 10, so n − 1 = 9])	25.33 kg^2
		Standard deviation	$\sqrt{25.33}$ kg^2 = 5.03 kg

all measured on the same set of 500 lambs: 8-week weight, scanning weight, muscle depth and fat depth. Read these data into your favourite spreadsheet program. Plot a distribution of each trait to see how they vary about the mean. Now try to calculate the mean, variance and standard deviation of each trait.

As mentioned earlier, many of the traits of interest in farm livestock follow a normal distribution. Calculating variances and standard deviations for these traits, as described above, allows some important predictions to be made about the proportions of animals expected in different 'bands' of performance. These predictions are based on some very useful characteristics of normal distributions that are worth noting here (see Fig. 2.23(a)):

- The mean is in the middle of the distribution – half of the records will be above the mean, and half below.
- About 68% of the records fall in the range −1 to +1 standard deviations from the mean; a characteristic which is complex to explain, but very useful in practice. For example, if the standard deviation (s.d.) of lamb 20-week weight is 5 kg, and the mean is 65 kg, then about 68% of the lamb weights are expected to fall in the range 60–70 kg (the mean −1 s.d. is 60 kg, the mean +1 s.d. is 70 kg). This is illustrated in Fig. 2.23(b).
- About 95% of the records fall in the range −2 to +2 s.d. from the mean. So, in the lamb weight example, we expect about 95% of lamb weights to fall between 55 kg and 75 kg.
- Over 99% of the records fall in the range −3 to +3 s.d. from the mean. So, in the lamb weight example, we expect over 99% of lamb weights to fall between 50 kg and 80 kg. In other words, when traits are normally distributed, the performance of most animals will be close to the average. Progressively fewer animals will have performance near either extreme.

If a trait of interest does not have a normal distribution, *transformation* of the data can be used to convert measured values into data with a normal distribution. There are a number of common transformations used with livestock data, including log, square root and cubed root. Some examples of these occur in later chapters on particular species. Also have a look at the data you plotted using Spreadsheet 2.2. Are there any traits that do not look normally distributed?

Variances or standard deviations provide a valuable tool for comparing variation in the same trait in different groups of animals, e.g. animals in different herds or flocks, or belonging to different breeds. A higher variance or standard deviation indicates a greater spread from the mean of the trait, which may be the result of a wider variation in genetic merit, or a wider variation in environment, or both. It is difficult to directly compare variances or standard deviations for different traits, such as growth rate and fatness. But this can be done by calculating the *coefficient of variation* – this is the standard deviation, divided by the mean

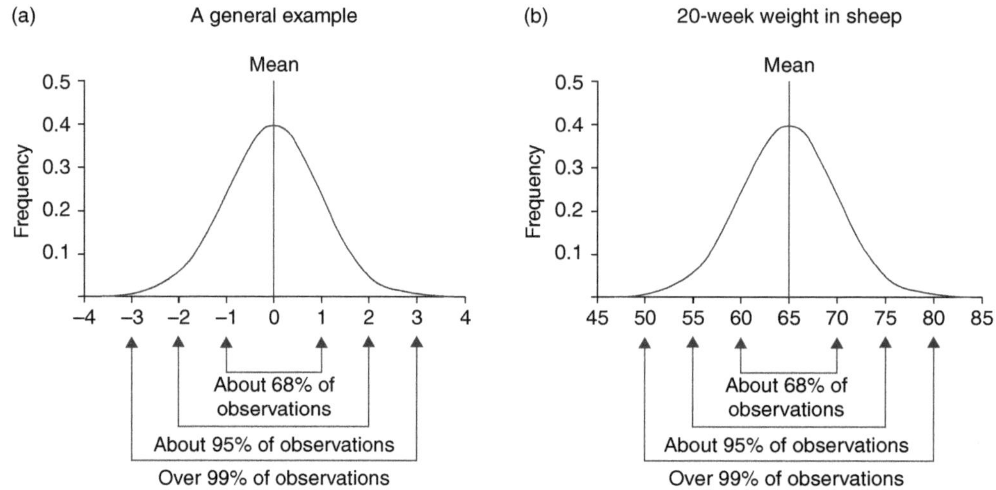

Fig. 2.23. Some properties of the normal distribution, which are useful in predicting the proportions of animals which fall in different 'bands' of performance. (a) A general example: the vertical axis shows the expected frequency of observations, and the horizontal axis is in standard deviation units. (b) An example of 20-week weight in sheep, which is assumed to have a standard deviation of about 5 kg; the horizontal axis is in kilograms.

for the trait concerned in a population. The coefficient of variation is often expressed as a percentage, i.e. multiplied by 100. Table 2.9 shows the means, standard deviations and coefficients of variation for 20-week weights and ultrasonic fat and muscle depths in a group of Suffolk ram lambs. This table shows that, proportionately, there is most variation in fat depth, and slightly more variation in weight than in muscle depth. You might like to calculate the coefficient of variation of the four traits in the lamb data set using Spreadsheet 2.2. How do your results compare to those in Table 2.9, bearing in mind these results are from different groups of sheep?

The principle of splitting the individual animal's phenotype into genotype and environment was explained above using a simple mathematical model. The same principle can be extended to groups of animals, so that the total variation observed (phenotypic variance, or VAR_P for short) may be split into a component due to variation in the genotype of the animals (genetic variance, VAR_G), and a component due to variation in their environment (environmental variance, VAR_E). (The fact that variation from different sources can be split and added together in this way is another reason why variances are such a useful tool in animal breeding.) To summarize, the total phenotypic variance in a population of animals, for a particular trait, is the sum of the genetic and environmental variance (after Lush, 1945):

$$VAR_P = VAR_G + VAR_E$$

The split between genetic and *environmental variation* is illustrated in Fig. 2.24. The narrower, taller distribution in the centre of the curve represents the genetic variation in this particular population. The environmental variation adds to this genetic variation, to create the wider, flatter curve, which represents the total phenotypic variation. In practice, what we see and measure directly when we record animal performance is the wider distribution, or phenotypic variation. However, it is important to remember that this results from underlying distributions of genetic and environmental variation.

As before, the genetic part of the variation can be split into parts due to *additive genetic variance* (variance in breeding values) and variance due to the non-additive (VAR_{NA}) genetic effects of dominance and epistasis:

$$VAR_G = VAR_A + VAR_{NA}$$

and

$$VAR_P = VAR_A + VAR_{NA} + VAR_E$$

Table 2.9. Means, standard deviations and coefficients of variation of live weight, ultrasonic fat depth and ultrasonic muscle depths in a group of SAC Suffolk ram lambs.

Trait	Mean	Standard deviation	Coefficient of variation = s.d./mean
Live weight (kg)	69.4	7.1	0.10 (10%)
Fat depth (mm)	7.3	1.3	0.18 (18%)
Muscle depth (mm)	28.5	2.3	0.08 (8%)

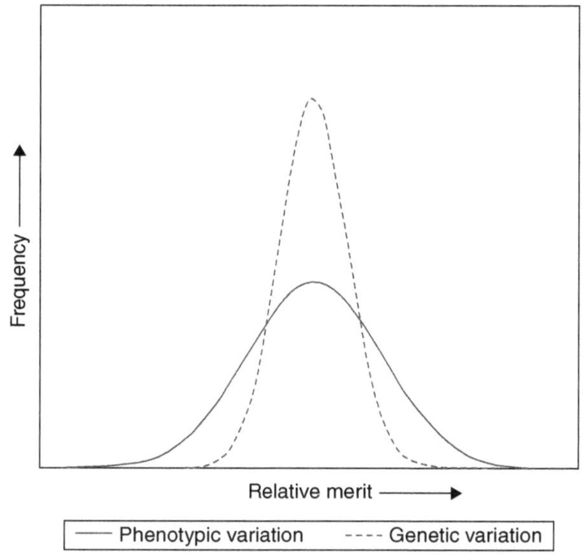

Fig. 2.24. A typical distribution showing the variation in performance of farm livestock. The distribution has been split into its genetic and environmental components. The narrower distribution in the centre of the curve represents the genetic variation in this particular population. The environmental variation adds to this genetic variation, to create the wider outside curve, which represents the total phenotypic variation. In practice, what we see and measure directly when we record animal performance is the wider distribution, or phenotypic variation.

How we attempt to split the distribution into its components, and the rôle these have in practical genetic improvement is discussed in more detail in later chapters. However, Fig. 2.25 gives a simple example. This diagram shows distributions of estimated genetic merit of bulls for milk yield, based on the performance of their daughters, along with distributions of the yield of their daughters in a sample of herds.

You may be wondering why we use this rather complicated way of looking at genetics. In farmed livestock one of the key features of the traits we may want to improve is the extent to which they will be passed on, or inherited, from one generation to the next. So, if we have a herd of sows that produces many piglets, will their female offspring also produce many piglets? After all, if this is not the case then there is no point in trying to use genetics to improve the herd. The way we measure this 'ability to pass on similar levels of performance' is using a measure called the *heritability* of the trait. In simple English, this is the level of genetic control of a trait compared to the influence of the combined genetic and *environmental effects* on performance (feeding, management, health, etc.). The heritability is defined as the ratio of VAR_A to VAR_P, i.e. VAR_A/VAR_P. As you can see above, VAR_P contains VAR_A so the value of the heritability of a trait must lie between 0 and 1. If a trait had a heritability of 0 there would be no point in attempting to improve that trait by selective breeding since it is not influenced by genetics. We will see in Chapter 6 how to

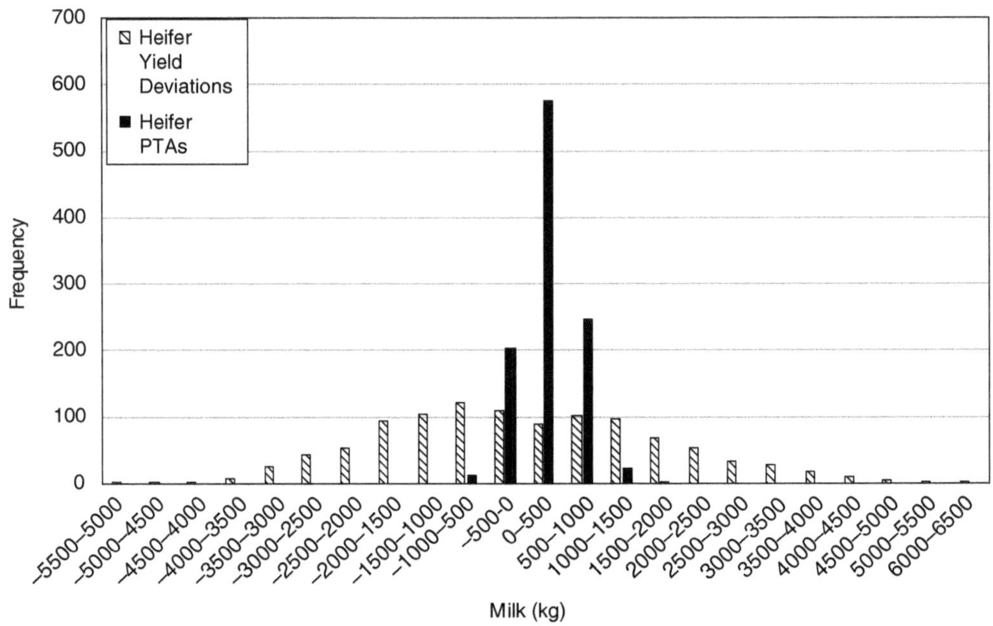

Fig. 2.25. Distribution of the first lactation yield of about 1000 Holstein Friesian heifers from a sample of UK herds, together with a distribution of their estimated genetic merit for milk yield. The heifers' yields are expressed as deviations from the mean yield. The distribution of yields estimates VAR_P. The heifers' genetic merit is expressed as the 'predicted transmitting ability' (PTA) – the expected deviation in yield due to additive genetic effects (VAR_A). (EGENES, Scotland's Rural College.)

calculate the heritability of a trait, and in other chapters we will see how we use the heritability of a trait in breeding programmes.

Measuring Associations Between Traits and Between Animals

Within breeds of farm livestock there are often associations between traits. For example, higher-yielding dairy cows tend to have a lower milk protein percentage; faster-growing meat animals tend to be fatter; and sheep with higher body weight tend to have slightly larger litter sizes. These associations are caused mainly by pleiotropy – that is, the same gene (or genes) influences the two traits – or by environmental conditions which affect one trait also affecting the other. Linkage of genes can also cause an association between traits, but this association will be broken down by recombination over time, unless the genes concerned occur very closely together on the same chromosome.

It is often easiest to see any association between traits by plotting a graph of the measurements of two characteristics for each animal. Fig. 2.26 illustrates this. When there is a positive association between two characters, an upward-sloping line (from left to right) through the points produces the best fit. If there is no association between the traits, the points appear to be scattered randomly all over the graph, and it is impossible to see any pattern at all. With a negative association, the points appear to be gathered around a downward-sloping line.

It is important to be able to measure the direction and strength of associations between traits for a number of purposes in animal breeding. For instance, if we select on one trait we might want to know how other traits will change. Or, we may wish to choose among alternative measurements as predictors of the trait of interest, e.g. different live animal measurements as predictors of carcass composition. Also, measuring the degree of similarity in performance among related animals provides valuable information on the extent to which the measured character is under genetic control. The degree of association between two characters, or between the same character measured at different times, or

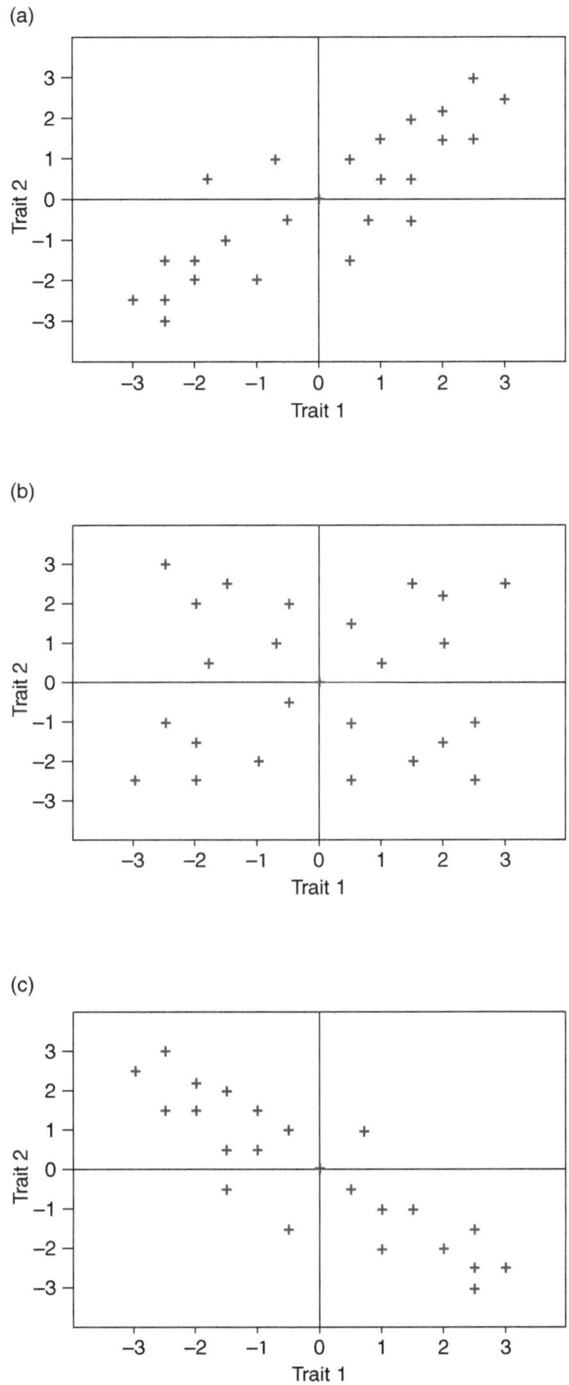

Fig. 2.26. Scatter diagrams illustrating (a) positive, (b) zero and (c) negative associations between traits.

between the same character on related animals is usually measured by one of two closely related statistics – the *regression coefficient* and the *correlation coefficient* (regression and correlation for short).

Regressions measure the extent to which changes in one character are associated with changes in another, in the units of measurement. For example, a regression coefficient would express the association between milk protein percentage and milk yield in terms of the percentage unit change in protein per kilogram increase in milk yield. This is useful if we want to predict an animal's milk protein percentage from its yield. It also tells us about the direction of the association between traits (slightly negative in this case; protein percentage goes down as yield goes up) but it is not easy to tell at a glance whether the association between the two traits is strong or weak. As we shall see in Chapter 6, the regression of offspring performance on parent performance is often used to estimate the heritability of a trait, i.e. the extent to which it is under genetic control.

Correlation coefficients also measure the association between traits, but they do so on a scale from –1, through 0, to +1, rather than in units of measurement. Correlations are more useful than regressions if we want to tell at a glance the strength and direction of the association between two traits, or if we want to compare the strength of associations between different pairs of traits. A correlation which is greater than zero indicates that as one character increases, the other generally increases too (as in the example of live weight and fatness in growing animals). A correlation of zero indicates that there is no apparent association between the two characters. A negative correlation indicates that as one character increases, the other generally decreases (as in the example of milk yield and milk protein percentage). The size of the correlation, either positive or negative, indicates how closely the individual points are clustered around the line drawn through them. If the correlation is +1 or –1, then all of the points will be on the line. With weaker positive or negative correlations then the points are more widely spread out around the line.

It is worth noting that the use of the terms 'positive' and 'negative' when dealing with correlations refers to their mathematical properties (i.e. the slope of the regression line between two traits) *but not their biological properties*. For example, the negative correlation between growth rate and feed conversion ratio (kg feed per kg live weight) in chickens is often considered a good thing since it implies that faster-growing birds are more efficient at converting feed to meat. The mathematical negative correlation arises because a smaller value of feed efficiency implies a more efficient bird which in many situations is preferred. As an alternative example, we observe that milk yield in cows is often positively correlated with calving interval, a common measure of fertility. However, in many situations, this is not a good thing and so a positive correlation is not helpful. Hence, it is important to think of correlations in terms of their biological meaning and not just their mathematical one.

Regression and correlation coefficients are calculated from the variance of one or both of the two characters concerned, and the *covariance* between the two characters. The covariance is calculated in a similar way to the variance, as shown in the last section. However, instead of calculating squared deviations from the mean for a single trait, the deviations from the means of the two traits measured on the same animal are multiplied together to give cross products. Unlike squared deviations, which are always positive, cross products (and covariances) can be positive or negative. To calculate the covariance these cross products are summed, and then divided by $n - 1$, where n is the number of animals. Table 2.10 and Spreadsheet 2.3 (see online resources) give an example data set for the calculation of a covariance. In this case, it is the covariance between fat depth and live weight, for the ten sheep included in Table 2.8. (NB these examples are for illustration only – substantially larger numbers of animals are needed to get reliable estimates of variances and covariances.)

The regression of one trait on another is calculated from the covariance between the two traits and the variance of one of them:

$$\text{regression of trait 2 on trait 1} = \frac{\text{covariance between traits 1 and 2}}{\text{variance of trait 1}}$$

This expresses the change in trait 2, in units of measurement, for each unit change in trait 1. (Conversely, the regression of trait 1 on trait 2 is simply the covariance between the two traits divided by the variance of trait 2.) For example, using the information in Spreadsheet 2.3 and Table 2.10, we can calculate the regression of ultrasonic fat depth on 20-week weight in this group of sheep as:

Table 2.10. Calculation of the covariance between two traits (lamb weight and ultrasonic fat depth at 20 weeks of age). The unshaded cells show the records, the calculations are shown in the shaded areas.

Animal identity	20-week weight (kg)	Deviation from mean (kg)	Ultrasonic fat depth at 20 weeks (mm)	Deviation from mean (mm)	Cross products (column 3 × column 5; kg × mm)
1	70	+5	8.0	+1.1	+5.5
2	73	+8	8.7	+1.8	+14.4
3	61	−4	5.7	−1.2	+4.8
4	58	−7	5.6	−1.3	+9.1
5	63	−2	6.1	−0.8	+1.6
6	67	+2	6.4	−0.5	−1.0
7	60	−5	7.3	+0.4	−2.0
8	68	+3	7.8	+0.9	+2.7
9	69	+4	6.2	−0.7	−2.8
10	61	−4	7.2	+0.3	−1.2
Total	650	0	69	0	31.1
Mean	65 kg		6.9 mm	**Covariance** (total from column 6 divided by 9 (*n* − 1))	3.456 (approx.)

$$\text{regression of fat depth on live weight} = \frac{\text{covariance between fat depth and live weight}}{\text{variance of live wight}}$$

$$= \frac{3.456}{25.33}$$

$$= 0.136 \text{ mm fat per kg live weight (approx.)}$$

In other words, in these sheep, fat depth increases, on average, by about 0.136 mm for each 1 kg increase in 20-week weight.

Correlation coefficients are calculated from the covariance between two traits and the standard deviations of each of them:

$$\text{correlation between traits 1 and 2} = \frac{\text{covariance between traits 1 and 2}}{\text{s.d. trait 1} \times \text{s.d. trait 2}}$$

If we repeat the calculations in Spreadsheet 2.2 for the fat depth measurements, we get a value of 1.11 mm^2 (approx.) for the variance of fat depth, which gives a standard deviation of 1.05 mm. Substituting this into the formula above gives:

$$\text{correlation between weight and fat depth} = \frac{3.456}{5.03 \times 1.05}$$

$$= +0.65$$

Correlations express the relationship between two characters in standard deviation units. For example, a correlation of +1 indicates that an animal which is 1 s.d. above average in one trait is expected to be 1 s.d. above average in the second. Similarly, an animal 2 s.d. better than average in one trait is expected to be 2 s.d. better in the second. A correlation of +0.65 such as that calculated above, indicates that an animal which is 1 s.d. above average in one trait is expected to be 0.65 s.d. above average in the second. Similarly, a correlation of −1 or −0.5 indicates that animals which are 1 s.d. above average in one trait are expected to be 1 s.d. or 0.5 s.d. below average in the other, and so on.

See if you get the same answer using Spreadsheet 2.3 and the functions in your software. If you have been successful, go to the data in Spreadsheet 2.2 and see if you can repeat the regression and correlation calculations between these four traits.

Phenotypic, Genetic and Environmental Associations

There are three types of correlation that are widely used in animal breeding: *phenotypic*, *genetic* and *environmental correlations* (abbreviated r_P, r_G and r_E respectively). There are also equivalent regressions, of which the phenotypic and genetic regressions are the most commonly used (b_P and b_G).

Phenotypic correlations or regressions measure the direction and strength of the association between observed performance, or phenotype, in two characters, e.g. the correlation between live weight and fat depth measured on the same animals. The example calculations in Spreadsheet 2.2 were for phenotypic correlations or regressions.

(a)

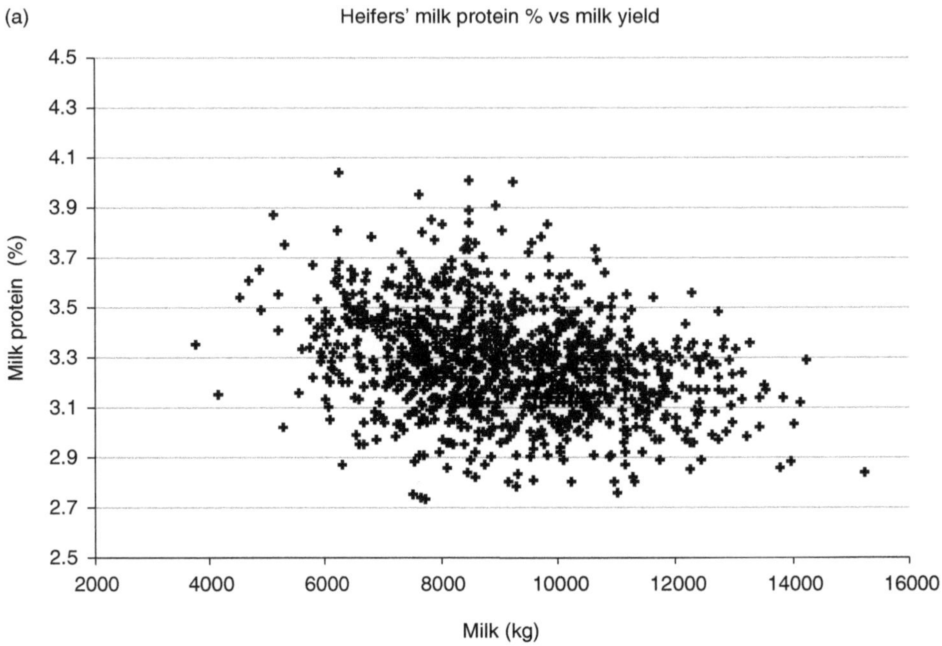

(b)

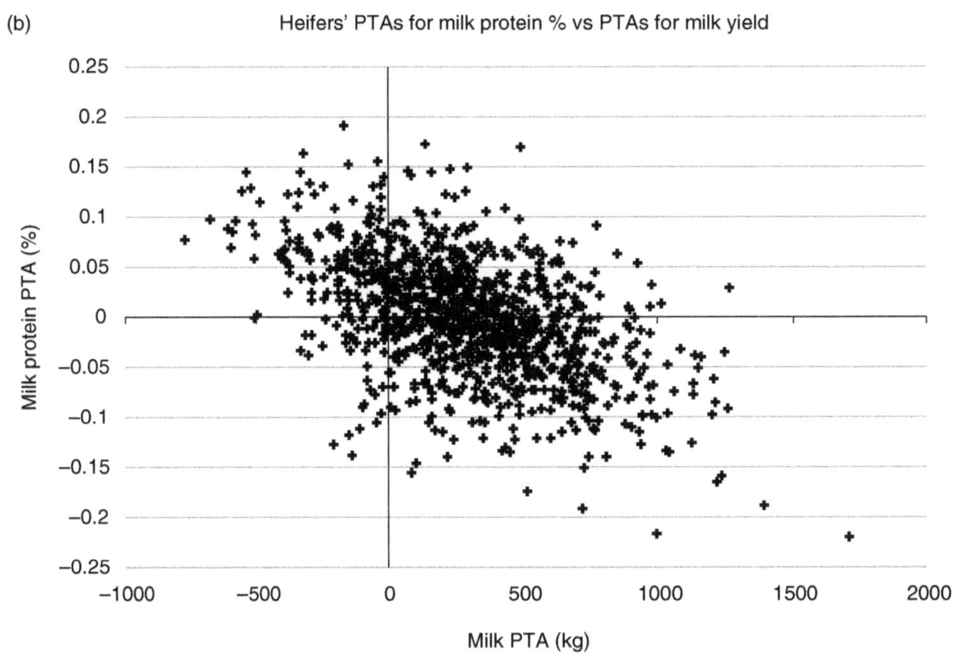

Fig. 2.27. Scatter diagrams illustrating (a) the phenotypic association between milk yield and milk protein % in about 1000 Holstein Friesian heifers, and (b) the association between estimated genetic merit (PTAs) for milk yield and milk protein % of these heifers. Since plot (b) uses predicted rather than true genetic merit, this is not strictly a genetic association. However, since the PTAs are from large scale analyses, they are expected to be close to true genetic merit. (EGENES, Scotland's Rural College.)

Genetic correlations or regressions measure the direction and strength of the association between genetic merit (also known as breeding value) for the two characters – strictly speaking these are *additive* genetic correlations or regressions, abbreviated r_A or b_A. Genetic correlations and regressions are calculated from covariances and variances of breeding values, rather than covariances and variances of phenotypic measurements. A genetic correlation (or regression) between two traits implies that they are affected directly or indirectly by the same genes (either positively or negatively). Often the phenotypic and genetic correlations between two traits are similar, e.g. for many growth traits. They are less similar for traits separated across time, e.g. milk production traits in first and later lactations. Figure 2.27 illustrates the phenotypic association between milk yield and milk protein percentage in dairy cattle and the association between breeding values for milk yield and milk protein percentage.

A positive environmental correlation indicates that environmental conditions which increase one character also increase the second. For instance, feeding a high energy diet *ad libitum* may favour both weight gain and fat deposition, and so create an environmental correlation between them. A negative environmental correlation indicates that environmental conditions which increase one character decrease the second. For example, there is a positive genetic correlation but a negative environmental correlation between mature size and litter size within several species. The negative environmental correlation can arise because the growth of females which are born in large litters is often permanently stunted because of the competition they face for space in the uterus as they develop from an embryo, and the competition they face after birth for a limited supply of milk from their mother. So, although they carry the genes for both high body size and high litter size, they are prevented from fully expressing their genes for body size because of the 'poor' environment they experienced in early life. It is not always easy to define causes of environmental correlations, and they do not often act in the opposite direction to genetic correlations, as in the weight and litter size example. However, it is important to recognize that they exist, and that they lead to differences in the scale, and occasionally the direction, of genetic and phenotypic correlations.

With estimates of any two of these types of correlations, and of the heritabilities of the traits concerned, it is possible to calculate the third (e.g. see Falconer and Mackay, 1996); unlike the situation with the equivalent variances, the phenotypic correlation is *not* simply the sum of the genetic and environmental correlations. Some examples of the three types of correlation in dairy cattle are shown in Table 2.11. More examples of phenotypic and genetic correlations in the various species covered in this book are given in the later chapters on different species of farmed livestock.

Correlations, regressions, variances and covariances are used in animal breeding to:

- predict the changes in one trait which are expected following selection on another;
- construct *selection indexes* which allow simultaneous selection for several characters;
- predict genetic merit or breeding value for single or multiple traits (when there is a positive or negative genetic correlation between two traits, records on one trait can help in predicting genetic merit in the other, e.g. if we had a dairy bull with a high predicted breeding value for milk production, but no records on his daughters' protein percentage, we would predict that he would have a relatively poor breeding value for protein percentage, because of the negative genetic correlation between milk yield and protein percentage);
- measure the *accuracy of predicted breeding values* for individuals;
- measure the *repeatability* of a trait (the correlation between repeated records on the same animal); and
- measure the *accuracy of selection* in a population (the accuracy of selection is the correlation between the criterion on which selection is based, e.g. the animal's own performance, or average performance of a group of *sibs* or progeny, and the true breeding value).

Table 2.11. Examples of phenotypic, genetic and environmental correlations in dairy cattle. (After Visscher and Thompson, 1992.)

Correlations between	r_P	r_A	r_E
Milk yield and protein % (1st lactation)	–0.42	–0.50	–0.36
Milk yield in 1st and 2nd lactations	0.58	0.87	0.42

The first of these uses is discussed in Chapter 4. The others are discussed in more detail in Chapter 7.

Summary

- Modern methods of livestock improvement are founded on the principles of genetics. Hence, an understanding of some of these principles helps in understanding approaches to the genetic improvement of livestock.
- The unit of inheritance is the gene. Genes occur in sequences on the chromosomes which are present in the nuclei of cells. In body cells the chromosomes occur in pairs – the number of pairs is a characteristic of the species concerned. However, the sex cells or gametes – sperm and eggs – contain only a single member of each pair of chromosomes. Hence, every animal receives one member of each pair of chromosomes from its mother, via the egg, and the other from its father, via the sperm. As a result, progeny receive half of their genes from each parent.
- Chromosomes and genes are made up of deoxyribonucleic acid, or DNA. DNA has a ladder-like structure, with rungs of the ladder formed by pairs of bases. This structure, together with the fact that these bases always pair in the same way, provides a very reliable mechanism for copying DNA during cell division - this occurs as part of the growth and development of an animal (mitosis) or during the formation of gametes (meiosis).
- Genes are made up of sequences of bases down one side of the 'ladder', which form a template for the production of proteins. These proteins are either used directly in growth and repair of the body tissues, or they act as signals controlling body functions. Coding regions of genes (exons) account for only around 3% of the total DNA in chromosomes – the rest is involved in controlling the expression of genes, or has an unknown function or no function.
- The site or 'address' of a gene on a chromosome is known as a locus (though the words gene and locus get used interchangeably). Alternative sequences of bases at a locus are termed alleles or genes. There may be many alternative alleles at a locus, but any individual animal will either have two copies of the same allele (one on each member of the pair of chromosomes concerned) or will have a copy of two different alleles.
- Although sperm and eggs receive only one member of each pair of chromosomes, each of these carries genes from both the father and mother of the animal producing the sperm or egg (i.e. the grandparents of the animal which is created when a sperm fertilizes an egg), as a result of recombination. Unless loci occur very close to each other on the same chromosome (i.e. they are linked), genes at different loci are effectively inherited independently, because of recombination and the independent assortment of chromosomes at meiosis.
- Usually DNA gets copied faultlessly during cell division, or errors are corrected by special repair enzymes. However, occasionally mistakes are made which do not get corrected. If these gene mutations occur in cells producing sperm and eggs they lead to changes in the genetic code of offspring. Often these mutations have little or no effect, but sometimes they have favourable or deleterious effects. Mutations which have occurred over many generations are responsible for much of the genetic variation we see today. New mutations are largely responsible for most selected populations continuing to change, even after many generations of selection.
- The particular combination of alleles or genes which an animal inherits is called its genotype (e.g. RR, RW or WW). Animals which have two copies of the same allele (e.g. RR or WW) are homozygous, while those with a copy of two different alleles (e.g. RW) are heterozygous. What we observe when we look at animals, or measure them in some way, is called the phenotype (e.g. red, roan or white coat colour). In some cases, we can infer the genotype from the phenotype (e.g. as with Shorthorn coat colour). In many others we cannot do so, either because of the type of gene action, or because many genes or many genes plus non-genetic effects influence the phenotype for the character concerned.
- The genotype frequencies expected in offspring from matings between two animals of known genotype can be predicted by using a Punnett square. The actual genotype frequencies observed can depart quite widely from these expectations, especially when the number of matings is small. When more than two parents are involved this method of predicting offspring genotypes can be repeated for each type of mating and weighted according to the proportion of each type of mating. However, at a herd, flock or breed level it is

easiest to work with gene frequencies rather than genotype frequencies.

- In large, random-mating populations with no selection, no movement of animals in or out of the population, and ignoring mutation, gene frequencies are expected to stay the same from one generation to the next. However, these conditions are rarely met in farm animals. For instance, chance changes in gene frequency can occur because populations are subdivided into smaller inter-breeding groups. Also, the frequency of genes which have a favourable effect on the trait of interest is expected to increase as a result of selection, while the frequency of those with an unfavourable effect is expected to decrease.
- Genetic improvement depends on genetic variation. The most important sources of genetic variation between individuals or groups of animals are differences in gene frequencies, segregation of genes, recombination and mutation. To use a card-playing analogy, the first three of these sources of genetic variation work by shuffling and splitting the existing pack. However, mutation can create completely new cards.
- Genes or alleles can act in several different ways. With co-dominance, heterozygotes show characteristics of each of the homozygous types. The equivalent type of gene action on measured traits, when heterozygotes are exactly intermediate to homozygotes, is called additive gene action. Complete dominance occurs when the presence of one allele completely masks the effect of another allele at the same locus. Partial dominance occurs when the performance of heterozygotes is closest to that of animals homozygous for one of the alleles concerned. Overdominance occurs when the performance of heterozygous animals exceeds that of both homozygous types.
- The action of some genes depends on the sex of the animal. If the locus is on one of the sex chromosomes, it is said to be sex linked; if the trait of interest is only ever seen in one sex, but the locus is not on one of the sex chromosomes, it is said to be sex limited; other traits, which are neither sex linked nor sex limited, may be sex influenced. Genomic imprinting occurs when the expression of a gene in offspring depends on which sex of parent contributed the gene. Pleiotropy occurs when an allele at a single locus influences more than one characteristic of the animal. Epistasis occurs when the presence of an allele at one locus masks the effect of an allele at another locus. When a character is entirely controlled by a single gene, but not all animals of a given genotype show the expected phenotype, this is termed incomplete penetrance. The equivalent type of gene action when animals show the expected phenotype, but to varying degrees, is called variable expressivity. Small amounts of genetic information are passed from mothers to daughters via mitochondrial DNA. This may influence animal performance to a small extent. This is termed cytoplasmic or mitochondrial inheritance.
- Many traits of interest in farm animals are influenced not only by genes, but also by the environment in its widest sense (including feeding and management). For these traits it is useful to think of an animal's phenotype being comprised of its genotype (which can be further subdivided into an additive genetic component, termed its breeding value, and a non-additive genetic component) and an environmental component. Modern methods of livestock improvement attempt to disentangle these components as far as possible. Selection between and within breeds acts largely on additive genetic merit, while crossbreeding may be used to benefit from additive or non-additive genetic differences between animals, or both of these.
- There are quite a few traits of interest in farm animals under the control of single genes (e.g. coat colour, polledness, many genetic disorders). However, most traits of interest are affected by genes at many different loci, as well as by non-genetic factors. Although Mendelian segregation is at work at each of these loci, it is difficult to distinguish different phenotypes. Instead, the performance of animals tends to show continuous variation. Often the performance of animals follows a bell-shaped curve, or 'normal distribution', with most animals near the middle, and only a few at either extreme.
- Many of the 'tools' used in livestock improvement rest on properties of this bell-shaped distribution of performance. The variation in performance in a group of animals can be measured using a statistic called the variance, or its square root the standard deviation. From these statistics, we can predict the proportions of animals with different levels of performance. The variance in performance in a group of animals can

also be split into additive genetic, non-additive genetic and environmental components. This allows comparisons of the relative importance of these different sources of variation and is useful when deciding on a strategy for genetic improvement, and for predicting responses to selection.

- There are often associations between traits in livestock. These associations are caused mainly by pleiotropy or by environmental conditions that affect one trait also affecting the other. Linkage of genes can also cause an association between traits, but this association is soon broken down by recombination, unless the genes concerned occur very closely together on the same chromosome.
- It is important to be able to measure the direction and strength of associations between traits. This is achieved using regression or correlation coefficients, which are calculated from the covariance between the two traits and the variances of one or both traits. Regressions express the association between two traits in units of measurement. Correlations fall in the range –1 to +1. The sign indicates the direction of the association between traits. The size of the coefficient indicates the strength of the association; the closer to 1 the correlation, the stronger the association between the traits.
- There are three types of correlation which are widely used in animal breeding: phenotypic correlations, genetic correlations and environmental correlations (abbreviated to r_P, r_G and r_E). Similarly, phenotypic and genetic regressions are widely used (b_P, b_G). Phenotypic correlations or regressions measure the degree of association between observed performance, or phenotype, in two characters. Additive genetic correlations or regressions measure the degree of association between breeding values for two characters (r_A or b_A). A positive environmental correlation indicates that environmental conditions which are favourable for one character are also favourable for the second. A negative environmental correlation indicates that environmental conditions which favour one character are unfavourable for the second.
- Correlation, regressions, variances and covariances, are used in animal breeding to predict the changes in one trait which are expected following selection on another, to construct selection indexes which allow simultaneous selection for several characters, to predict breeding values, and to measure the accuracy of selection or the accuracy of predicting breeding values.

References

Aiello, D., Patel, K. and Lasagna, E. (2018) The myostatin gene: an overview of mechanisms of action and its relevance to livestock animals. *Animal Genetics* 49, 505–519. DOI: 10.1111/age.12696.

Ansari, H.A., Pearce, P.D., Maher, D.W., Malcolm, A.A. and Broad, T.E. (1993) Resolving ambiguities in the karyotype of domestic sheep (*Ovis aries*). *Chromosoma* 102, 340–347. DOI: 10.1007/BF00661277.

Biotechnology and Biological Sciences Research Council (1996) *The New Biotechnologies – Opportunities and Challenges*. BBSRC, Swindon, UK.

Boulanger, L., Pannetier, M., Gall, L., Allais-Bonnet, A., Elzaiat, M. *et al.* (2014) FOXL2 is a female sex-determining gene in the goat. *Current Biology* 24, 404–408. DOI: 10.1016/j.cub.2013.12.039.

Cockett, N.E, Jackson, S.P., Shay, T.L., Farnir, F., Berghmans, S. *et al.* (1996) Polar overdominance at the ovine callipyge locus. *Science* 273, 236–238. DOI: 10.1126/science.273.5272.236.

Comber, S.C. and Smith, C. (2004) Polyploidy in fishes: patterns and processes. *Biological Journal of the Linnean Society* 82, 431–442. DOI: 10.1111/j.1095-8312.2004.00330.x.

Davis, G. H. (2004) Fecundity genes in sheep. *Animal Reproduction Science* 82–83, 247–53. DOI: 10.1016/j.anireprosci.2004.04.001.

Falconer, D.S. and Mackay, T.F.C. (1996) *Introduction to Quantitative Genetics*, 4th edn. Longman, Harlow, UK.

Fogarty, N.M. (2009) A review of the effects of the Booroola gene (FecB) on sheep production. *Small Ruminant Research* 85, 75–84. DOI: 10.1016/j.smallrumres.2009.08.00.

Georges, M., Charlier, C. and Hayes, B. (2019) Harnessing genomic information for livestock improvement. *Nature Reviews Genetics* 20, 135–156. DOI: 10.1038/ s41576-018-0082-2.

Gibson, J.P., Freeman, A.E. and Boettcher, P.J. (1997) Cytoplasmic and mitochondrial inheritance of economic traits in cattle. *Livestock Production Science* 47, 115–124. DOI: 10.1016/S0301-6226(96)00023-1.

Gutiérrez-Gil, B., Wiener, P. and Williams, J.L. (2007) Genetic effects on coat colour in cattle: dilution of eumelanin and phaeomelanin pigments in an F2-Backcross Charolais × Holstein population. *BMC Genetics*, 8, 56. Available at: https://bmcgenet.biomedcentral.com/articles/10.1186/1471-2156-8-56. (accessed 27 August 2020).

Houston, R.D., Haley, G.S., Hamilton, A., Guy, D.R., Mota-Velasco, J.C. *et al.* (2010) The susceptibility of Atlantic salmon fry to freshwater infectious pancreatic necrosis is largely explained by a major QTL. *Heredity* 105, 318–327. DOI: 10.1038/hdy.2009.171.

Hu, Z., Reecy, J.M., McCarthy, F.M. and Park, C.A. (2014) Standard Genetic Nomenclature. Available at: http://lib.dr.iastate.edu/ans_pubs (accessed 1 February 2019).

Innovate UK (2019) *How to Manage or Remove Inherited Diseases from Animal Populations using "Homozygosity Mapping".* Technical manual, RIDGENE. Available at: https://connect.innovateuk.org/documents/3285671/31025255/RIDGENE%20Manual (Accessed 10 January 2019).

Lush, J.L. (1945) *Animal Breeding Plans,* 3rd edn. Iowa State College Press, Ames, Iowa.

Maniatis, N. and Pollott, G.E. (2002) Nuclear, cytoplasmic and environmental effects on growth, fat and muscle traits in Suffolk lambs from a sire referencing scheme. *Journal of Animal Science* 80, 57–67. DOI: 10.2527/2002.80157x.

Martínez. P., Viñas, A.M., Sánchez, L., Díaz, N., Ribas, L. and Piferrer, F. (2014) Genetic architecture of sex determination in fish: applications to sex ratio control in aquaculture. *Frontiers in Genetics* 5, 340. DOI: 10.3389/fgene.2014.00340.

Mendel, G. (1865) Experiments in plant hybridization. *Paper read at the February 8th, and March 8th, 1865, meetings of the Brünn Natural History Society.* Available at: http://www.esp.org/foundations/genetics/classical/gm-65.pdf (accessed 3 January 2019).

Nicholas, F.W. (1987) *Veterinary Genetics.* Oxford University Press, Oxford.

Nicholas, F.W. (2010) *Introduction to Veterinary Genetics*, 3rd edn., Wiley-Blackwell, UK.

OMIA (Online Mendelian Inheritance in Animals) (2019) Sydney School of Veterinary Science. Available at: https://omia.org/home/ (accessed 3 January 2019).

Patrushev, L.I. and Kovalenko, T.F. (2014) Functions of noncoding sequences in mammalian genomes. Originally published in *Uspekhi Biologicheskoi Khimii*, 54, 39-102. English version available at *Biochemistry (Moscow)* 79, 1442–1469. DOI: 10.1134/S00062 97914130021.

Piper, L.R., Bindon, B.M. and Davis, G.H. 1985. The single gene inheritance of the high litter size of the Booroola Merino. In: Land, R.B. and Robinson, D.W. (eds.) *Genetics of Reproduction in Sheep.* Butterworths, London. pp. 115–125.

Pollott, G. E. (2018) Invited review: Bioinformatic methods to discover the likely causal variant of a new autosomal recessive genetic condition using genome-wide data. *Animal* 12, 2221–2234. DOI: 10.1017/S1751731118001970.

Simm, G. (1998). *Genetic Improvement of Cattle and Sheep*. Farming Press, Ipswich, UK.

Simm, G., Bünger, L., Villanueva, B. and Hill, W.G. (2004) Limits to yield of farm species: genetic improvement of livestock. In: Sylvester-Bradley, R. and Wiseman, J. (eds) *Yields of farmed species. Constraints and opportunities in the 21st century.* Nottingham University Press, Nottingham, UK, pp. 123–141.

Singh, M., Ma, X., Amoah, E. and Kannan, G. (2011) In vitro culture of fibroblast-like cells from postmortem skin of Katahdin sheep stored at 4°C for different time intervals. *In Vitro Cellular and Developmental Biology - Animal* 47, 290–293. DOI: 10.1007/s11626-011-9395-6.

Surani, M.A. and Allen, N.D. (1990) Genomic imprinting: epigenetic control of gene expression, phenotypic variations and development. *Proceedings of the 4th World Congress on Genetics Applied to Livestock Production,* Vol XIII, pp. 27–34. Available at: http://www.wcgalp.org/proceedings/1990 (accessed 3 January 2019).

Visscher, P.M. and Thompson, R. (1992) Univariate and multivariate parameter estimates for milk production traits using an animal model. I. Description and results of REML analyses. *Genetics, Selection, Evolution* 24, 415–430. DOI: 10.1186/1297-9686-24-5-415.

Willis, M.B. (1991) *Dalton's Introduction to Practical Animal Breeding*, 3rd edn. Blackwell Scientific Publications, Oxford.

Xue, Y., Wang, Q., Long, Q., Ng, B.L., Swerdlow, H. *et al.* (2009) Human Y chromosome base-substitution mutation rate measured by direct sequencing in a deep-rooting pedigree. *Current Biology* 19, 1453–1457. DOI: 10.1016/j.cub.2009.07.032.

Zimin, A.V., Delcher, A.L., Florea, L., Kelley, D.R., Schatz, M.C. *et al.* (2009) A whole-genome assembly of the domestic cow, *Bos Taurus. Genome Biology* 10, R42. DOI: 10.1186/gb-2009-10-4-r42.

Recommended Reading

Lush, J.L. (1945) *Animal Breeding Plans,* 3rd edn. Iowa State College Press, Ames, Iowa.

Lynch, M. and Walsh, B. (1998) *Genetics and Analysis of Quantitative Traits*. Sinauer Associates, Sunderland, Massachusetts.

Nicholas, F.W. (1987) *Veterinary Genetics.* Oxford University Press, Oxford.

Nicholas, F.W. (2010) *Introduction to Veterinary Genetics*, 3rd edn., Wiley-Blackwell, UK.

Online Mendelian Inheritance in Animals. Available at: https://omia.org/home/ (accessed 03 January 2019).
Orel, V. (1996) *Gregor Mendel: The First Geneticist*. Oxford University Press, Oxford.
Schafberg, R. and Swalve, H.H. (2015). The history of breeding for polled cattle. *Livestock Science* 179, 54–70. DOI: 10.1016/j.livsci.2015.05.017.
Walsh, B. and Lynch, M. (2018) *Evolution and Selection of Quantitative Traits*. Oxford University Press, Oxford.

3 Strategies for Genetic Improvement

Introduction

For thousands of years humans have attempted to alter populations of animals to make them more suitable for the production of food and fibre, as providers of transport, draught power, etc. These attempts have been increasingly effective over the last couple of centuries, especially since the mid-1900s. Generally, improved breeds of livestock produce food, fibre or other products, which are of higher quality, or are better matched to modern requirements than their predecessors. Also, improved breeds usually have higher efficiency of production than unimproved breeds, and so the relative cost of production is lower. For example, in many countries genetic improvement of pigs and poultry has contributed to the change in status of pig and poultry meat from being luxury foods, to being the cheapest meats available. In many countries, the price of milk has fallen in real terms over the last few decades, partly as a result of genetic improvement of yield and overall efficiency of production. Selection for reduced fibre diameter and increased fleece weight in specialized sheep breeds has been important in allowing wool to continue to win a share of the market for clothing fabrics. Genetic improvement is particularly valuable because it is permanent, it is cumulative when selection is continuous, and it is usually highly cost effective (we give examples in later chapters on different farmed species).

The aim of this chapter is to describe the strategies which are employed to achieve genetic improvement. Some more detailed examples of both the benefits and, importantly, the possible negative consequences of selection, and how these can be avoided or reduced, are discussed in later chapters. Traditionally three main strategies have been used for the genetic improvement of livestock. These are:

- *Selection between breeds* or breed types – comparing two or more breed types and selecting the most appropriate, or substituting one breed type for another.
- *Selection within breeds* or breed types – choosing better parents within a particular breed type.
- *Crossbreeding* – mating parents of two or more different breed types or species together.

We use the terms breed type here to cover conventional pure breeds, strains within breeds, *composite* or synthetic lines, and populations recently derived from wild stock, as in the case of finfish.

These strategies are discussed in more detail below. Developments in molecular and reproductive biology are augmenting these approaches, e.g. the growing use of markers in *genomic selection* within breeds or strains. These developments are also allowing new strategies, still largely in experimental use in livestock, including the ability to transfer genes within or between species, to 'edit' genes, and to regulate or modify the expression of existing or introduced genes. These new possibilities are discussed in more detail in Chapter 5.

For any genetic improvement strategy to be effective, it is important to have a clear view of what the economically – or otherwise – important animal characteristics (traits) are. Then it is logical to choose the most appropriate breed type or cross, based on their performance in these traits. It is then sensible to consider whether this pure breed, or component breeds of the chosen cross, can be improved further by *within-breed selection*. In practice, the availability of information on the performance of different breeds and crosses, the financial and physical resources available, the current breeds or crosses in use, local traditions, local market demands and personal preferences also influence the choice of breed or cross, and the extent to which within-breed selection is practised, at least in the short term.

Before discussing the different strategies for genetic improvement in detail, it will be helpful to

Genetic Improvement of Farmed Animals (G. Simm *et al.*)
DOI: 10.1079/9781789241723.0003

consider the structure of the livestock breeding industries in which they are applied.

The Structure of Livestock Breeding Industries

The structure of livestock breeding industries in most industrialized nations is often described schematically as a pyramid with *elite* (or *nucleus, seedstock* or *stud)* populations or breeders at the top, one or more middle tiers of purebred or *crossbred* multipliers, and a final tier of commercial herds or flocks, or end users (see Fig. 3.1). In this generalized model, the elite breeders' rôle is to produce breeding stock (particularly males, as fewer of these are needed to produce a given number of offspring) for use within the top tier and in multipliers' herds or flocks. The elite populations are the main focus for genetic improvement. The main rôle of multipliers, as the name suggests, is to take improved stock from the tier above, and to create larger numbers of breeding animals for sale to the tier below. In most industries, there are purebred multipliers involved in producing greater numbers of purebred animals, particularly males, for the tiers below. However, in some industries there are also crossbred multipliers, who produce crossbred animals, particularly females, for use in the commercial tier. Usually flocks or herds in the commercial tier are primarily involved in the production of eggs, meat, milk or fibre, and have little or no involvement in selling stock for further breeding. Hence, genetic improvement flows down the pyramid, or is disseminated, from elite, through multiplier, to commercial tiers. The difference in genetic merit of different tiers of the pyramid is termed the *improvement lag*.

In the pig and poultry industries in many countries, the elite and multiplier tiers are mainly in the hands of a small number of multinational breeding companies. They maintain elite purebred or synthetic lines, often in several countries, in which most of the selection is practised. Breeding stock from these lines then moves to the company's own multiplier herds or flocks, or to herds or flocks contracted by them, to produce both males and females for sale to commercial producers. These pigs and poultry produced for the commercial tier are usually crossbred. (In some countries there is further 'vertical integration', with companies being involved from nucleus breeding, multiplication through to commercial production and processing.)

For the most advanced aquaculture sectors, such as Atlantic salmon, the supply of genetically improved stock is largely controlled by few, large multinational breeding companies (in some cases, the same companies that produce elite pigs and poultry lines). There is less need for multiplication tiers for aquaculture species, and large breeding nuclei can supply siblings of elite *broodstock* for production, or they have a single multiplication layer. The companies do not typically produce specialized lines, nor is crossbreeding common, but some companies do offer *marker-assisted* or genomic selection for specific characteristics (e.g. resistance to specific pathogens). For the aquaculture sectors that are less advanced, the status of breeding programmes and the commercial interest varies dramatically within a single species. For example, Nile tilapia is arguably the world's most

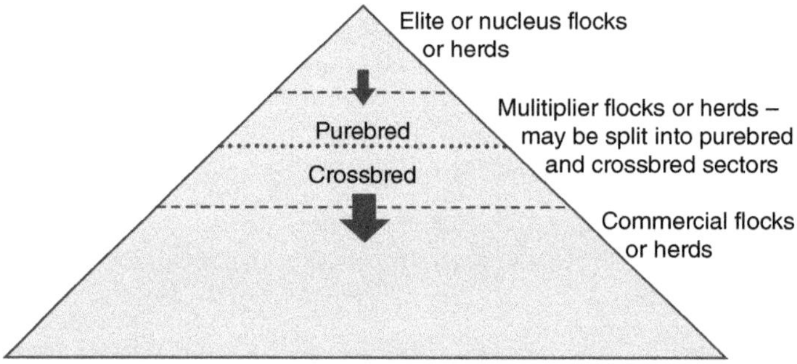

Fig. 3.1. Diagram illustrating the structure of livestock breeding industries in many industrialized nations. This is a pyramid with elite or nucleus populations at the top, one or more middle tiers of purebred or crossbred multipliers, and a final tier of commercial herds or flocks, or end users. (After Nicholas, 1987.)

important food fish, and while some genetically improved lines are bred and disseminated globally by major multinational breeding companies, the majority of production is via local hatcheries and smallholder farmers. In these systems the breeding is less well controlled and can be a mix of commercial and public sector suppliers of stock. Across most sectors, there is a mix of specialized breeding companies with core business in supply of genetically improved eggs and juveniles and also integrated companies who perform both selective breeding and production via vertical integration, as observed in some pig and poultry companies.

The very widespread use of artificial insemination (AI) in the dairy industries of most countries has effectively removed the middle tier from the breeding pyramid. That is, the commercial tier has direct access to elite animals via AI. The elite tier in dairy cattle breeding is usually owned by a mixture of private breeders and breeding companies – the former own most of the elite cows, and the latter own most of the elite bulls. Unlike the situation in the pig and poultry industries, in most temperate countries the commercial tier in the dairy industry is made up largely of purebred animals (New Zealand is a notable exception).

In most countries, all tiers of the pyramid in the sheep, goat and beef cattle breeding industries are in the hands of individual breeders, rather than breeding companies. (A few sheep and beef breeding companies have emerged in the last few years and have gained a significant market share in New Zealand, North and South America.) However, the structures of the breeding industries vary quite markedly from country to country. For instance, the Australian finewool industry is based on purebred Merino sheep in all tiers. The middle and lower tiers of the Merino industry also act as crossbred multipliers for some sectors of the lamb meat industry, by producing half-bred Merinos (crosses between Merino ewes and, usually, Border Leicester rams). These, in turn, are mated to rams from *terminal sire* or meat breeds (especially the Poll Dorset). The New Zealand sheep industry was based largely on purebred dual-purpose ewes in all tiers. These included the Romney, Coopworth, Perendale and Corriedale breeds which had been selected to produce both meat and wool. In commercial flocks a proportion of these pure dual-purpose ewes were often crossed to terminal sires. With stronger market demand for meat than wool in the last few decades, there has been a shift in both Australia and New Zealand towards more specialized meat-producing breeds or crosses, including newly created crosses or composites. In the UK, hill sheep flocks in all tiers are usually purebred. As in the Merino example, many of these UK hill flocks act as crossbred multipliers, producing crossbred ewes for the commercial tier of the sheep industry in the lowlands and uplands. These are usually produced from *draft* hill ewes – those which have had about four lamb crops on the hill and have been moved to a less extreme environment for crossing, usually to rams from one of the longwool breeds. The resulting crossbred ewes are generally mated to purebred rams from a terminal sire or specialized meat breed, to produce lambs for meat production.

The pastoral beef industries of many temperate countries or regions are based on purebred cows of the traditional British beef breeds – Hereford, Aberdeen Angus and Shorthorn, or crosses between them. Often these are mated to purebred bulls from the larger continental European breeds, such as the Charolais, Simmental or Limousin. Purebred animals are the norm in all tiers of the French beef industry. In contrast, much of the commercial tier in Britain and Ireland has been based traditionally on beef × dairy crossbred cows. Until recently, the popularity of these crossbred cows was partly because of the plentiful supply of replacement beef × dairy heifers from dairy herds – a by-product of the practice of crossing dairy heifers, and those cows not required for breeding replacement dairy heifers, to a beef bull. In these cases, dairy herds act as multipliers of crossbred cows for the beef industry. (These cows kept for rearing calves for beef production are called *suckler cows*.) Table 3.1 gives some examples of where some typical livestock enterprises fit on the breeding and dissemination pyramid.

The terms purebred and pedigree require further explanation. Purebred or straightbred animals are those produced from several or many generations of matings between animals of the same breed. Strictly speaking, any purebred animal whose parentage, or more distant ancestry, is known can be described as a *pedigree animal*. However, pedigree is often used to mean *pedigree registered* – in other words an animal whose ancestry, and other details, are officially recorded by a *breed society* or other organization set up for this purpose. In Britain, most sheep in the elite tier, except in some hill breeds, and virtually all beef and dairy cattle in the elite tier are pedigree registered. This is also true for a significant

Table 3.1. Examples of enterprises in various tiers of the 'breeding pyramid'. Several tiers may be present in a single farm or business. (After Simm *et al.*, 1994 and Simm, 1998.)

Tier	Dairy cattle	Beef cattle	Sheep	Pigs	Poultry
1. Elite or nucleus breeders	Breeding companies 'contract mating' top AI bulls to elite cows often in private ownership. Pedigree Holstein Friesian breeders selling heifers to other breeders in this tier, or to the tier below.	Pedigree terminal sire (or other) beef breeders, selling bulls to other elite pedigree herds (tier 1), and purebred multiplier herds (tier 2).	Pedigree terminal sire or longwool sheep breeders, selling rams to other elite pedigree flocks (tier 1) and multiplier pedigree flocks (tier 2). Purebred 'stud' breeders of Merinos selling rams within this tier and to purebred multipliers.	Breeding companies selecting sire and dam lines. Pedigree breeders.	Breeding companies selecting egg laying and broiler strains of chicken. Pedigree breeders.
2. Purebred multipliers	Pedigree or other breeders producing heifers for sale to commercial herds.	Pedigree terminal sire herds buying bulls from tier 1, and selling bulls for crossing in commercial herds (tier 4).	Pedigree terminal sire flocks buying rams from tier 1, and selling rams for crossing in commercial flocks (tier 4). Pedigree longwool breeders selling rams to crossbred multipliers.	Breeding companies multiplying sire and dam lines for sale to tier 4. Pedigree breeders.	Breeding companies multiplying egg laying and broiler strains. Pedigree breeders.
3. Crossbred multipliers	-	Dairy herds buying beef bulls from tier 2 or beef semen from tier 1 or 2, and selling beef x dairy heifers to suckler herds in tier 4. Pure beef herds (e.g. Galloway) crossing to another beef breed (e.g. White Shorthorn) and selling crossbred heifers (e.g. Blue Grey) to suckler herds in tier 4.	Draft ('retired') hill ewes (e.g. Scottish Blackface) crossed to longwool sires (e.g. Bluefaced Leicester) to produce crossbred breeding females (e.g. Scottish Mule) for use in tier 4. Draft Merino ewes crossed to Border Leicester rams to produce crossbred females for tier 4.	Breeding companies or their partners/agents creating crosses for sale to tier 4 producers.	Breeding companies or their partners/agents creating crosses for sale to tier 4 producers.
4. Commercial or end users	Purebred Holstein Friesian (or other) dairy herds, using AI with semen from bulls in tier 1.	Crossbred suckler cow herds (e.g. Hereford or Simmental × Holstein Friesian; Blue Grey) buying replacement females from tier 3, and bulls from tier 2.	Crossbred ewe flock (e.g. Scottish Mule, Border Leicester × Merino) buying replacement females from tier 3, and rams from tier 2.	Commercial pig farmers buying replacement gilts and boars from multipliers in tier 3.	Commercial egg producers buying point-of-lay pullets from multipliers; commercial broiler producers buying day old chicks from multipliers/hatcheries in tier 3.

proportion of 'commercial' dairy cattle. Most purebred beef cattle and sheep in the multiplier tier are pedigree registered; others have unofficial records of ancestry but are not registered with a breed society. In the commercial tier most beef and sheep are crossbred, though a few are purebred but not pedigree registered. Traditionally, great status has been attached to animals which are officially pedigree registered. In many cases pedigree-registered animals have a higher monetary value than non-registered animals, though this does not always reflect their genetic merit. Breed societies have generally provided a valuable service in maintaining accurate records of animals' pedigrees – a service which is valued by both breeders and potential buyers of pedigree livestock. However, until relatively recently, fewer societies have actively promoted performance recording, and the use of both pedigree and performance records to assist selection decisions. The combination of performance and pedigree records is one of the factors which makes modern methods of genetic improvement so effective. Increasingly, breed societies have recognized this, and many have broadened their services to provide detailed information on performance as well as ancestry, and have improved their members' access to, and understanding of, selection tools.

In the idealized model of a livestock breeding industry, strong market signals ought to go up this pyramid from one tier to the next, resulting in a clearly defined *breeding goal* in each tier. This is an accurate reflection of what happens in most pig, poultry, finfish and dairy cattle breeding industries in industrialized countries. It is also increasingly the case in beef cattle and sheep breeding industries, though in some breeding goals are still set 'top down' instead of 'bottom up'. In other words, breeding goals for elite animals are influenced much more by market signals from within the top tier (e.g. by the high prices other breeders pay for show-winning or 'fashionable' animals), rather than from tiers below. Frustration with this situation led to the formation of *group breeding schemes* in several sheep and beef cattle breeds in New Zealand in the 1960s (Parker and Rae, 1982). The farmers concerned were not satisfied that the tiers above were producing breeding stock relevant to their needs, and so they established co-operative breeding schemes to produce their own replacement breeding stock, especially males. In most cases, this involved the formation of nucleus flocks or herds. These are elite flocks or herds formed by screening the best cows or ewes from co-operators' own herds or flocks. Comprehensive recording and rigorous selection in the nucleus results in genetic improvement of commercially important traits in the nucleus animals, which is then disseminated to members' own flocks or herds when they obtain replacement rams and bulls (or females) from the nucleus (see Fig. 3.2). While these schemes have become less common in industrialized countries, they are being applied to good effect in some lower-income countries, circumventing the lack of industry-wide infrastructure for breeding programmes. They often form the basis of community-based breeding programmes in these countries (see e.g. Mueller *et al.*, 2015 and later chapters).

A number of factors are involved in diluting the signals between tiers in livestock industries. The many links in the chain connecting primary producers to consumers often leads to imperfect communication, and so the signals reaching commercial producers may be weak in the first place. In some countries, direct or indirect subsidies may mask 'true' market signals. There may be a lack of understanding of, or low availability of, objective information on the genetic merit of breeds, crosses or individual animals within breeds. Also, social factors are often important – for instance, especially historically, some breeders preferred to breed show winners than to follow strict market signals. For a small and decreasing number of elite breeders there are still niche markets which are based mainly on show performance. At least in the short term, it is probably more profitable for this minority of breeders to breed for show performance, than to breed for the traits of most economic or other importance in the tiers below. Unfortunately, other breeders may be lured by the potentially big rewards from these small niche markets and neglect the larger markets. A further complication occurs if the animals produced in some tiers are by-products of other primary activities. For example, the main concerns of most dairy farmers crossing to a beef bull is the bull's effect on calving ease in their dairy herd, and then the potential sale value of the calf. They are less concerned about the possible use of some daughters of the beef bull as suckler cows, and so most of them pay little attention to the performance traits which might be useful in that rôle (e.g. intermediate mature size and good maternal performance) when choosing a beef bull.

It will be apparent now that the number of tiers present in the breeding pyramid, and their relative importance, will vary between species and countries.

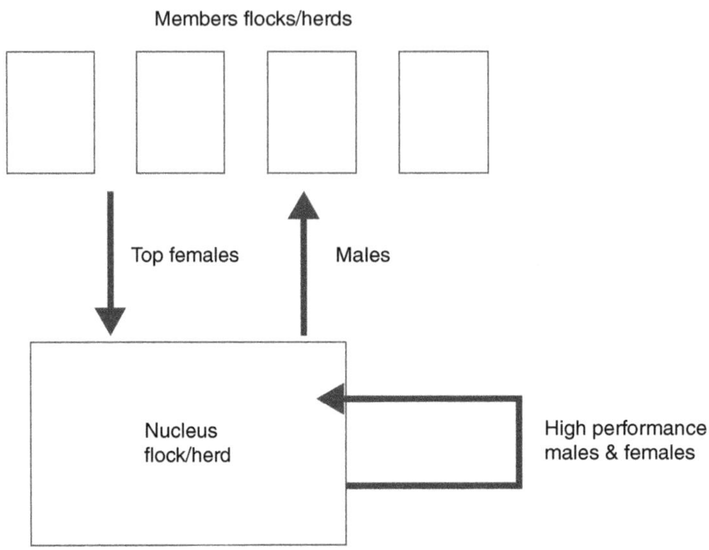

Fig. 3.2. A diagram illustrating the principles of group breeding schemes. These include (i) formation of a central nucleus herd or flock, from the best females available in members' own herds or flocks; (ii) comprehensive recording and rigorous selection for commercially-important traits in the nucleus; (iii) the best males produced in the nucleus are retained there for breeding, while the next best group (or ex-nucleus males) are the main source of breeding males for members' herds or flocks – this is the main route for dissemination of genetic improvement from the nucleus to the base herds or flocks; (iv) elite females may continue to be 'promoted' to the nucleus from base herds or flocks, on the basis of genetic merit (this only takes place in 'open' nucleus schemes – in some cases 'closed' nucleus schemes are preferred, for example to minimize risks of transfer of disease to the nucleus, or because of a lack of recording in base herds or flocks).

The most relevant strategy for genetic improvement for any individual breeder will depend on the breeder's position in the breeding pyramid. Most elite breeders and purebred multipliers will be interested in within-breed selection, and occasionally in *between-breed selection*, if the market changes substantially and their current breed becomes less relevant. Crossbred multipliers will be interested mainly in crossbreeding. Commercial producers will probably be interested in several or all of the strategies for genetic improvement. Although they are users, rather than creators, of genetically improved stock, a knowledge of the techniques involved should allow them to make better decisions on which breed, cross or individual animals to use.

Selection Between Breeds or Breed Types

Selection between breeds or breed types can achieve dramatic and rapid genetic change when there are large genetic differences between populations in characteristics of economic and other importance. *Breed substitution* has led to major step changes in genetic improvement in numerous livestock production systems. However, this benefit is achieved only once per breed substitution, unlike the improvement brought about by continuous within-breed selection.

It is obviously costly to replace whole flocks or herds of breeding females at once. In practice, changes are often made more gradually. If replacement females (i.e. females brought into the breeding herd or flock to replace those that have died of natural causes, or have been *culled*) are usually purchased, then the switch to the new breed type can be made gradually by buying replacements from the new breed. If replacement females are normally homebred, then the composition of the herd or flock can be changed gradually by *grading up* or repeated *backcrossing* to the new breed. Grading up or backcrossing involves repeated mating of the current females, and subsequently their female offspring, to sires of the new breed. Table 3.2

Table 3.2. The proportion of genes from each of two breeds following successive generations of backcrossing, and the time taken to achieve these proportions in cattle and sheep. The letters A and B are used as abbreviations for the two breeds here (not as abbreviations for alleles, as in the previous chapter). In the first cross exactly half of each animal's genes come from each of the two breeds. In subsequent generations of backcrossing the proportions of genes shown are the averages expected – individual animals may have greater or smaller proportions than shown because of segregation and recombination.

Breed composition of:			Number of years after initial cross to produce offspring of the composition shown, assuming females first leave offspring at:		
Sire	Dam	Offspring	1 year old (some sheep breeds)	2 years old (sheep and some cattle breeds)	3 years old (cattle)
A	B	½ A, ½ B	–	–	–
A	½ A, ½ B	¾ A, ¼ B	1	2	3
A	¾ A, ¼ B	⅞ A, ⅛ B	2	4	6
A	⅞ A, ⅛ B	15/16 A, 1/16 B	3	6	9

shows the proportion of genes coming from each of two breeds of cattle or sheep, following successive generations of backcrossing – on average each generation of crossing halves the proportion of genes from the original breed, compared to that in the previous generation. Table 3.2 also shows the minimum time required to achieve particular proportions of genes from each breed. Many pedigree breed societies allow registration of crossbred animals in a separate register, with eventual acceptance as purebred animals once they are 7/8 (the EU legal standard) or 15/16 purebred. Modern pig, poultry and fish (and increasingly cattle and sheep) breeding operations are not subject to these strictures or traditions.

The first important criterion for choosing between breeds, strains or crosses is that the choice ought to be made on the basis of objective comparisons of performance *in the relevant environment* and at a relevant endpoint. There are some dramatic examples of the cost of ignoring this rule – high-performing temperate breeds of livestock have been introduced often to the tropics without this sort of trial, and have then succumbed to diseases or to nutritional deprivation, to which local breeds were tolerant. See Marshall (2014) and the International Livestock Research Institute (ILRI) and partners' African Chicken Genetic Gains (ACGG, 2019) and African Dairy Genetic Gains (ADGG, 2019) projects, for more on this.

Less dramatically, there are important economic benefits to be gained, in any country, from matching breeds or crosses to particular production systems – as indicated by the old adage 'horses for courses' (see Fig. 3.3). The concept that genotypes do not always rank the same in different environments, or that the advantage to a particular genotype in one environment may be smaller or greater in another, is an important one in livestock improvement. In general, this is called a *genotype × environment (G×E) interaction*, or in this particular case, a *breed × production system interaction.* Figure 3.4 illustrates two types of genotype × environment interaction. The genetic correlation between the performance of related animals in two environments can also be used to detect genotype × environment interactions. In theory, if the genetic correlation between performance in the two environments is less than 1, then there is an interaction. However, correlations have to be substantially less than 1 before an interaction is of practical importance.

In wealthier countries, a great deal of research has been done on comparing the performance of different genotypes (breeds, strains, crosses, or animals of different genetic merit within a breed) in different environments (countries, production systems, feeding levels) to help livestock producers choose the most appropriate breed type for their circumstances. In lower-income countries, however, much work remains to be done (Marshall, 2014). At first sight the results of many G×E studies are in conflict – many of them appear to deny the existence of interactions, while others firmly support their existence. It is probably fair to say that if there is a big enough difference in performance between the genotypes, or a big enough difference between the environments in which they are compared, or both, then there will be an interaction. For example, several classical studies indicate that small- or medium-sized beef and sheep breeds have higher

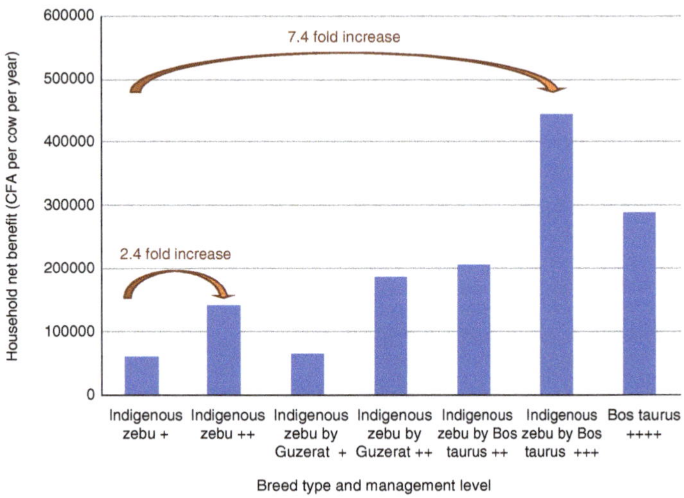

Fig. 3.3. Results of a survey on the impact of choice of dairy breed type and management level on household income in Senegal. The graph shows net benefit in West African CFA Franc per cow per annum, assuming a herd size of eight cows, with management level ranging from + (the lowest level of management) to ++++ (the highest level of management). (After Marshall *et al*., 2016, 2020.)

overall productivity or profitability in extensive grazing systems than larger breeds. But larger breeds tend to do best in more intensive systems with high levels of concentrate feeding (Dickerson, 1978; Cartwright, 1982). There are several possible explanations for this. The more extensive the production system, the greater the effort animals will have to make to harvest the resources they require for maintenance and growth. Hence, smaller breeds may have an advantage in extensive systems, because they have lower requirements for maintenance and growth than larger breeds, and so their requirements are more in balance with the effort they expend in meeting them. An alternative explanation is that the larger sheep and beef breeds are probably the ones which have been subjected to the greatest artificial selection. At the same time, there may have been modifications to their environment, which have reduced natural selection for adaptation to extensive conditions. As a consequence of these two factors, favourable attributes for extensive systems (e.g. high mobility, particular patterns of grazing behaviour, cold or heat tolerance, drought tolerance, disease resistance and strong maternal behaviour) may have been lost, or may have diminished in larger, more intensely selected sheep and beef cattle breeds. (The results of some experiments investigating interactions are given in later chapters.)

Another important criterion for breed or breed type comparisons is that the samples of animals compared should be sufficiently large and representative of the breeds concerned to allow inferences to be drawn about these breeds in general, and not just the sample itself. In other words, the breed comparisons need plenty of animals from different sires and dams (though dams are usually automatically well represented in the less prolific species), and these sires themselves need to be sampled randomly, or in a balanced way, from several to numerous different flocks or herds. This criterion is often violated – newly introduced breeds are often promoted on the basis of very flimsy comparisons, or no objective comparisons at all. The size of the sample required depends on the minimum difference between breeds that is considered to be of economic importance. It also depends on the amount of variation that exists in the trait concerned.

For example, let us assume that a 25 kg advantage in the 18-month weight of Charolais-cross beef calves was the minimum that would justify a producer switching from Simmental crosses. If the standard deviation of 18-month weight is about 50 kg in both crosses, then we would need to compare about 70 animals of each cross to be 90% sure that Charolais crosses were really better,

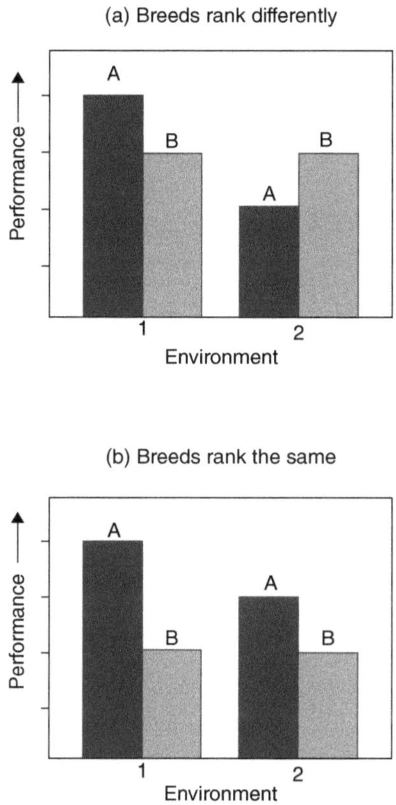

Fig. 3.4. A diagram illustrating two types of genotype x environment interaction. (a) Breeds A and B rank differently in the two environments. (b) Breeds A and B rank the same in the two environments, but the advantage to breed A is much less in environment 2 than in environment 1.

and about 85 animals of each cross to be 95% sure. (See Snedecor and Cochran (1989) or other standard statistics textbooks, for details of how to calculate the numbers of animals required for this sort of test.)

Generally, the higher the degree of genetic control of a trait (i.e. the higher the heritability – this is the ratio of additive genetic to total phenotypic variation in the trait of interest), the greater the number of sires that should be used in a breed comparison. As a rough guide, five or more sires should be used if the traits of interest are lowly heritable, and ten or more should be used if the trait is highly heritable. (This seems odd at first sight, but there is proportionally more variation between sire families for highly heritable traits than for lowly heritable traits. This means that there is a greater risk of mistakenly choosing one breed over another, as a result of the chance sampling of one or two exceptional sires, when the heritability of the trait is high.) Ideally, sires should be from different flocks or herds. References to examples of well-designed breed comparisons are given at the end of this chapter. Tables 3.3 and 3.4 summarize the results of two of these. These results are presented here for illustration only. It is important to remember that breeds change over time as a result of within-breed selection. So, the results of breed comparisons can become outdated fairly quickly, particularly if some breeds are pursuing effective improvement programmes and others are not, or if breeds are selecting for different characteristics.

There are many recent examples of selection between breeds in the livestock industries. In Britain, many dairy herds of Shorthorn, Ayrshire and Channel Island breeds (Jersey and Guernsey) changed to Friesians in the 1950s and 1960s. In the 1980s and 1990s, the local strains of black-and-white dairy cattle in many European and other countries were partly or wholly substituted by North American Holstein strains (see Fig. 3.5). (Most of these different black-and-white strains originate from importations of Dutch Black Pied animals at some time in the last few hundred years, but they have been selected for different objectives, with different rates of progress in different countries, since then.) Typically, the breed substitutions have been prompted by the higher total milk yield of the incoming breed or strain. In many temperate beef-producing countries the traditional British beef breeds have been replaced, at least as terminal sires, by the larger, leaner, continental European breeds such as the Charolais, Limousin and Simmental. In the British sheep industry, many rams from the Border Leicester breed have been replaced by rams from the more prolific Bluefaced Leicester breed for mating to draft hill ewes to produce crossbred breeding females for commercial flocks. Over the last few decades, some commercial dam lines of pigs have been influenced by importations of the prolific Meishan breed from China, while many sire lines have included importations from the Duroc and Pietrain breeds because of their carcass and meat attributes. Table 3.5 shows examples of breed introductions in Africa and South/South-East Asia.

Table 3.3. Results of a comparison between different sire breeds of sheep, mated to Mule (Bluefaced Leicester × Swaledale) ewes. These results are from just a sample of the breeds involved in a large trial run by the Meat and Livestock Commission in Britain. The results here are from 'late flocks' producing lambs off grass, forage crops and roots. The sire breed means are for lambs at the same estimated level of subcutaneous fatness. The superscripts show whether or not sire breeds differ significantly. Within a row, sire breeds with different superscripts differ significantly; those with the same superscript do not differ significantly, e.g. Oxford Down cross lambs were significantly older at slaughter than Southdown crosses, but were not significantly different in age from Suffolk or Texel crosses. (After Kempster *et al.*, 1987.)

	Sire breed mean			
Trait	Oxford Down	Southdown	Suffolk	Texel
Age at slaughter (days)	258^{c}	214^{ab}	228^{bc}	262^{c}
Carcass weight (kg)	19.7^{c}	17.0^{a}	18.6^{b}	19.2^{c}
Daily gain of carcass lean (g)	46^{bc}	50^{c}	49^{c}	46^{bc}
Daily gain of carcass fat (g)	23^{bc}	25^{cd}	23^{bc}	20^{ab}

Table 3.4. Results of a comparison between different sire breeds of beef cattle, mated to Hereford × Friesian and Blue Grey suckler cows. These results are from just a sample of the breeds involved in a large trial run by the Meat and Livestock Commission in Britain. The results here are from winter fattening systems. The sire breed means are for steers at the same estimated level of subcutaneous fatness. The superscripts show whether or not sire breeds differ significantly. Within a row, sire breeds with different superscripts differ significantly; those with the same superscript do not differ significantly, e.g. Charolais crosses were older at slaughter than Aberdeen Angus or Hereford crosses, but were not significantly older than Limousin or Simmental crosses. (After Kempster *et al.*, 1982; Southgate *et al.*, 1982.)

	Sire breed mean				
Trait	Aberdeen Angus	Charolais	Hereford	Limousin	Simmental
Age at slaughter (days)	477^{c}	520^{a}	492^{b}	517^{a}	517^{a}
Carcass weight (kg)	205^{e}	268^{a}	214^{de}	247^{c}	258^{b}
Conformation (15-point scale)	9.9^{b}	11.2^{a}	8.7^{cd}	11.0^{a}	9.9^{b}
Saleable meat in carcass (g/kg)	725^{bc}	727^{b}	719^{cd}	733^{a}	720^{cd}
Fat trim in carcass (g/kg)	96^{abc}	90^{c}	97^{abc}	92^{bc}	93^{abc}

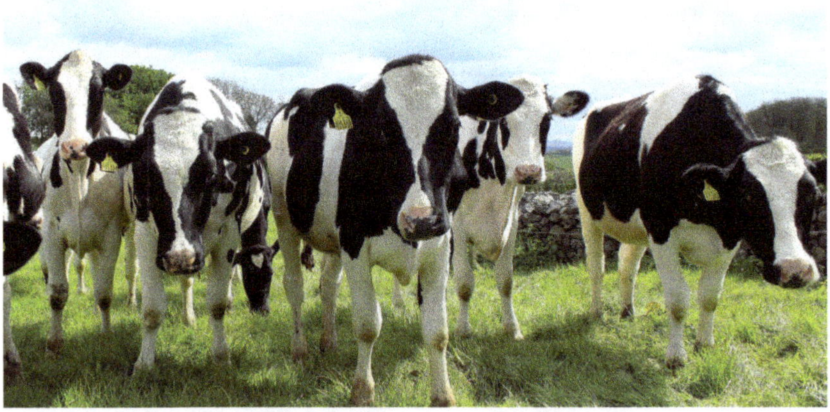

Fig. 3.5. North American Holstein Friesians have had a dramatic impact on the populations of dairy cattle in most temperate countries over the last few decades. (Available at: https://pixabay.com/photos/holstein-cattle-cows-heifers-field-2318436/, accessed 8 December 2019.)

Table 3.5. Examples of breed introduction in livestock production systems in Africa and South/South-East Asia. For most livestock types two examples are given: one where the breed originated in a higher income country, and one where the breed originated in a lower-income country. (After Marshall, 2014; Data from FAO, 2007 and according to the Domestic Animal Diversity Information System (DAD-IS: http://dad.fao.org/) accessed September 2012.)

Livestock type	Example
Cattle – dairy	European dairy breeds (including Holstein Friesian and Jersey, amongst others) in 26 African and 12 South and South-East Asian countries
	The Sahiwal dairy breed of Pakistan/India in 12 African and 6 other South and South-East Asian countries
Cattle – meat or dual-purpose	The Brahman, developed in North America from Indian stock, in 15 African and 3 South and South-East Asian countries
	The Boran of Kenya and Ethiopia in 7 other African countries
Sheep	The Suffolk from UK in 6 African and 2 South and South-East Asian countries
	The Blackhead Persian from Somalia in 12 other African and 1 South and South-East Asian country
Chicken	The Rhode Island Red of North America in 16 African and 8 South and South-East Asian countries
	The Aseel from India in 2 other South and South-East Asian countries
Goat	The Saanen dairy goat of Europe in 17 African and 6 South and South-East Asian countries
	The Jamnapari of India in 7 other South and South-East Asian countries
Pig	The Large White of Europe in 24 African and 10 South and South-East Asian countries

Selection Within Breeds or Breed Types

Selection within breeds or breed types involves comparing animals of the same breed type and mating the preferred animals to produce the next generation. This process is usually repeated each generation, and as long as there is genetic variation in the characters under selection, this produces changes in successive generations (compared to between-breed selection, where the changes occur only once per breed substitution).

In any population of farm (or wild) animals, the size of the population can only be maintained if adults produce enough offspring in their lifetime to replace themselves when they die or are culled. The capacity to produce potential replacements varies between species and between sexes. For instance, pigs, poultry and especially fish, produce far more potential replacements per adult than cattle, sheep and goats, and in all species there are generally far fewer replacement males needed than females, since each male is usually mated to several or many females. It is this production of more replacements than needed to maintain population size which provides the opportunity for selection within breeds.

Whenever a group of animals is reproductively isolated, and some animals are allowed to breed while others are not, then within-breed selection is being practised. When the choice of animals to breed is based on their performance or other characteristics, this is also known as *assortative mating*. In livestock breeding, this is usually *positive* assortative mating, i.e. animals are chosen for breeding based on them having similar characteristics – typically their performance in one or more traits of economic or other importance. The phenomenon of positive assortative mating is often observed in humans and wild animals too. (Negative assortative mating, where parents show dissimilar characteristics, is rarer.)

As discussed in Chapter 1, assortative mating and within-breed selection have occurred for many centuries during and following the creation of distinct breeds. However, the use of within-breed selection as a tool for genetic improvement became widely recognized following its successful application in improving racehorses in the 17th century and farm livestock breeds in the 18th century.

It was common in those times to mate closely related animals in an attempt to 'concentrate' desirable characteristics in the offspring. For example, strains of animals would be created from a series of father–daughter or mother–son matings. This practice of mating close relatives, called linebreeding, is much less common in livestock breeding today. Linebreeding is an extreme form of *inbreeding* – the mating of animals which have one or more ancestors in common. Eventually inbreeding occurs whenever selection is practised in a closed population, but steps are usually taken to limit it by deliberately avoiding matings between close relatives.

Related animals have more genes in common than unrelated animals, and the closer the relationship, the more genes they have in common. This means that animals of outstanding genetic merit, for any characteristic, are likely to have relatives which have higher merit than average. For these reasons, it appears entirely logical to breed from closely related animals, but there is a 'downside'. As well as having more favourable genes in common, related animals also have more unfavourable genes in common, on average. For instance, there are many recessive genes which cause genetic diseases, or adversely affect reproduction, survival or the overall 'fitness' of animals. Because these genes generally act recessively, they only cause problems in animals that carry two copies of the gene (homozygous recessive animals). Across a breed as a whole, there may be very few animals which are homozygous for these particular genes, but the genes are still there, undetected, in heterozygous or carrier animals. Matings between related animals are more likely to produce offspring which are homozygous for some of these genes, than matings between unrelated animals. So, in some cases breeders may be lucky, and they may only see the benefits of mating related animals of high genetic merit. However, in other cases there may be very unfavourable consequences because of infertility or genetic disease in the offspring.

Today we tend to hear only about the past success stories which resulted from linebreeding or close inbreeding, but for each of these there were probably several failures. In plant breeding, and to a lesser extent in poultry breeding, breeders can afford to try linebreeding or close inbreeding in many different lines, and only continue to breed from those which show favourable responses. However, in other livestock species, because of the longer *generation intervals*, the lower reproductive rate, and the higher value of the individual breeding animals, it is not practical to keep many different lines, and the risks from linebreeding usually outweigh the potential benefits. A more gradual, but inevitable and cumulative increase in inbreeding occurs whenever selection is practised in a closed population (e.g. a breed or a closed herd or flock) over a long period of time. This, too, can result in the same unfavourable effects as linebreeding. The effects of inbreeding, and methods of controlling inbreeding in selection programmes are discussed further in Chapter 4.

Requirements for within-breed selection

The choice of animals to breed from may be based solely on their appearance, or on a subjective assessment of their own, or their relatives' performance. For example, selection may be based on visual appraisal of the breed characteristics of an animal – its shape, colour, etc. – or on subjective estimates of the amount of wool or milk produced, or the size of animals. Alternatively, objective records of the performance of the animal itself, or its relatives, may be used. That is, actually weighing the fleeces or the animals, or measuring the volume of milk produced rather than guessing the production. Often a combination of objective and subjective information is used. Objective methods of within-breed selection (i.e. those that rely on recording performance, rather than making subjective judgements about the merit of animals) have become widely used in pig, poultry and dairy cattle breeding since the 1960s. They have been used to a lesser extent in fish, sheep, goat and beef cattle breeding until recently, but this situation is changing in many countries.

Objective selection within breeds or strains is intended to increase the average level of additive genetic merit (termed breeding value) of the population. Ideally, the steps involved are:

1. Deciding what to improve – termed the breeding goal or *selection objective*. For example, a simple breeding goal could be to increase daily weight gain, while a more complicated breeding goal could be to increase lean content of a carcass. As mentioned before, it is sensible to identify the breed or cross which has the highest merit in this trait or combination of traits, and to decide on the most appropriate breeding strategy (e.g. *pure* or crossbreeding) before embarking on within-breed selection in the best breed, or in component breeds of the best cross. Also, there must be genetic variation in this trait or combination of traits within the breed if any improvement is to be made – in other words, there need to be differences between animals in each of these traits, and at least part of these differences need to be inherited.
2. Deciding what to measure and select on within the breed (the *selection criterion*) in order to make improvements in the breeding goal. In some cases, the selection criterion or criteria may be the same as the goal; in others some indirect measurement is needed, for example when the goal trait can only be measured in one sex or after slaughter.

3. Designing the breeding programme (e.g. numbers of males and females to be selected annually; ages at mating).
4. Implementing the programme, i.e. doing the routine recording, evaluation and mating of animals.
5. Monitoring progress and redesigning the programme if necessary.

These steps are summarized in Fig. 3.6. In practice, most breeding schemes evolve in a less planned way than this, but it is useful to have this ideal structure in mind when attempting to optimize breeding scheme design.

In most circumstances, unique and permanent identification of individual animals is a requirement for successful within-breed selection. This may sound obvious, but it is harder to achieve than it first seems – particularly when the identities of animals have to be unique across herds, flocks, years or countries. The small size of juvenile fish make this particularly challenging. There are several reasons why unique identification is important. Firstly, it is important to be able to assign records of performance to the right animal, each time its performance is recorded. Secondly, modern methods of *genetic evaluation* make full use of information from relatives, so it is important to be able to establish how recorded animals are related to each other. Thirdly, having recorded and evaluated animals and decided which ones to use for breeding, it is important to be able to find them again! In some special cases, there is justification for simplified recording of identification. For example, in some extensive production systems, animals may be identified only as members of a particular sire family, rather than individually identified. Molecular genetic techniques now allow retrospective identification of parents where identification of young animals is impractical – such as in some extensive sheep systems or in fish farming. This is achieved using DNA samples from the animals of interest and all of the possible parents to identify the most likely parents.

Objective selection depends on having records of performance on the candidates for selection, or their relatives, or both. In principle, there is no reason why each breeder should not devise their

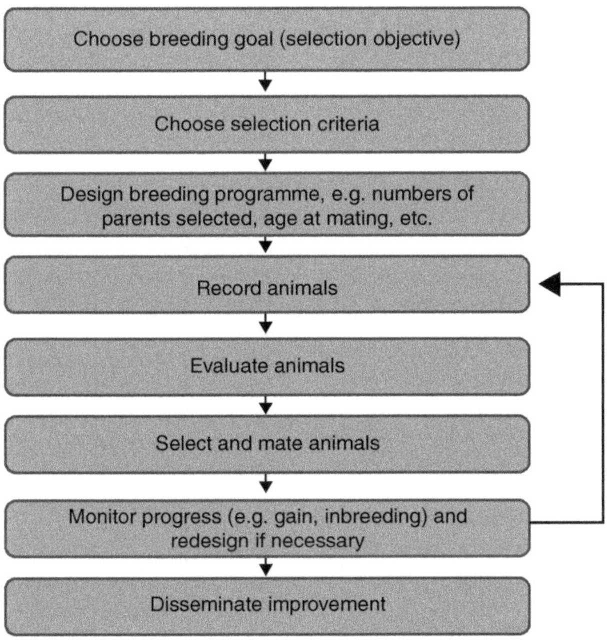

Fig. 3.6. A diagram showing the steps ideally involved in a within-breed improvement programme based on objective measurement of performance. Once the breeding goal is established, different breeds and crosses should be compared in this character, and then within-breed improvement should be used in the best breed, or in component breeds of the best cross. (After Harris *et al*., 1984.)

own method for recording performance in traits relevant to their own breeding goal. Most major pig, poultry and fish breeding companies do this. However, in practice cattle, sheep and goat breeders often use recording schemes which are operated by regional or national agencies that specialize in recording and evaluation. (The difference between the species has probably arisen for a number of reasons. These include the relatively small number of pig, poultry and fish breeders in the elite tier compared to the situation in cattle, sheep and goat breeding, so there are fewer 'products' for commercial producers to be aware of. Also, many pig and poultry companies aim to fulfil both elite and multiplier rôles, so the breeding companies can communicate directly with their final customers and there is less need for a nationally recognized recording system.) For example, in many countries there are milk recording agencies which visit dairy farms at regular intervals to record the yield and other traits of individual cows, and to sample the milk for analysis of fat and protein content. This information is used to assist management decisions and, when accumulated and analysed, it is used to provide estimates of the genetic merit of cows in the herd and their sires. In the beef and sheep sectors, this performance-recording rôle may be fulfilled by government or industry-funded agencies, breed societies or by breeders themselves. In many countries, the recording agencies adopt the recognized international standards of the *International Committee on Animal Recording* (ICAR) for recording and evaluation methods.

There are several advantages to using regional or national systems in species, like cattle and sheep, with many dispersed breeding flocks or herds:

- they encourage discipline and consistency in which traits are recorded, and how and when they are recorded;
- they often provide some type of authentication of the records of performance – either by supervising some of the recordings or, more commonly now, simply by checking that performance records fall into expected ranges, and that details from different sources (e.g. breeder and breed society) match;
- they usually allow access to more sophisticated methods of data storage, processing and evaluation than is feasible on most farms;
- depending on the method of evaluation and the population structure, they can allow direct comparison of the estimated genetic merit of animals across many herds or flocks – this increases the pool of animals available for selection by breeders, and also allows customers to identify individual animals, or flocks and herds of high genetic merit; and
- there are often benefits when it comes to selling breeding stock, because large recording schemes can achieve a stronger 'identity' and better communication about their purposes and products than individual breeders could achieve.

There are also disadvantages to membership of large regional or national recording schemes. There is usually a greater (apparent) cost than with 'home-grown' schemes, and often there is less flexibility to tailor breeding goals to individual breeders' requirements. However, on balance, the advantages to co-ordinated regional or national schemes usually far outweigh the disadvantages.

Factors affecting rates of improvement

As discussed in Chapter 2, many traits of economic or other importance in farm livestock are under the control of a large number of genes and show continuous variation. The response to selection (R) *per generation* in these polygenic traits depends on the *selection differential* (S) and the heritability of the trait under selection (h^2) (after Lush, 1945):

$$R = S \times h^2$$

This is known as the 'breeder's equation', attributable to Jay Lush in the 1930s, one of the founders of animal breeding theory.

The selection differential is the difference between the mean performance of selected animals (i.e. those identified to become parents of the next generation) and the overall mean of the group of animals from which they were selected. This itself depends on two factors – the amount of phenotypic variation in the traits concerned and the *selection intensity* achieved. This is related to the proportion of animals selected to become parents, based on their own performance or that of their relatives. The lower the proportion of animals selected, the higher the selection intensity and hence the better the selected animals will be, on average.

The heritability can also be defined as the proportion of superiority of parents in a trait (i.e. the proportion of the selection differential) which, on average, is passed on to offspring.

Usually, it is helpful to be able to predict *annual* rates of response to selection, and this is achieved by dividing response per generation by the generation interval, so:

$$R\,(\text{per annum}) = \frac{S \times h^2}{L}$$

The generation interval is the average age of parents when their offspring are born. Essentially, this regulates the speed with which selected animals contribute their better genes to the flock or herd, via their offspring.

These factors are discussed in more detail in Chapter 4. Generally speaking, the higher the selection differential and heritability, and the lower the generation interval, the higher the annual rate of genetic improvement.

The main opportunities for breeders to accelerate rates of improvement are through choice of the most accurate methods of predicting breeding values – accuracy also depends on the heritability of the trait of interest and the amount of information available on the animal and its relatives – and by maintaining high selection intensities and low generation intervals. However, there are biological limits to the extent to which selection intensity and generation interval can be altered. It is possible to achieve much higher selection intensities in species or breeds with a high reproductive rate. Similarly, shorter generation intervals can be achieved in those species or breeds which reach sexual maturity at a younger age. These reproductive characteristics of different species are compared in Table 3.6. Largely because of biological advantages in these reproductive characteristics, higher rates of genetic change are possible in fish, pigs and poultry than in ruminants (see Fig. 3.7). However, the reproductive rate of female cattle and sheep can be altered dramatically (at a cost) by the use of reproductive technologies such as *multiple ovulation and embryo transfer*. This effectively makes cattle and sheep 'reproductively' more like poultry and pigs and enables higher rates of genetic gain. The use of these technologies is discussed in more detail in Chapter 5, and species-specific examples are given in Chapters 8 to 13.

Selection for more than one trait

In most livestock production systems profitability depends on several different animal characteristics rather than any single trait. For instance, in dairy cattle income often depends not only on yield, but also on fat and protein content of the milk, and often on somatic cell count too. Feed, health and rebreeding costs are important variable costs. In meat animals, returns per animal depend not only on carcass weight, but also on measures of carcass quality such as fatness and conformation, and on feed costs. In genetic improvement programmes it is important to reflect the fact that several traits influence profit, and so animals are usually selected (whether objectively or subjectively) on a combination of traits. This can be achieved in a number of ways.

One approach, called *tandem selection*, involves selection for one trait for one or more generations, followed by selection for a second trait for one or more generations, possibly followed by selection on more traits, eventually returning to selection on the first, and so on. It can be useful in some circumstances – for instance, if there is an urgent need to improve one trait and other traits need only very minor improvement, it might be appropriate to select only on the first trait until some economically important threshold was reached, and then to turn to the others. However, if the associations between traits of importance are unfavourable, the selection goes round in circles, improving one trait in one generation, and then wholly or partly cancelling

Table 3.6. Comparison of the reproductive characteristics of farm livestock species. Those for ruminants can be increased dramatically by the use of reproductive technologies such as embryo transfer, as discussed in Chapter 5.

Species	Typical age of females at birth of first offspring (limits generation interval)	Typical annual number of offspring per female (limits selection intensity)
Salmon	36–48 months	10,000–20,000
Chickens	7 months	120–280
Pigs	9–12 months	20–24
Sheep	12–24 months	1–3
Cattle	24–36 months	1

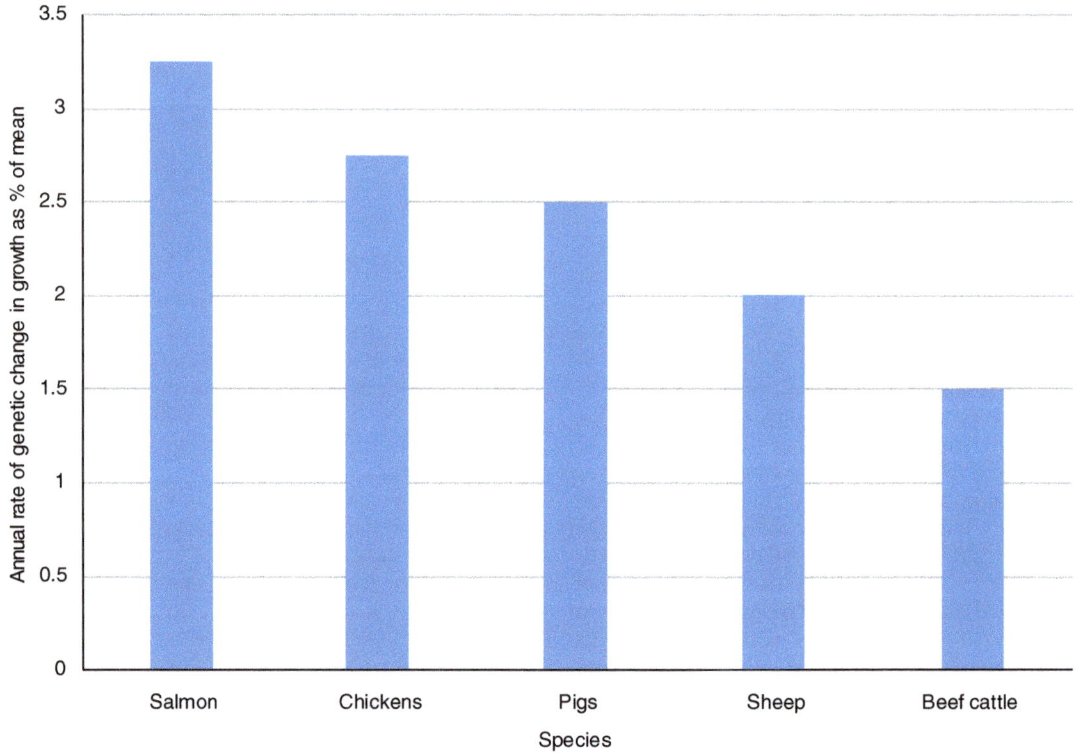

Fig. 3.7. Annual rates of genetic change possible in growth rate in different livestock species. The rates of genetic change are expressed in percentage units of the average growth rate of the species concerned. The differences in rates of change between species are largely due to differences in the natural reproductive characteristics of the species. NB this is for illustration only – few modern breeding programmes select for a single characteristic. (After Smith, 1984 and Simm, 1998; salmon data from Gjedrem and Rye, 2018.)

that improvement in the next generation when selection is for a second trait.

A more consistent method, called *independent culling levels*, is to set minimum qualifying standards, or thresholds, in several traits of interest. To qualify for selection, animals must then surpass the qualifying standard in each trait. There are methods available to allow the most appropriate qualifying standards, or cut-off points, to be calculated. Figure 3.8(a) illustrates this method of selection. In this example beef bulls are only selected if they achieve a 400-day weight above 560 kg, and a muscling score of over 12 points (on a scale of 1 to 15). An informal version of this approach is used by most breeders when they check candidates for selection for breed type or any 'functional' defects (such as overshot or undershot jaws, locomotion faults or small testicles) before breeding from them. This approach is probably a very efficient way of dealing with functional defects which occur irregularly but are suspected of having a genetic component, or traits of minor importance. A version of independent culling levels, or sequential or *two-stage selection*, may also be useful when one trait of interest is very difficult or expensive to measure. For example, it may not be cost effective to record and select on feed intake or feed efficiency on all animals in a selection programme, but it may well be effective to do so, say, on those with weaning weights in the top 25% of those tested.

In theory, the optimal method of selection when there are several traits of economic or other importance is to calculate a selection index. This is a score of overall genetic merit for each of the animals available for selection, based on their own or their relatives' performance in the traits of interest.

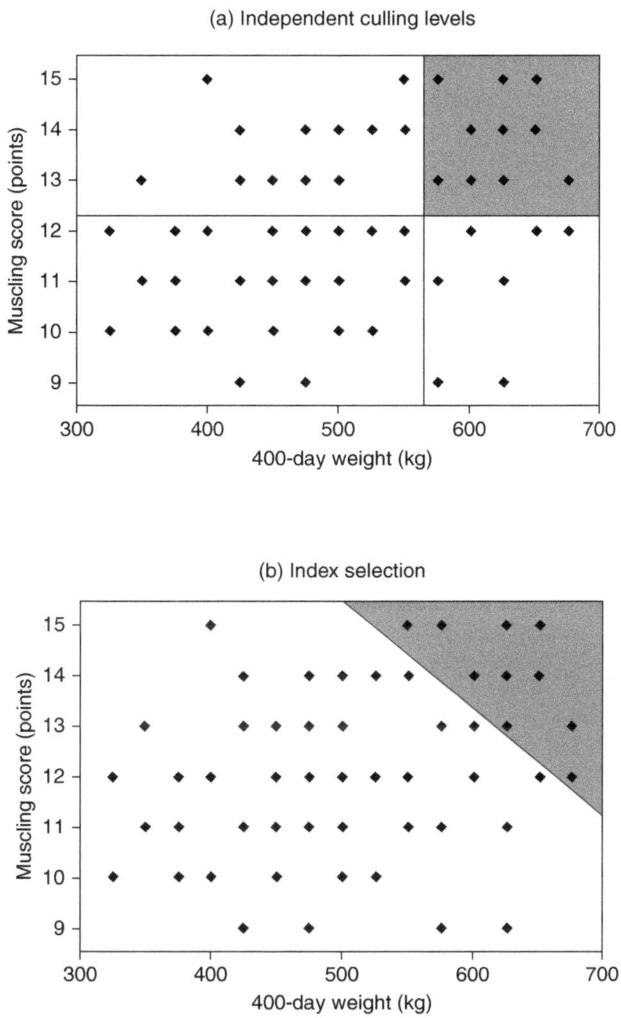

Fig. 3.8. The use of independent culling levels or index selection to select simultaneously for increased 400-day weight and increased muscling score. Each point on the two graphs shows the 400-day weight and muscling score of a single beef bull. (a) Independent culling levels involves setting minimum qualifying standards, or thresholds, in each trait of interest. To qualify for selection, animals must then surpass the qualifying standard in each trait, represented by the vertical and horizontal lines on the graph. In this example, bulls are only selected if they achieve a 400-day weight above 560 kg and a muscling score greater than 12 points (on a scale of 1–15). (b) A selection index scores animals based on all traits of interest, but there are no fixed cut-off points for individual traits – an animal can be selected with lower performance in one trait, providing that it excels in another. Animals above the diagonal line in the graph would be selected. In this example, eight of the ten selected animals would be the same whichever method was used; two of the ten selected animals would differ, depending on the method used.

In some respects, *index selection* is similar to independent culling levels – animals are selected for more than one trait simultaneously, and altering the emphasis on a trait in a selection index is broadly similar to moving the cut-off point for culling with independent culling levels. However, with index selection an animal can compensate for poor performance in one trait by excelling in another.

Although the individual animals that are selected may not have the ideal combination of characters, this is the most efficient way to move a whole population in the desired direction. Index selection is illustrated in Fig. 3.8(b).

Table 3.7 gives a simple example of how an index can help in selection. The table shows milk fat and protein yields for three dairy cows. If selection was based solely on protein yield, then cow A would be selected. If selection was based solely on fat yield, then cow B would be selected. However, if selection was based on fat plus protein yield – a simple index – then cow C would be selected. In this case, the index gives equal emphasis to protein and fat yields, so the two are simply added together. If the desired emphasis on protein:fat was 2:1, then animals could be selected on twice their protein yield, plus their fat yield, and so on. In practice, the traits of interest are often measured in different units, and they have different heritabilities, and so arriving at the most appropriate weighting factors is a bit more complicated than it seems at first sight. To derive these weighting factors, it is necessary to know: (i) how much additive genetic variation there is in the traits of interest; (ii) the direction and strength of associations among these traits; and (iii) their relative economic importance. Obtaining reliable estimates of the genetic variation in traits and associations among them requires comprehensive recording of hundreds or thousands of animals. When the traits of interest are already recorded in a large regional or national scheme then there should be plenty of records to obtain these estimates. However, it will be more difficult and costly to obtain them for traits which are not already recorded, which can be a major limitation to the wider use of index selection. Selection indexes are discussed further in Chapter 4 and applications are given in Chapters 8 to 13.

Table 3.7. An example of the use of a simple index to select cows on protein plus fat yield. The yields in bold type show which cow would be selected if selection was for protein yield only, fat yield only, or protein plus fat yield.

Cow	Protein yield (kg)	Fat yield (kg)	Protein + fat yield (kg)
A	**230**	280	510
B	200	**300**	500
C	225	295	**520**

Crossbreeding

Reasons for crossing

Crossbreeding involves mating animals of different lines, breeds, breed types or species. It is used usually for one or more of the following reasons:

- **To improve the overall efficiency of a production system by crossing breeds or breed types which have high genetic merit in different traits (*complementarity*).** The use of specialized sire and dam breeds or lines is a good example of this (Smith, 1964). It is common for commercial herds and flocks in all of the terrestrial meat-producing species to be made up of breeding females from small- or medium-sized breeds or crosses, which have relatively low maintenance costs, and good reproductive and maternal characteristics. These are mated to males from larger terminal sire breeds, with faster growth rate and better carcass characteristics. The use of different breed types with complementary characteristics usually results in production systems with much higher overall efficiency and profitability than those based entirely on small breeds with good reproductive and maternal traits, or those based entirely on large breeds with good growth and carcass traits (Dickerson, 1978).
- **To produce individual animals of intermediate performance between that of two more extreme parent breeds or breed types.** At first sight this is similar to the use of crossbreeding to exploit complementarity. However, the emphasis here is on creating individual animals of intermediate performance, rather than matching different breeds with different rôles in a crossing system. Beef × dairy suckler cows, such as Hereford or Angus × Holstein Friesians, provide a good example of this use of crossing – the crossbred cows have higher beef merit than pure dairy cows, but higher milk yield than pure beef cows. Also, beef × beef crosses, such as the Blue Grey, combine the hardiness of the Galloway with the faster growth and likely higher milk yield of the Shorthorn. In some smallhold livestock production systems in developing countries (e.g. dairy cattle, pigs), it is becoming more common to cross indigenous breeds (that are typically well adapted to the local environment conditions but have low productivity) to improved exotic breeds (that are typically poorly adapted to the local environmental conditions but highly productive), to create animals

that are intermediate in terms of both adaptation and productivity (Marshall *et al.*, 2016).

- **For grading up to a new breed or breed type.** As explained earlier, this involves mating animals (usually females) of an existing breed type to those (usually males) from a new breed type (see Table 3.2). The progeny from these matings are themselves mated to the new breed or strain, and this process continues for several generations. For example, the spread of North American Holsteins to many temperate and some tropical countries has been brought about largely by grading up indigenous populations of black-and-white (or other) dairy or dual-purpose cattle.
- **As an intermediate step in the creation of a new synthetic or composite breed type.** Creating a synthetic breed or line usually involves crossing two or more different breeds or breed types. If more than two breeds are involved, then this step can take several generations. For instance, if four breeds are involved (A,B,C and D), two different crossbred types could be produced in the first generation (AB and CD). In the second generation, these two crossbred types could be mated to each other, to produce offspring which have a quarter of their genes from each of the four original breeds. Males and females of these four-way crosses could then be mated to each other in subsequent generations.

When two breeds are crossed, the offspring (called the F_1 generation) are relatively uniform, since exactly half of each animal's genes come from each parent breed. However, if F_1 males are mated to F_1 females (i.e. if the F_1 generation is *interbred*), the resulting offspring, called the F_2 generation, show huge variation in appearance and performance. This is because segregation and recombination have now occurred, leading to a wide variation in the proportion of genes which individual animals inherit from the original breeds (as explained in Chapter 2). For any particular characteristic, some offspring will resemble one of the original parent breeds, while others will resemble the other parent breed, and most will be somewhere in the middle. Following this explosion of variation in the F_2 generation, it takes several generations of selection for the desired characteristics before the variation in performance and appearance is reduced, and a recognizable breed type emerges.

Most synthetic lines of pigs and poultry have been created in this way, although they are not regarded as new breeds since, in most cases, these lines are still open to the introduction of yet more breeds or other synthetic lines. However, there are several examples of synthetic breeds in cattle and sheep. The Luing cattle breed was created from crosses between Shorthorn and Highland cattle, subsequently interbred. There are several synthetic dairy cattle breeds in the tropics which have been created by crossing more productive *Bos taurus* dairy breeds with indigenous heat- and disease-tolerant *Bos indicus* breeds (e.g. the Australian milking Zebu, formed from the Sahiwal, Red Sindi and Jersey breeds and the Jamaica Hope formed from the Jersey, Friesian and Sahiwal breeds (Wiener, 1994)). The Coopworth dual-purpose sheep breed from New Zealand was created by crossing Border Leicester and Romney sheep, followed by interbreeding the crosses with intense selection for numbers of lambs born or weaned, weaning weight, fleece weight and quality and 'easy care' characters, such as lambing ease (Beatson, 1993; see Fig. 3.9). The Meatlinc is a synthetic terminal sire sheep breed, created in Britain by crossing animals from several breeds, including the Suffolk, Dorset Down, Ile de France, Berrichon du Cher and Charollais, and selecting for growth and carcass traits (Fell, 1979). As mentioned earlier, there has been a recent growth in interest in the use of composite beef and sheep breeds, to better meet changing market requirements (see, for example, Innovis (2019); Kelso (2019); Leachman (2019)). There are also examples of 'open composites' with ongoing introduction of new breeds, together with *ad hoc* crossing systems, that share some of the benefits of creating more formal composites, in both higher and lower-income countries (e.g. open beef composites in N America; ongoing *ad hoc* crossing among local Zebu × imported *Bos taurus* crosses in some African smallholder dairy systems; crossing of composite Red Dorper sheep (derived from the Dorset Horn and the Blackhead Persian) with local breeds in E Africa).

- **To introduce new variation to numerically small breeds or breed types.** In many numerically-small breeds it is difficult for breeders to find enough unrelated animals of sufficiently high genetic merit to sustain a genetic improvement programme. Often, these problems are exacerbated because the population is inbred and

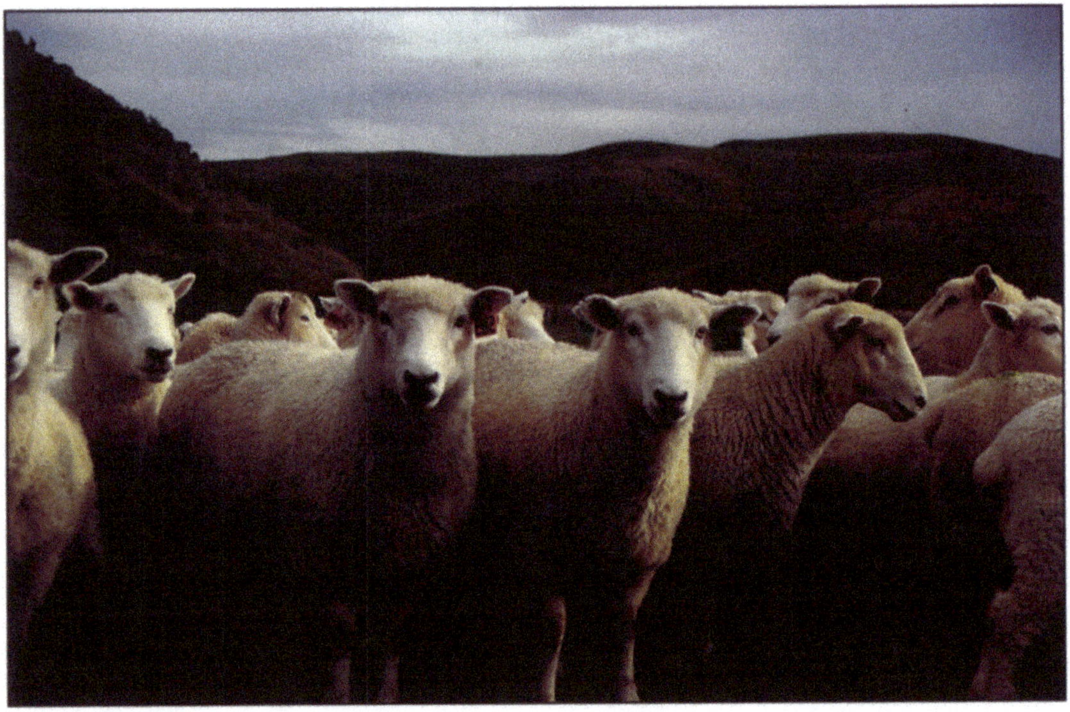

Fig. 3.9. Coopworth ewes near Wanganui, New Zealand. The Coopworth is a synthetic breed, the development of which has been based on objective performance recording.

genetic defects have emerged which need to be controlled. In these cases, it is quite common for animals from other breeds to be introduced, either officially or unofficially! This is similar to the creation of a synthetic breed, except that the long term aim is to have a much lower proportion of genes from the new breed.

- **To introduce a single gene for a favourable characteristic to an existing breed or breed type (*introgression*).** Crossing is sometimes used to introduce a single gene for a favourable characteristic to an existing breed. Good examples include the introgression of the gene controlling polledness into naturally horned cattle breeds, and the introgression of the Booroola gene affecting fecundity, originally found in Merino sheep, into other sheep breeds. Unlike the creation of a synthetic breed, the aim of introgression is usually to introduce and retain only the desired gene from the new breed, and to remove the other genes contributed by this breed by successive generations of backcrossing to the original breed. It is important in this case to ensure that as many as possible of the females retained for backcrossing carry the desirable gene. After several generations of backcrossing, carrier animals can be mated to each other, to create offspring which are homozygous for the newly introduced gene, but in other respects are similar to the original breed. (See Chapter 5 for more details on how molecular genetic techniques can assist in this process.)
- **To exploit *heterosis* or *hybrid vigour*.** When two breeds are crossed, intuitively we expect the performance of the crossbred offspring to fall midway between that of the parent breeds (i.e. at the mid-parent mean). However, in practice, the performance of crossbreds is often better than we expect. This advantage in performance above the mid-parent mean is called heterosis or hybrid vigour (see Fig. 3.10). It is measured either in the units in which the trait was originally

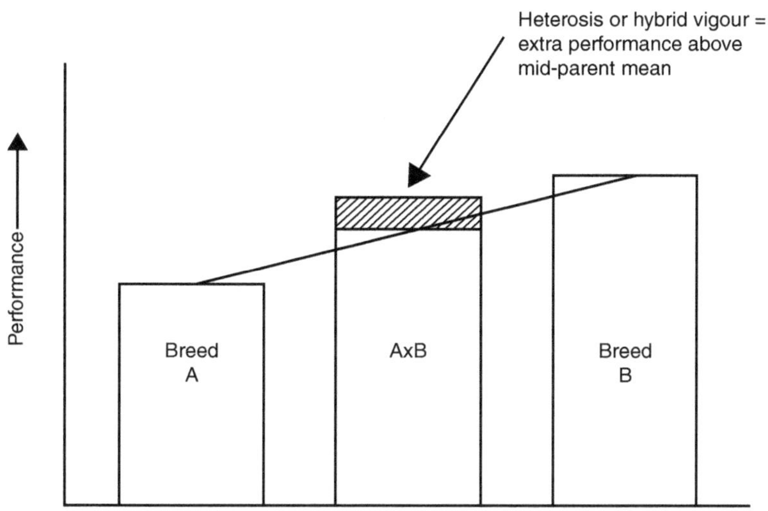

Fig. 3.10. A graph illustrating the phenomenon of heterosis or hybrid vigour. Heterosis is defined as the advantage in performance of crossbred animals above the mid-parent mean of the two parent breeds. In this case the amount of heterosis is the shaded part of the middle bar in the graph. Heterosis is most useful when it leads to the average performance of the crossbred animals exceeding that of the *best* parent breed in a single important trait or a combination of important traits.

measured, or as a percentage increase over the mid-parent mean. For example, if two sheep breeds have average litter sizes of 1.0 and 2.0 lambs, respectively, we expect crossbred ewes to have an average litter size of 1.5 (the mid-parent mean). If, in fact, the crosses have an average litter size of 1.6 lambs, this indicates that there is heterosis in litter size of 0.1 lamb (1.6 – 1.5) or 6.7% (0.1/1.5 × 100). Heterosis is usually greatest in traits associated with reproduction, survival and overall fitness. (Note that heterosis can sometimes be negative/detrimental as well as positive/beneficial; see, for example, Bunning *et al.* (2018).) There are many important examples of heterosis in animal breeding. The beneficial effects of heterosis occur for exactly the opposite reason that the detrimental effects of inbreeding occur. In other words, when two breeds or lines are crossed there is a much lower proportion of offspring which are homozygous for recessive genes affecting reproduction, survival and overall fitness, or causing genetic disease, than if animals of the same breed are mated. Crossbreeding creates animals which are heterozygous at more loci, whereas *purebreeding* creates animals which are homozygous at more loci.

Selection between breeds, selection within breeds, and the first four applications of crossbreeding listed above, all exploit differences in additive genetic merit between populations or individual animals. However, heterosis is the result of non-additive gene action. That is, it is a result of dominance at individual loci, or epistasis between loci, or both (see Chapter 2 for details). The fact that heterosis is a result of non-additive gene action means that it is difficult to predict the amount of heterosis to expect when particular breeds are crossed. Some crosses result in substantial heterosis and others do not. When a particular cross produces a large amount of heterosis, the parent breeds are sometimes said to *nick* well, or show good *combining ability*. Although it is difficult to predict the level of heterosis that will arise from crossing any two breeds, it is usually greater for crosses between genetically diverse breeds. For example, heterosis is usually greater in beef x dairy cattle crosses than in crosses between two dairy breeds, and it is usually greater in crosses between *Bos taurus* and *Bos indicus* cattle breeds, than in crosses between two European *Bos taurus* or two *Bos indicus* breeds; it appears to be greater still in crosses between tropical and European *Bos taurus* breeds (Bunning *et al.*, 2018). This is probably because the more distantly related the two breeds, the greater the proportion of loci at which different alleles are fixed in the two breeds, and hence the greater the number of loci at which the crossbred offspring are heterozygous. As mentioned above, heterosis is usually greatest for traits affecting reproduction, survival and overall fitness, and it is usually least for 'production' traits like growth and milk yield. Figure 3.11 shows the relative milk yield of indigenous *Bos indicus* cattle breeds, *Bos taurus* dairy breeds, F_1 crosses between indigenous and exotic dairy breeds, and subsequent generations of interbred animals from a review of many dairy cattle crossbreeding experiments in the tropics.

Heterosis is a useful bonus if there are other primary reasons for crossbreeding, for example, to exploit complementarity of breeds. However, crossbreeding solely to exploit heterosis is only really justified if the heterosis is sufficient to make the crossbred animals better, on average, than the best parent breed. In other words, having substantial heterosis is of no net benefit if the crossbred animals are still inferior to purebred animals of one of the parent breeds. So, any evaluation of crossbreeding as a strategy for genetic improvement needs to take into account the additive genetic merit of the pure breeds, as well as the non-additive 'bonus' that occurs when they are crossed.

There are numerous examples of experiments to compare both pure breeds and crosses of cattle and sheep. The results from one of these, an experiment to compare the reproductive and maternal performance of three different types of crossbred sheep in Britain, are shown in Table 3.8. Others include a large 'multi-breed' experiment, established at the Animal Breeding Research Organisation (ABRO) in Edinburgh in 1970, to estimate the extent of between-breed differences in traits affecting overall efficiency. The experiment involved 25 cattle breeds of different mature size and different levels of milk production. The results showed that at about 1 year of age, between-breed variation accounted for about 70% of the total variation in body weight and 60% of the total variation in cumulated food intake, which highlights the importance of selecting the most appropriate breed (Thiessen *et al.*, 1984). In the 1970s and 1980s, a series of large-scale experiments was done at the US Meat Animal Research Center in Nebraska, to compare the growth, carcass characteristics and reproductive performance of many beef breeds and crosses, to compare crossbreeding systems and to compare different synthetic strains (Cundiff *et al.*, 1982, 1986; Gregory *et al.*, 1982; see Leachman (2019) for industry application of these results). A similar experiment was established in the early 1990s at the Australian Beef Co-operative Research Centre in

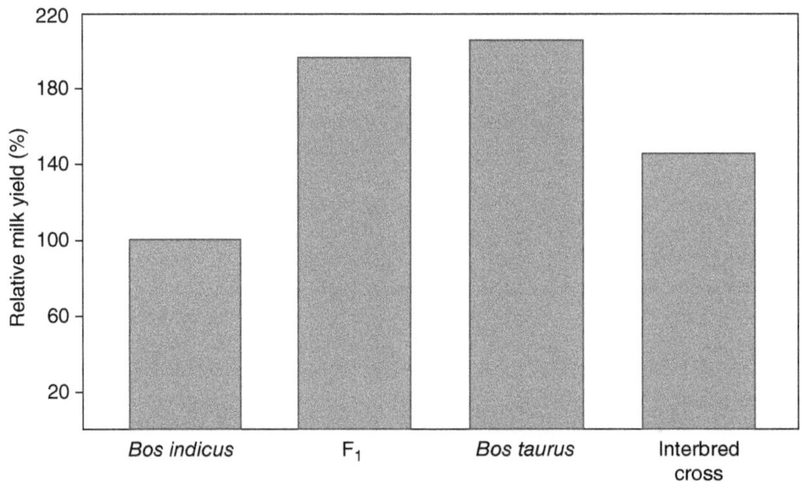

Fig. 3.11. The relative milk yield of indigenous *Bos indicus* cattle breeds, F_1 crosses between *Bos indicus* and *Bos taurus* dairy breeds, *Bos taurus* dairy breeds, and subsequent generations of interbred animals from a review of many dairy cattle crossbreeding experiments in the tropics. Yields are expressed in percentage units relative to that of the *Bos indicus* breeds. (After Cunningham and Syrstad, 1987; Davis and Arthur, 1994.)

Table 3.8. Results of a comparison between three different crossing breeds of sheep: the Border Leicester, Bluefaced Leicester and ABRO Damline. The table shows the average performance of crossbred ewes produced by mating rams from these three breeds to ewes of several hill breeds. The crossbred ewes were mated in their first year, which partly explains the relatively low levels of performance. Matings were to a terminal sire breed. The superscripts show whether or not the crossbred ewe types differ significantly. Within a row, crossbred means with different superscripts differ significantly; those with the same superscript do not differ significantly, e.g. significantly fewer Border Leicester cross ewes lambed in their first year, compared to the other two crosses, but there was no significant difference in the proportion of Bluefaced Leicester cross or Damline cross ewes lambing in their first year. (After Cameron *et al.*, 1983.)

	Crossbred ewe type		
Trait	Border Leicester ×	Bluefaced Leicester ×	ABRO Damline ×
Ewes lambing per ewe mated in first year of life	0.62[a]	0.73[b]	0.78[b]
Total number of lambs born per ewe mated (avg. of first three matings)	1.29[a]	1.40[b]	1.54[c]
Number of lambs born alive per ewe mated (avg. of first three matings)	1.16[a]	1.28[b]	1.37[c]
Estimated litter weight at 10 weeks, per ewe mated (kg)	25.94	31.10	28.68
Productivity relative to Border Leicester cross (=100) taking into account estimated ewe feed requirements	100	114	117

Armidale, with the emphasis on investigating differences in meat quality between breeds and crosses.

In most temperate dairy industries, there is very little systematic use of crossbreeding. A major reason for this is that the milk production of crossbreds rarely exceeds that of the pure Holstein Friesian, although there is heterosis for several important traits. In contrast, there is widespread use of systematic crossing, especially between Jerseys and Holstein Friesians, in the extensive pasture-based dairy industries of New Zealand and to a lesser extent Australia. (In 2017/18, Holstein Friesian-Jersey crosses, Holstein Friesians and Jerseys accounted for around 48%, 33% and 9%, respectively of dairy cows in New Zealand (Livestock Improvement Corporation Ltd and DairyNZ Ltd, 2018).) Both of these breeds have a long history of successful within-breed selection in New Zealand, and so have high additive genetic merit for production from grass. Additionally, crossbred animals appear to be particularly favoured when comparisons are made on the basis of milk production per hectare. Since heterosis for production is higher than that for liveweight, crossbred animals achieve the extra production above the parental mean without incurring the 'penalty' of higher live weight, and hence higher maintenance costs (Harris *et al.*, 1996).

Types of heterosis

When parents of two different breeds are mated, the crossbred progeny may show heterosis in a range of characteristics. These might include the time taken to get up and suck after birth, neonatal survival and early growth. Once the crossbred animals themselves mature and reproduce, heterosis may be evident in another set of traits associated with fertility and maternal ability. At this stage, some of the benefits of heterosis accrue to the offspring of the crossbred female, rather than to the female herself. So, it is useful to distinguish between:

- *Individual heterosis* – influencing performance as a result of animals themselves being crossbred.
- *Maternal heterosis* – influencing the reproductive and other maternal performance characteristics of crossbred females. The benefits in this case are often measured in the offspring (e.g. extra weight of offspring weaned by crossbred cows, compared to purebreds). Maternal heterosis occurs as a result of dams being crossbred.
- *Paternal heterosis* – influencing the reproductive performance of crossbred males. Paternal heterosis occurs as a result of sires being crossbred.

Although there may be paternal heterosis for traits such as libido and male fertility, individual and maternal heterosis are of most practical value.

Table 3.9 gives some examples of individual and maternal heterosis in economically important traits in crosses between breeds of sheep, beef and dairy cattle, pigs and poultry. There are several good examples of industry structures, or breeding schemes, which make good use of both individual and maternal heterosis, as well as complementarity. There is widespread, organized use of crossing in the pig and poultry industries. The aim is to produce breeding females for commercial herds and flocks which, as well as having high additive genetic merit for reproduction and associated characteristics, show maternal heterosis. Mating these females to males of a different breed or strain/line then maximizes individual heterosis in the offspring. For example, in the pig industry in the UK and elsewhere, commercial F_1 females are produced typically by crossing strains based on the Large White and Landrace breeds, which have been selected for high maternal performance. In commercial herds these sows, in turn, are mated to boars from breeds, or synthetic lines based on several breeds, including the Hampshire, Duroc and Pietrain, which have been selected for growth, carcass traits and feed conversion efficiency.

Crossbreeding schemes in sheep and beef cattle have often evolved over time in a less planned way than in the pig and poultry industries. For instance, some production systems based on crossbred animals have probably been stimulated by the availability of relatively cheap F_1 females as a by-product of other enterprises, for example the use of beef × dairy suckler cows in Britain and Ireland (see Fig. 3.12) and the use of longwool × Merino ewes or longwool × hill ewes for lamb production in Australia and the UK, respectively. Nonetheless, the benefits are still obtained.

The *stratified* system of sheep breeding in the UK provides a good example of the use of complementarity and both maternal and individual heterosis (see Fig. 3.13, Chapter 10 and Meat and Livestock Commission, 1988). Most hill sheep flocks in the UK are made up of purebred ewes of traditional hill breeds such as Scottish Blackface, Swaledale and Welsh Mountain. Typically, these ewes are bred pure in the hills for about four lamb crops. Then they are 'drafted' to better land on the same farm, or sold to other farms, for crossing – usually with a ram from a longwool breed, such as the Bluefaced Leicester or Border Leicester. The F_1 females resulting from these matings are widely used in commercial flocks in the uplands and lowlands (see Fig. 3.14). They, in turn, are mated to rams from the terminal sire breeds, such as the Suffolk and Texel, to produce lambs for slaughter. The use of F_1 longwool × hill females in commercial flocks makes full use of maternal heterosis. Crossing these to a third breed maximizes the benefits of individual heterosis in the slaughter generation. Additionally, there are benefits from complementarity, because of the use of medium-sized F_1 breeding females with good reproductive and maternal characteristics, but much larger terminal sires with good growth and carcass characteristics.

Similarly, the use of large terminal sire beef breeds in herds of cows made up of crosses between traditional British beef breeds, or crosses between beef and dairy breeds, makes full use of complementarity and both maternal and individual heterosis. Figure 3.15 illustrates the cumulative benefits of individual and maternal heterosis in beef cattle.

Systems of crossing

The simplest type of cross is that between two breeds. For obvious reasons this is called a *two-way cross*. The progeny resulting from a two-way cross are called F_1 or first cross animals. In the previous section there were several examples of this type of cross, including longwool × hill breed commercial ewes, and beef × dairy suckler cows.

If animals from this two-way cross are then mated back to one of the parent breeds, this is termed a *backcross*, as mentioned earlier. When F_1 crossbred animals are mated back to one of the parent breeds, heterozygosity, and so individual heterosis of the resulting offspring, is halved on average, compared to that in the F_1 generation. This is also true in all subsequent generations of backcrossing. Individual heterosis is at its maximum in the F_1 generation and is halved in every subsequent generation of backcrossing to the same parent breed. (This happens because each generation of backcrossing halves the number of loci which are heterozygous, on average). Similarly, when F_1 animals are interbred to produce an F_2 generation, heterosis is expected to halve compared to that in the F_1 generation (though experimental results sometimes depart from this expectation – possibly because of differences in the relative contribution of epistatic compared to dominance effects; see Falconer and Mackay, 1996). No further reduction in heterosis is expected in the F_3 and F_4 generations until inbreeding occurs.

Table 3.9. Examples of heterosis in traits of economic importance in livestock. Values shown are specific for the combination of breeds concerned. (After Simm *et al.*, 1994.)

Species/type of animal	Breeds crossed	Trait	Type of heterosis	Amount of heterosis in units of measurement or as a % of the mid-parent mean	Source
Sheep	Galway, Border	Fertility	Maternal	7.3%	Timon (1974)
	Leicester, Cheviot and	Litter size	Maternal	2.3%	
	Blackface	Lambs/ewe mated	Maternal	10.0%	
		Lamb wt/ewe mated	Maternal	11.8%	
		Lamb mortality	Maternal	2.0%	
	Several breeds	Lamb daily gain	Individual	2–4%	Mayala (1974)
Beef cattle	Hereford, Angus,	Weight calf weaned per cow	Maternal	14.8%	Cundiff *et al.* (1982)
	Shorthorn	exposed	Individual	8.5%	
	Several breeds	Age at puberty	Individual	–9.4%	Cundiff *et al.* (1986)
		Post-weaning gain	Individual	11.0%	
		Carcass weight	Individual	15.0%	
		Fat thickness	Individual	0.1%	
Dairy cattle	Holstein Friesian,	Milk	Individual	129 litres (3.9%)[a]	Harris *et al.* (1996)
	Jersey	Fat	Individual	6.8 kg (4.1%)[a]	
		Protein	Individual	5.0 kg (4.1%)[a]	
		Survival from 1st to 2nd lactation	Individual	4.7%	
		Liveweight	Individual	7.2 kg (1.9%)[b]	
Pigs	Yorkshire, Landrace,	Average daily gain 70-154 days	Individual	7.3%	Cassady *et al.*
	Large White, and	Average daily feed intake	Maternal	1.1%	(2002)
	Chester White	Carcass backfat	Individual	10.8%	
			Maternal	0%	
			Individual	–0.2%	
			Maternal	2.2%	
Chickens	High and low body	Body weight 266 days	Individual	13%	Williams *et al.*, 2002
	weight selected lines of	Age at first egg	Individual	–23%	
	White Plymouth Rock	Hen-day ovulations	Individual	34%	

[a]% heterosis derived from mean performance of the two pure breeds in 1995/96 (Livestock Improvement, 1996).
[b]% heterosis derived from assumed mid-parent mean liveweight of 375 kg.

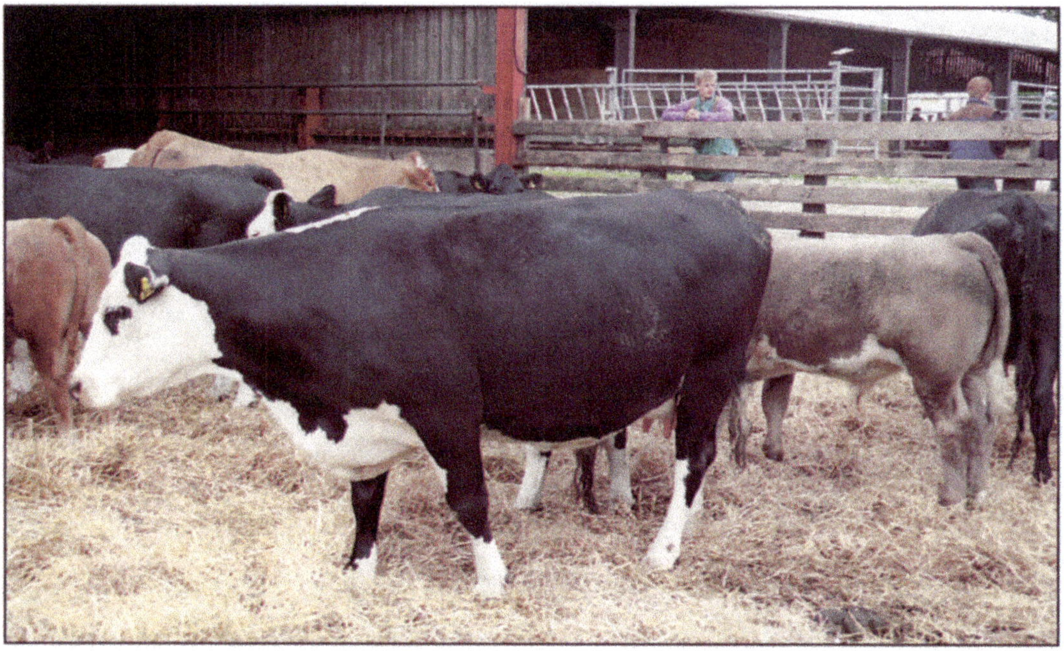

Fig. 3.12. Beef × dairy suckler cows have been very important historically in Britain and Ireland. However increasing specialization in the dairy herd, and reduced dairy cow numbers, means that more beef producers in these countries are breeding their own beef x beef replacements.

The performance of later generations of crossbred animals, after the F_1, may also be reduced as a result of *recombination loss* (Dickerson, 1973). This is believed to occur as the result of the breakdown of favourable 'epistatic blocks' of alleles from parental breeds, where these blocks have been established by many generations of selection.

Table 3.10 shows the fractions of individual, maternal and paternal heterosis which are expected to be maintained in different types of crossbreeding schemes, *relative to that in the F_1*. For example, a value of 1 in the table indicates that a particular type of cross maintains the full amount of heterosis seen in the F_1; a value of ½ indicates that heterosis is halved compared to that in the F_1. As mentioned before, the value of a particular cross depends on its average merit compared to that of the best parent breed, i.e. it is a function of the additive genetic merit of both of the parent breeds, as well as heterosis.

One way of maintaining heterosis after producing a two-way cross is to mate to a third breed, to produce a three-way cross. The progeny of terminal sire sheep or beef breeds out of the type of F_1 ewes and cows described above are three-way crosses. New breeds can be added to the mix, in an attempt to maintain heterosis, but unless additional breeds have high additive genetic merit, the benefits of keeping heterosis high will soon be outweighed by the use of inferior breeds. Also, although three-way crosses maintain the *relative* level of heterosis compared to that in the F_1 generation, the *absolute* amount will depend on the specific breeds concerned – some combinations of breeds will lead to high absolute levels of heterosis, and other combinations will not.

Systems based on specific crosses can be very efficient, especially if specialized sire and dam breeds are used. However, as illustrated above, in cattle and sheep breeding these systems usually depend on a readily available external supply of replacement F_1 females. Otherwise, substantial numbers of at least one of the constituent breeds will need to be kept alongside the crossbred commercial herd or flock, just to breed sufficient replacement females.

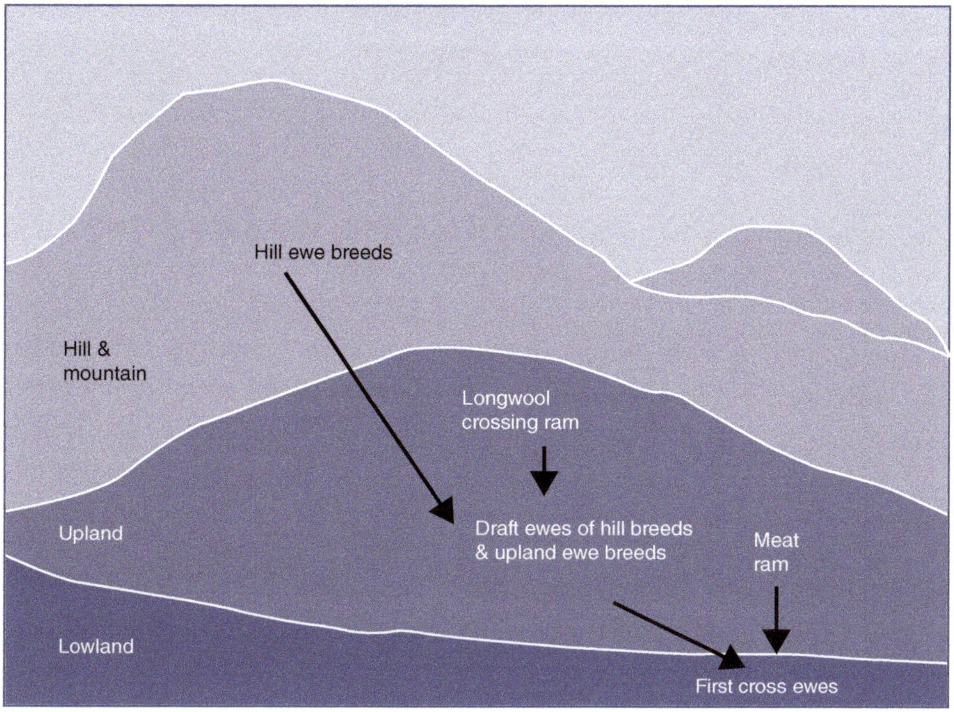

Fig. 3.13. A diagram illustrating the stratified system of sheep breeding in the UK. This system makes use of complementarity of different breeds and of both maternal and individual heterosis. (After Meat and Livestock Commission, 1988.)

An alternative to the use of specific crosses is *rotational crossing*. This involves the use of the same two or three (or more) breeds in rotation. In a two-breed rotational cross, breeds A and B would be mated to produce F_1 offspring with 50% of the genes of each parent breed (abbreviated to AB here). These would be mated to sire breed A, to produce a second generation (abbreviated A(AB)) of offspring with an average of 3/4 A genes and 1/4 B genes. These, in turn, would be bred to sires from breed B, producing offspring with an average of 3/8 A genes and 5/8 B genes. This process continues until the proportions of genes from the two breeds stabilizes at an average of about 1/3A, 2/3B and 2/3A, 1/3B in successive generations (see Table 3.11). In a three-breed rotational cross the proportions of genes from the three breeds stabilizes at an average of about 1/7, 2/7, 4/7, with the highest proportion of genes coming from the sire breed used to produce the most recent generation, and *vice versa*. In practice, most farmed livestock species live for varying lengths of time, and produce offspring at a range of ages, and so generations overlap rather than being discrete. This means that herds or flocks are soon made up of animals with different proportions of genes from the breeds involved, and several sire breeds need to be used each year. This can lead to additional difficulties in recording, arranging mating groups, and in managing and feeding animals of different genetic make-up if they differ markedly in size or productivity. Two- and three-breed rotational crossing maintains about 2/3 and 6/7, respectively, of the level of heterosis seen in the F_1 generation. However, as mentioned already, it is the combined effect of additive genetic merit and heterosis in the particular crosses or crossbreeding systems concerned that needs to be evaluated.

Rotational crossing is used in the pastoral beef industries of several countries – particularly to breed replacement females which are two- or three-way crosses between the traditional British beef breeds (Aberdeen Angus, Hereford, Shorthorn).

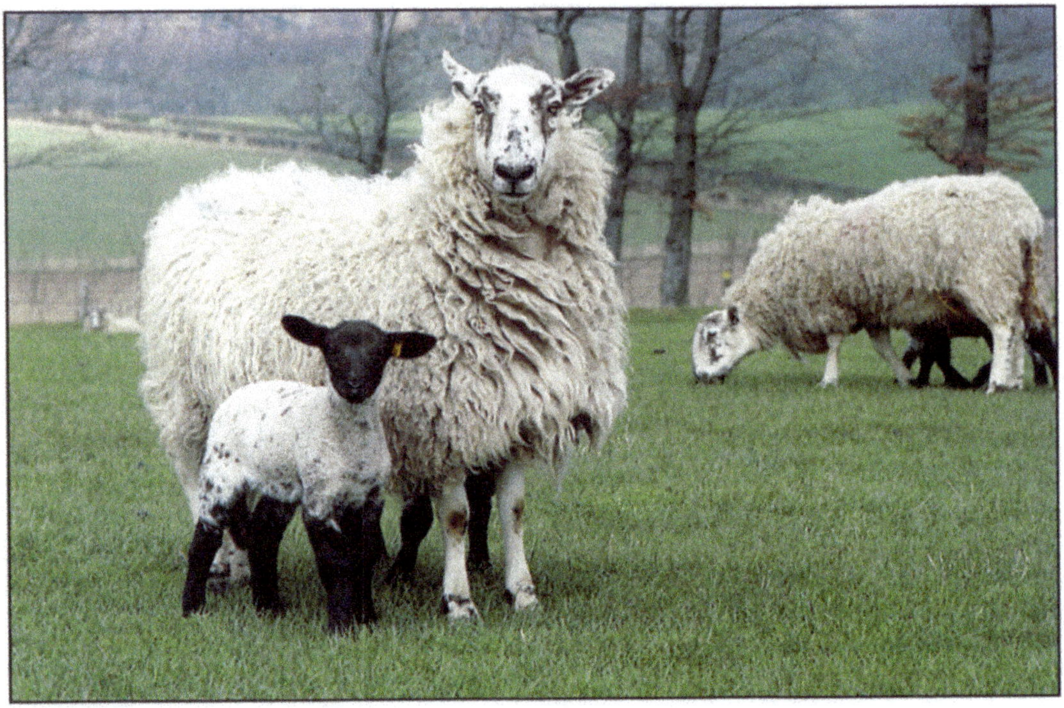

Fig. 3.14. Crossbred ewes such as these Scottish Mules (Bluefaced Leicester × Scottish Blackface) form the backbone of the commercial sheep industry in Britain.

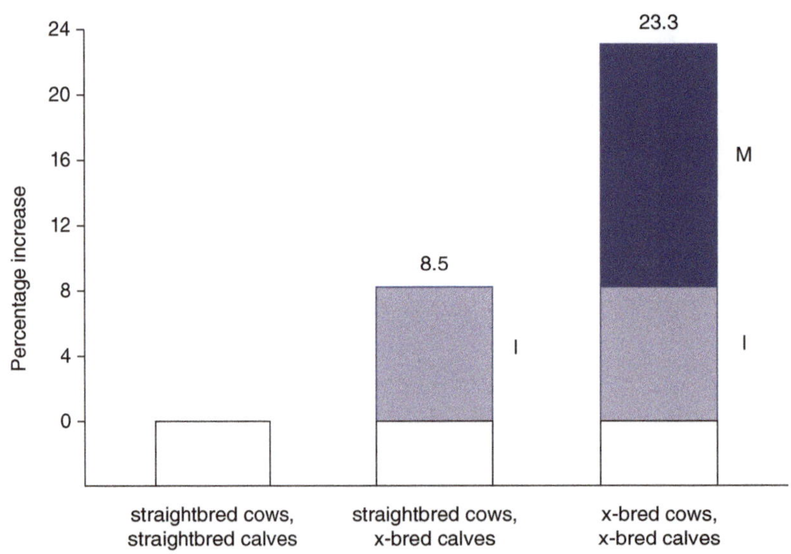

Fig. 3.15. A diagram illustrating the cumulative benefits of individual (I) and maternal (M) heterosis on weight of calf weaned per beef cow exposed to breeding. (After Cundiff and Gregory, 1977; Nicholas, 1987.)

Table 3.10. Fractions of heterosis expected to be maintained in different crossing systems. (After Dickerson, 1974; Nicholas, 1987.)

Type of crossing system (breed of male is given first)	Fraction of heterosis relative to that in the F_1		
	Individual heterosis (e.g. in survival of the crossbred animal itself)	Maternal heterosis (e.g. in fertility, or total weight of calf weaned by cows)	Paternal heterosis (e.g. in male fertility or libido)
Pure breed	0	0	0
Two-breed cross			
A × B	1	0	0
Backcross			
A or B with AB	1/2	1	0
AB with A or B	1/2	0	1
Three-breed cross			
C × AB	1	1	0
AB × C	1	0	1
Four-breed cross			
AB × CD	1	1	1
Rotational cross			
2 breed	2/3	2/3	0
3 breed	6/7	6/7	0
Composite[a]			
2 breeds, equal contribution	1/2	1/2	1/2
4 breeds, equal contribution	3/4	3/4	3/4
8 breeds, equal contribution	7/8	7/8	7/8

[a]Retention (compared to F_1) = approx. $1-\Sigma_i^n P_i^2$ where: P_i = proportion of each of n breeds used to create composite (Gregory *et al.*, 1993).

Table 3.11. The average proportion of genes from two breeds in offspring following successive generations of rotational crossing. (After Nicholas, 1987.)

Breed of parents (sire breed shown first)	Proportion of genes in offspring from:	
	Breed A	Breed B
A × B	1/2 (0.5)	1/2 (0.5)
A × (AB)	3/4 (0.75)	1/4 (0.25)
B × [A(AB)]	3/8 (0.375)	5/8 (0.625)
A × (B[A(AB)])	11/16 (0.688)	5/16 (0.313)
B × [A(B[A(AB)])]	11/32 (0.344)	21/32 (0.656)
A × (B[A(B[A(AB)])])	43/64 (0.672)	21/64 (0.328)
B × [A(B[A(B[A(AB)])])]	43/128 (0.336)	85/128 (0.664)

There is also interest in this type of system in countries traditionally dependent on beef × dairy replacements, as increasingly specialized dairy breeds, such as Holsteins, usually have poorer beef characteristics than the dairy breeds they replaced.

Composite breeds are sometimes preferred as an alternative to rotational crossing, as they can maintain relatively high levels of heterosis (though lower than with rotational crosses among the same component breeds), while avoiding the variability in performance seen in herds or flocks with different generations of rotational crosses, and reducing complexity of management. For example, composites made up of equal proportions of two, four or eight breeds will retain 50%, 75% and 87.5%, respectively, of the heterosis seen in the F_1. These proportions of heterosis retained will decline as a result of inbreeding in the population.

Some of the long-established cattle and sheep composite breeds mentioned earlier are now treated effectively as pure breeds, in that they are closed to the introduction of new breeds. Often in pig and poultry breeding, and with some of the newer beef and sheep composites, there is a much more fluid concept of the composite, with new breeds or crosses being added if they are expected to enhance overall performance.

Conservation of Genetic Resources

Conservation of animal, plant and microbial genetic resources used in agriculture is vital for future food security and resilience of food systems. All of the strategies for genetic improvement discussed in this chapter depend on genetic variation, so it is important for the success of future improvement programmes that genetic variation is used in a sustainable way. It is useful to consider two types of conservation of genetic variation in domestic animals, although they overlap. The first is the conservation of rare breeds or strains of livestock, which are in danger of extinction. The second is conservation of genetic variation within breeds involved in active improvement programmes. The first of these is discussed below. Conservation of variation within breeds is discussed further in Chapter 4, in the context of designing within-breed improvement programmes.

Why conserve rare breeds?

In several industrialized countries, interest in breed conservation was stimulated from the 1960s onwards by farmers and breed enthusiasts who were concerned that the increasing use of a few specialized breeds was leading to a severe decline in the numbers of animals in many traditional breeds. Organizations like the Rare Breeds Survival Trust (RBST) in the UK and the American Minor Breeds Conservancy (now the American Livestock Breeds Conservancy) were set up to promote conservation of those breeds thought to be at risk. In many lower-income countries, interest in conservation was stimulated, at about the same time, by the widespread crossing of indigenous breeds to imported breeds.

There are a number of economic, social and cultural reasons to conserve rare breeds. Farm animal genetic resources (FAnGR) are the foundation for livestock production, which is responsible for around 40% of the value of agricultural output globally (FAO, 2019). So, there are strong economic arguments to protect FAnGR. Livestock have a particularly important rôle in supporting livelihoods of many of the world's poorest people. Breeds and crosses that can prosper in harsh conditions may make a particularly important contribution to feeding those humans most in need. Rare breeds are reservoirs of genetic variation that are being overlooked and may become important in future, especially in response to the challenges of climate change, food insecurity, and so on. In addition to this utilitarian view, FAnGR are part of wider biodiversity, which many argue has intrinsic value. Also, the wide variety of livestock breeds we have today is part of our cultural heritage and deserves protection for this reason too.

Scientific support for breed conservation has a rather chequered history. The subject received relatively little scientific attention until the late 1900s, perhaps because support for conservation originated largely from 'grassroots' enthusiasts, and bypassed most scientists. However, there is also a counter argument to conservation on biological grounds. This is that the markets for animal products do not usually change dramatically, and so there is scope for popular breeds to keep pace with new markets by changing the emphasis in selection, without the need to return to rare breeds for new genetic variation. There is already wide genetic variation in most breeds, which permits short- and medium-term responses to selection. In the longer term, new variation is created by mutation, and so current breeds should be able to adapt to new markets indefinitely, provided that population sizes are large. While this argument probably holds for breeds that are not that much different from each other in the first place, it is probably not true globally. Many of the breeds or strains most at risk have evolved over a long time in very harsh or specialized environments. It would be difficult and time consuming to reinstate in 'improved' breeds some of the traits, like tolerance to disease, heat and nutritional deprivation, which some breeds at risk already possess. Hence, the case for conservation is widely accepted.

Over the last few decades, the Food and Agriculture Organization of the United Nations (FAO) has had a key rôle in informing international policy and coordinating national efforts on conservation and sustainable use of genetic resources. The FAO website (FAO, 2019) has links to many key reports and other resources relevant to conservation of animal genetic resources, including periodic reports on the *State of the World's Animal Genetic Resources,* global action plans and the Domestic Animal Diversity Information System (DAD-IS).

Many breeds or lines of economic or other importance in many countries are imported or have been developed with contributions from foreign breeds or lines. As part of the Convention on Biological Diversity (CBD), *The Nagoya Protocol on Access and Benefits Sharing* is an international agreement intended to ensure that the benefits arising from the utilization of genetic resources, as well as traditional knowledge associated with them, are shared in an equitable manner (see CBD, 2019). Over 116 countries are parties to the Nagoya Protocol. These parties are obliged to establish legislative and/or other measures regarding access to genetic resources. Implementation of the Nagoya Protocol is co-ordinated by an international body known as the Access and Benefits Sharing Clearing House (https://absch.cbd.int/).

Which breeds should be conserved?

If the case for conserving breeds is accepted, the next decision is which breeds to conserve. There are around 8800 breeds or strains of livestock globally, belonging to 38 species (FAO, 2019). Seventeen percent of these breeds are believed to be extinct or at risk of extinction, and for another 58% the risk status is unknown. With limited resources to devote to conservation, priorities must be set. International co-operation is important if resources are to be used efficiently. For instance, there is no point in two countries devoting their scarce resources to the conservation of the same or closely related breeds, while others get neglected. (Though the vast majority of breeds are reported in only one country.) Hence, collecting information on the status of different breeds has been a priority for organizations involved in conservation. (See Wainwright *et al.* (2019) for one approach to prioritizing breeds for conservation.)

The FAO DAD-IS system mentioned above (FAO, 2019) collates available information on:

- breeds and strains that exist in each member country;
- whether the breeds exists in other countries (transboundary breeds);
- numbers of breeding animals in each population and risk status;
- conservation programmes in operation;
- genetic and production characteristics of each breed;
- typical production systems; and
- cultural importance.

This information helps in the identification of breeds or strains which are declining in numbers rapidly, though large gaps and errors in the data (as reported by countries) remain. Table 3.12 shows the 'headline' threshold population sizes used by FAO to assign risk status to livestock breeds. These are further refined, depending on the species reproductive rate, trends in population size, and extent of pure breeding. Other institutions or countries use higher population thresholds to declare populations at risk, recognizing that it may be more cost effective to act sooner where populations are declining. This is especially true in countries with constrained resources or infrastructure. It is also important to note that breeds may be at risk not just because of numerical scarcity, but also because of low genetic variability, because of geographical concentration or because of adaptation to a specific environment. The UK considers native breeds to be at risk when populations of breeding females fall below 5000 (equines), 7500 (cattle), 10,000 (sheep and goats), 15,000 (pigs) or 25,000 (poultry). For more information on this, on UK National Action Plans and other resources, see Defra (2019).

Historically, the degree of similarity between breeds has been estimated from knowledge of the history of the breed, or from variation in the blood groups present. However, molecular genetic tools can be used to measure the diversity or *genetic distance* between breeds more objectively, to ensure that the most diverse breeds are conserved, and that the conserved population is based on individuals which are as dissimilar as possible. These techniques can also be used to target breeds or individuals carrying particularly rare or important alleles, where these are known (see, for example, FAO, 2015).

Genes conferring resistance to viruses, resistance to insects and herbicide tolerance have been transferred into plants from viruses, bacteria and other plant species. This supports the need for wider conservation efforts across phyla and species, not just those of

Table 3.12. FAO threshold breed population sizes for assigning risk status. (After FAO, 2015.)

Risk status	No. of breeding females	No. of breeding males
Extinct	0	0
Critical	≤ 100	≤ 5
Critical Maintained	As above, but with actively managed conservation programme	
Endangered	101–1000	6–20
Endangered Maintained	As above, but with actively managed conservation programme	

immediate concern. While these techniques have yet to be applied widely to animals for agricultural purposes, this remains a future possibility. However, this approach may be supplanted by *gene editing* techniques, outlined in Chapter 5, that allow targeted changes in base sequence within the breed and species concerned.

Methods of conservation

The main methods of conservation which have been proposed or used are:

- **Maintaining breeds in a commercial farm environment.** The advantages of this approach are that the genetic resources are still being utilized, they can be seen and enjoyed, the performance characteristics can be properly recorded, and the breeds have the opportunity to evolve, e.g. to develop resistance to new disease challenges, or to adapt to changes in husbandry. The disadvantages are that selection and genetic drift (the chance change in gene frequency which occurs across generations due to small population size) may result in unfavourable genetic changes, there is a risk of increasing inbreeding and hence homozygosity which is associated with reduced fitness, and the animals are at risk from disease or other natural disasters. Also, they are likely to be less productive, and so more costly to maintain than more popular breeds. This may increase the risk of individual breeders ceasing to keep rare breeds. Grants to farmers keeping rare breeds are used in some countries as a way of promoting this type of conservation.
- **Maintaining breeds in farm parks or other collections.** Many of the pros and cons are similar to the method above. However, there is potentially more control over the management of the population. Also, there may be greater opportunities for education, and to recoup some of the costs of conservation, by promoting public access. This approach, pioneered by the RBST, has become very popular in several countries.
- **Creating a *gene pool*.** This involves crossing several rare breeds together, then breeding them to maintain genetic variability (Maijala, 1970). It is probably an effective way of conserving genetic variation from two or three populations, but there is a greater risk of losing useful genes when more populations are combined. Although useful genes may be conserved with this approach, the 'identity' of different breeds is lost.
- **Frozen storage (*cryopreservation*) of semen, embryos, oocytes, somatic cells, *primordial germ cells* or DNA from breeds at risk.** These methods have the advantage that, after the initial investment, they are relatively inexpensive. Also, the population being conserved is free from unintended genetic change. During storage, frozen genetic material is at less risk from disease and natural disasters than live animals, but obviously at risk from technological failures. These risks can be minimized by splitting the material collected from a particular population and storing it in different locations. The disadvantages are that reproductive technologies are not uniformly successful for all individuals or all species, and the expertise is not always available in the places where it is needed most for collection or reinstatement. Also, cryopreservation prevents adaptation to changes in the production environment and to new disease challenges. If frozen semen is used as the only method of conservation, then several generations of backcrossing are needed to reinstate the breed concerned. In contrast, breeds can be reinstated rapidly from frozen embryos. At the time of writing, techniques for recreating populations from somatic (body) cells, primordial germ cells (cells that give rise to eggs) or DNA are either still at an experimental stage or yet to be tested. For instance, scientists at the Roslin Institute, University of Edinburgh, have demonstrated experimentally an approach for regenerating rare breeds of chicken. This involves collecting and freezing primordial germ cells from rare breeds and transplanting these into eggs from hens genetically modified to be infertile, giving rise to chicks with DNA entirely from the rare breed. This so-called 'frozen aviary' provides a potentially efficient method of conserving avian genetic resources (Liu *et al.*, 2017).
- ***In silico* conservation.** Sequencing the whole genomes of breeds at risk provides a form of *in silico* conservation, potentially allowing reconstruction at a future date, by means yet to be tested.

When the costs of different current methods of conservation are compared, as well as their effectiveness in avoiding inbreeding, the combined use of live animals and frozen semen or embryos appears to be the best strategy (Lömker and Simon, 1994; FAO, 2019). However, integrating the use of some of the newer techniques is likely to be cost effective in the medium term. When conservation is based on live animal populations, or a combination of live animals and frozen genetic material, there are useful guidelines which help to maintain genetic variation in the population (de Rochambeau and Chevalet, 1990; Frankham, 1994; FAO, 1998, 2015, 2019). In summary, these are:

- Start with as variable a population as possible.
- Start with as large a population as possible.
- Turn over generations as slowly as possible.
- Use enough parents (especially males) to keep inbreeding at acceptable levels (what acceptable levels of inbreeding are, the effect of number of parents on rates of inbreeding, and mating designs to minimize inbreeding are discussed in more detail in Chapter 4).
- Minimize the variation in family sizes to reduce inbreeding – ideally each male parent should be replaced by a son, and each female by a daughter.
- Subdivide the breeding population to reduce inbreeding and genetic drift. In small populations it may be most effective to practice a form of *within-family selection*, i.e. to organize the population into 'families' in a notional circle, and keep female replacements in the family in which they were born, but move replacement males from the family in which they were born, to the next family in the circle, in the same sequence each year (see Fig. 3.16). In slightly larger populations it is more effective to mate males from one group to females of different groups in successive years.

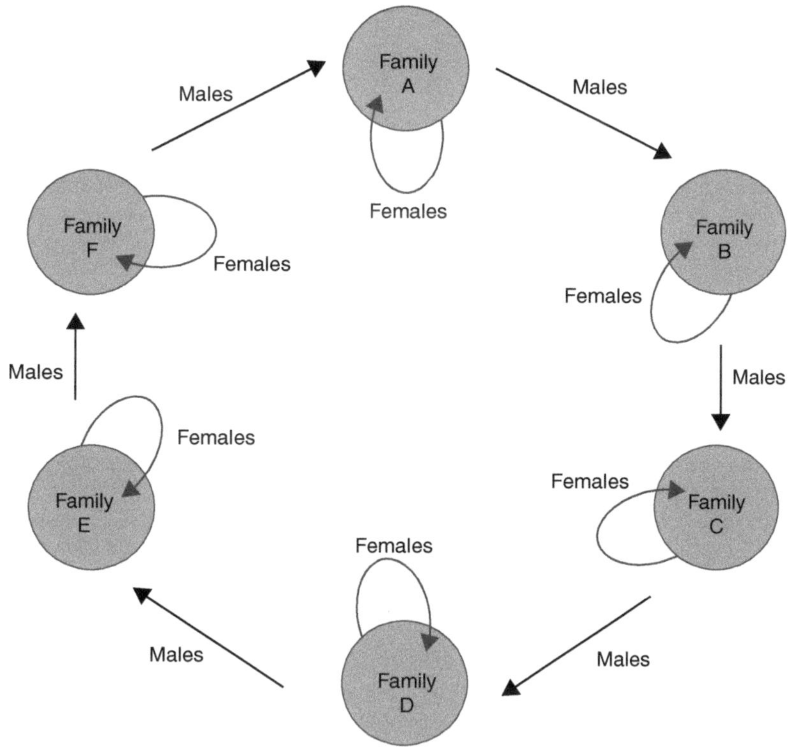

Fig. 3.16. A diagram illustrating the use of within-family selection to limit inbreeding. Female replacements remain in the family in which they were born, while males born in one family move to the next for mating. (This method was used to limit inbreeding in the unselected 'control' line in an SAC selection experiment using Suffolk sheep. The control line was maintained to allow estimation of response to selection by comparing the performance of animals in the two lines each year. The control line comprised 75 breeding females divided into 6 families, and 6 males were used per annum. After 10 years the level of inbreeding in this flock was similar to that in the selection line which was over double the size of the control line but did not use within-family selection.)

Sometimes, unselected 'control' populations of animals are maintained as a benchmark against which to measure response to selection in an experimental or industry breeding scheme. The guidelines above are also helpful in establishing and maintaining such a population.

Summary

- Traditionally, three main strategies have been used for the genetic improvement of livestock. These are (i) selection between breeds or breed types; (ii) selection within breeds or breed types; and (iii) crossbreeding. New strategies, such as the ability to transfer genes within or between species, and gene editing, are becoming available as a result of developments in molecular genetics and reproductive biology.
- For any genetic improvement strategy to be effective, it is important to have a clear view of what the economically-important traits are. Then it is logical to choose the most appropriate breed or cross, based on their performance in these traits. It is then sensible to consider whether this pure breed, or component breeds of the cross, can be improved further by within-breed selection.
- The structure of livestock breeding industries in most industrialized nations is often described schematically as a pyramid with *elite* or *nucleus* breeders at the top, one or more middle tiers of purebred or crossbred *multipliers*, and a final tier of *commercial herds* or *flocks*, or end users. Ideally, market signals from commercial herds or flocks influence breeding decisions in the tiers above.
- Selection between breeds or strains can achieve dramatic and rapid genetic change when there are large genetic differences between populations in characteristics of economic or other importance. It is costly to replace whole flocks or herds of breeding females at once. In practice, changes are often made more gradually by grading up to the new breed. It is important that choices among breeds are made on the basis of well-designed objective comparisons of performance in the relevant production environment.
- Selection within breeds involves comparing animals of the same breed and mating the preferred animals to produce the next generation. This process is usually repeated each generation, and as long as there is genetic variation in the characters under selection, this produces changes in each generation.
- Objective selection within breeds or strains is intended to increase the average level of additive genetic merit or breeding value of the population. Ideally, the steps involved are: (i) deciding on the breeding goal; (ii) deciding on the selection criterion; (iii) designing the breeding programme, e.g. numbers of males and females selected annually, ages at mating; (iv) implementing the programme, i.e. doing the routine recording, evaluation and mating of animals; and (v) monitoring progress and redesigning the programme, as necessary.
- Objective selection depends on having records of performance on the candidates for selection, or their relatives, or both. In most industrialized countries, the majority of cattle and sheep breeders use recording schemes which are operated by regional or national agencies who specialize in recording and evaluation. Although these schemes are sometimes less flexible and more expensive than 'home-grown' schemes, they encourage discipline and consistency in recording, they often allow access to more sophisticated methods of evaluation, and they can improve communication with customers.
- Annual rates of genetic improvement in polygenic traits depend on the *selection differential*, the *heritability* of the trait under selection, and the *generation interval*. Generally speaking, the higher the selection differential and heritability, and the lower the generation interval, the higher the annual rate of genetic improvement.
- Profitability usually depends on several different animal characteristics rather than any single trait. Hence, in genetic improvement programmes animals are usually selected on a combination of traits. This can be achieved by tandem selection, the use of independent culling levels or, most efficiently, by index selection.
- Crossbreeding involves mating animals of different breeds, lines or species. It is usually used for one or more of the following reasons: (i) to improve the overall efficiency of a production system by crossing breeds which each have high genetic merit in different traits (complementarity); (ii) to produce individual animals of intermediate performance between that of two more extreme parent breeds; (iii) for grading up to a new breed or strain; (iv) as an intermediate step in the creation of a new synthetic or composite breed; (v) to introduce new variation to numerically small breeds; (vi) to introduce a single gene for a favourable characteristic to an existing breed

(introgression); or (vii) to exploit heterosis or hybrid vigour.

- Heterosis is defined as the advantage in performance above the mid-parent mean. It is most useful when it leads to the average performance of crossbred animals exceeding that of the best parent breed. Individual heterosis directly influences the performance of crossbred animals themselves. Maternal and paternal heterosis arise when dams or sires are crossbred, and the effects are often measured in terms of improved reproductive efficiency or improved performance of offspring.
- Different systems of crossing lead to different proportions of individual, maternal and paternal heterosis being maintained. However, the most appropriate system of crossing depends not only on this, but also on the additive merit of the breeds available, and the absolute level of performance of crossbreds.
- Each of the strategies for genetic improvement depends on genetic variation, so it is important for the success of future improvement programmes that genetic variation is used in a sustainable way. However, there are aesthetic as well as biological reasons for conservation of genetic resources.
- It is difficult to decide which breeds should be conserved. International organizations, such as the FAO, are attempting to identify those breeds most in need of conservation programmes and provide guidelines to implement these. Molecular genetic tools may help to ensure that the most diverse breeds and individuals are conserved.
- The main methods of conservation which have been proposed or used are: (i) maintaining breeds in their normal farm environment; (ii) maintaining breeds in farm parks or other collections; (iii) creating a gene pool; and (iv) frozen storage of semen, embryos, oocytes, somatic or primordial germ cells or DNA from rare breeds. When the costs of these different methods of conservation are compared, as well as their effectiveness in avoiding inbreeding, the combined use of live animals and frozen semen or embryos is usually the best current strategy.
- When conservation is based on live animal populations, it helps in maintaining genetic variation to: (i) start with as variable a population as possible; (ii) start with as large a population as possible; (iii) turn over generations as slowly as possible; (iv) use enough parents (especially males) to keep inbreeding at acceptable levels; (v) minimize the variation in family sizes to reduce inbreeding; and (vi) subdivide the breeding population to reduce inbreeding and genetic drift.

References

ACGG (2019) African Chicken Genetic Gains project. Available at: https://africacgg.net/ (accessed 17 May 2019).

ADGG (2019) African Dairy Genetic Gains project. Available at: https://africadgg.wordpress.com/ (accessed 17 May 2019).

Beatson, P.R. (1993) Coopworths: making a concept happen. In: Blair, H.T. and McCutcheon, S.N. (eds) *Proceedings of the A.L. Rae Symposium on Animal Breeding and Genetics,* Massey University, Palmerston North, New Zealand, pp. 154–159.

Bunning, H., Wall, E., Chagunda, M.G.G., Banos, G. and Simm, G. (2018) Heterosis in cattle crossbreeding schemes in tropical regions: Meta-analysis of effects of breed combination, trait type and climate on level of heterosis. *Journal of Animal Science* 97, 29-34. DOI: 10.1093/jas/sky407.

Cameron, N.D., Smith, C. and Deeble, F.K. (1983) Comparative performance of crossbred ewes from three crossing sire breeds. *Animal Production* 37, 415-421. DOI: 10.1017/S0003356100002038.

Cartwright, T.C. (1982) Objectives in beef cattle improvement. In: Barton, R.A. and Smith, W.C. (eds) *Proceedings of the World Congress on Sheep and Beef Cattle Breeding,* Vol. II. Dunmore Press, New Zealand, pp. 19–27.

Cassady, J.P., Young, L.D. and Leymaster, K.A. (2002) Heterosis and recombination effects on pig growth and carcass traits. *Journal of Animal Science* 80, 2286–2302.

CBD (2019) The Nagoya Protocol on Access and Benefit-sharing. Available at: https://www.cbd.int/abs/ (accessed 19 May 2019).

Cundiff, L.V. and Gregory, K.E. (1977) *Beef Cattle Breeding.* United States Department of Agriculture, Agriculture Information Bulletin No. 286. USDA, Washington, DC.

Cundiff, L.V., Gregory, K.E. and Koch, R.M. (1982) Effects of heterosis in Hereford, Angus and Shorthorn rotational crosses. In: *Beef Research Program Progress Report No. 1. (ARM-NC-21)* pp. 3–5. Roman L. Hruska U.S. Meat Animal Research Center, Nebraska.

Cundiff, L.V., Gregory, K.E., Koch, R.M. and Dickerson, G.E. (1986) Genetic diversity among cattle breeds and its use to increase beef production efficiency in a temperate environment. *Proceedings of the 3rd World Congress on Genetics Applied to Livestock Production* Vol. IX, pp. 271–282. Available at: http://www.wcgalp.org/proceedings/1986 (accessed 25 June 2020).

Cunningham, E.P. and Syrstad, O. (1987) *Crossbreeding* Bos indicus *and* Bos taurus *for Milk Production in the Tropics.* FAO Animal Production and Health Paper No. 68, Food and Agriculture Organization of the United Nations, Rome. Available at: http://www.fao.org/3/t0095e/T0095E00.htm (accessed 28 August 2020).

Davis, G.P. and Arthur, P.F. (1994) Crossbreeding large ruminants in the tropics: current knowledge and future directions. *Proceedings of the 5th World Congress on Genetics Applied to Livestock Production*, Vol. 20, pp. 332–339. Available at: http://www.wcgalp.org/proceedings/1994 (accessed 25 June 2020).

Defra (2019) Farm Animal Genetic Resources Committee. Available at: https://www.gov.uk/government/groups/farm-animal-genetic-resources-committee-fangr (accessed 10 January 2019).

de Rochambeau, H. and Chevalet, C. (1990) Genetic principles of conservation. *Proceedings of the 4th World Congress on Genetics Applied to Livestock Production*, Vol. XIV, pp. 434–442. Available at: http://www.wcgalp.org/proceedings/1990 (accessed 25 June 2020).

Dickerson, G.E. (1973) Inbreeding and heterosis in animals. *Journal of Animal Science* 1973, 54–77. DOI: 10.1093/ansci/1973.Symposium.54.

Dickerson, G.E. (1974) Evaluation and utilization of breed differences. *Proceedings of Working Symposium on Breed Evaluation and Crossing Experiments in Farm Animals.* Instituut voor Veeteeltkundig Onderzoek, 'Schoonoord', Zeist, Netherlands, pp. 7–23.

Dickerson, G.E. (1978). Animal size and efficiency: basic concepts. *Animal Production* 27, 367–379. DOI: 10.1017/S0003356100036278.

Falconer, D.S. and Mackay, T.F.C. (1996) *Introduction to Quantitative Genetics*, 4th edn. Longman, Harlow, UK.

FAO (1998) Secondary Guidelines for Development of Farm Animal Genetic Resources Management Plans: Management of small populations at risk. Available at: http://www.fao.org/3/a-w9361e.pdf (accessed 08 January 2019).Food and Agriculture Organization of the United Nations, Rome.

FAO (2007) The State of the World's Animal Genetic Resources for Food and Agriculture. Rischkowsky, B. and Pilling, D. (eds). FAO, Rome. Available at: http://www.fao.org/3/a-a1260e.pdf (accessed 26 October 2019).

FAO (2015) The Second Report on the State of the World's Animal Genetic Resources for Food and Agriculture. Food and Agriculture Organization of the United Nations, Rome. Available at: http://www.fao.org/3/a-i4787e.pdf (accessed 10 January 2019).

FAO (2019) Genetic Resources. Food and Agriculture Organization of the United Nations, Rome. Available at: http://www.fao.org/genetic-resources/en/ (accessed 10 January 2019).

Fell, H.R. (1979) *Intensive Sheep Management.* Farming Press, Ipswich, UK.

Frankham, R. (1994) Conservation of genetic diversity for animal improvement. *Proceedings of the 5th World Congress on Genetics Applied to Livestock Production*, Vol. 21, pp. 385–392. Available at: http://www.wcgalp.org/proceedings/1994 (accessed 28 August 2020).

Gjedrem, T. and Rye, M. (2018) Selection response in fish and shellfish: a review. *Reviews in Aquaculture* 10, 168–179. DOI: 10.1111/raq.12154.

Gregory, K.E., Cundiff, L.V. and Koch, R.M. (1982) Comparison in crossbreeding systems and breeding stocks used in suckling herds of continental and temperate areas. *Proceedings of the 2nd World Congress on Genetics Applied to Livestock Production*, Vol. V. pp. 482–503. Available at: http://www.wcgalp.org/proceedings/1982 (accessed 28 August 2020).

Gregory, K., Cundiff, L.V. and Koch, R.M. (1993) Composite breeds – what does the research tell us? *Range Beef Cow Symposium* 207. Available at: http://digitalcommons.unl.edu/rangebeefcowsymp/207 (accessed 17 May 2019).

Harris, B.L., Clark, J.M. and Jackson, R.G. (1996) Across breed evaluation of dairy cattle. *Proceedings of the New Zealand Society of Animal Production* 56, pp. 12–15. Available at: http://www.nzsap.org/system/files/proceedings/1996/ab96005.pdf (accessed 10 January 2019).

Harris, D.L., Stewart, T.S. and Arboleda, C.R. (1984) *Animal Breeding Programs: A Systematic Approach to their Design*. Advances in Agricultural Technology, Publication No. AAT-NC-8, Agricultural Research Service, North Central Region, US Department of Agriculture, Peoria, Illinois.

Innovis (2019) Innovis – Breeding Sheep. Available at: www.innovis.org.uk (accessed 1 August 2019).

Kelso (2019) Kelso. Available at: http://kelso.co.nz/ (accessed 1 August 2019).

Kempster, A.J., Cook, G.L. and Southgate, J.R. (1982) A comparison of different breeds and crosses from the suckler herd. 2. Carcass characteristics. *Animal Production* 35, 99–111. DOI: 10.1017/S0003356100000866.

Kempster, A.J., Croston, D., Guy, D.R. and Jones, D.W. (1987) Growth and carcass characteristics of crossbred lambs by ten sire breeds, compared at the same estimated subcutaneous fat proportion. *Animal Production* 44, 83–98. DOI: 10.1017/S0003356100028099.

Leachman (2019) Leachman Stabilisers. Available at: https://www.leachman.com/leachman-stabilizers (accessed 1 August 2019).

Liu, C., Chang, I.-K., Khazanehdari, K.A., Thomas, S., Varghese, P. *et al.* (2017) Uniparental chicken offsprings derived from oogenesis of chicken primordial germ cells (ZZ). *Biology of Reproduction* 96, 686–693. DOI: 10.1095/biolreprod.116.144253.

Livestock Improvement (1996) *Dairy Statistics 1995-1996*. Livestock Improvement Corporation Limited, New Zealand Dairy Board, Hamilton, New Zealand.
Livestock Improvement Corporation Ltd and DairyNZ Ltd (2018). *New Zealand Dairy Statistics 2017-18*. LIC, Private Bag 3016, Hamilton 3240, New Zealand; DairyNZ, Private Bag 3221, Hamilton 3240, New Zealand.
Lömker, R. and Simon, D.L. (1994) Costs of and inbreeding in conservation strategies for endangered breeds of cattle. *Proceedings of the 5th World Congress on Genetics Applied to Livestock Production*, Vol. 21, pp. 393–396. Available at: http://www.wcgalp.org/proceedings/1994 (accessed 23 August 2020).
Lush, J.L. (1945) *Animal Breeding Plans,* 3rd edn. Iowa State College Press, Ames, Iowa.
Maijala, K. (1970) Need and methods of gene conservation in animal breeding. *Annales de Génétique et de Sélection Animale*2, 403–415. DOI: 10.1186/1297-9686-2-4-403.
Marshall, K. (2014) Optimizing the use of breed types in developing country livestock production systems: A neglected research area. *Journal of Animal Breeding and Genetics* 131, 329–340. DOI: 10.1111/jbg.12080.
Marshall, K., Tebug, S., Juga, J., Tapio, M. and Missohou, A. (2016) Better Dairy Cattle Breeds and Better Management Can Improve the Livelihoods of the Rural Poor in Senegal. ILRI Research Brief 65. ILRI, Nairobi. https://cgspace.cgiar.org/handle/10568/72865.
Marshall, K., Salmon, G.R., Tebug, S., Juga, J., MacLeod, M. *et al.* (2020) Net benefits of smallholder dairy cattle farms in Senegal can be significantly increased through the use of better dairy cattle breeds and improved management practices. *Journal of Dairy Science* 103, 8197–8217.
Mayala, K. (1974) Breed evaluation and crossbreeding in sheep. A summarising report. *Proceedings of Working Symposium on Breed Evaluation and Crossing Experiments in Farm Animals.* Instituut voor Veeteeltkundig Onderzoek, 'Schoonoord', Zeist, Netherlands, pp. 389–405.
Meat and Livestock Commission. (1988) *Sheep in Britain*. MLC, Milton Keynes, UK.
Mueller, J., Rischkowsky, B., Haile, A., Philipsson, J., Mwai, O. *et al.* (2015) Community-based livestock breeding programmes: essentials and examples. *Journal of Animal Breeding and Genetics* 132, 155–168. DOI: 10.1111/jbg.12136.
Nicholas, F.W. (1987) *Veterinary Genetics.* Oxford University Press, Oxford.
Parker, A.G.H. and Rae, A.L. (1982) Underlying principles of co-operative group breeding schemes. In: Barton, R.A. and Smith, W.C. (eds) *Proceedings of the World Congress on Sheep and Beef Cattle Breeding*, Vol. II. Dunmore Press, New Zealand, pp. 95–101.
Simm, G. (1998). *Genetic Improvement of Cattle and Sheep*. CAB International, Wallingford, UK.
Simm, G., Conington, J. and Bishop, S.C. (1994) Opportunities for genetic improvement of sheep and cattle in the hills and uplands. In: Lawrence, T.L.J, Parker, D.D. and Rowlinson, P. (eds) *Livestock Production and Land Use in Hills and Uplands.* Occasional Publication No. 18, British Society of Animal Production, pp. 51–66. DOI: 10.1017/S0263967X00001506.
Smith, C. (1964) The use of specialised sire and dam lines in selection for meat production. *Animal Production* 6, 337–344. DOI: 10.1017/S0003356100022133.
Smith, C. (1984) Rates of genetic change in farm livestock. *Research and Development in Agriculture* 1, 79–85.
Snedecor, G.W. and Cochran, W.G. (1989) *Statistical Methods*, 8th edn. Iowa State University Press, Ames, Iowa.
Southgate, J.R., Cook, G.L. and Kempster, A.J. (1982) A comparison of different breeds and crosses from the suckler herd. 1. Live-weight growth and efficiency of food utilization. *Animal Production* 35, 87–98. DOI: 10.1017/S0003356100000854.
Thiessen, R.B., Hnizdo, E., Maxwell, D.A.G., Gibson, D. and Taylor, C.S. (1984) Multibreed comparisons of British cattle. Variation in body weight, growth rate and food intake. *Animal Production* 38, 323–340. DOI: 10.1017/S0003356100041520.
Timon, V.M. (1974) The evaluation of sheep breeds and breeding strategies. *Proceedings of Working Symposium on Breed Evaluation and Crossing Experiments in Farm Animals.* Instituut voor Veeteeltkundig Onderzoek, 'Schoonoord', Zeist, Netherlands, pp. 367–387.
Wainwright, W., Ahmadi, B., McVittie, A., Simm, G. and Moran, D. (2019) Prioritising support for cost effective rare breed conservation using multi-criteria decision analysis. *Frontiers in Ecology and Evolution* 7, 110. DOI: 10.3389/fevo.2019.00110.
Wiener, G. (1994) *Animal Breeding*. The Tropical Agriculturalist series. Macmillan, London and CTA, Wageningen, Netherlands.
Williams, S.M, Price, S.E. and Siegel, P.B. (2002) Heterosis of growth and reproductive traits in fowl. *Poultry Science* 81, 1109–1112. DOI: 10.1093/ps/81.8.1109.

Recommended Reading

Amer, P.R., Kemp, R.A. and Smith, C. (1992) Genetic differences among the predominant beef cattle breeds in Canada: An analysis of published results. *Canadian Journal of Animal Science* 72, 759–771. Available at: https://www.nrcresearchpress.com/doi/pdfplus/10.4141/cjas92-088 (accessed 28 August 2020).
Baker, R.L. and Rege, J.E.O. (1994) Genetic resistance to diseases and other stresses in improvement of ruminant livestock in the tropics. *Proceedings of the 5th World Congress on Genetics Applied to Livestock Production*, Vol. 20, pp. 405–412. Available at: http://www.wcgalp.org/proceedings/1994 (accessed 25 June 2020).

Barker, J.D., Smith, C. and Bateman, N. (1985) Crossbred ewes for hill conditions. In: Maxwell, T.J. and Gunn, R.G. (eds) *Hill and Upland Livestock Production*. Occasional Publication No. 10, British Society of Animal Production, Edinburgh, p. 164.

Bichard, M. (1971) Dissemination of genetic improvement through a livestock industry. *Animal Production* 13, 401–411. DOI: 10.1017/S0003356100010606.

Falconer, D.S. and Mackay, T.F.C. (1996) *Introduction to Quantitative Genetics*, 4th edn. Longman, Harlow, UK.

FAO (2019). Genetic Resources. Food and Agriculture Organization of the United Nations, Rome. Available at: http://www.fao.org/genetic-resources/en/ (accessed 10 January 2019).

Gregory, K.E., Cundiff, L.V. and Koch, R.M. (1992) *Composite Breeds to Use Heterosis and Breed Differences to Improve Efficiency of Beef Production* United States Department of Agriculture, Agricultural Research Service, Roman L. Hruska U.S. Meat Animal Research Center, Nebraska.

Gregory, K.E., Cundiff, L.V. and Koch, R.M. (1994) Germplasm utilization in beef cattle. *Proceedings of the 5th World Congress on Genetics Applied to Livestock Production*, Vol. 17, pp. 261–268. Available at: http://www.wcgalp.org/proceedings/1994 (accessed 28 August 2020).

Guy, D.R. and Smith, C. (1981) Derivation of improvement lags in a livestock industry. *Animal Production* 32, 333–336. DOI: 10.1017/S0003356100027239.

Hazel, L.N. (1943) The genetic basis for constructing selection indexes. *Genetics*, 28, 476–490. Available at: https://www.genetics.org/content/28/6/476 (accessed 28 August 2020).

Lush, J.L. (1945) *Animal Breeding Plans,* 3rd edn. Iowa State College Press, Ames, Iowa.

OMIA (Online Mendelian Inheritance in Animals) (2019) Sydney School of Veterinary Science. Available at: https://omia.org/home/ (accessed 03 January 2019).

Proceedings of Working Symposium on Breed Evaluation and Crossing Experiments in Farm Animals, 1974. Instituut voor Veeteeltkundig Onderzoek, 'Schoonoord', Zeist, Netherlands.

The Ark. (Quarterly journal of the Rare Breeds Survival Trust. Includes a list of UK breeds at risk of extinction.)

4 What Affects Response to Selection Within Breeds?

Introduction

Over the last few decades, in higher-income countries, objective selection within breeds has been practised widely in pig and poultry breeding, and to a slightly lesser extent in dairy cattle and finfish breeding. It has been used less widely still in beef cattle, sheep and goat breeding. There are several reasons for this. These include the 'biological advantages' that allow faster rates of genetic improvement in pigs and poultry, as outlined in Chapter 3, and so higher rates of return on investment. Pig and poultry breeding in higher-income countries has become concentrated in a small number of global companies, which sell breeding stock into a large and very competitive sector that sends clear market signals. So, setting breeding goals has been more straightforward. In contrast, market signals have often been less clear in beef cattle and sheep production, and in some countries commercial breeding objectives have been obscured by fashions in the show ring, until recently. Those responsible for breeding decisions in pig and poultry breeding companies have been committed to objective methods, and less influenced by traditional breeding practices than cattle and sheep breeders. In contrast, beef and sheep breeding is often in the hands of individual breeders, many of whom have a long family history in the profession. Some have been sceptical about new approaches, which is understandable if traditional methods have served them well from a financial perspective. However, this is changing, with much wider recognition of the value of objective methods. This tradition was particularly strong in Britain, where so many breeds of livestock were developed and exported world-wide – though history shows the dangers of 'resting on your laurels' in livestock breeding. Many breeds which were very popular even a few decades ago are minority breeds today.

Dairy cattle breeding has fallen between these two extremes. Perhaps this is because market signals have been clearer than in beef cattle and sheep production, and because breeders, and their customers, are confronted each milking time with visible evidence of the link between their breeding decisions and profitability. For commercial beef and sheep producers, selection between breeds and crossbreeding have been easier strategies for improvement, because there are often more obvious differences between breeds and crosses than between individual bulls or rams of the same breed at a sale. Also, there are often easily identified 'markers', like coat colour, for particular breeds or crosses of proven merit.

Objective breeding programmes are a newer concept in finfish farming, and especially in shellfish farming. However, they have been adopted rapidly in some species (e.g. salmon) and are being adopted in others, benefiting from experience in terrestrial species. In several species, especially salmon, there is a growing trend towards a small number of broodstock producers operating across major production countries, as in pigs and poultry. In some cases, the same companies are involved in multiple species.

It would be too simplistic to set up pig and poultry breeding as a model to which other breeders should aspire, without qualification. There is no doubt that pig and poultry breeders have employed objective breeding techniques very successfully to improve major performance traits. However, at least in their earlier years, it is fair to say that most had rather narrow breeding goals. In some cases, this contributed to problems of 'functional fitness', such as leg weakness in pigs and poultry, and the inability of the males of some strains of turkey to mate naturally because of excessive breast muscle development. There is now a growing awareness that there are animal welfare, ethical and economic arguments against the pursuit of very narrow breeding goals. While this increases the importance of choosing appropriate breeding goals, and paying

Genetic Improvement of Farmed Animals (G. Simm *et al.*)
DOI: 10.1079/9781789241723.0004

attention to the functional fitness of selected animals, it should not detract from the value of objective selection. The success of objective selection methods in pigs and poultry is sometimes attributed to the intensive systems in which they are often kept. Although performance recording may be easier in these systems, intensive production systems are not a prerequisite for successful selection programmes. If cattle and sheep breeders are going to meet the more exacting demands of their local customers, and if animal agriculture is going to help to meet the demands of a growing global population, then it is vital that there is wider use of relevant objective methods of within-breed selection. The key to this will be a better understanding of the procedures involved, their value and their limitations.

Hence, the purpose of this and the next three chapters is to expand on the introduction to within-breed improvement given in Chapter 3. This chapter deals with predicting response to selection and designing breeding programmes to achieve the maximum response to selection. Chapter 5 examines tools and technologies used in breeding, while Chapter 6 covers analysing genetic variation. Chapter 7 deals with predicting the breeding values of individual animals – a vital component in achieving responses once the overall design of a breeding scheme has been decided.

Factors Affecting Rates of Genetic Gain

The factors affecting rates of genetic gain were introduced in Chapter 3. These are easiest to understand if we consider the special case where animals are selected on a single measurement of their own performance in one trait, ignoring information from relatives. This is often called *individual* or *mass selection*. It is also simplest to consider the process of selection in a single closed flock or herd – that is, a flock or herd which is producing all of its own replacement breeding stock, rather than buying these in from other flocks or herds. Each year new animals are born, their performance is recorded, and the best performing animals are selected and retained. Once they reach normal breeding age, they replace those adult males or females in the breeding herd or flock which have died of natural causes, or which the breeder wishes to cull and replace by superior animals. Although this is an annual process, it is easiest to follow if we concentrate initially on a single group of recorded animals and their offspring.

For example, let us consider a group of lambs of both sexes, each with a record of 20-week weight (generation 1). From this group, the lambs of each sex with the highest 20-week weight are selected for breeding to each other. The same performance trait, 20-week weight, is recorded eventually in their offspring (generation 2). The *response* is measured by comparing the average performance of all the lambs in generation 1 with the average performance of all of the lambs in generation 2 (i.e. the offspring of those animals selected for breeding from generation 1). In this case, the response to selection (R) *per generation* depends on just two things: the *selection differential* achieved (S), and the *heritability* of the trait selected on (h^2), as we saw in Chapter 3 (after Lush, 1945):

$$R = S \times h^2$$

Selection differential

The selection differential is the difference between the mean performance of selected animals (i.e. those identified to become parents of the next generation) and the overall mean of the group of animals from which they were selected. To continue the example above, it is the difference between the mean performance of selected animals in generation 1, and the overall mean of generation 1 animals. This is illustrated in Fig. 4.1. Because there are usually unequal numbers of male and female parents selected, but each sex eventually contributes half of the genes to the offspring, it is important to calculate selection differentials separately for males and females, and then average them to get an overall selection differential. In this example, the selection differential achieved in males is +10 kg, while that achieved in females is +2 kg, so the average selection differential achieved is +6 kg ([10 + 2] / 2). Figure 4.1 illustrates that the fewer animals selected for high performance, the further away from the mean they will be, and so the higher the selection differential will be. A further point to note is that the wider the variation in performance of the group, the higher the selection differential which can be achieved. (Although, as we will see later, this is only of value if there is a lot of genetic, rather than environmental, variation).

Heritability

The second factor affecting the response to selection per generation is the heritability of the trait concerned.

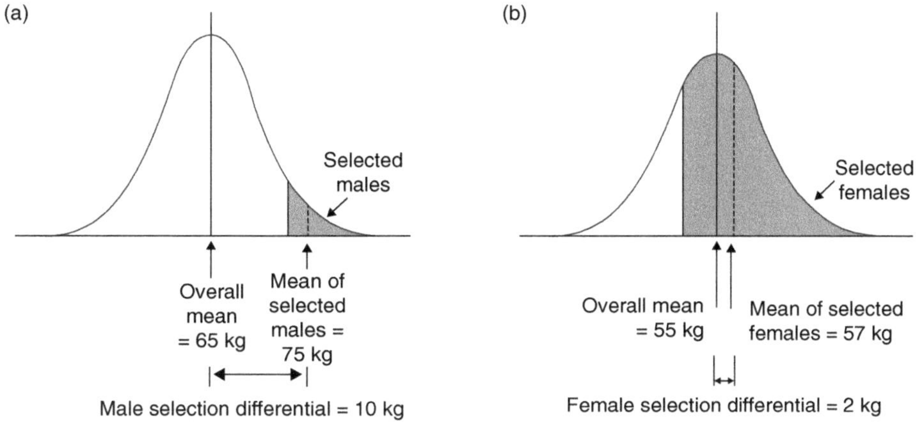

Fig. 4.1. (a) The selection differential achieved in males by selecting the heaviest ram lambs from a performance-recorded group at 20 weeks of age. The selection differential among males is the average weight of selected males minus the average of the group of males as a whole. (b) The selection differential achieved by selecting a larger proportion of ewe lambs from a recorded group, at the same age.

There are several ways of defining heritability. As mentioned in the last chapter, the simplest definition is that the heritability is the proportion of superiority of parents in a trait (i.e. the proportion of the selection differential) which, on average, is passed on to offspring. So, if the heritability of a trait is high, a lot of the superiority of the parents is a result of the genes they carry and we can expect much of this superiority to be passed on to offspring. If the heritability of a trait is low, only a little of the superiority of parents is a result of the genes they carry, and so only a little of this superiority will get passed on to offspring. Heritabilities are expressed as proportions from 0 to 1, or as percentages from 0 to 100%.

It will be easiest to understand selection differentials and heritabilities, and how they act together to influence response, by returning to the sheep example. In the case above, the average selection differential achieved across both sexes was +6 kg. If the heritability of live weight at 20 weeks of age is 0.3 or 30%, then we expect 30% of this 6 kg superiority to be passed on to offspring, on average. So, in this example we expect a 1.8 kg improvement in 20-week weight of the next generation (0.3 × 6 kg). This is illustrated in Fig. 4.2. It is important to note that selection achieves an increase in the *average* performance of the next generation – it does *not* add 1.8 kg to the weight of every lamb.

So how do we know what the heritability of a particular trait is in the first place? It may sound circular, but the simplest way of estimating the heritability for a particular trait is to select parents on this trait, measure the selection differential achieved, mate them, measure the same trait in their offspring and then calculate, using the regression techniques outlined in Chapter 2, how much of the superiority of parents was passed on to offspring. There are other more sophisticated methods which involve measuring the degree of resemblance in performance between different classes of relatives; these are discussed in Chapter 6.

Also, there is an alternative definition of heritability, which follows from the discussion of different types of variation in Chapter 2. The heritability of a trait is the additive genetic variation in that trait (or the variation in breeding values), expressed as a proportion of the total phenotypic variation in that trait. The fact that the heritability is the ratio of two variances explains why it is abbreviated to h^2. The square root of the heritability, abbreviated to h, is the ratio of the *additive genetic standard deviation* of a trait to the phenotypic standard deviation. Using the abbreviations introduced in Chapter 2 (after Lush, 1945):

$$\text{Heritability} = VAR_A \,/\, VAR_P$$

Distributions of VAR_A and VAR_P for two traits with different heritabilities are shown in Fig. 4.3. The inner distributions show the proportion of the total phenotypic variation which is a result of additive genetic variation, or variation in breeding

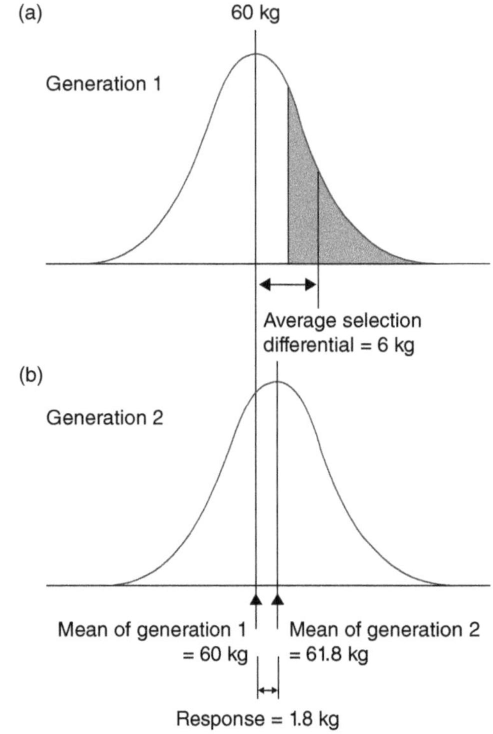

Fig. 4.2. Expected response to selection on 20-week weight in sheep, with an average selection differential of +6 kg, and a heritability of 0.3.

values. In one case, additive genetic variation accounts for 10% of the total phenotypic variation so, as we have seen, the heritability is 10%. In the other case a higher proportion of the total variation, 50%, is additive genetic variation, so the heritability is 50%. The graphs illustrate that when the heritability of a trait is low, the distribution of breeding values will be narrower, relative to phenotypic variation, than when the heritability of the trait is high. Table 4.1 shows typical examples of heritabilities for some traits of interest in cattle and sheep.

The ability to predict response to selection is important in planning breeding programmes, and especially in comparing alternative schemes. The problem with the approach described so far is that it predicts response per generation, but generations can be of variable length. For instance, in the sheep example, if the selected males and females had been mated at 7 months of age, the earliest age possible in most breeds, then their offspring would be born when they were about a year old. If, on the other hand, the selected animals were mated at 19 months of age, the offspring would be born a year later, when the parents were 2 years old. So, two breeders may be achieving equal selection differentials and equal responses per generation, but achieving these responses in quite different lengths of time. The solution to this problem is to express predicted responses *per annum* rather than per generation. To do this, we need to know the *generation interval* in the flock or herd concerned.

Generation interval

The generation interval (abbreviated L) is the average age of parents when their offspring are born. Because there are unequal numbers of male and female parents, and they often breed at different ages, generation intervals have to be calculated separately for each sex of parent, and then averaged. An additional complication is that in most flocks or herds there are different proportions of animals in each age group. Also, if the fertility of parents of different age groups differs, then this too must be taken into account. This means that we cannot simply average the parents' age classes, we must weight them according to the number of offspring produced by each age class. For example, if we had a flock of ewes comprising 50% 2-year olds and 50% 3-year olds, the average age would simply be 2.5 years. If, as is usually the case, we had a higher proportion of young animals in the flock to allow for natural wastage, then we could not simply average the age classes. If we had 60% 2-year olds and 40% 3-year olds, the average age of the ewes would be $(0.6 \times 2) + (0.4 \times 3) = 2.4$ years. If these two age groups produce equal numbers of offspring per ewe, then the female generation interval would simply be 2.4 years. If the youngest ewes are less prolific than older ones, so that 55% of lambs come from two year old ewes, and 45% from three year old ewes, then the female generation interval would be 2.45 years $([0.55 \times 2] + [0.45 \times 3] = 2.45)$. A more realistic example is given in Table 4.2. As the generation interval can differ for males and females, but each contribute equally to the next generation, it is averaged over these.

To predict responses to selection *per annum*, rather than per generation, we simply divide the formula shown above for response per generation by the average generation interval (L):

$$R(\text{per annum}) = \frac{S \times h^2}{L}$$

Table 4.1. Typical heritabilities for some traits of economic importance. See Chapters 8 to 13 for average values for these and many other traits from comprehensive literature searches.

Species/breed	Trait	Typical heritability values
Dairy cattle	Milk yield	25–40%
	Milk fat %	50–60%
	Milk protein %	50–60%
	Various measures of fertility	1–5%
	Incidence of various production diseases	0–25%
Beef cattle	Birth weight	25–35%
	Weaning weight	20–30%
	Yearling weight	30–40%
	Carcass fat depth	35–50%
	Calving ease	5–15%
Sheep	Birth weight	10–25%
	Weaning weight	15–25%
	Yearling weight	20–35%
	Carcass fat depth	25–35%
	Various combined measures of fertility and lamb output	5–15%
	Fleece weight	30–40%
	Fibre diameter	45–55%
Chickens	Growth rate	30–60%
	Feed conversion ratio	15–30%
	Resistance to range of diseases	5–50%
	Egg number	15–60%
	Egg weight	30–70%
Pigs	Litter size	5–10%
	Average daily gain	10–30%
	Backfat depth	40–65%
	Feed conversion ratio	15–30%
Atlantic salmon	Growth rate	40–60%
	Carcass characteristics	10–50%
	Resistance to range of diseases	10–60%

So, if we selected on 20-week weight each year in a flock with the age structure shown in Table 4.2, and achieved the selection differentials shown in Fig. 4.1 each year, we would have:

$S = 6$ kg,

$h^2 = 0.3$, and

$L = 2.67$ years.

So, we would expect to get a response *per annum* of:

$$R = \frac{6 \times 0.3}{2.67}$$

= 0.67 kg *per annum* (approximately).

A more useful formula for predicting response

As mentioned already, it is very useful to be able to predict rates of response to selection, in order to compare alternative breeding programmes – for example, to choose the design likely to maximize annual response. At first sight it appears that we need to know quite a lot of information in advance in order to predict response. We need to know the heritability of the trait under selection, but for most traits there are already estimates available which we can use. We also need to know the generation interval, but usually this can be predicted accurately from the expected age distribution of parents, together with typical levels of reproductive performance for parents of each age group. A greater limitation of the formula used so far is that

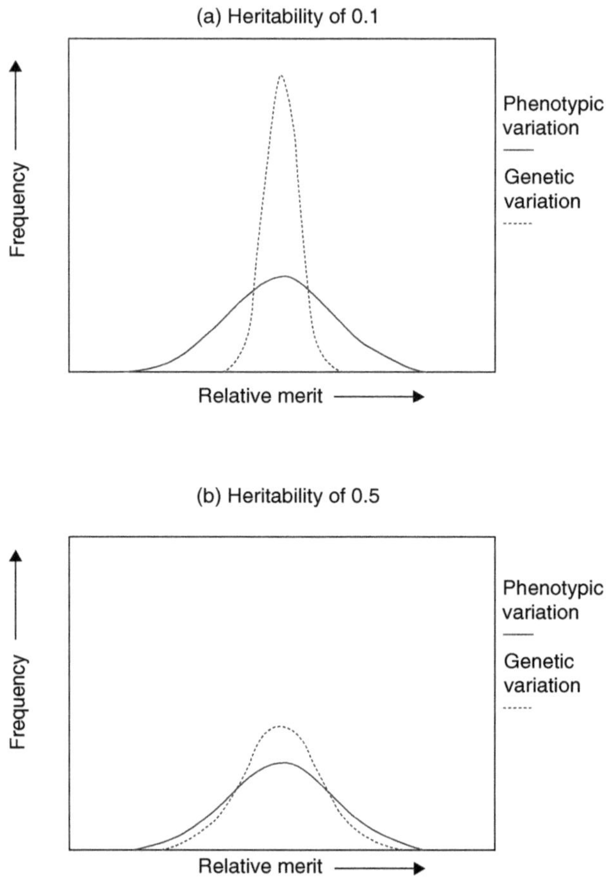

Fig. 4.3. Distributions of additive genetic variation (VAR_A) and phenotypic variation (VAR_P) for two traits with different proportions of additive genetic variation, and hence different heritabilities. (a) Heritability of 0.1 or 10%. (b) Heritability of 0.5 or 50%.

we need to know the selection differential in advance in order to predict response. It is easy to calculate a selection differential once animals have been performance recorded and parents have been selected, but how can we predict what selection differential is likely to be achieved before embarking on a breeding programme?

We saw in Chapter 2 that one of the features of normal distributions is that we can predict remarkably accurately what proportion of animals will fall in different ranges of performance around the mean. For example, about 68% of animals will have performance in the range from 1 standard deviation below the mean to 1 standard deviation above the mean, 95% of animals fall in the range –2 to +2 standard deviations, and so on. So, if we know how many standard deviations better than average our selected animals are, and we know the standard deviation of the trait of interest (i.e. how many kg of live weight or litres of milk each standard deviation is 'worth'), we can predict the selection differentials achieved.

If we know the total number of animals recorded, and the number selected from this group, there are standard statistical tables which allow us to express the merit of selected animals in standard deviation units above the mean. A table of these values is shown at the end of the book. Table 4.3 shows part of it. This table shows, for example, that if we select the best 5 rams out of a total of 75 that are performance recorded, on average they are expected to be 1.893 standard deviations above the mean of all 75 rams. If the standard deviation of 20-week weight

Table 4.2. Calculating the average generation interval in a flock of sheep of mixed ages.
(a) Calculating the female generation interval. In this example, the 100-ewe flock has a typical age distribution, with progressively fewer ewes in successive age groups, as a result of natural wastage. The average litter size is 1.6 lambs, but prolificacy is lowest in the youngest ewes, it is highest in ewes of intermediate age, and then declines slightly in the oldest ewes. Calculating the female generation interval involves recording the number of ewes in each age group at lambing (column 2), calculating the number of lambs (column 3) and then the proportion of lambs (column 4) from ewes in each age group. Each ewe age is then multiplied by the relevant proportion of lambs (column 1 × column 4 = column 5), to get the contribution of this age group to the average weighted age. These values are then summed over all age groups to get a weighted average age, which is the female generation interval.

Age of ewes at lambing (years)	Number of ewes in this age group	Number of lambs from ewes in this age group	Proportion of lambs from ewes in this age group (approx.)	Contribution of ewes in this age group to weighted average age (col. 1 × col. 4)
2	25	35	0.22	0.44
3	22	37	0.23	0.69
4	20	34	0.21	0.84
5	18	30	0.19	0.95
6	15	24	0.15	0.90
Total	100	160	1.00	3.82

Weighted average age of ewes = 3.82 years (approx.)
Female generation interval = 3.82 years (approx.)

(b) Calculating the male generation interval. In this example four rams are used in the flock, and they are mated to groups of ewes of mixed ages. Hence the two age groups of rams have roughly equal numbers of lambs born. Weighted average ages are calculated as described above for ewes.

Age of rams at birth of their offspring (years)	Number of rams in this age group	Number of lambs from rams in this age group	Proportion of lambs from rams in this age group (approx.)	Contribution of rams in this age group to weighted average age (col. 1 × col. 4)
1	2	78	0.49	0.49
2	2	82	0.51	1.02
Total	4	160	1.00	1.51

Weighted average age of rams = 1.51 years (approx.)
Male generation interval = 1.51 years (approx.)

(c) Calculating the average generation interval.

Female generation interval = 3.82 years (approx.)
Male generation interval = 1.51 years (approx.)
Average generation interval = 2.67 years (approx.)

is about 5 kg, then we expect the average weight of the five selected rams to be about 9.5 kg heavier than the average of all 75 recorded rams (1.893 × 5 kg = 9.465 kg).

The superiority of animals selected, expressed in standard deviation units, is called the standardized selection differential or *selection intensity* (abbreviated **i**). Table 4.3 shows that the selection intensity is largely a function of the proportion of animals selected – the lower the proportion selected, the higher the selection intensity. This is also illustrated in Fig. 4.4. However, with a fixed proportion of animals selected, selection intensities increase slightly as the total number of animals tested rises. For instance, compare the selection intensity when 10 animals are selected from 50 tested (1.372) with that when 20 animals are selected from 100 tested (1.386). As for selection differentials, selection intensities have to be calculated separately for each sex, then averaged.

Table 4.3. Examples of the selection intensity achieved, in standard deviation units, by selecting different numbers of animals from groups of 25, 50, 75 or 100 animals in total. See the table at the end of this book for a fuller set of selection intensities from the same source. (After Becker, 1984.)

	Total number of animals from which they were selected:			
	25	50	75	100
Number of animals selected	Selection intensity (i)			
1	1.965	2.249	2.403	2.508
5	1.345	1.705	1.893	2.018
10	0.936	1.372	1.588	1.730
15	0.624	1.139	1.381	1.536
20	0.336	0.951	1.217	1.386
25	0	0.786	1.079	1.259
35	–	0.488	0.843	1.050
50	–	0	0.539	0.792
75	–	–	0	0.420
100	–	–	–	0

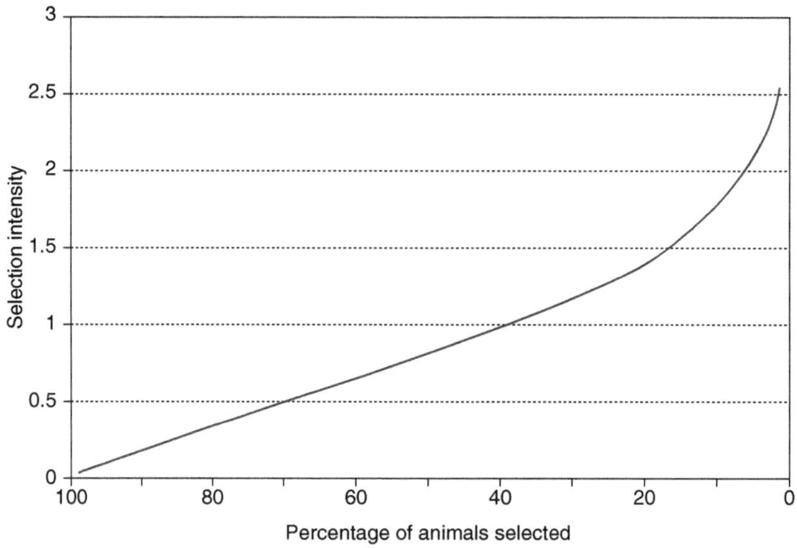

Fig. 4.4. The relationship between the proportion of animals selected and selection intensity – the selection intensity is measured in standard deviation units. The values shown assume that animals are selected from a very large total number of animals tested.

We can calculate the phenotypic variance (VAR_P) or phenotypic standard deviation (sd_P) of the trait under selection in the initial population of animals, as explained in Chapter 2. Alternatively, we could use published estimates of variation from similar animals to those we are interested in, kept in a similar production system (usually variances for the same trait are relatively constant within a given breed and level of production). Putting this together, we can predict selection differentials by multiplying the selection intensity, which tells us how many s.d. units better than average our selected animals are, by the phenotypic s.d., which tells us how much each s.d. unit is worth in kg of live weight, litres of milk, etc. So (after Lush, 1945):

$$S = i \times sd_P$$

Substituting **i** × $\mathbf{sd_p}$ instead of **S** in the formula used before gives a new formula for predicting response *per annum* (after Lush, 1945):

$$R = \frac{i \times sd_p \times h^2}{L}$$

It is easiest to see the connection with the earlier formula when the terms are presented as above, but most commonly the terms are re-ordered and the formula is shown as:

$$R = \frac{i \times h^2 \times sd_p}{L}$$

To illustrate the use of this formula, let us consider a beef cattle breeding programme to improve calf weaning weight (200-day weight) in a herd of 120 Simmental cows. Let us assume that there are 100 calves reared *per annum*, so on average there are 50 calves of each sex available for selection each year. We estimate that the phenotypic standard deviation of weaning weight in the Simmental breed is 35 kg. If we pick the top five bull calves each year, based on their own weaning weight, then we predict a male selection intensity of 1.705 standard deviations (see Table 4.3). If we select the top 35 heifers each year from 50 recorded, then the female selection intensity will be 0.488 standard deviations (see Table 4.3). This gives an average selection intensity across both sexes of 1.097. If the bulls are mated once only, at 15 months of age, then their progeny will be born when they are 2 years old, and the male generation interval will be 2 years. If the herd is made up of 35 heifers (3 years old), 30 4-year-old cows, 25 5-year-old cows, 20 6-year-old cows and 10 7-year-old cows, and they have equal calving rates, then the weighted average age of dams, and hence the female generation interval, is 5.5 years. The male and female generation intervals together give an average generation interval of 3.25 years. The heritability of weaning weight in beef cattle is usually about 25%. Putting these values into the new formula gives:

$$i = 1.097 \text{ s.d. units}$$

$$sd_p = 35 \text{ kg}$$

$$h^2 = 0.25$$

$$L = 3.25 \text{ years}$$

and so:

$$R = \frac{1.097 \times 35 \times 0.25}{3.25} \text{ kg per annum}$$

$$R = 2.95 \text{ kg } \textit{per annum} \text{ (approximately)}$$

The link between selection intensity and generation interval

The formula above shows that the annual response to selection will be highest when the selection intensity is high, the heritability is high, and the generation interval is low. There is little that breeders can do about the heritability of a trait – this is largely a biological characteristic of the trait concerned. But, within biological limits, breeders can increase selection intensities and decrease generation intervals, although these two measures are linked. The strength of that link varies between both species and sexes. For any breeding herd or flock to remain the same size, the breeding animals have to be replaced at least when they die of natural causes or are culled for unavoidable reasons. Because relatively few males are required for breeding, there is a plentiful supply of potential replacement males in all farmed species. This means that it is usually possible to keep male generation intervals short and, at the same time, keep male selection intensities high. But this is not the case for females in all species. The females of most breeds of cattle and sheep rear less than two offspring *per annum*, and so less than one female offspring *per annum* on average. This automatically sets an upper limit to the number of breeding females which can be replaced each year in these species. This is far less of a constraint in prolific species like pigs, poultry and fish.

It is easiest to see the link between selection intensity and generation interval by considering two extreme examples of a herd or flock replacement policy. At one extreme, all of the available young replacement females could be brought into a herd or flock to replace older females. In this case, the average age of the herd or flock would be low, and female generation intervals would be short. However, there would be no selection at all among female replacements (i.e. the female selection intensity would be 0). At the other extreme, if breeding females were only replaced when they died of natural causes, then the average age of the herd or flock would be high, and the female generation interval would be long. However, in this case few replacement females would be needed, so they could be highly selected, and selection intensities would be high. These two extreme situations, and some of the intermediate ones, are illustrated in Table 4.4.

The optimum flock or herd age structure to maximize response is often intermediate to the two extremes described. This is illustrated in Table 4.5 and Fig. 4.5. The table and graph show the predicted annual rate of response in 20-week weight for the different female replacement rates shown in Table 4.5. In all cases it is assumed that 5 ram lambs are selected from 75 available in each flock each year, and so a male selection intensity of 1.893 standard deviations is achieved. Each ram is used for 1 year only, so the male generation interval is 1 year in all cases. In this example the maximum rate of gain is achieved by replacing 45 females *per annum*, though the difference between alternative schemes is fairly small. The difference between schemes would be more marked if more males were selected, so reducing male selection intensity, or if male generation intervals were longer.

In the past, optimizing generation intervals and selection intensities was central to the design of breeding programmes. Deciding on the optimum proportion of animals to select from each

Table 4.4. Female generation intervals and selection intensities achieved in six flocks of 100 ewes when different proportions of available female replacements are brought into each flock. The extreme cases are in flock 1, where females are retained for as long as possible (up to 5 lamb crops), and in flock 6, where all available females are brought into the flock, displacing older ewes. In all cases natural wastage of about 10% is assumed, and ewes are assumed to lamb first at 2 years of age, and to rear an average of 1.5 lambs, of which half are males and half females (for simplicity, it is assumed that ewes of different ages have the same reproductive rate). Selection intensities can be converted to selection differentials by multiplying them by the standard deviation of the trait concerned. For example, if selection is for 20-week weight, the selection intensities would be multiplied by the standard deviation of 20-week weight, assumed to be about 5 kg. So, the female selection differential achieved in flock 1 would be about 5.4 kg (1.079 × 5 = 5.395 kg); that in flock 2 would be about 4.2 kg, and so on.

	Number of ewes in each age group					
Ewe age at lambing (years)	Flock 1	Flock 2	Flock 3	Flock 4	Flock 5	Flock 6
2	25	35	45	55	65	75
3	22	31	40	45	35	25
4	20	27	15	–	–	–
5	18	7	–	–	–	–
6	15	–	–	–	–	–
Female generation interval (weighted average age)	3.76 years	3.06 years	2.70 years	2.45 years	2.35 years	2.25 years
Female selection intensity achieved in 20-week weight (in standard deviation units)	1.079	0.843	0.637	0.443	0.244	0

Table 4.5. Predicted annual response to selection on 20-week weight in sheep, with different female replacement policies. Female generation intervals and selection intensities are those shown in Table 4.4. The heritability of 20-week weight is assumed to be 0.3 and the phenotypic standard deviation of 20-week weight is assumed to be 5 kg. Responses are calculated from the formula shown in the text.

	Flock 1	Flock 2	Flock 3	Flock 4	Flock 5	Flock 6
Female generation interval (years)	3.76	3.06	2.70	2.45	2.35	2.25
Male generation interval (years)	1.00	1.00	1.00	1.00	1.00	1.00
Average generation interval (years)	2.38	2.03	1.85	1.725	1.675	1.625
Female selection intensity	1.079	0.843	0.637	0.443	0.244	0
Male selection intensity	1.893	1.893	1.893	1.893	1.893	1.893
Average selection differential (kg)	1.486	1.368	1.265	1.168	1.069	0.947
Predicted annual response to selection (kg *per annum*)	**0.94**	**1.01**	**1.03**	**1.02**	**0.96**	**0.88**

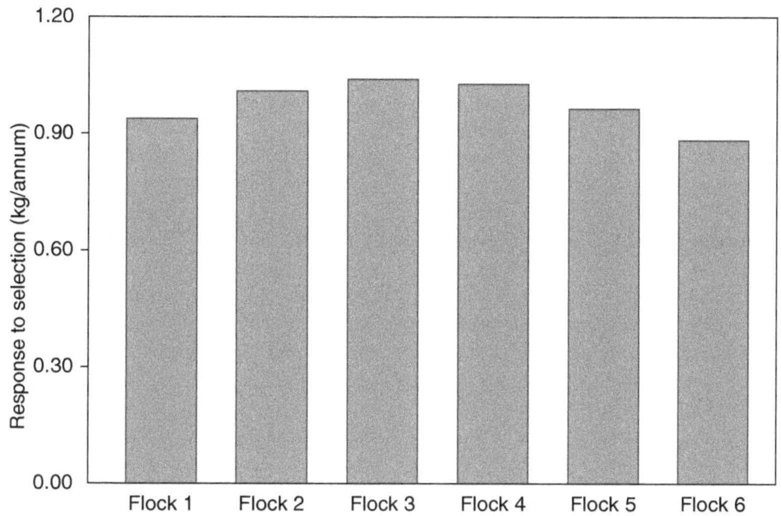

Fig. 4.5. Predicted annual response to selection on 20-week weight in sheep, with different female replacement policies, as shown in Table 4.4.

age group was important because animals were evaluated usually only once, and the results of these evaluations could only be compared within age groups. The modern methods of genetic evaluation described in Chapter 7 allow comparison of animals of different age groups. Also, advances in the methodology for evaluation and the power of computers means that it is feasible to do evaluations much more often than in the past. When these modern evaluation methods are available, genetic progress will be maximized by selecting animals with the highest predicted breeding value, regardless of age, rather than aiming for a fixed proportion of animals in each age group. The age structure of a flock or herd will still end up close to the optimum calculated as described above. However, there will be some additional gains as a result of keeping animals which are better than expected for their particular age group longer, and culling animals which are poorer than expected for their particular age group sooner.

Using information from relatives

So far, we have considered only a single measurement of performance on the animal itself as the selection criterion. However, this is only one of a number of sources of information which are commonly used in animal breeding. These include records of performance from:

- **The animal's ancestors**. Selection on ancestors' information is called *pedigree selection*. An index combining information on ancestors' performance is usually called a *pedigree index*, and selection on pedigree indexes is common in young animals until they get a record of performance themselves.
- **The animal itself**. Selection on the animal's own performance is the simplest method of selection. Historically, many farm livestock breeding schemes aimed at improving growth have been based on this source of information alone (individual selection or mass selection). When animals' performance is recorded consistently according to a defined protocol (e.g. specific feeding regimes to a target age or weight) this is usually termed a performance test.
- **The animal's full or half *siblings*** (*sibs* for short – these are the animal's brothers and sisters). Full sibs are animals which have both parents in common; half sibs are animals which have only one parent in common. In early population genetics experiments with fruit flies and mice, selection was often practised between families (*family selection*) or within families (*within-family selection*). Family selection involves selection of entire

families with the best average performance, from which to breed the next generation of animals. Within-family selection involves selection of the best individual animal in each family, from which to breed the next generation. Family selection can be especially useful in selecting for low heritability traits. However, it can lead to rapid rates of inbreeding, which become difficult to manage with the more constrained sizes of breeding populations of most farmed animal species. However, modifications of family selection were used in early livestock breeding practice and are still useful in establishing breeding programmes for new species. A selection programme based on information from siblings is called *sib selection* or a *sib test*. Sib tests are particularly useful if the trait of interest is only measurable on one sex. For instance, milk records from full sisters are helpful when selecting young dairy bulls. Similarly, early pig breeding programmes intended to improve carcass composition were based on sib selection, following carcass dissection of a full sib. This approach is less common now, because of the widespread use of ultrasonic scanning to assess carcass characteristics in live animals, although it is still used in meat poultry (broiler) breeding. Conversely to the situation in family selection, some form of within-family selection can help to limit rates of inbreeding, and so is often used in conservation of rare breeds, or in maintaining control populations in selection experiments.

- **The animal's progeny.** A breeding programme based on the performance of an animal's offspring is termed a progeny test. Again, information on the performance of progeny is particularly useful when the trait of interest can be measured in only one sex. In most countries, selection for milk production in dairy cattle is based on progeny testing. Bulls undergoing tests are used in many milk-recording herds through artificial insemination. They are then selected for wider use, or culled, on the basis of the milk production records of their daughters, compared with those of *contemporary animals*.
- **Any other relatives of the animal.**
- **Combinations of the classes of relatives listed above.** Modern livestock breeding schemes use information from all available relatives, weighted appropriately, to predict breeding values as accurately as possible. Chapter 7 describes how this is achieved.

Records of performance from relatives are useful in selection because related animals have genes in common, and so the performance of relatives can provide clues to the genetic merit or breeding value of the candidates for selection. Figure 4.6 shows the proportion of genes in common between the bull marked X, and various classes of relatives. (These proportions are the same for animals of the same relationship in all species.)

Offspring always have exactly one-half of their genes in common with each parent (apart from the slight inequalities caused by the different size of the X and Y chromosomes). This is because every animal develops from an embryo that has one member of each pair of its chromosomes from the father, via the sperm, and one member from the mother, via the egg. However, for other classes of relatives the proportion of genes in common are averages. This is because segregation and recombination lead to chance variation in the proportion of genes from ancestors (as explained in Chapter 2). Each sperm and each egg carry copies of half of the genes of the animals that produced them. Which sample of genes make up this half is determined entirely by chance. So, some pairs of full sibs have more than half of their genes in common, by chance, and others have less. (While we have known about this sampling for many years, it has not been easy to measure until recently. However, we can now estimate the proportion of genes in common in any pair of related animals, using the molecular genetic techniques described in Chapter 5.) Each generation, or link in the pedigree diagram, which separates two relatives leads to a halving of the genes they have in common, on average.

In order to predict response to selection using these new sources of information, we need a modified version of the formula used so far:

$$R = \frac{i \times h^2 \times sd_P}{L}$$

For reasons which are explained in the appendix at the end of this chapter, this can be rewritten as (after Falconer and Mackay, 1996):

$$R = \frac{i \times h \times sd_A}{L}$$

In this formula the **R**, **i** and **L** have exactly the same meaning as before. The new terms are **h**, which is the square root of the heritability, also referred to as the accuracy of selection on a single record of the animal's own performance, and **sd_A**, which is an

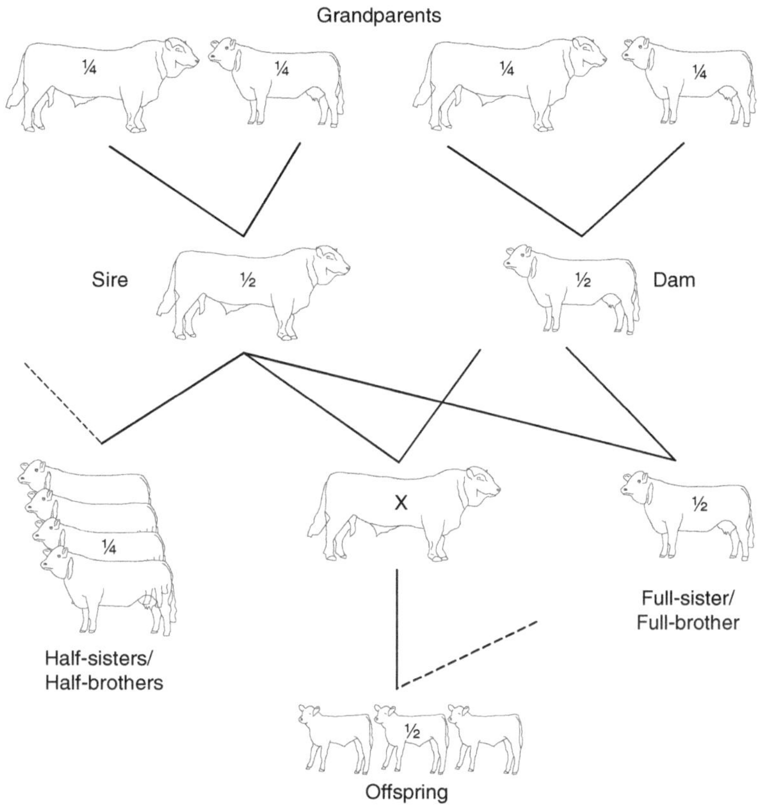

Fig. 4.6. The proportion of genes in common between the bull marked X, and various classes of relatives. Parents and offspring have exactly half their genes in common. The proportions of genes in common between other classes of relatives are expected average proportions. (After Wray and Simm, 1991.)

abbreviation for the additive genetic standard deviation, or *standard deviation of true breeding values*.

This formula still refers to the special case when selection is on the animal's own performance. There is a more general version in which **h** is substituted by **r**, which is the accuracy of selection on any combination of records from the animal and its relatives:

$$R = \frac{i \times r \times sd_A}{L}$$

As mentioned in Chapter 2, the symbol r is usually used to denote a correlation. In this case the accuracy is the correlation between animals' true breeding values for the trait(s) under selection, and the measurement(s) on which selection is based.

Accuracy of selection

The accuracy of selection itself depends mainly on three things: (i) the heritability of the trait concerned – the higher the heritability, the higher the accuracy; (ii) the source of information on which selection is based, e.g. the class of relative – the closer the relatives on whose records selection is based, the higher the accuracy of selection; and (iii) the amount of information available from relatives – the more relatives of a given class recorded (and the more often they are recorded, if the trait can be measured repeatedly), the higher the accuracy, although there are diminishing returns as the numbers of relatives increase. Table 4.6 shows the relationship between accuracy and the square root of the heritability, for different classes of relatives, assuming that selection is based on a single record of performance from that type of relative. To predict response to selection on such a record, we simply use the appropriate value of r in the formula above. So, for example, if selection is on a single record on the animal itself, the accuracy of selection is equal to the square root of the heritability of the trait concerned (r = h). To continue an example used earlier, the heritability of weaning weight in beef cattle is about 0.25, so its square root, h, is 0.5. Hence the accuracy of selection for weaning weight, when selection is based on a single record of the animal's own performance, is 0.5, or 50%. If selection is based on a single measurement from one parent, or one offspring, then the accuracy is only half that when selection is based on a record on the animal itself. In the beef cattle example, selection on a single parent or offspring record would give an accuracy of 0.25 or 25%.

Table 4.6 shows that the accuracy of selection on a single record of performance for different types of relative is directly related to the proportion of genes they have in common. This is a very important principle in objective animal breeding. In subjective selection, it is easy to overplay the importance of a particular favourite ancestor, or other relative, in making selection decisions (e.g. if it has won prizes in major shows or was sold for a very high price). In objective selection, the aim is to give each performance record from a relative its proper emphasis, and this emphasis depends on the expected proportion of genes in common between the relative and the candidate for selection.

Table 4.6. The accuracy of selection on a single record of performance on the candidate animal itself, or on a single record from a relative. Accuracies are presented as proportions of h, the square root of the heritability of the trait under selection. So, for example, if $h^2 = 0.25$, h = 0.5, the accuracy of selection on the animal's own performance is 0.5, the accuracy of selection on one parent's record, or one full sib's record, or one progeny's record is 0.25 (½ × 0.5 = 0.25), the accuracy of selection on one grandparent's record, or one half sib's record, is 0.125 (¼ × 0.5 = 0.125), and so on. (After Nicholas, 1987.)

Single measurement of performance on:	Accuracy (r)
Animal itself	h
One parent	½ h
One grandparent	¼ h
One great-grandparent	⅛ h
An identical twin	h
One full sib	½ h
One half sib	¼ h
One progeny	½ h

Calculating the accuracy of selection with records from greater numbers of relatives is slightly more complicated, although the results are easy to understand. Figure 4.7 shows the accuracy of selection on records from varying numbers of half or full sibs and progeny.

These graphs illustrate that:

- The closer the relative, the more valuable the record. For example, a single record from an offspring is twice as valuable as a single record from a half sib, other things being equal (i.e. the accuracy of selection is twice as high).
- As the number of progeny increases, the accuracy of selection tends towards 1. As the number of full sibs increases, the accuracy tends towards 0.7. With half sibs, the accuracy tends towards 0.5 as numbers increase.
- A single record from a full sib is of equal value to a single progeny record, but thereafter records from progeny are more valuable in terms of increasing the accuracy of selection.
- Initially, the more relatives of a given class, the higher the accuracy, although there are diminishing returns.
- Initially, the higher the heritability, the higher the accuracy.
- Initially, the lower the heritability, the greater the proportional contribution which records from relatives make (e.g. compared to the accuracy of selection on a single record on the animal itself, selection on records from 50 progeny increases the accuracy of selection by a factor of about 5 when the heritability is 0.1, but only by a factor of about 1.6 when the heritability is 0.3).

Additive genetic standard deviation

The value of the additive genetic standard deviation or standard deviation of breeding values can be derived from the heritability of the trait concerned, and its phenotypic standard deviation. We have already seen that:

$$\text{Heritability}\left(h^2\right) = \frac{VAR_A}{VAR_P}$$

Standard deviations are the square root of variances, and so we can take the square root of all terms in this equation to get:

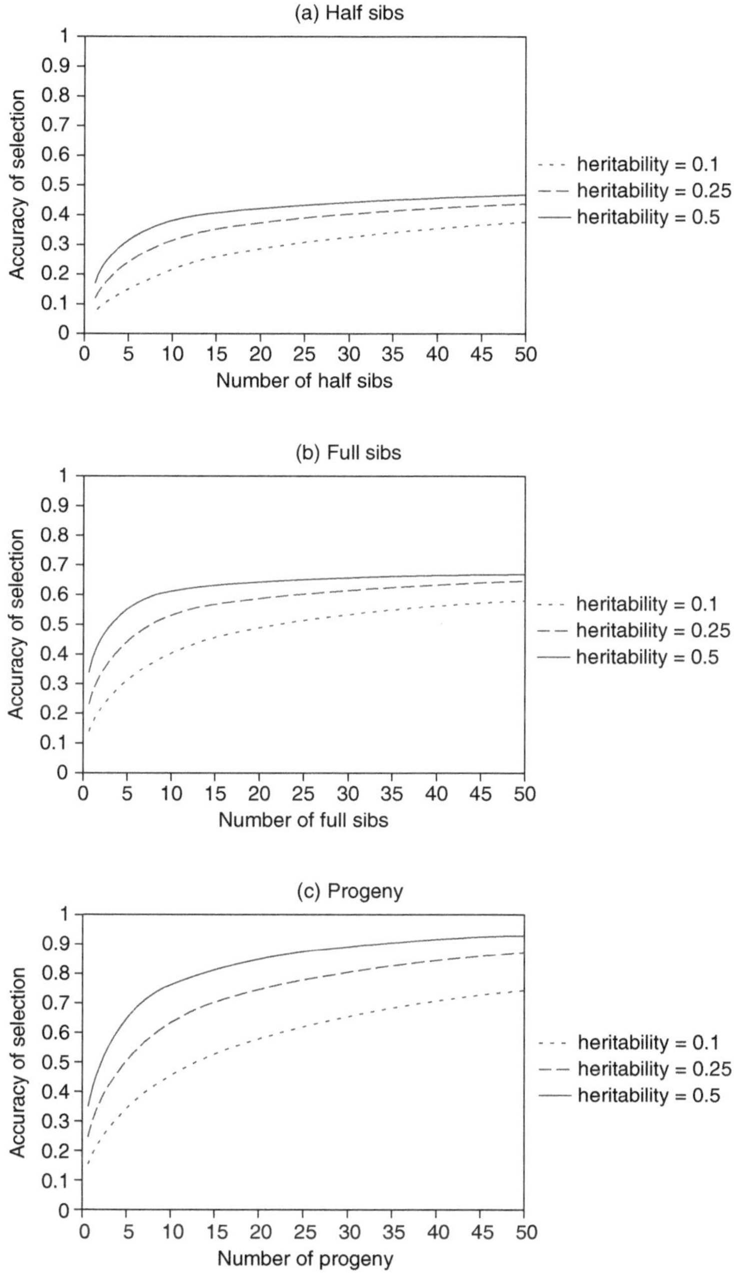

Fig. 4.7. The accuracy of selection on performance records from relatives with varying numbers of records, and traits of different heritability. In graph (a) the records are from half sibs, in graph (b) they are from full sibs, and in graph (c) they are from progeny. (After Nicholas, 1987.)

$$h = \frac{sd_A}{sd_P}$$

We can re-arrange the terms in this equation (by multiplying both sides by sd_P, then cancelling out the two sd_Ps which appear on the right-hand side of the equation) to give:

$$sd_A = h \times sd_P$$

So, the additive genetic standard deviation is simply the phenotypic standard deviation multiplied by the square root of the heritability.

A practical example

Although using records of performance from relatives can increase the accuracy of selection, it is important to recognize that this benefit can be outweighed by increases in the generation interval. For example, if we want to select for increased 400-day weight in a 120-cow herd of beef cattle, we might consider two main options, performance testing and progeny testing. For simplicity, let us assume that selection is based on males only, and that all available replacement females enter the herd, giving a female generation interval of 3.85 years and a female selection intensity of 0. Also, let us assume that progeny testing takes place in several separate crossbred herds. In each case, if we select 5 males from a total of 50 which are either performance recorded in the pure herd, or progeny tested in the crossbred herds, then the selection intensity among males is 1.705. The average selection intensity is then 0.8525 ([1.705 + 0]/2).

The heritability of 400-day weight is about 0.4, so if we select bulls on their own performance alone, the accuracy of selection is about 0.632 (the square root of the heritability). Subject to them reaching sexual maturity, we should be able to mate bulls at about 15 months of age, giving a male generation interval of 2 years. This means that in the herd using performance testing the average generation interval is 2.925 years ([3.85 + 2]/2). If we select bulls on the records from 20 progeny, the accuracy is higher – about 0.830 – but the crossbred progeny do not reach 400 days of age until the bulls are over 3 years old. So, the minimum male generation interval possible in the purebred herd is approaching 4 years (it is safest to assume 4 years exactly if we want to maintain a seasonal pattern of calving). This means that in the herd using progeny testing the average generation interval is 3.925 years ([3.85 + 4]/2).

To predict annual response to selection in the two schemes, we also need to know the additive genetic standard deviation of 400-day weight. This is about 28.4 kg for the larger beef breeds. (This is calculated from the phenotypic standard deviation of 400-day weight (about 45 kg) multiplied by the square root of the heritability of 400-day weight (square root of 0.4 = 0.632); so 45 × 0.632 = 28.4 kg. Table 4.7 summarizes the characteristics of the two breeding schemes.

The predicted annual response to selection can then be calculated from these characteristics, using the formula introduced in the last section. This is illustrated below for the scheme based on performance testing:

$$i = 0.8525$$

$$r = 0.632$$

$$sd_A = 28.4\,kg$$

$$L = 2.925$$

and so:

$$R = \frac{0.8525 \times 0.632 \times 28.4}{2.925}$$

$$R = 5.23\,kg\ \textit{per annum}\ (\text{approx.}).$$

The equivalent response for the scheme based on progeny testing is 5.12 kg *per annum*. In this example, the

Table 4.7. Characteristics of the two beef cattle breeding schemes described in the text – one based on performance testing, the other on progeny testing. In both cases selection is to increase 400-day weight.

	Performance testing	Progeny testing
Average selection intensity (i)	0.8525	0.8525
Approx. accuracy of selection (r)	0.632	0.830
Additive genetic standard deviation (sd_A in kg)	28.4	28.4
Average generation interval (L in years)	2.925	3.925
Predicted response (kg *per annum*, approx.)	5.23	5.12

gains in accuracy from progeny testing are outweighed by the longer generation interval among males which is necessary to obtain records of performance on progeny. However, with a lower heritability, or more progeny records, the reverse could be true. So, it pays to check the expected responses from different types of selection, using the relevant values for the heritability and number of relatives to derive the accuracy, before embarking on selection. Usually records from ancestors and at least some sibs (or other *collateral relatives* – those from the same generation as the animal itself) can be used to increase accuracy of selection without lengthening the generation interval. Using records from descendants usually increases the generation interval, and so there is a trade-off between increasing accuracy and increasing generation interval. The methods of combining information from different types of relative are discussed in later sections. As we will see later, genomic information is revolutionizing animal breeding, by increasing the accuracy of selection with the same, or shorter, generation intervals.

Comparisons of different breeding schemes also need to consider the resources needed, as well as predicted responses. Even when it appears justified by higher predicted responses, it would be very expensive to maintain crossbred herds solely for progeny testing. In some cases, equivalent responses could be achieved at lower cost from performance testing, by expanding the purebred herd to increase selection intensity. Also, in most cases it would be quite wasteful to progeny test all available bulls. If the number tested is reduced arbitrarily, then this will lead to lower selection intensity than that possible from performance testing. In practice, it makes sense to use all available information in selection – in the example above it would have been more efficient to progeny test only those bulls which themselves had high 400-day weight (a process called two-stage selection). Also, records from half sibs are generated as a by-product of most performance testing schemes, so these can often increase accuracy at no extra cost in money or time. (See Weller (1994) for methods of comparing the cost-effectiveness of different breeding schemes.)

Using repeated records of performance

So far, we have considered only single records of performance on candidates for selection, or their relatives. However, many traits of interest can be measured more than once over an animal's lifetime. For example, growing meat animals can be weighed on several occasions, most dairy cows have about four lactations during their lifetime, breeding pigs usually have multiple litters of piglets during their lifetime, most beef cows would wean six or seven calves during their lifetime, and sheep would have four or five litters during their lifetime and be shorn annually for four or five years.

Often there are very strong genetic associations between performance at different stages in an animal's life. In these cases, it is safe to assume that performance at these different stages is being influenced by the same genes. Hence, repeated records of performance can give additional clues to the breeding value of animals and enhance the accuracy of selection. If repeated measurements are influenced by exactly the same genes, then any differences in performance from contemporaries, for example in yield in different lactations, is due to differences in the environment or management experienced by the animal. We have already seen that the performance of an animal can be split into genetic and environmental components (after Falconer and Mackay, 1996):

$$\text{Phenotype}\,(P) = \text{Genotype}\,(G) + \text{Environment}\,(E)$$

Splitting the genetic part down further into additive genetic merit (breeding value), plus non-additive genetic effects, as explained in Chapter 2, gives:

$$\begin{aligned}\text{Phenotype}\,(P) = {} & \text{Additive genetic}\,(A) + \\ & \text{Non-additive genetic}\,(NA) + \\ & \text{Environment}\,(E)\end{aligned}$$

However, the environmental component of performance can also be split further into permanent (E_p) and temporary (E_t) environmental effects. This gives:

$$P = A + NA + E_p + E_t$$

Like the genes, *permanent environmental effects* stay with the animal for life but, unlike the genes, they do not get passed on to offspring. *Temporary environmental effects* have a much shorter impact, for example affecting only one lactation or one weight record. If a dairy heifer suffered a severe mastitis infection in one-quarter of her udder, and as a result of damage to the secretory tissue in that quarter, never produced milk from it again, that would be a permanent environmental effect. Yield in the other quarters may rise slightly to compensate, but the animal would produce less milk in total in each successive lactation, than if it had not been affected by mastitis. In a single lactation, the yield of the same animal may be temporarily depressed because it happened to be housed in a group of cows which was fed very poor-quality silage. However, when the animal was fed on better silage in subsequent lactations, this effect would disappear. So, this would be classified as a temporary environmental effect.

The value of repeated records in selection depends on a measure called the *repeatability*. This is the correlation between repeated records from the same animal. It is defined as the proportion of the total phenotypic variation which is explained by the combined effects of the genes and the permanent environmental variation (after Falconer and Mackay, 1996):

$$\text{Repeatability} = \frac{\text{VAR}_{\text{G}} + \text{VAR}_{\text{Ep}}}{\text{VAR}_{\text{P}}}$$

or, in full:

$$\text{Repeatability} = \frac{\text{VAR}_{\text{A}} + \text{VAR}_{\text{NA}} + \text{VAR}_{\text{E}_{\text{P}}}}{\text{VAR}_{\text{P}}}$$

This looks similar to the equation used earlier to calculate the heritability, except that there are a few extra terms on the top of the equation. The heritability is concerned only with the 'predictable' additive genetic part of the equation, whereas the repeatability also includes the variation due to non-additive genetic and permanent environmental effects, which are specific to individual animals, and hence difficult to predict. As a result, the repeatability sets an upper limit to the heritability. Like heritabilities, repeatabilities range from 0 to 1, or from 0 to 100%. Some examples of the repeatability of different traits are shown in Table 4.8.

It may seem counter-intuitive at first sight, but the higher the repeatability of a trait, the lower the value of repeated records in selection for that trait. In other words, if the repeatability is high, the first record of performance gives a good indication of the animal's genetic merit, and adding subsequent records only improves the accuracy slightly. If the repeatability is low, the first record of performance gives a poor indication of subsequent performance. Here, repeated records help to build up a more accurate estimate of the animal's genetic merit, but the law of diminishing returns applies. This is illustrated in Fig. 4.8, which shows the accuracy of selection for traits with different repeatability, depending on the number of repeated records available. As with the use of information from relatives, it is important to take into account any time lag in obtaining repeated records. In principle, the benefits of higher accuracy are often outweighed by the penalty from increases in generation interval. However, in practice, selection is usually based on a single record initially, with subsequent records being used to refine later estimates of genetic merit.

Repeatabilities measure the similarity between repeated records of the same trait, assuming that performance measured in different years (or at other intervals) is controlled by exactly the same genes. However, there are often associations between different traits which are not likely to be influenced by exactly the same genes. For instance,

Table 4.8. Estimates of the repeatabilities of some traits of economic importance in livestock.

Breed/species	Trait	Repeatability	Source
Dairy cattle	Milk yield	0.55	Animal Data Centre (1997)
	Days to first service	0.08	Hayes *et al.* (1992)
	Days open	0.10	Hayes *et al.* (1992)
	No. services per conception	0.07	Hayes *et al.* (1992)
Beef cattle	Cows calving per cow pregnant	0.06	Morris *et al.* (1993)
	Calves weaned per cow calving	0.05	Morris *et al.* (1993)
	Cow weight pre-mating	0.57	Morris *et al.* (1993)
	Calf weaning weight (age adjusted)	0.37	Morris *et al.* (1993)
Sheep	Greasy fleece weight	0.58	Fogarty (1995)
	Wool fibre diameter	0.70	Fogarty (1995)
	Ovulation rate across years	0.31	Fogarty (1995)
	No. lambs weaned per ewe mated	0.08	Fogarty (1995)
Chickens	Egg shell stiffness	0.41–0.59	Wolc *et al.* (2017)
Pigs	Prenatal survival of piglets	0.19–0.23	Blasco *et al.* (1998)

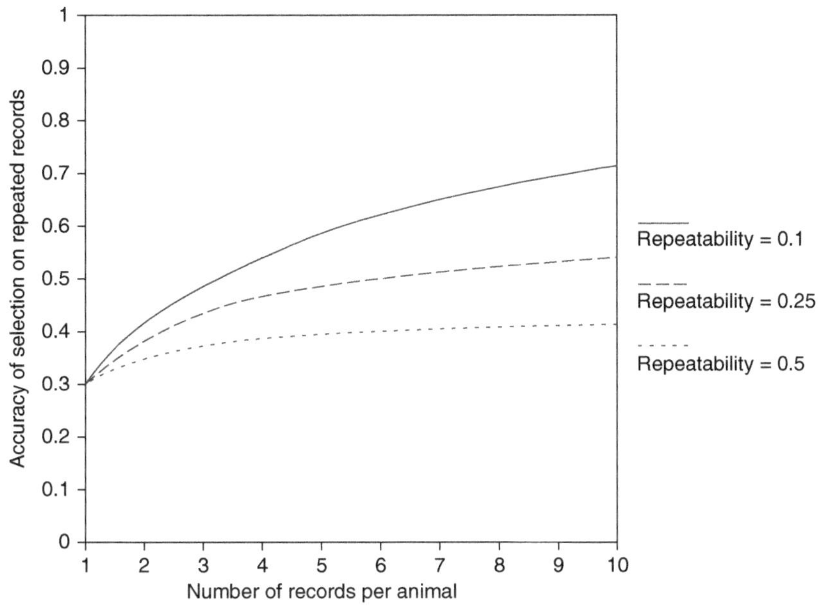

Fig. 4.8. The effect of different numbers of repeated records on the accuracy of selection, for traits with different repeatabilities. In this example the heritability of the trait is 0.1. (After Nicholas, 1987.)

animals that are heavier than their contemporaries at a given age tend to be fatter too; and higher yielding cows generally have lower milk protein percentage. Even when the same trait is measured at different times, different genes may influence the trait at different times. For example, animals which are heavier than average at an early age are often heavier at later ages, but not all the genes influencing early weight also influence mature weight. Similarly, heifers which have a high milk yield compared to contemporaries, often have comparatively high yields in later lactations, and *vice versa*, but not all the genes which influence early lactations also influence later lactations. The degree of association between different characteristics is measured by the correlation coefficient, as explained in Chapter 2.

Predicting correlated responses to selection

Before embarking on a selection programme, it is useful to predict what the consequences will be, not only in the trait under selection, but also in other associated traits. Providing that the heritabilities of the trait under selection and other traits of interest are known, their phenotypic variances (or standard deviations) are known, and the genetic correlation between them is known, the *correlated response* to selection can be predicted. It is easiest to think of this as a three-step procedure:

1. Calculate the predicted annual response in the trait under selection (trait X). If we want to predict correlated responses it is simplest if we first predict the direct response in the trait under selection *in additive genetic standard deviation units*, rather than units of measurement. If selection is based on a single record of the animal's own performance, this becomes:

$$R_X = \frac{i \times h_X}{L} \text{ (in additive genetic s.d. units of X } \textit{per annum}\text{)}$$

(Note that this formula is identical to the one presented earlier, except that the term sd_A is omitted, in order to express the response in additive genetic s.d. units, rather than units of measurement.)

2. Multiply the predicted annual response from (1) by the genetic correlation between the traits under selection and the second trait of interest (trait Y), to get the predicted correlated response in the second trait, *expressed in additive genetic standard deviation units*:

$CR_Y = R_X \times r_{AXY}$ (in additive genetic s.d. units of Y *per annum*)

3. Multiply the predicted correlated response in standard deviation units from (2) by the additive genetic standard deviation of the second trait (sd_{AY}) to express the predicted correlated response *in the units of measurement per annum*:

$CR_Y = R_X \times r_{AXY} \times sd_{AY}$ (in units of measurement *per annum*)

Writing this out in full gives (after Falconer and Mackay, 1996):

$$CR_Y = \frac{i \times h_X \times r_{AXY} \times sd_{AY}}{L}$$

To extend an example used before, if we select for 20-week weight in sheep, we expect an increase in fat depth as a result of a positive genetic correlation between these two traits. We can predict the direct response in weight (in units of measurement) from one of the formulae presented earlier in this chapter, and the correlated response in fat depth using the formula above. If we assume that:

$$i = 1.4$$

$$h^2_X = 0.3$$

$$h_X = 0.55$$

$$h^2_Y = 0.3$$

$$h_Y = 0.55$$

$$r_A = 0.4$$

$$sd_{AX} = 2.75$$

$$sd_{AY} = 0.715$$

$$L = 2.0$$

then the predicted response in 20-week weight is:

$$R_X = \frac{i \times h_X \times sd_{AX}}{L} \quad \text{(in kg } \textit{per annum}\text{)}$$

$$R_X = \frac{1.4 \times 0.55 \times 2.75}{2.0}$$

$$R_X = 1.06\,\text{kg} \quad \textit{per annum}\,\text{(approx.)}$$

and the correlated response in fat depth is:

$$CR_Y = \frac{1.4 \times 0.55 \times 0.4 \times 0.715}{2.0}$$

$$CR_Y = 0.11\,\text{mm } \textit{per annum.}$$

Limitations of these predictions

Reduction in variation following selection

There are several limitations to the methods of predicting response described above which need to be mentioned. The first concerns the amount of variation in the trait under selection. Selection itself causes a reduction in the amount of genetic variation in the first few generations. In other words, choosing parents with performance at one end of the distribution results in a narrower distribution in the performance and breeding values of their offspring. The reduction in variation depends on the heritability of the trait concerned and the intensity of selection. The higher the heritability, and the higher the selection intensity, the greater the reduction in variation from one generation to the next. As a result of this, predictions of long-term responses to selection based on the initial variation in the population may be too high. For example, with intense selection for a trait with a high heritability, there may be a loss of about 20% in response to the second generation of selection, compared to that obtained in the first generation (Falconer and Mackay, 1996). This reduction in genetic variation happens in the first few generations of selection, and then the amount of variation stabilizes, or approaches equilibrium. Typically, the loss in response to selection compared to that in the initial generation, stabilizes at about 25%. There are two ways to deal with this problem. The first is to re-estimate the amount of variation and the heritability after the first few generations of selection, and then re-calculate predicted responses from these equilibrium values. The second, which is less costly, is to use more complex formulae to predict long-term response to selection, which account for the fact that heritability and genetic variation were estimated from populations in which selection had not been practised (Dekkers, 1992; Villanueva *et al.*, 1993).

Selection limits

After many generations of selection, the variation in the trait of interest may become exhausted – for example, if each animal in the population has copies of only those alleles that have a favourable effect on performance. As a result, no further response to selection can be achieved. While these *selection limits* or *plateaux* have been reached in some selection experiments with fruit flies and other laboratory species, they are rarely of practical concern in farm animals (see Simm *et al.* (2004) for a review). This is because they occur after many generations of selection, which implies many decades of selection for the same trait in farm livestock. Over this time span it is unusual for market requirements to remain the same, and so it is unlikely that selection is for exactly the same animal characteristics. Also, livestock populations are rarely closed over this length of time – the introduction of new animals introduces new variation and hence delays the approach to the selection limit. Even in a closed population, with selection for the same trait, new mutations prolong the period over which responses to selection are achieved. So, in theory, predictions of response do not hold true indefinitely. But, in practice, they are usually satisfactory over the lifetime of a particular breeding programme.

Variation in response

The final limitation which needs to be mentioned concerns the variation in response that may be achieved in different selection programmes. The formulae presented earlier predict the average response to selection. However, if several identical breeding programmes were started at the same time, they would not achieve identical responses. Some schemes would achieve lower responses than predicted, others would achieve higher responses, but on average the response should match that predicted. It is usually too expensive to demonstrate this variation in response by running identical experimental breeding programmes in farm livestock, but there are many good examples of this in laboratory animal selection experiments. However, for fairly simple breeding programmes, it is possible to predict the variation in response.

The variation in the response achieved occurs because there is an element of chance as to which genes are present in the initial group of animals. There is also an element of chance in which genes are lost and which ones are retained each time parents are selected. (These elements of chance are fundamental to the study of genetic improvement of livestock and help to make it such a fascinating subject for scientists and practical breeders alike.) The main factors affecting the variation in response from that predicted are: (i) the size of the population – the smaller the population, the greater the risk of a difference between predicted and achieved responses; and (ii) the number of parents selected each generation – the smaller the number of parents selected, particularly males as there are usually fewer of these needed in the first place, the greater the risk of a difference between predicted and achieved responses.

Controlling Inbreeding

As explained earlier, inbreeding is the mating of two related animals. Sometimes breeders pursue a deliberate policy of mating related animals, with the aim of increasing the frequency of favourable genes. However, even when steps are taken to avoid it, inbreeding is inevitable in closed populations. Sooner or later, matings will occur between related animals. In smaller populations this will tend to occur sooner, and in larger populations it will tend to occur later. The chances of related animals mating are increased when selection is practised in a closed population. This is because related animals have genes in common and hence their performance and breeding values are more alike than those of unrelated animals. As a result, selection for a particular characteristic increases the frequency of matings between related animals and hence increases inbreeding compared to that in a random mating population.

There are two main reasons for wishing to limit inbreeding. The first is that inbreeding reduces the amount of genetic variation in a population, and so can reduce response to selection (and increase variation in response to selection). The second is that inbreeding can lead to a decline in performance in traits associated with fitness, such as reproductive rate and disease resistance. This decline in performance is known as *inbreeding depression*. Table 4.9 gives some examples of inbreeding depression in a range of characteristics in farm livestock. Inbreeding depression is thought to be the result of an increase in the frequency of recessive genes which adversely affect those characters

Table 4.9. Examples of inbreeding depression in traits of economic importance.

Animals	Breed	Trait	Inbreeding depression expressed as change in trait per 1% increase in inbreeding	Source
Dairy cattle	Holstein	Milk yield	–25 kg (–0.37%)[a]	Miglior *et al.* (1995b)
		Fat yield	–0.9 kg (–0.35%)	Miglior *et al.* (1995b)
		Protein yield	–0.8 kg (–0.36%)	Miglior *et al.* (1995b)
		Fat %	+0.05% (+1.32%)	Miglior *et al.* (1995b)
		Protein %	+0.05% (+1.55%)	Miglior *et al.* (1995b)
		Somatic cell score	+0.012 (+0.51%)	Miglior *et al.* (1995a)
Beef cattle	Hereford	Pregnancy rate (2 y.o. cows)	–0.23% (–0.33%)[b]	MacNeil *et al.* (1989)
		Prenatal survival (2 y.o.)	–1.67% (–1.73%)	MacNeil *et al.* (1989)
		Weaning rate (2 y.o.)	–1.24% (2.26%)	MacNeil *et al.* (1989)
		Weaning weight (as trait of cow; all ages)	–0.47 kg (0.24%)	MacNeil *et al.* (1989)
Sheep	S. Blackface, Cheviot, W. Mountain	Gross lifetime income per ewe	–£1.27 (1.16%)[b]	Wiener *et al.* (1994a)
		Greasy fleece weight	–0.01 kg (0.53%)	Wiener *et al.* (1994b)
	Many breeds	Greasy fleece weight	–0.017 kg	Lamberson and Thomas (1984)
		Weaning weight	–0.111 kg	Lamberson and Thomas (1984)
		Ewe fertility (ewes lambing/ewe joined)	–0.014	Lamberson and Thomas (1984)
		Lamb survival (lambs weaned/lambs born)	–0.028[c] / –0.012[d]	Lamberson and Thomas (1984)
Pigs	Iberian (Guadyerbas strain)	Total number piglets born	–0.012 to –0.023	Saura *et al.* (2015)
		Total number piglets born alive	–0.012 to –0.023	Saura *et al.* (2015)
Chickens	White Leghorn (lines selected for egg number, weight or mass)	Age at first egg	+0.83 to +1.08%	Sewalem *et al.* (1999)
		Egg number at 63 weeks	–1.67 to –2.75%	Sewalem *et al.* (1999)
		Egg weight at 63 weeks	0 to –0.94%	Sewalem *et al.* (1999)

[a] All figures in brackets express inbreeding depression as a percentage of the mean of the trait concerned when the mean was presented;
[b] figures in brackets express inbreeding depression as a percentage of the mean performance of crosses between inbred and control lines;
[c] per 1% increase in inbreeding of lamb;
[d] per 1% increase in inbreeding of dam.

associated with survival and overall 'fitness'. These are generally the same sort of traits which show heterosis as a result of crossbreeding. So, it is helpful to think of inbreeding and inbreeding depression as being the opposite of crossbreeding and heterosis, respectively.

The decline in genetic variation following inbreeding, and the amount of inbreeding depression, both depend on the amount of inbreeding. The closer the relationship between two animals which are mated, the greater the amount of inbreeding in the resulting offspring. Hence, it is important to be able to measure the amount of inbreeding of existing animals, as well as the animals which could be produced from a particular future mating. It is also important to be able to predict the rate at which inbreeding will accumulate over time in a herd, flock or breed involved in a particular breeding programme.

The amount of inbreeding is measured by the *inbreeding coefficient* (abbreviated F). The inbreeding coefficient is formally defined as the probability that two alleles at any locus are *identical by descent*. This is not as complicated as it sounds. Consider two calves, both of which inherit two genes for black coat colour (BB). The first calf is the result of a mating between an unrelated bull and cow. It has two alleles which are *identical by state* (i.e. they are both B alleles, and they have the same effect, but they originated in unrelated ancestors). The second calf is the result of a mating between two heterozygous black half sibs (Bb). The pedigree of the second calf is shown in Fig. 4.9. In this example the bull and cow that are mated are paternal half sibs, i.e. they have the same sire (the calf's grandsire). If this is a heterozygous black bull (Bb), and the calf's granddams are both homozygous red cows (bb), then the calf must have obtained both copies of his B allele from the common grandsire. In this case the two B alleles are identical by descent, i.e. they are copies of a single allele in a common ancestor. The inheritance of segments of chromosome that are identical by descent (IBD) is illustrated in Fig. 4.10.

Figure 4.11 shows an abbreviated version of a pedigree of an animal which is the result of a mating between two half sibs (such as the calf in the previous example). The inbreeding coefficient of the animal at the bottom of the pedigree (animal D) can be calculated from pedigrees like this by counting the number of individuals in each path through the pedigree which leads from the animal whose inbreeding coefficient is being calculated, through a common ancestor and back to the original animal. This is easiest to follow by referring to Fig. 4.11. If we start with animal D, we can trace a path through B to the common ancestor A and back through C to D again. In other words, there are three animals in the common path excluding D itself – these are B, A and C. If there is more than one common ancestor, then this process is repeated for each one. The inbreeding coefficient can be calculated from the formula (after Lush, 1945):

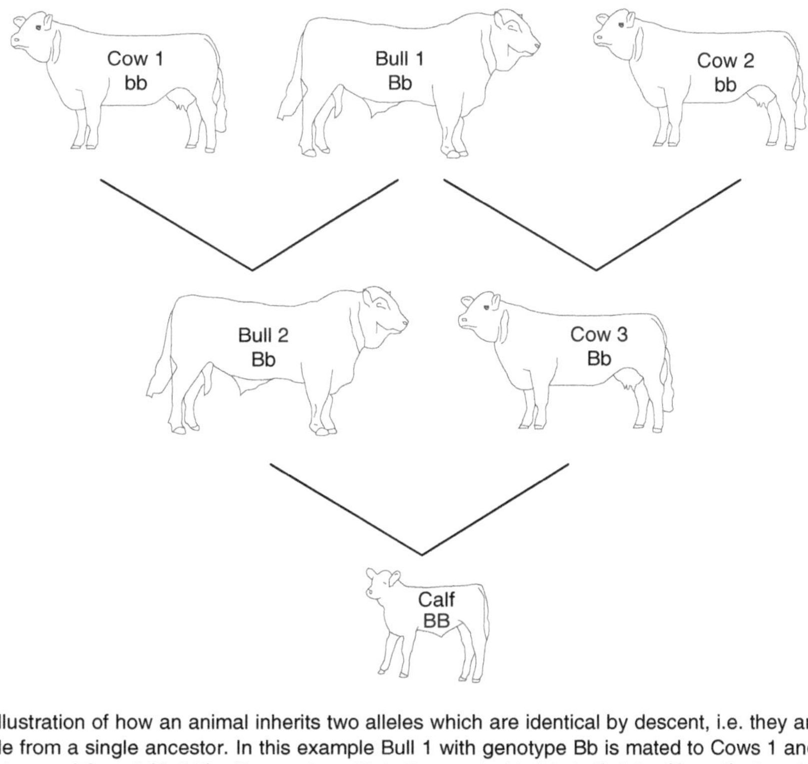

Fig. 4.9. An illustration of how an animal inherits two alleles which are identical by descent, i.e. they are copies of the same allele from a single ancestor. In this example Bull 1 with genotype Bb is mated to Cows 1 and 2, both with genotype bb. A son of Cow 1 (Bull 2) with genotype Bb is then mated to his half-sister (Cow 3) also of genotype Bb. The resulting calf has the genotype BB. This calf must have inherited both copies of the B allele from Bull 1, as this bull is the only animal in the grandparent generation to carry a copy of this allele.

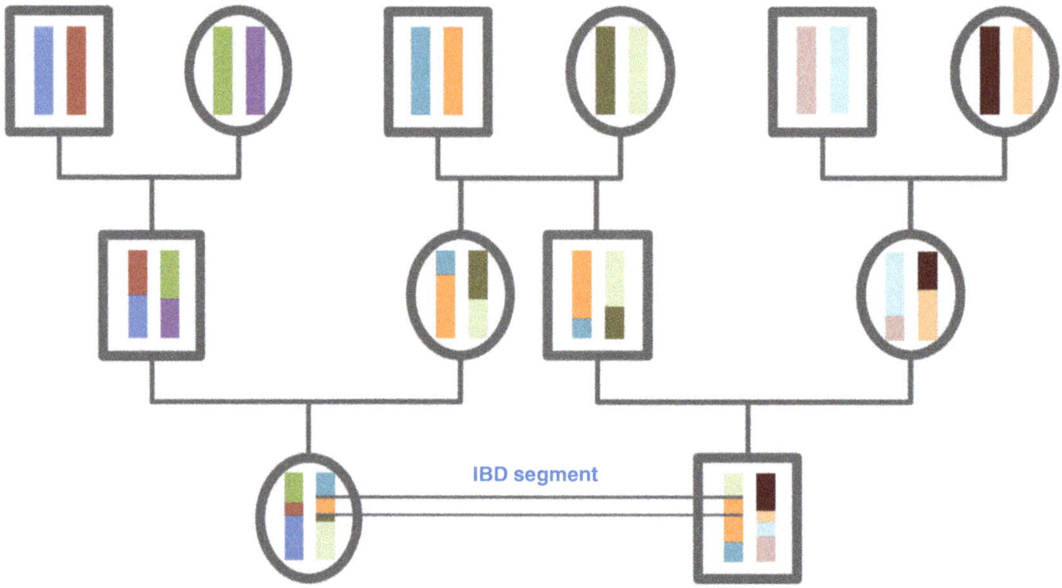

Fig. 4.10. The inheritance of segments of chromosome that are identical by descent (IBD). (Available at: https://commons.wikimedia.org/wiki/File:Pedigree,_recombination_and_resulting_IBD_segments,_schematic_representation.png, by Gklambauer, CC-BY-SA 3.0, accessed 8 December 2019.)

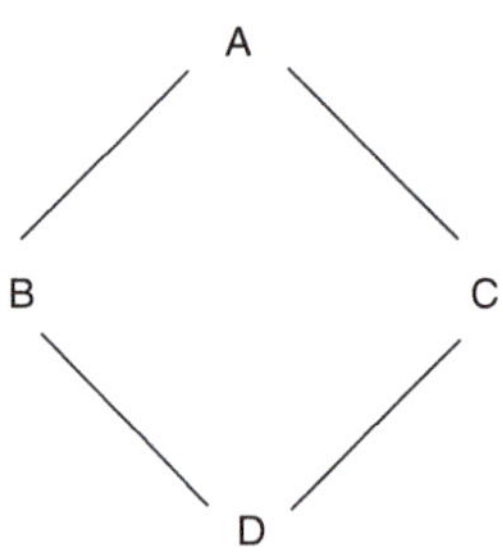

Fig. 4.11. An abbreviated and more general version of the pedigree shown in Fig. 4.9, where two half sibs are mated together. Animal A is the common ancestor, i.e. the father of both animals B and C if they are paternal half sibs, or their mother if they are maternal half sibs. Animals B and C are of opposite sex and they are mated to produce animal D.

$$F_D = \Sigma(½)^n (1 + F_A)$$

where:

the symbol Σ indicates that the results are summed for each path through a common ancestor;

n is the number of individuals in each path (the ½ appears in the formula to account for the fact that only 50% of sperm or eggs get a copy of the allele being traced from the common ancestor; the other 50% will get a copy of an allele from other unrelated ancestors). The formula shows ½ 'raised to the power of n' – so if n = 2, the ½ is squared (½ × ½), if n = 3, the ½ is cubed (½ × ½ × ½), and so on;

F_D is the inbreeding coefficient of animal D; and

F_A is the inbreeding coefficient of animal A.

If the inbreeding coefficient of animal A is unknown, then it is assumed to be 0, and the formula simplifies to:

$$F_D = \Sigma(½)^n$$

So, in the example above where there is only a single common ancestor, and three individuals in the path, the inbreeding coefficient of animal D is calculated from:

$$F_D = (½)^3$$

$$F_D = 0.125 \text{ or } 12.5\%.$$

In other words, there is a 12.5% chance that the two alleles at any locus are IBD in an animal which results from a mating between half sibs. This example also illustrates the fact that, generally, the inbreeding coefficient of an animal is one-half of the additive relationship between its parents. In this case the parents were half sibs, which are expected to have 25% of their genes in common, so they are said to have an additive relationship of 25%. So, when half sibs are mated to each other we expect their offspring to have inbreeding coefficients of 12.5%. Table 4.10 shows pedigrees and inbreeding coefficients for some other types of mating between close relatives.

If pedigrees could be traced back far enough, then all animals in a species would be related to

Table 4.10. Calculating the inbreeding coefficient for animals resulting from matings between different types of close relative. In each case it is assumed that the common ancestor is not inbred itself, so the simpler version of the formula is used.

Type of mating	Number of individuals in pathway through common ancestor	Inbreeding coefficient (F)
Father - daughter 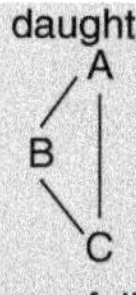	2 (B, A)	$F_C = (½)^2$ $F_C = 0.25$ or 25%
Full bother - full sister 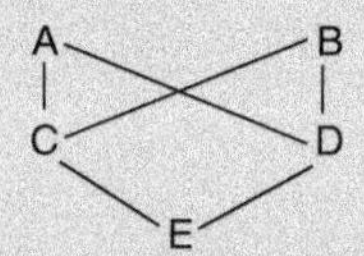	3 (C, A, D) + 3 (C, B, D)	$F_E = (½)^3 + (½)^3$ $F_E = 0.125 + 0.125$ $F_E = 0.25$ or 25%
Half-brother – half-sister 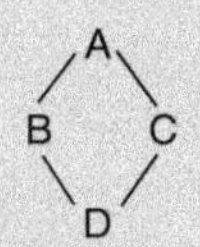	3 (B, A, C)	$F_D = (½)^3$ $F_D = 0.125$ or 12.5%
Full cousins 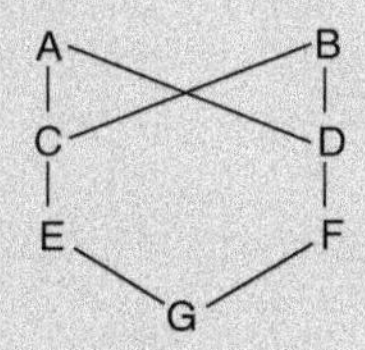	5 (E, C, A, D, F) + 5 (E, C, B, D, F)	$F_G = (½)^5 + (½)^5$ $F_G = 0.03125 + 0.03125$ $F_G = 0.0625$ or 6.25%
Half uncle - niece 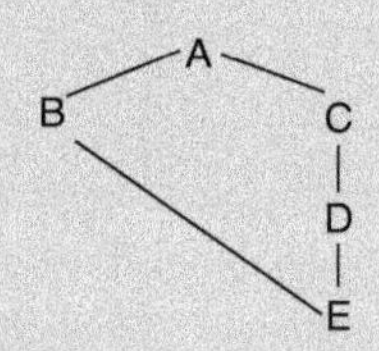	4 (B, A, C, D)	$F_E = (½)^4$ $F_E = 0.0625$ or 6.25%
Half cousins 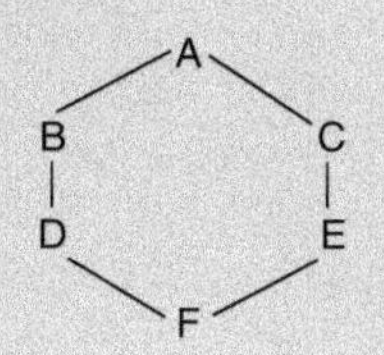	5 (D, B, A, C, E)	$F_F = (½)^5$ $F_F = 0.03125$ or 3.125%

each other, though the relationship would be very distant in most cases. It is not practical, or necessary, to go this far back in calculating inbreeding coefficients in livestock breeding, but it is important to define the reference population from which coefficients are calculated. For example, we might define the first generation of animals recorded in a herd or flock book, or animals born in some other significant year, as the initial reference population. Then, in calculating inbreeding coefficients, we assume that none of the animals in this initial population are inbred themselves. If the reference population chosen is too recent, or if there is a lot of missing information in pedigrees, then inbreeding coefficients may be severely underestimated.

Matings between close relatives are relatively uncommon in farmed animal breeding today, because of the recognition of the high risk of undesirable side effects from high levels of inbreeding. However, high levels of inbreeding can occur also as a result of matings between less closely related animals for several generations. It is important to recognize this in designing breeding programmes. In this case the average inbreeding coefficient across a herd, flock or breed, and the rate at which this changes, are useful measures. Inbreeding coefficients can be calculated for large numbers of animals by a number of methods which are more amenable to computer programming than the method outlined above (Meuwissen and Luo, 1992; Mrode, 2014).

It is also useful to be able to predict the rate of inbreeding in advance, for example when comparing alternative designs for a breeding programme. Although it is relatively easy to predict rates of inbreeding for unselected populations, it is very difficult to do so accurately for populations under selection. Similarly, it is easier to predict rates of inbreeding when family sizes are equal than when they are not. Many of the simpler formulae underpredict rates of inbreeding, and so can give misleading results. There are more accurate formulae; however, these are too complex to describe here. (See Caballero (1994) and Villanueva *et al.* (1996) for more information on this problem.) The formulae below are reasonably simple, and illustrate some important points about rates of inbreeding, but they should be used with caution because they depend on assumptions which are rarely met in livestock breeding (equal family sizes, no selection, discrete generations).

The rate of inbreeding (usually abbreviated to ΔF) *per generation* can be calculated from (after Lush, 1945):

$$\Delta\text{F per generation} = \frac{1}{8\text{M}} + \frac{1}{8\text{F}} \text{ (approx.)}$$

where:

M = the total number of males entering the population *each generation*; and

F = the total number of females entering the population *each generation*.

Since the number of females used is usually much larger than the number of males used in most livestock breeding programmes, it is the number of males that influences the rate of inbreeding most.

The rate of inbreeding *per annum* can be calculated from a modified version of this formula:

$$\Delta\text{F per annum} = \frac{1}{8\text{mL}^2} + \frac{1}{8\text{fL}^2} \text{ (approx.)}$$

where:

m = the total number of males entering the population *each year*;

f = the total number of females entering the population *each year*; and

L^2 = the average generation interval in years, squared (i.e. multiplied by itself).

So, for example, in a closed flock of 100 sheep with 5 different rams and 35 new females entering the flock each year, and an average generation interval of 2 years:

$$m = 5$$

$$f = 35$$

$$L = 2$$

$$L^2 = 4$$

and

$$\Delta F = \frac{1}{8\times5\times4} + \frac{1}{8\times35\times4} = \frac{1}{160} + \frac{1}{1120}$$

$$= 0.00625 + 0.00089$$

= approximately 0.007 *per annum*, or 0.7% *per annum* (of which 0.625% is due to males).

Table 4.11 shows the expected annual rates of inbreeding for several other breeding schemes, calculated using this formula. These results show that the number of parents selected *per annum*, and especially the number of sires selected, has a major impact on rates of inbreeding, as mentioned above. The values shown assume that selected animals are unrelated. However, in practice, related animals are often selected together because their breeding values are more alike than those of unrelated animals. This is particularly true when modern methods of predicting breeding values are used, which maximize the use of performance information from relatives. (These methods are explained in Chapter 7.) This co-selection of relatives increases the rate of inbreeding further. It is important in designing breeding programmes to achieve a balance between selecting fewer parents to achieve high selection intensities, which maximizes response, and using enough parents to keep inbreeding at acceptable levels. Traditionally, these two objectives have been pursued separately. However, the concept of optimizing genetic contributions of parents allows these goals to be pursued jointly (for a review, see Woolliams *et al.*, 2015). Statistical methods and software packages are available now to implement this approach (e.g. Wellmann, 2019).

The results in Table 4.11 also show that shorter generation intervals increase the annual rate of inbreeding. This explains why turning over generations slowly is a useful method of minimizing inbreeding in conservation programmes, as explained in Chapter 3. Although there is little hard evidence available, it is generally accepted that absolute levels of inbreeding below 10%, or annual rates of inbreeding below 1% are unlikely to result in serious inbreeding depression. There is evidence that achieving a given level of inbreeding quickly through close matings is likely to be more harmful than achieving the same level of inbreeding more slowly through successive matings between less closely related animals – possibly because faster inbreeding allows fewer opportunities for deleterious alleles to be removed by natural selection (e.g. Pekkala *et al.*, 2014).

Table 4.11. Predicted rates of inbreeding with different numbers of males and females selected. The generation intervals assumed are rounded versions of those shown in Table 4.5.

Number of males used *per annum*	Number of females used *per annum*	Predicted rate of inbreeding (% *per annum*)
1	35	3.21
5	25	0.53
5	35	0.71
5	75	1.01
10	35	0.40
20	35	0.25

Summary

- It is important to be able to predict response to selection, in order to compare alternative breeding programmes, and so choose those which will achieve a high response to selection in a cost-effective way.
- When animals are selected on a single measurement of their own performance in one trait, the response to selection (R) per generation can be predicted by multiplying the selection differential (S) achieved by the heritability (h^2) of the trait selected on. The selection differential is the difference between the mean performance of selected animals and the overall mean of the group of animals from which they were selected. The heritability is the proportion of superiority of parents in a trait (i.e. the proportion of the selection differential) which, on average, is passed on to offspring. Alternatively, it can be defined as the additive genetic variation in that trait (or the variation in breeding values), expressed as a proportion of the total phenotypic variation in that trait. Heritabilities are expressed as proportions from 0 to 1, or as percentages from 0 to 100%.
- The ability to predict response to selection is important in planning breeding programmes and comparing alternative schemes. It is usually more useful to predict responses *per annum* rather than per generation. To do this, we have to divide the response per generation by the generation interval (the weighted average age of parents when their offspring are born; L) in the flock or herd concerned:
- From properties of the normal distribution, if we know what proportion of animals are selected as parents, we can predict their superiority in standard deviation units. This is called the standardized selection differential or selection intensity (i).

- The annual response to selection will be highest when the selection intensity is high, the heritability is high, and the generation interval is low. There is little that breeders can do about the heritability of a trait – this is largely a biological characteristic of the trait concerned. Within biological limits, breeders can increase selection intensities and decrease generation intervals.
- Records of performance from relatives are useful in selection. This is because related animals have genes in common, and so the performance of relatives can provide clues to the genetic merit or breeding value of the candidates for selection. Records of performance are often used from the animal's ancestors, the animal itself, the animal's full or half sibs, the animal's progeny, other more distant relatives of the animal, or combinations of these classes of relatives.
- To predict the response to selection when using information from relatives, a more general version of the formula is used. This involves the accuracy of selection (r) on any combination of records from the animal and its relatives. The accuracy is the correlation between animals' true breeding values for the trait(s) under selection, and the measurement(s) on which selection is based.
- The accuracy of selection on a single record of performance from a relative is calculated as the product of the proportion of genes they have in common and the square root of the heritability of the trait under selection. With records from greater numbers of relatives, in general: (i) the closer the relative the more valuable the record, (ii) initially, the more relatives of a given class, the higher the accuracy, although there are diminishing returns, (iii) initially, the higher the heritability, the higher the accuracy, and (iv) initially, the lower the heritability, the greater the proportional contribution which records from relatives make.
- Using records of performance from relatives can increase the accuracy of selection, but this benefit can be outweighed by increases in the generation interval. Usually records from ancestors and collateral relatives can be used to increase accuracy of selection without lengthening the generation interval. Using records from descendants usually increases the generation interval, and so there is a trade-off between increasing accuracy and increasing generation interval. Comparisons of different breeding schemes also need to consider the resources required, as well as predicted responses.
- Many traits of interest can be measured more than once over an animal's lifetime. Repeated records of performance can give additional clues to the breeding value of animals and enhance the accuracy of selection. The value of repeated records in selection depends on the repeatability. This is the correlation between repeated records from the same animal.
- The repeatability sets an upper limit to the heritability. Like heritabilities, repeatabilities range from 0 to 1, or from 0 to 100%. The higher the repeatability of a trait, the lower the value of repeated records in selection for that trait. As with the use of information from relatives, it is important to take into account any time lag in obtaining repeated records.
- Repeatabilities measure the similarity between repeated records of the same trait, assuming that performance measured in different years (or at other intervals) is controlled by exactly the same genes. However, there are often associations between different traits which are not likely to be influenced by exactly the same genes. The degree of association between these characteristics is measured by the correlation coefficient.
- Correlated response to selection can be predicted from the direct response if the genetic correlation between the two traits and the additive genetic standard deviation of the second trait are known.
- There are several limitations to the methods of predicting response outlined. The first is that selection itself causes a reduction in the amount of genetic variation in the first few generations of selection, so predictions of long-term responses to selection based on the initial variation in the population may be too high. However, there are more complex formulae to predict long-term response to selection. The second limitation is that after many generations of selection the variation in the trait of interest may become exhausted. But, predictions of response are usually satisfactory over the lifetime of most livestock breeding programmes. The final limitation is that the formulae presented predict the average response to selection. Individual breeding programmes may achieve higher or lower responses than this, by chance.
- Inbreeding is the mating of two related animals. Even when steps are taken to avoid it, inbreeding

is inevitable in closed populations. There are two main reasons for wishing to limit inbreeding: (i) it reduces the amount of genetic variation in a population, and so can reduce response to selection; and (ii) it can lead to a decline in performance in traits associated with fitness, known as inbreeding depression. Effectively inbreeding and inbreeding depression are the opposite of crossbreeding and heterosis, respectively.

- The decline in genetic variation following inbreeding, and the amount of inbreeding depression, both depend on the amount of inbreeding. The closer the relationship between two animals which are mated, the greater the amount of inbreeding in the resulting offspring. Hence it is important to be able to measure the amount of inbreeding of existing animals, or the animals which could be produced from a particular mating. The amount of inbreeding is measured by the inbreeding coefficient (abbreviated F). The inbreeding coefficient is formally defined as the probability that two alleles at any locus are 'identical by descent'.
- The inbreeding coefficient of an animal can be calculated from its pedigree by counting the number of individuals in each path through a common ancestor and back to the original animal. If there is more than one common ancestor, then this process is repeated for each one.
- It is also useful to be able to predict the rate of inbreeding in advance, e.g. when comparing alternative designs for a breeding programme. Many of the simpler formulae underpredict rates of inbreeding. However, the more accurate formulae are complex. The rate of inbreeding (ΔF) *per generation* can be calculated approximately from the total number of males and females entering the population *each generation*. The rate of inbreeding *per annum* can be calculated approximately from the total number of males and females entering the population *each year*.
- The number of parents selected *per annum*, and especially the number of sires selected, has a major impact on rates of inbreeding. It is important in designing breeding programmes to achieve a balance between selecting fewer parents to achieve high selection intensities, which maximize response, and using enough parents to keep inbreeding at acceptable levels. The co-selection of relatives increases the rate of inbreeding further. Also, shorter generation intervals increase the annual rate of inbreeding. Absolute levels of inbreeding below 10%, or annual rates of inbreeding below 1% are unlikely to result in serious inbreeding depression.

Appendix: The Connection Between the Two Formulae Presented to Predict Response to Selection

The original formula presented early in this chapter is:

$$R = \frac{i \times sd_P \times h^2}{L}$$

This can be converted to the second, more general formula in several steps. Firstly, we can expand the heritability to become:

$$h^2 = \frac{sd_A \times sd_A}{sd_P \times sd_P}$$

Substituting this in the formula above, instead of $\mathbf{h^2}$ gives:

$$R = \frac{i \times sd_P \times sd_A \times sd_A}{L \times sd_P \times sd_P}$$

The $\mathbf{sd_P}$ on the top of the equation cancels out with one of the $\mathbf{sd_P}$ values on the bottom (i.e. both can be removed, to simplify the formula). Also, one of the $\mathbf{sd_A}$ values on the top of the equation, and the remaining $\mathbf{sd_P}$ value on the bottom can be removed, and rewritten as **h**, giving (after Falconer and Mackay, 1996):

$$R = \frac{i \times h \times sd_A}{L}$$

This formula is appropriate if selection is on a single record of performance of the animal itself (i.e. r = h). For other types of selection **h** is replaced by **r**, the more general value of accuracy. If you do not follow the algebra involved in deriving these formulae, but want to prove that they really do mean the same thing, then re-calculate the response to selection for weaning weight in Simmental cattle, as in the earlier example, but using the new formula, with **h** = 0.5 (from $\mathbf{h^2}$ = 0.25) and $\mathbf{sd_A}$ = 17.5 kg (from **h** × $\mathbf{sd_P}$ = 35 × 0.5).

References

Animal Data Centre. (1997) *UK Statistics for Genetic Evaluations (Dairy)*. February 1997. ADC, Rickmansworth, UK.

Becker, W.A. (1984) *Manual of Quantitative Genetics,* 4th edn. Academic Enterprises, Pullman, Washington.

Blasco, A., Sorensen, D. and Bidanel, J.P. (1998) Bayesian inference of genetic parameters and selection response for litter size components in pigs. *Genetics* 149, 301–306.

Caballero, A. (1994) Developments in the prediction of effective population size. *Heredity* 73, 657–679.

Dekkers, J.C.M. (1992) Asymptotic response to selection on best linear unbiased predictors of breeding values. *Animal Production* 54, 351–360. DOI: 10.1017/S0003356100020808.

Falconer, D.S. and Mackay, T.F.C. (1996) *Introduction to Quantitative Genetics*, 4th edn. Longman, Harlow, UK.

Fogarty, N.M. (1995) Genetic parameters for live weight, fat and muscle measurements, wool production and reproduction in sheep: a review. *Animal Breeding Abstracts* 63, 101–143. (Also, see erratum in Volume 63, No. 12.)

Hayes, J.F., Cue, R.I. and Monardes, H.G. (1992) Estimates of repeatability of reproductive measures in Canadian Holsteins. *Journal of Dairy Science* 75, 1701–1706. DOI: 10.3168/jds.S0022-0302(92)77927-2.

Lamberson, W.R. and Thomas, D.L. (1984) Effects of inbreeding in sheep: a review. *Animal Breeding Abstracts* 52, 287–297.

Lush, J.L. (1945) *Animal Breeding Plans,* 3rd edn. Iowa State College Press, Ames, Iowa.

MacNeil, M.D., Dearborn, D.D., Cundiff, L.V., Dinkel, C.A. and Gregory, K.E. (1989) Effects of inbreeding and heterosis in Hereford females on fertility, calf survival and preweaning growth. *Journal of Animal Science* 67, 895–901.

Meuwissen, T.H.E and Luo, Z. (1992) Computing inbreeding coefficients in large populations. *Genetics, Selection and Evolution* 24, 305–313. DOI: 10.1186/297-9686-24-4-30.

Miglior, F., Burnside, E.B. and Dekkers, J.C.M. (1995a) Nonadditive genetic effects and inbreeding depression for somatic cell counts of Holstein cattle. *Journal of Dairy Science* 78, 1168–1173.

Miglior, F., Burnside, E.B. and Kennedy, B.W. (1995b) Production traits of Holstein cattle: estimation of nonadditive genetic variance components and inbreeding depression. *Journal of Dairy Science* 78, 1174–1180.

Morris, C.A., Baker, R.L., Hickey, S.M., Johnson, D.L., Cullen, N.G. and Wilson, J.A. (1993) Evidence of genotype by environment interaction for reproductive and maternal traits in beef cattle. *Animal Production* 56, 69–83. DOI: 10.1017/S0003356100006176.

Mrode, R.A. (2014) *Linear Models for the Prediction of Animal Breeding Values*, 3rd edn. CAB International, Wallingford, UK.

Nicholas, F.W. (1987) *Veterinary Genetics*. Oxford University Press, Oxford.

Pekkala, N., Knott, K.E., Kotiaho, J.S., Nissinen, K. and Puurtinen, M. (2014) The effect of inbreeding rate on fitness, inbreeding depression and heterosis over a range of inbreeding coefficients. *Evolutionary Applications* 7, 1107–1119. DOI: 10.1111/eva.12145.

Saura, M., Almudena Fernández, A., Varona, L., Fernández, A.I., de Cara, M.A.R. *et al.* (2015) Detecting inbreeding depression for reproductive traits in Iberian pigs using genome-wide data. *Genetics Selection Evolution* 47, 1–9. DOI: 10.1186/s12711-014-0081-5. hal-01341281.

Sewalem, A., Johansson. K., Wilhelmson, M. and Lillpers, K. (1999) Inbreeding and inbreeding depression on reproduction and production traits of White Leghorn lines selected for egg production traits. *British Poultry Science* 40, 203–208. DOI: 10.1080/00071668.2014.989490.

Simm, G., Bünger, L., Villanueva, B. and Hill, W.G. (2004) Limits to yield of farm species: genetic improvement of livestock. In: Sylvester-Bradley, R. and Wiseman, J. (eds) *Yields of Farmed Species. Constraints and Opportunities in the 21st Century*. Nottingham University Press, Nottingham, UK, pp. 123–141.

Villanueva, B., Wray, N.R. and Thompson, R. (1993) Prediction of asymptotic rates of response from selection on multiple traits using univariate and multivariate best linear unbiased predictors. *Animal Production* 57, 1–13. DOI: 10.1017/S0003356100006541.

Villanueva, B., Woolliams, J.A. and Gjerde, B. (1996) Optimum designs for breeding programmes under mass selection with an application in fish breeding. *Animal Science* 63, 563–576. DOI: 10.1017/S1357729800015459.

Weller, J.I. (1994) *Economic Aspects of Animal Breeding*. Chapman and Hall, London.

Wellmann, R. (2019) Optimum contribution selection for animal breeding and conservation: the R package optiSel. *BMC Bioinformatics,* 20, 25. DOI: 10.1186/s12859-018-2450-5.

Wiener, G., Lee, G.J. and Woolliams, J.A. (1994a) Consequences of inbreeding for financial returns from sheep. *Animal Production* 59, 245–249. DOI: 10.1017/S000335610000773X.

Wiener, G., Lee, G.J. and Woolliams, J.A. (1994b) Effects of breed, rapid inbreeding, crossbreeding and environmental factors on fleece weight and fleece shedding in sheep. *Animal Production* 59, 61–70. DOI: 10.1017/S0003356100007510.

Wolc, A., Arango, J., Settar, P., O'Sullivan, N.P. and Dekkers, J.C.M. (2017) Repeatability vs. multiple-trait models to evaluate shell dynamic stiffness for layer chickens. *Journal of Animal Science* 95, 9–15. DOI: 10.2527/jas.2016.0618.

Woolliams, J.A, Berg, P., Dagnachew, B.S. and Meuwissen, T.H.E. (2015) Genetic contributions and their optimization. *Journal of Animal Breeding and Genetics* 132, 89–99. DOI: 10.1111/jbg.12148.

Wray, N.R. and Simm, G. (1991) *BLUP for Pedigree Beef and Sheep Breeders*. SAC Technical Note T265. The Scottish Agricultural College, Perth, UK.

Recommended Reading

Becker, W.A. (1984) *Manual of Quantitative Genetics,* 4th edn. Academic Enterprises, Pullman, Washington.

Cameron, N.D. (1997) *Selection Indices and Prediction of Genetic Merit in Animal Breeding*. CAB International, Wallingford, UK.

Dickerson, G.E. and Hazel, L.N. (1944) Effectiveness of selection on progeny performance as a supplement to earlier culling of livestock. *Journal of Agricultural Research* 69, 459–476. Available at: https://naldc.nal.usda.gov/download/IND43969888/PDF (accessed 29 August 2020).

Falconer, D.S. and Mackay, T.F.C. (1996) *Introduction to Quantitative Genetics,* 4th edn. Longman, Harlow, UK.

Goddard, M.G. and Smith, C. (1990) Optimum number of bull sires in dairy cattle breeding. *Journal of Dairy Science* 73, 1113–1122. DOI: 10.3168/jds.S0022-0302(90)78771-1.

Lush, J.L. (1945) *Animal Breeding Plans,* 3rd edn. Iowa State College Press, Ames, Iowa.

Meuwissen, T.H.E. and Woolliams, J.A. (1994) Response versus risk in breeding schemes. *Proceedings of the 5th World Congress on Genetics Applied to Livestock Production*, Vol. 18, pp. 236–243. Available at: http://www.wcgalp.org/proceedings/1994 (accessed 29 August 2020).

Nicholas, F.W. (2010) *Introduction to Veterinary Genetics*, 3rd edn, Wiley-Blackwell, UK.

Rendel, J.M. and Robertson, A. (1950) Estimation of genetic gain in milk yield by selection in a closed herd of dairy cattle. *Journal of Genetics* 50, 1–8. Available at: https://link.springer.com/article/10.1007/BF02986789 (accessed 29 August 2020).

Weller, J.I. (1994) *Economic Aspects of Animal Breeding*. Chapman and Hall, London.

5 Tools and Technologies in Animal Breeding

Introduction

Genetic improvement is one of the most effective strategies available for enhancing the performance of farmed animals. Some approaches, such as within-breed selection, are relatively slow compared to some other methods, such as improved feeding, but it is permanent and cumulative, and in most cases, it is highly cost effective and sustainable. Populations of animals of high genetic merit are needed to achieve high efficiency, competitiveness, and both economic and environmental sustainability, in any livestock industry. Genetic improvement has generally been used very effectively in the pig, poultry and dairy industries of many wealthier countries, and increasingly so in certain aquaculture sectors. However, it has been used less effectively until recently in other ruminant sectors. The use of objective genetic improvement of farmed animals has been much less widespread in low- and middle-income countries to date, and this represents a major opportunity for improving productivity and livelihoods. The aim of this chapter is to discuss some of the tools and technologies which are being used, or could be used, to lead to more effective genetic improvement programmes in farmed animals. While most of these tools and technologies are relevant in all species, they are likely to be applied in a species-specific manner. Some such applications are described in later chapters.

Rates of genetic improvement depend on four main factors, as outlined in Chapter 4: (i) the selection intensity achieved; (ii) the accuracy with which genetic merit in the trait of interest is predicted; (iii) the amount of genetic variation in the trait of interest; and (iv) the generation interval. Generally speaking, the greater the selection intensity, accuracy and genetic variation, and the shorter the generation interval, the greater the annual rate of genetic improvement. The main opportunities for breeders to accelerate rates of improvement are through choice of the most accurate methods of predicting breeding values, and by maintaining high selection intensities and short generation intervals. However, there are often biological limits on the extent to which selection intensity and generation interval can be altered. As a result of their earlier sexual maturity, and their higher reproductive rates, it is possible to achieve greater selection intensities and shorter generation intervals in pigs, poultry and some aquaculture species than in ruminants. Largely as a result of this, annual rates of genetic improvement in pigs, fish and poultry are often up to double those predicted or achieved in ruminants (Smith, 1984; Gjedrem and Rye, 2018).

The scope for increasing rates of genetic gain through the wider use of BLUP and genomic methods of predicting breeding values is discussed in later chapters. Rates of genetic gain in overall economic merit will be maximized by ensuring that breeding goals include all heritable traits which are of major economic importance, and include none that are of very minor importance, or are not heritable. Similarly, selection indexes should include all the available measurements that make a significant contribution to predicting merit in breeding goal traits. There is considerable scope for the use of more comprehensive breeding goals and criteria in most livestock breeding programmes. For instance, including traits affecting longevity, health and greenhouse gas emissions in dairy cattle breeding indexes is likely to make an increasingly important contribution to overall economic progress, cow welfare, and the sustainability of breeding programmes. Also, the inclusion of traits related to leg health and reduced mortality in addition to growth rate in broiler birds could improve sustainability of the breeding programme and increase public acceptability. Similarly, a better understanding of the relationships between production traits and traits conferring adaptation to harsh environments could help in the production of more sustainable breeding programmes for hill or tropical sheep and beef cattle in these environments.

Genetic Improvement of Farmed Animals (G. Simm *et al.*)
DOI: 10.1079/9781789241723.0005

In most cases the tools to achieve these improvements are already available but they need to be finetuned and applied more widely. For instance, the methodology for producing more comprehensive breeding goals and indexes is well developed. However, indexes need to be tailored to the particular goal, by obtaining estimates of the relevant *genetic parameters* and *economic values*. Although the methodology is available, this is by no means a trivial task. In other cases, new technologies can contribute to accelerating genetic improvement. For example, new scanning techniques can improve rates of progress in carcass characteristics, by providing more accurate predictions of the carcass composition of candidates for selection. New techniques for automatic identification of animals and data capture could improve the accuracy of selection for a range of performance traits in many livestock species; these are especially useful in difficult-to-measure traits such as feed intake and disease incidence. Similar techniques could provide vast amounts of additional information on the carcass weights and grades of commercial meat animals. This could be of considerable value in increasing the accuracy of evaluation of related purebred animals. Methods to estimate greenhouse gas emissions from individual ruminant animals will contribute greatly to selection programmes seeking to incorporate reduction of emissions in their breeding goals.

In addition to data capture tools, the other types of new technologies which can have a major impact on rates of genetic improvement include reproductive and genomic technologies. The current and potential future reproductive, genetic and data capture technologies, together with their possible impact on genetic improvement of livestock, are discussed in detail in the next three sections. Any new technique needs to have a favourable cost–benefit ratio to be widely adopted. These issues are not discussed in detail here, partly because many of the techniques are at an early stage of development, and so both success rates and costs are difficult to estimate. However, it is worth making two general comments about the cost–benefits of new technologies. Firstly, it will usually be easier to justify the use of more expensive technologies in order to accelerate genetic improvement programmes in elite populations, than to justify their use for dissemination of improvement to commercial tiers. This is because of the higher average value of animals produced from elite populations. Secondly, it will be easier to justify the use of more expensive technologies in species with a higher average *per capita* value of elite and commercial animals or those species where reproductive rates are high, such as pigs, poultry and aquaculture species.

In many industrialized countries over the last few years there has been growing public interest in methods of food production, and particularly in the welfare of farmed animals. Particular concerns are expressed about the potential animal welfare or ethical implications of some of the reproductive and genetic technologies outlined in this chapter, and these issues are discussed in Chapter 14.

Reproductive Technologies

It is possible to achieve much higher selection intensities in species or breeds with a high reproductive rate than in those with lower reproductive rates. Similarly, shorter generation intervals can be achieved in those species or breeds which reach sexual maturity at a younger age. It is largely because of biological advantages in these reproductive characteristics that higher rates of genetic change are possible in fish, poultry and pigs than in ruminants. In dairy cattle the main traits of interest are sex-limited and measured fairly late in life, which compounds the disadvantage that cattle suffer in reproductive rate. There are several reproductive technologies which can accelerate progress in genetic improvement programmes in livestock. These include artificial insemination (AI), multiple ovulation and embryo transfer (MOET), *in vitro production of embryos* (i.e. production by laboratory culture), sexing of semen or embryos, and *cloning* (i.e. mass production of identical embryos). These techniques are outlined briefly below, and their potential impacts are discussed. More details on the techniques themselves are given in reviews or books by Woolliams and Wilmut (1989), Wilmut *et al.* (1992), Robinson and McEvoy (1993), Gordon (1994, 1996, 1997), Luo *et al.* (1994), Hernandez Gifford and Gifford (2013), Rutten *et al.* (2013) and Niemann and Wrenzycki (2018).

In addition to their potential value in accelerating response to selection in breeding programmes, many of these techniques also have the potential to accelerate dissemination of genetic improvement from the elite to the commercial tiers of livestock industries. Techniques of value in selection will generally be useful in dissemination but their cost and ease of use may limit their rôle in dissemination.

However, not all techniques of value in dissemination will be useful in selection programmes. So, the value of each of the techniques in dissemination is also discussed.

Artificial insemination

Artificial insemination has been available to cattle breeders for many years, to enhance the reproductive rate of males (see Foote (2002) for a review of AI development). The development of reliable techniques for extending (i.e. diluting to allow wider use) and freezing cattle semen has augmented this benefit. AI allows much higher selection intensities amongst males than those possible with natural mating. Also, the desired number of progeny can often be produced sooner by AI than by natural mating, so male generation intervals can be reduced. AI can contribute to more accurate evaluation of genetic merit as well, by permitting large-scale progeny testing in many herds or flocks. As a result, substantial rates of genetic improvement have been achieved in many countries through the use of AI in well-designed dairy cattle breeding schemes. Progress has been particularly high when the use of AI has been coupled with accurate techniques for predicting breeding value, as outlined in Chapter 7.

Although the use of AI is less widespread in beef cattle breeding than in dairy cattle breeding, the technique can have a similar impact. In many countries, one of the major contributions of AI to beef breeding programmes is to create *genetic links* between herds, which allow across-herd genetic evaluations.

The fact that AI in cattle is relatively cheap and simple, and often allows access to very reliably proven, high genetic merit animals means that it is currently the most effective method of dissemination of genetic improvement to commercial herds. This is particularly true in dairying, where commercial herds rely heavily on AI, and have as good access as elite breeders to high genetic merit bulls. Most commercial beef cows are kept in more extensive production systems than dairy cows. This makes oestrous detection more difficult and hence limits the use of AI for dissemination. However, there is growing use of oestrus synchronization in commercial beef herds to make AI more practical, and so allow access to bulls of higher merit.

To date, AI has had a much smaller impact in most sheep breeding programmes than in cattle breeding programmes. This is largely because of the poor conception rates which usually accompany the cervical insemination of frozen semen. However, the technique has had an important impact in schemes where the use of fresh semen is practical, including dairy sheep breeding programmes, or in schemes involving the laparoscopic intra-uterine insemination of frozen semen. (With laparoscopic AI, the uterus is viewed, and semen is inserted into the uterus via small incisions in the abdomen.) For instance, the strategic use of laparoscopic AI, and in some cases cervical AI, to create genetic links across flocks, has been central to the success of sheep sire referencing schemes, as outlined in Chapter 10. There is no doubt that new techniques which produce high conception rates, and use less invasive insemination methods than laparoscopy, could have a major impact on both the rates of genetic gain and the dissemination of genetic improvement in the sheep industries of many countries. The use of objective selection in sheep breeding programmes and the evidence of high rates of improvement achieved in several large co-operative breeding schemes, make the development and application of improved techniques for dissemination particularly timely.

In lower income countries, especially in sub-Saharan Africa, AI has been of limited use, even in dairy cattle breeding. Some of the major challenges include lack of reliable plants to produce the liquid nitrogen needed for freezing semen, high cost, lack of trained AI technicians, and small farms that are widely dispersed and often inaccessible. In a review of world statistics on AI in cattle, Thibier and Wagner (2002) reported 646 bulls in semen collection centres in Africa compared to 9627 bulls in North America and 20,785 in Europe. In an attempt to address some of the constraints, the Bill and Melinda Gates Foundation are currently implementing a project called PAID (Public Private Partnership for AI Delivery, 2019) in collaboration with private AI companies to increase the efficiency of AI usage in several African countries.

Multiple ovulation and embryo transfer

Over the last few decades, increasingly reliable procedures have been developed for superovulation, embryo recovery, embryo freezing and embryo transfer in cattle (Woolliams and Wilmut, 1989). Similar procedures have been developed for sheep but, unlike the situation in cattle, embryo recovery and transfer techniques are only practicable at present with laparoscopy or surgery (Dingwall and

McKelvey, 1993; Gordon, 1997). A number of applications of embryo procedures have been proposed or practised in cattle and sheep breeding. These include uses in: (i) within-breed genetic improvement programmes; (ii) the international trading of genetic material (offering potential advantages in economy, animal welfare and disease control); (iii) accelerating breed substitution by multiplication of newly introduced breeds; and (iv) conservation of genetic material by freezing embryos from valuable individual animals, or from rare or endangered breeds or species. Additionally, several of the new reproductive or genetic procedures discussed in this chapter hinge on the use of embryo transfer.

MOET potentially offers similar benefits in selection of females to those offered by AI in males (though in practice the benefits are often smaller). That is, female selection intensities can be increased, female generation intervals can be reduced, and the accuracy of evaluating embryo donors, or full sibs created by MOET, can be increased. Since the mid-1970s there have been several studies on the potential impact of MOET on the rates of genetic improvement in ruminants. The earliest of these studies predicted that rates of improvement in beef cattle, dairy cattle and sheep could be increased up to twofold compared to conventional breeding schemes (Land and Hill, 1975; Nicholas, 1980; Nicholas and Smith, 1983; Smith, 1986).

As a result of the early work, commercial dairy cattle breeding schemes based on MOET were initiated in several countries in the mid- to late 1980s. Experimental breeding schemes involving MOET were also established in beef cattle and sheep at about the same time. However, further theoretical work from the mid-1980s onwards showed that the initial results were very sensitive to alterations in some key assumptions. For example, most of the early studies used optimistic success rates for MOET, and these have been difficult to achieve on a 'field scale' in practice. Also, the early studies usually ignored the fact that genetic variation, and hence response to selection, is reduced by the process of selection, and by inbreeding – the latter being a usual consequence of effective selection in domestic animals. These factors appear to be particularly important in small, closed nucleus populations such as those in which the use of MOET was first envisaged. The large variability in numbers of transferable embryos recovered per flush was also ignored in many early studies. This variability is expected to have an unfavourable impact on rates of genetic gain and, especially, on rates of inbreeding, since fewer animals make a bigger contribution to the genetic makeup of the next generation. Advances in the theory of predicting rates of inbreeding also showed that these had been significantly underestimated in most of the early studies (Villanueva and Simm, 1994; Nicholas, 1996).

Much effort has been directed at the design of breeding schemes to overcome these high rates of inbreeding, and several successful techniques have been identified (Toro *et al.*, 1988; Woolliams, 1989; Grundy *et al.*, 1994; Villanueva and Simm, 1994; Wray and Goddard, 1994a; Caballero *et al.*, 1996; Meuwissen, 1997). These include:

- the use of factorial mating designs (mating each donor female to different selected males in successive matings, rather than to the same male);
- using selected parents only once;
- equalizing family sizes (this will be easier to achieve with new techniques producing higher yields of embryos);
- using more than one male from each selected full sib family;
- deliberately choosing less closely related animals; and reducing the emphasis on ancestors' performance when calculating BLUP EBVs (because BLUP methods use records of relatives they tend to lead to selection of more closely related animals, and so to higher rates of inbreeding; this effect can be reduced by altering the emphasis on records from relatives); and
- minimizing the average coancestry (or half the average *additive genetic relationship*) among selected parents or maximizing genetic improvement while restricting the average coancestry among selected parents.

Use of some of these techniques, either alone or in combination, is expected to reduce inbreeding substantially, with little or no change in genetic gain. So, with appropriate modifications to design, MOET schemes can probably offer increased rates of response compared to conventional schemes. However, these rates of response are still unlikely to be as high as first predicted. For example, in beef MOET schemes, rates of gain may be 30% higher than in conventional schemes, at acceptable levels of inbreeding, rather than 100% higher, as first predicted (Villanueva *et al.*, 1995). In future, the advantage to MOET schemes may be augmented as a result of the use of techniques which result in improved yields of transferable embryos, or through the use of some of the new reproductive or genetic technologies outlined below. For example, Pryce and Daetwyler (2012) and Granleese *et al.* (2015) examined the incorporation of genomic selection into MOET schemes by using or reviewing simulation studies. The latter authors estimated that the use of genomic selection with MOET schemes should result in increases in the rates of genetic gain of between 38% and 76%, depending on the level of inbreeding modelled, when compared to using AI or natural mating.

There have been few recent studies of the benefits of MOET in sheep. However, for meat breeds, it is probably reasonable to expect similar benefits to those in beef MOET schemes. In wool breeds, the benefits appear to be similar to those outlined for beef cattle too (Wray and Goddard, 1994b; Bergstein-Galan *et al.*, 2019).

In theory, MOET could be a highly effective technique for the dissemination of genetic improvement to commercial sectors of the livestock industries. Since embryos have already passed the hurdle of fertilization, they have the potential to produce higher calving or lambing rates than AI, though this potential is still far from being realized. Similarly, embryos already contain the full complement of chromosomes necessary for their development. So, MOET can deliver populations of commercial animals with 100% of their genes from elite sector parents, whereas AI used on commercial females produces animals with only 50% of their genes from the elite sector. However, with current MOET techniques, each donor female produces relatively few embryos, at least compared to the number of doses of semen which can be produced by each male. Partly for this reason, but also because of the more complex techniques involved, MOET remains far more expensive than AI, and so less attractive as a means of dissemination. Some newer techniques that have the potential to allow the wider use of embryo transfer are discussed next.

In vitro production of embryos

Over the last few decades, a great deal of effort has gone into developing techniques for the *in vitro* maturation, fertilization and culture of eggs from farm animals, as well as humans. *In vitro* literally means in glass, as opposed to in the body. The rationale for this research in humans is to allow certain types of infertility to be overcome (e.g. that due to blocked Fallopian tubes), or to allow the use of donor semen or eggs in cases of complete infertility of one partner. The main aim of developing these techniques in farm animals is to allow the use of the thousands of eggs present in the ovaries of female animals at birth, most of which never develop to the point of ovulation (Betteridge *et al.*, 1989; Gordon and Lu, 1990; Wilmut *et al.*, 1992; Gordon, 1994).

One of the earliest intended uses of *in vitro*-produced embryos was to improve the beef merit of calves from dairy or suckler cows, by creating a supply of embryos with 3/4 or 7/8 beef genotype. Initially, the main source of eggs was the ovaries of slaughtered beef heifers. Companies were established in several countries, including Britain and Ireland, to collect eggs from beef heifers with a high proportion of continental beef breeds in their genetic makeup, and to produce embryos from these by maturing them and then fertilizing them with semen from high merit, proven bulls. These embryos were then marketed for transfer into beef suckler cows or dairy cows. Transfers were made either singly or to create twins by transferring an *in vitro*-produced embryo into cows already carrying a natural embryo or by transferring two *in vitro*-produced embryos. Despite a ready supply of ovaries from slaughtered heifers, early techniques produced few transferable embryos per ovary. Also, some *in vitro* culture techniques are implicated in the birth of very large calves, generally with associated calving difficulties (Kruip and den Daas, 1997). Partly for these reasons, some of the original companies are no longer in business.

All purebred cows are slaughtered or die of natural causes at some stage, but most are no longer prime candidates for selection by the time this happens, so recovering eggs *post mortem* is not so beneficial. Hence, the method outlined above using slaughtered heifers is particularly suitable for the dissemination of genetic improvement. The majority of donors are likely to be crossbred animals of unknown genetic merit, with high performance in commercial beef traits. Despite the lack of predictions of genetic merit of donors, selection on the basis of breed or crossbred type, or crude selection on phenotype, should be sufficient to ensure that their merit for beef production is better than that of most dairy cows, and many suckler cows. Also, the technique requires semen from only a small number of very highly selected bulls to fertilize eggs, so it allows very high male selection intensities and accuracies to be achieved. This will usually compensate for possible deficiencies in the selection procedures for donor females. With improvements in the techniques involved, and selection of appropriate parents, the *in vitro* production of embryos could improve both quality and uniformity of beef production in future.

Techniques have been developed to allow the recovery of unfertilized eggs directly from the ovaries of live cows. These involve collection of eggs through an ultrasonically guided needle inserted into the ovary, usually via the vagina (Kruip, 1994; Boni, 2012). This type of recovery is called *in vivo* aspiration of oocytes, or *ovum pick up* (OPU). It has several potential advantages compared to recovery of eggs from slaughtered cows, or to conventional embryo recovery techniques:

- Purebred animals of high genetic merit can be used as donors, so the technique is of potential benefit in genetic improvement and not just in dissemination.
- The technique can be applied to produce embryos in a more planned manner than with *post-mortem* recovery.
- It is possible to collect oocytes from younger donors in this way than with conventional embryo recovery techniques.
- It is possible to collect oocytes from donors in the early stages of pregnancy.
- Eggs can be collected from donors on a weekly basis, allowing tens or potentially hundreds of embryos to be produced from the same donor.

Because it is an invasive technique it does require skilled veterinary input. However, there appears to be no evidence of injury to the donor, nor any adverse effects on subsequent reproductive performance.

OPU is being used in several countries to produce a higher number of transferable embryos than that produced by conventional MOET. Increasing the yield of transferable embryos in this way could have a major impact on the rate of gain achievable in MOET breeding schemes, possibly allowing rates of gain up to 34% above those possible in conventional progeny testing schemes (Lohuis, 1993). Also, high yields of *in-vitro*-produced embryos make some of the methods of controlling inbreeding more practical (e.g. equalizing family sizes, use of factorial mating designs). Embryos produced by OPU are likely to be used in genetic improvement programmes in elite herds, rather than for mass dissemination of improvement to the commercial sector, unless the yield of transferable embryos increases dramatically, or it is combined with other new reproductive technologies such as embryo cloning.

In theory, *in-vitro*-produced sheep embryos would have many of the advantages already mentioned for cattle embryos. However, the techniques are less well developed for sheep, and the lower value of the end product is likely to limit applications in sheep breeding and especially in commercial sheep production.

Semen and embryo sexing

Sexing semen has been a major aim of reproductive technologists for decades. A major breakthrough came with the publication of the paper by Johnson *et al.* (1989) reporting success with rabbits. Most of the methods tested have used real or assumed physical differences between sperm bearing X and Y chromosomes as the basis for separation. For example, separation methods aimed at exploiting differences in mass, surface charge, antigenic properties and buoyant density of X- and Y-bearing sperm have been investigated, but success rates and repeatability have usually been low (White, 1989; Cran and Johnson, 1996). In the last few years, a more reliable technique for *semen sexing* has been developed. The technique uses the fact that sperm bearing the X and Y chromosomes differ slightly in their DNA content. Using a technique called flow cytometry, it is possible to detect these differences in size, and to sort sperm into two groups accordingly. The technique involves staining sperm with a fluorescent stain (e.g. a DNA-staining solution such as Hoechst 33342) and using differences in fluorescence when the cells pass through a laser beam to identify and sort X- and Y-bearing sperm. A number of reviews of this technology are available (Seidel and Garner, 2002; Seidel, 2012; de Graaf *et al.*, 2014). Currently, the method of sexing mammalian sperm using a flow cytometer and measuring DNA content of sperm through the fluorescence of the DNA-bound Hoechst 33342 is the only commercially viable method to sex-sort mammalian sperm and obtain pregnancies. Recently, the process has undergone several improvements both in sperm handling and preparation for sorting. Also, significant enhancements in sorter technology such as advanced digital processing, multiple sensor heads and automation has made this process more efficient and conception rates now compare favourably with conventional semen (Sharpe and Evans, 2009; Evans, 2010; Vishwanath and Moreno, 2018). This methodology is now used in several livestock species, including dairy and beef cattle, pigs, sheep, goats, deer and horses.

Several approaches have been taken to develop techniques for sexing embryos (van Vliet *et al.*, 1989; White, 1989; Woolliams and Wilmut, 1989). These are based on removing a small number of cells from embryos at the 16-cell stage or later stages of development. In some cases, the sex of the embryo can be determined by direct observation of a preparation of chromosomes using a microscope (karyotyping), to confirm the presence of either two X chromosomes or one Y and one X chromosome. Alternative approaches include the use of an immunological test for the H-Y antigen produced only by male embryos, using sex-linked differences in enzyme activity, or using some of the molecular techniques described later in this chapter to detect sequences of DNA specific to the Y chromosome (Zoheira and Allam, 2010; Kageyama and Hirayama, 2012). Perhaps the sector most in need of embryo sexing is the egg-laying chicken industry where the production of many unwanted males continues to be a welfare problem. (Unlike mammals, in birds females are the heterogametic sex so sexing semen is not relevant.) Invasive methods based on identifying sections of the sex chromosomes taken from biopsies of the eggs look promising to solve this long-term problem (He *et al.*, 2019).

In genetic improvement programmes, sexing of either semen or embryos could be useful to increase the selection intensity applied to females by producing more of them. This appears to be of little value when performance records are available on both sexes, and where the total number of animals tested is fixed, as an increase in the number of females implies a reduction in the number of males, and therefore a reduction in male selection intensities. However, when performance recording is sex-limited, as with milk production, there may be benefits in creating more animals of the recorded sex. This may be especially beneficial in nucleus schemes, if they already have access to high genetic merit males which have been accurately tested in a separate population (Colleau, 1991; Villanueva and Simm, 1994).

The use of relatively cheap, reliable techniques for sexing semen in large enough quantities for widespread conventional AI should lead to major improvements in the dissemination of genetic improvement and in the efficiency of animal production. In meat production systems there is interest in using 'female' semen to breed replacement animals from the highest merit females in the herd or flock. Since males usually show higher growth rates and leaner carcasses, there may be a preference for 'male' semen to produce animals for slaughter. However, so-called once-bred heifer systems, using only 'female' semen, may produce the highest overall efficiency (Taylor *et al.*, 1985). In these systems, each heifer leaves a replacement female calf before being slaughtered for beef production. In conventional dairy cattle systems, 'female' semen is used to breed replacements from the best heifers or cows, releasing a higher proportion of the herd for mating to 'male' semen from a beef breed, or for crossing to a beef bull. This is happening increasingly in the dairy sector in many countries.

Similarly, the development of techniques for the production of large numbers of cheap, sexed embryos could lead to the use of high merit female embryos to produce replacements, and cloned male embryos to produce slaughter animals, or the development of once-bred heifer systems based only on female embryos. In dairy herds, elite female embryos could be used to produce replacements, and male embryos of high beef merit and a proven record for calving ease, could be used in the majority of cows. Also, improved techniques for embryo multiplication could increase the benefits and practicality of crossbreeding. In cattle and sheep, crossbreeding is sometimes impractical because the low reproductive rate of these species means that many purebreds are needed to produce a regular supply of F_1 females. In some cases, there are too few breeds with high genetic merit in the traits of interest to sustain a rotational crossing scheme. However, improved reproductive techniques could allow a plentiful supply of F_1 (or other) embryos to produce replacement females, from a relatively small population of elite animals of the component pure breeds. This could lead to replacement policies in cattle and sheep similar to those already employed by conventional means in the commercial tier of the pig and poultry industries, where most replacement females are purchased crossbreds. So far this has had little impact on any livestock industry but the newer DNA-based methodologies for embryo sexing look promising for both cattle and chickens.

Embryo cloning

The production of groups of identical embryos from a single original embryo is often termed embryo cloning, or embryo multiplication. This can be achieved in one of two ways at present. The first involves physically splitting embryos into two halves (or four quarters). If the original embryo was at an early stage of development, the resulting halves need to be inserted into an empty *zona pellucida* or 'egg shell', before transfer. If the embryo is at a later stage of development, the halves can be transferred without this procedure (Woolliams and Wilmut, 1989). Splitting into more than four parts is not successful, as there are too few cells for normal development. Also, repeated bisection of embryos after further culture is not successful because it leads to too great a disparity between the physical composition and true chronological stage of development of the embryos. Embryo bisection can be employed to increase the yield of transferable embryos, particularly when donors are rare or very valuable, or in MOET *nucleus breeding schemes* where a target number of embryos is needed from each donor.

A larger number of identical embryos can be produced by the procedure of *nuclear transfer*. This involves removing the *zona pellucida* from a 16-, 32- or 64-cell embryo, and separating the identical cells within. Each of the resulting cells can be inserted into an unfertilized egg from which the nucleus containing the single copy of chromosomes has been removed. An electric current causes fusion of the introduced embryonic cell and the unfertilized egg, and the new embryo then develops as if newly fertilized (Woolliams and Wilmut, 1989). The advantage of this technique is that it produces larger numbers of identical animals, although the techniques involved are more complex. Initially, nuclear transfer was only accomplished using early embryos, or cells from early embryos. However, in 1996 it was reported that viable cloned embryos, and subsequently live cloned lambs, had been produced by transferring cells which were originally derived from embryos, but had been cultured and multiplied in the laboratory (Campbell *et al.*, 1996; Campbell and Wilmut, 1997). The ability to multiply embryonic cells in the laboratory, and achieve successful development of the resulting embryos following nuclear transfer, obviously gives the potential for far greater numbers of identical animals to be produced from a single pair of elite parents. It also creates potential opportunities for the rapid multiplication of embryos which have been genetically modified in some way (e.g. by *gene transfer* or editing).

In 1997 it was reported that a viable lamb ('Dolly') had been produced following nuclear transfer from a cultured cell originating in an adult ewe – the first time that a mammal has been produced from a cell derived from an adult (Fig. 5.1; Wilmut *et al.*, 1997). This presents new opportunities for adult cloning, since clones can be derived from a single animal of proven performance, rather than from embryos produced by two proven parents. By the year 2007, 10 years after Dolly's birth, an additional 18 mammalian species including pigs, cattle, goats and horses had been cloned from adult cells using somatic cell nuclear transfer (Baguisi *et al.*, 1999; Wells *et al.*, 1999; Polejaeva *et al.*, 2000; Galli *et al.*, 2003). The ability to create clones created great interest in agriculture and the biomedical industry, and Dolly's birth in particular, stimulated both commercial and wider public interest in cloning.

In genetic improvement programmes, cloning has the potential to be used to produce many animals of the same genotype in order to improve the accuracy of evaluation, or to allow evaluation of traits normally measured post slaughter on some members of the cloned group. This would involve implanting some embryos from each cloned line to produce animals for testing, and freezing others to allow subsequent use (or further cloning) of the best tested cloned lines in breeding or dissemination programmes. Cloning could theoretically be of value in breeding programmes under certain circumstances, for example in dairy cattle nucleus schemes, if there are elite males available which are tested in a separate population. One potential advantage of the use of cloning would be better utilization of non-additive genetic variation. Conventionally, selection for quantitative traits within breeds attempts to identify animals with the highest additive genetic merit. It is difficult to make use of non-additive genetic variation in selection since particular combinations of non-additive genes which lead to the high merit of parents get split up and mixed between one generation and the next. However, comparison of cloned lines created from different parents would allow selection of those lines with the best combination of additive and non-additive genetic merit. Since the animals produced from the same cloned line have identical

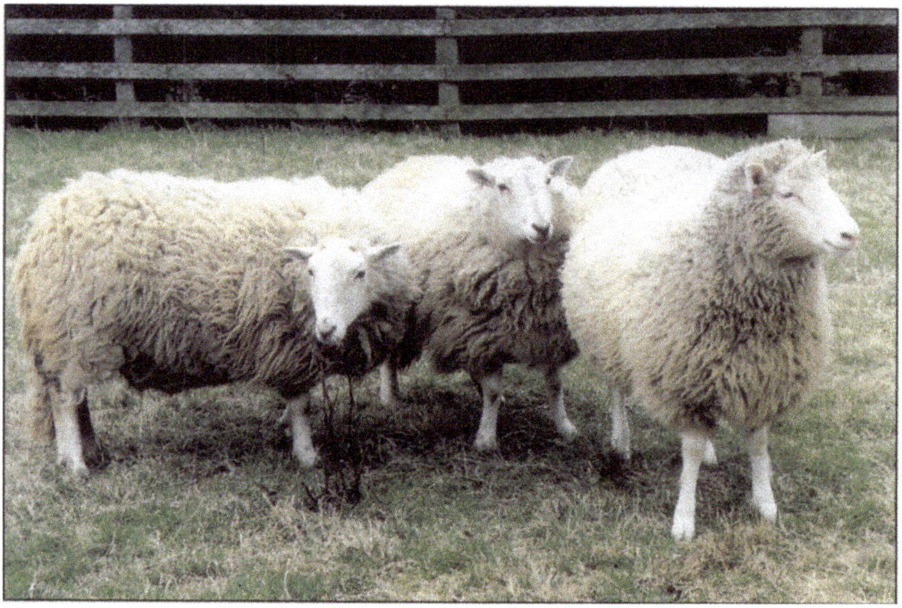

Fig. 5.1. Cloned sheep. The two sheep on the left (Megan and Morag) were produced by nuclear transfer of cultured cells originally derived from an embryo. The sheep on the right (Dolly) was produced by nuclear transfer of a cultured cell originating from an adult ewe – the first time that a mammal had been produced from a cell derived from an adult. (Courtesy of Professor Sir Ian Wilmut.)

genotypes, the favourable genotype could be recreated exactly by further cloning. Similarly, cloned lines could be produced from crosses between breeds to exploit heterosis if this is important for the traits of interest. Clones with the optimum proportion of each parent breed could be produced, so minimizing the problems seen with rotational crossing, which inevitably produces many animals with sub-optimal proportions of the different breeds involved. However, if cloning is considered only in the context of closed breeding schemes, with fixed numbers of animals tested, then the expected benefits generally diminish or disappear, as keeping more identical animals means that fewer different families can be kept, and so selection intensities will be reduced (de Boer *et al.*, 1994; Villanueva and Simm, 1994).

While the benefits of cloning in genetic improvement may be limited, the potential of the technique to accelerate dissemination of genetic improvement to commercial herds or flocks is great. However, a number of drawbacks have prevented this becoming a commercial reality to date. Firstly, fully reliable, cost effective and scalable methods for cloning and delivery are not yet available. Further, a disadvantage of the technique is the risk of producing very large numbers of animals which subsequently turn out to be susceptible to disease or to be unsuitable to new production methods. However, it should be possible to reduce such risks by maintaining reasonable genetic diversity in the conventionally bred elite populations and producing several or many separate cloned lines from these.

The future use of cloning may be in combination with other emerging technologies, such as genomic selection and gene editing, as discussed further below (Watson, 2018). For example, Carlson *et al.* (2016) combined gene editing with cloning to substitute the polled allele from Angus cattle into a Holstein cell line. Gene editing was used to introduce the Angus allele into a Holstein cell line and those cells in which the desired allele was present were selected for cloning. This approach significantly reduced the time it would take to introduce the trait through conventional breeding alone.

Kasinathan *et al.* (2015) reported the use of several reproductive technologies, cloning and genomic selection, in combination, to reduce the generation interval in cattle. They treated Jersey dairy cows to stimulate oocyte production. Oocytes were collected and used to produce IVF embryos. Multiple IVF embryos were transferred into surrogate mothers and allowed to develop for 21 days then flushed and collected. Cell lines were generated from the collected material and sent for DNA analysis to identify those of high genetic merit using genomic selection. The high genetic merit cell lines were used to produce cloned calves using nuclear transfer.

Surrogate sire technology

Surrogate sire technology can achieve some of the benefits of cloning, but is potentially more suitable for large-scale application. Surrogate sire technology is based on the creation of males that lack their own germline cells, for example, via genome-editing-targeted silencing of the genes essential for germ cell development (Fig. 5.2). Instead, they possess transplanted spermatogonial stem cells from other donor males (Gottardo *et al.*, 2019; Ciccarelli *et al.*, 2020). The recipient males have their germline ablated, which could be via genome-editing-targeted knockout of the genes essential for germ cell development. The surrogate sires can then be used widely, resulting in single elite male donors giving rise to huge numbers of progeny. The advantages of this are that it can reduce the genetic lag between the elite nucleus animals and the production animals, it can enable tailoring of specific animals for specific environments or management schemes, and it can improve protection of intellectual property of breeding companies via the more limited release of elite males (Gottardo *et al.* 2019).

The value of reproductive technologies in genetic improvement

The current or potential future value of these reproductive technologies in genetic improvement programmes, and in the dissemination of genetic improvement, is summarized in Table 5.1.

Table 5.1. The current or potential future value of reproductive technologies in genetic improvement programmes, and in the dissemination of genetic improvement. The technologies are rated on a scale from one to four ticks, with one tick representing little or no value, and four ticks representing high value.

Reproductive technology	Value in genetic improvement programmes	Value in dissemination of improvement to commercial tier
Artificial insemination	✓✓✓✓	✓✓✓✓
Multiple ovulation and embryo transfer	✓✓✓	✓
In vitro production of embryos	✓✓✓	✓✓✓
Sexing of semen and embryos	✓✓	✓✓✓
Cloning of embryos	✓✓	✓✓✓✓
Surrogate sires	✓✓	✓✓✓✓

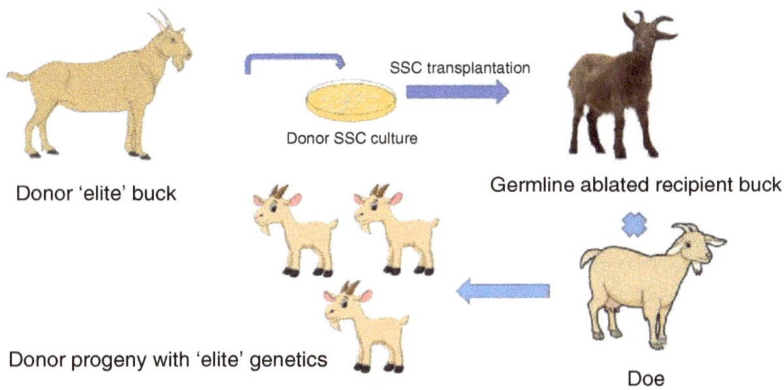

Fig. 5.2. How a surrogate sire scheme would work, showing the application of spermatogonial stem cell (SSC) transplantation methodology in goats. Indigenous germ line ablated bucks carry the sperm of 'elite' bucks. Instead of having one elite buck there would be many. This allows the dissemination of 'elite' semen without changing the existing infrastructure (Courtesy of Dr Emily Clark, Roslin Institute, University of Edinburgh and Prof Mike Coffey, SRUC; after Oatley, 2017 and Gottardo *et al.,* 2019; artwork from kambing animasi png 2).

Molecular Genetic Tools

Since the first detailed description of DNA by Crick, Watson, Franklin and Gosling in the early 1950s, scientists have been looking for ways to incorporate this information into breeding programmes. This was given fresh impetus in 1995 when the first free-living organism, the bacterium *Haemophilus influenza*, had its genome completely sequenced. The first complete sequence of the human genome was produced in the early 2000s. This was followed over the next 15 years by most of the commonly farmed species having their genome sequenced and mapped. The developments around this molecular genetic revolution are many and varied. Some have led to applications in the animal breeding industry and these will be discussed here. Needless to say, this is a rapidly changing field and so the molecular genetic tools used today, or in the recent past, may well be superseded soon by newer applications.

Many new subjects have been developed from the 21st century molecular genetic revolution. These often end in the term '*omics*' and relate to the different stages of biochemistry and physiology between the genome and the phenotype (see Fig. 5.3). So, for example, proteomics relates to the initial products from transcription and translation of the genome into proteins. It is beyond the scope of this book to describe in detail all the various 'omic' sciences. However, we will highlight those which most directly relate to animal breeding as well as other key laboratory methods which play an important rôle in some aspects of genetic improvement.

Bioinformatics is the umbrella term for any methodology used to record, store and analyse the vast wealth of molecular genetic data being generated by the 'omics'. It could be said that bioinformatics is to molecular genetic data what statistics is to numerical data; a means of making order out of them and being able to answer biological questions from them. Of course, modern bioinformatic methods are only limited by human imagination and computing power. As both develop, new and exciting applications in animal breeding will no doubt follow.

To date, most selection in livestock has been practised with little or no knowledge of what is happening at the DNA level. Selection has been based on the effects of the genes, rather than directly on the genes themselves. Some traits are controlled by a single gene, and have a large visible effect, e.g. coat colour, polledness, double muscling. In these cases, there is a fairly close association between the one (homozygotes) or two (heterozygotes) versions of the gene (alleles) an animal inherits, and their effects, although non-additive gene action, such as dominance and epistasis, can still

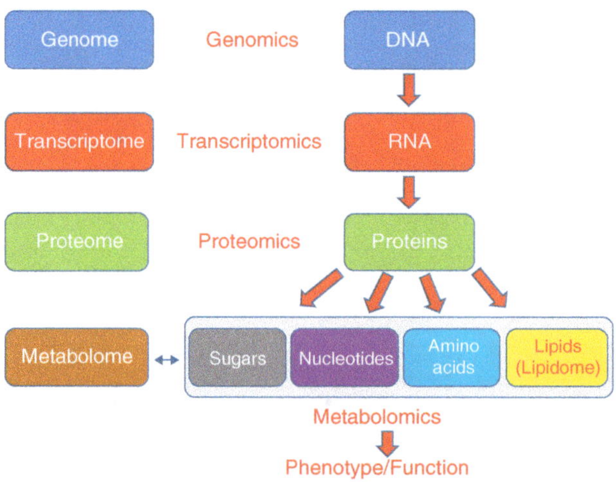

Fig. 5.3. The relationship between the various 'omics' and the biological pathway from DNA to trait. (Source: Lmaps under licence http://www.gnu.org/copyleft/fdl.html.)

cause difficulties in determining the true genotype of an animal. As described in Chapter 2, for most traits of economic importance the performance of animals is affected by their genotype at many different loci. Also, in most cases, the effects of these genes are influenced by environmental effects on the traits of interest, so the link between particular genes and performance is obscured even further.

Despite these complications, very effective methods have been developed to identify animals with favourable predicted breeding values, as discussed in Chapter 7. These work by removing as many environmental influences as possible (through management practices, statistically or both) and using clues from the performance of candidates for selection, and their relatives, to estimate the additive effect of all loci affecting the trait of interest. They are good at predicting the average genetic merit of offspring but cannot distinguish between them until the offspring get performance records of their own, or performance records from their progeny or siblings. These techniques have been applied with considerable success in most livestock species, as outlined earlier in this book and discussed more extensively in the species-focused Chapters 8 to 13. However, molecular technologies are increasingly being used to improve on existing methods. The aim in this section is to briefly review some of these technologies which have an impact on the genetic improvement of livestock, or which may have such an impact in the future. The related molecular technologies considered are genome mapping, the use of molecular markers in selection, genetic engineering and gene editing. First, some background information will help in understanding these technologies.

Linkage disequilibrium and haplotypes

Two related genetic phenomena are fundamental to understanding some of the applications in molecular genetics, namely *linkage disequilibrium* and *haplotypes*. Genes positioned close to one another on a chromosome have been recognized for many years, since certain versions of each gene can be observed in the population appearing together. This led to the two genes being described as being 'linked'. In fact, recombination, or crossing over, will ultimately split up these combinations of gene versions but the closer they are together, the less likely this is to happen. Sequences of the genome which are inherited together because of linkage are said to be haplotypes and if an organism has identical haplotypes on both chromosomes of a pair at a particular genome location it is said to be homozygous. Conversely if the two haplotypes are not identical then the organism is heterozygous at this location.

Being able to measure linkage is clearly an important aspect of genetics. *Linkage equilibrium* describes the situation in which the haplotype frequencies in a population have the same value that they would have if the genes at each locus were combined at random. The alternative concept, and much more widely used in modern genetics, is linkage disequilibrium (LD). This is the occurrence of combinations of linked genes in non-random proportions, due to them being positioned near to each other on the same chromosome. It is possible to measure LD using known haplotypes, with values close to 1 indicating that alleles are always inherited together and a value of 0 indicating that they are never inherited together (see Lin *et al.*, 2012).

Laboratory methodology

The isolation, amplification and study of DNA in the laboratory has become a cornerstone of modern molecular biology. There are certain key properties of DNA which allow it to be studied at the molecular level in the laboratory. Many of the initial technologies used to study DNA were covered in the previous version of this book (Simm, 1998) but have since receded from the mainstream of molecular genetics.

Phenotypic markers of variation at the DNA level, such as variation in coat colour, the presence or absence of horns and variation in animal size and shape, have probably been used in livestock selection since domestication began. A few decades ago, variation in blood groups and milk proteins was used as physiological markers of variation at the DNA level. However, it is only in more recent years that we have had the tools to directly measure this variation at the DNA level. These tools, known as *molecular genetic markers*, are basically alternative segments of DNA at a particular site on a chromosome which are identifiable by a laboratory test. Molecular genetic markers have been used to refine animal selection programmes in some cases or change them dramatically in others. They are also of value in checking the identity and parentage of animals, estimating breeding values, checking the origin of animal products, improving our understanding of evolution, and paving the way to a fuller understanding of the structure and function of genes, and their modification or transfer. It is quite possible to find an association between a particular molecular marker and an animal characteristic of interest, without knowing which chromosome, or which part of a chromosome, the marker is located on. However, the search for useful molecular markers is being guided increasingly by the burgeoning information coming from genome-sequencing projects. Hence, in this section *genome sequencing* is discussed before outlining the use of molecular markers in selection. The more recent advent of the possibility of targeted gene editing to create minor changes in livestock genomes also has potential to be transformative, and is discussed later. Each of these technologies depends on fairly recent advances in molecular and cell biology, so the most important of these advances are summarized briefly first of all. More details can be found in the texts listed at the end of the chapter.

As outlined in Chapter 2, the existence and gross structure of chromosomes has been known since the early 1900s, and the chemical structure of DNA and its rôle in inheritance have been known since the 1950s. However, it is only relatively recent advances in molecular and cell biology that have allowed the identification and location of individual functional genes, or other sequences of DNA, on chromosomes, and provided the molecular tools to assist conventional selection procedures, and to allow gene transfer or editing. Briefly, these advances include:

- **The discovery of restriction enzymes.** Bacteria produce a large number of enzymes called *restriction enzymes*, which are capable of 'cutting up' sequences of DNA. These enzymes act like microscopic scalpels, to protect the bacteria by attacking viral or other foreign DNA (Roberts, 2005). Different restriction enzymes 'recognize' different sequences, typically between four and eight base pairs, in DNA and make their cuts whenever they come across these sequences of bases in a strand of DNA. For example, one commonly used restriction enzyme recognizes the sequence GAATTC, and cuts the strand between the G and the adjacent A (the letters are abbreviations for the four bases in DNA: adenine (A), thymine (T), guanine (G) and cytosine (C), as explained in Chapter 2). This property of restriction enzymes has been widely used in the study of the DNA of livestock species. Treating (or digesting) identical sequences of DNA with the same enzyme(s) produces identical sets of fragments, each of a specific size. Conversely, treating different sequences of DNA with the same restriction enzyme produces different sets of fragments, of different sizes. Hence, these enzymes are useful in detecting similarities and differences in the DNA sequences of different animals (see Fig. 5.4). The same principles underlie genotyping-by-sequencing technologies (described below), but these technologies typically use high-throughput sequencing of genomic regions flanking the restriction enzyme digestion sites.

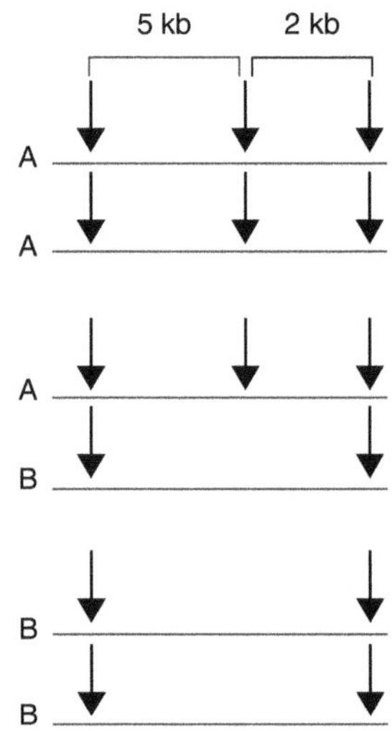

Fig. 5.4. Differences in the DNA sequences of different animals can be detected using restriction enzymes. The diagram shows fragments of DNA from each member of a pair of chromosomes from three different animals. Each DNA fragment has either two or three restriction sites – sequences between four and eight bases – recognized and cut by a particular restriction enzyme. Treatment of these fragments with the appropriate restriction enzyme will produce only DNA fragments 7 kilobases (kb) long when only two restriction sites are present but will produce fragments 5 and 2 kb long when there are three restriction sites present. Hence, three genotypes are distinguishable. Those with two restriction sites on one strand and three on the other produce fragments 7, 5 and 2 kb long (genotype AB). (After Womack, 1996.)

- **The development of techniques to allow DNA fragments of different lengths to be separated and detected.** Fragments of DNA of different lengths (e.g. resulting from digestion with restriction enzymes) can be separated by applying a sample of the fragments of mixed sizes to one end of a thin film of gel, and applying an electric current to the gel (*electrophoresis*). The fragments then move across the gel at different rates, depending on their size. Large fragments move slowly, and small fragments move quickly. The gel can be stained or treated in a variety of ways to show up a series of bands, with each band representing DNA fragments of a particular size. When different samples (e.g. DNA from different animals) are applied side by side to the same gel, a series of bands can be detected in a column arising from each sample. By comparing the patterns of bands across columns, it is possible to tell whether or not different samples contain DNA fragments of a similar length (see Fig. 5.5 and Alberts *et al.*, 2002). In addition, this early work on restriction-enzyme-based genotyping set the scene for the use of restriction-enzyme-based genotyping-by-sequencing technology, such as RAD-Seq (Baird *et al.*, 2008). This is a method now applied to generate population-scale, genome-wide *single-nucleotide polymorphism* (*SNP*; pronounced 'snip') marker genotypes without the need for prior investment in creating SNP arrays (see below for full descriptions), or where the population of interest is genetically distinct from the SNP discovery population (a different group of animals used for creating SNP arrays).

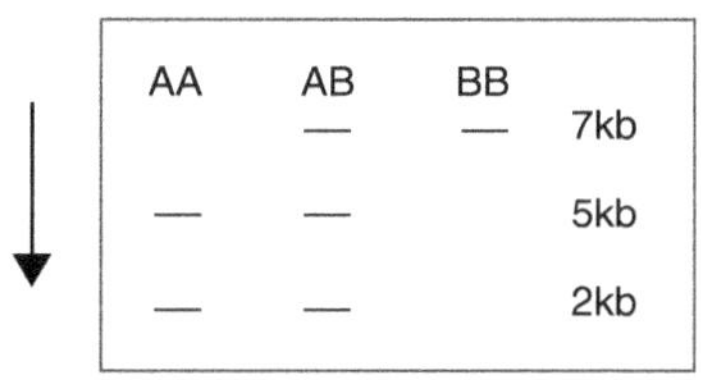

Fig. 5.5. Differences in the length of DNA fragments can be detected by applying DNA samples from different animals to a film of gel and applying an electric current to the gel to separate fragments of different length. This is called gel electrophoresis – smaller fragments move further away from the point at which the original sample was applied to the gel. The gel is then stained or treated in some other way (e.g. using a *DNA probe*), to allow the positions of bands, which represent fragments of different size, to be detected. The diagram shows the pattern of bands expected if samples of DNA from the three genotypes shown in Fig. 5.4 were treated with restriction enzymes, and then subjected to gel electrophoresis. (After Womack, 1996.)

- **The development of techniques to multiply sequences of DNA rapidly.** The *polymerase chain reaction*, or PCR for short, was discovered in the mid-1980s and involves DNA multiplication 'in a test tube'. Polymerase is an enzyme involved in the normal replication of DNA in the cell. However, sequences of DNA can be multiplied in the laboratory by adding a heat-stable version of this enzyme, together with two *primers* (short fragments of DNA which start off the replication of a specific sequence of DNA) and a supply of the four DNA bases (A, T, G and C). Heating this mixture up denatures the DNA in the fragments of interest, causing the strands to separate. Subsequent cooling of the mixture causes the primers to 'home in' on complementary sequences of DNA, and to initiate the process of copying the sequences of interest on each of the two separated strands. Each cycle of heating and cooling produces a doubling of the number of copies of the original DNA sequence, so in a matter of hours it is possible to produce sufficiently large quantities of DNA for characterization. Other important properties of PCR are that: (i) it multiplies *specific* sequences of DNA, which depend on the primers used; (ii) it is most effective for relatively short DNA sequences; and (iii) only very small amounts of DNA are needed initially, e.g. from hair follicles.
- **The development and automation of techniques to determine the sequence of bases on strands of DNA.** Several techniques exist to enable the sequence of bases on a strand of DNA to be determined from short strands up to whole genomes. This is a rapidly advancing field and a review of these methods is outside the scope of this book. However, a number of methods are available commercially to sequence genomes or short sequences (sometimes known as short reads). Some of these are described in the subsequent section on whole-genome sequencing methods.
- **The development of DNA probes and labelling techniques.** DNA *probes* are single-stranded molecules of DNA, of a known base sequence.

Like all strands of DNA, under the right circumstances these probes will bind to complementary sequences or fragments of DNA (as outlined in Chapter 2). Hence they can be used to detect the presence of a complementary DNA strand in samples of DNA (e.g. obtained by 'blotting' from a gel in a manner equivalent to blotting ink with absorbent paper – see Fig. 5.6), or in intact chromosomes. Probes can be 'labelled', which means that they can be made either radioactive or, more recently, fluorescent. This allows them to be readily detected later, when they have bound to a complementary DNA sequence. The use of sophisticated microscopes, cameras and computer-aided analysis systems allows rapid location of fluorescently labelled probes.

- **The development of markers for variation at the DNA level.** Any identifiable segment of DNA in the genome, which shows variation between animals, can be used as a marker. Hence, markers may be all or part of a 'functional' gene, or they may be a part of the rest of the genome which does not code directly for the production of a protein. Several different types of marker have been developed, based on some of the methods described above, for detecting variation at the DNA level. These markers are of value in genome mapping, marker-assisted selection, parentage verification, genomic selection, genome-wide association studies and product identification. Historically, several different types of molecular genetic markers have been developed including *restriction fragment length polymorphisms* (RFLPs) and *microsatellites*. Note that the word polymorphism literally means 'different forms'. RFLPs are differences between animals in the number and position of sites at which a given restriction enzyme will cut the DNA. They can be used to detect variation in the DNA sequence of different animals, and hence they can be used as markers in genome mapping. A region in the genome where the same sequence of base pairs is repeated several times, end to end, is called a microsatellite. The repeated sequences are between two and six (or more) base pairs long. The number of times a given sequence of bases is repeated varies greatly between alleles but is typically between 5 and 50 times. Because of this variation, microsatellites can be used as

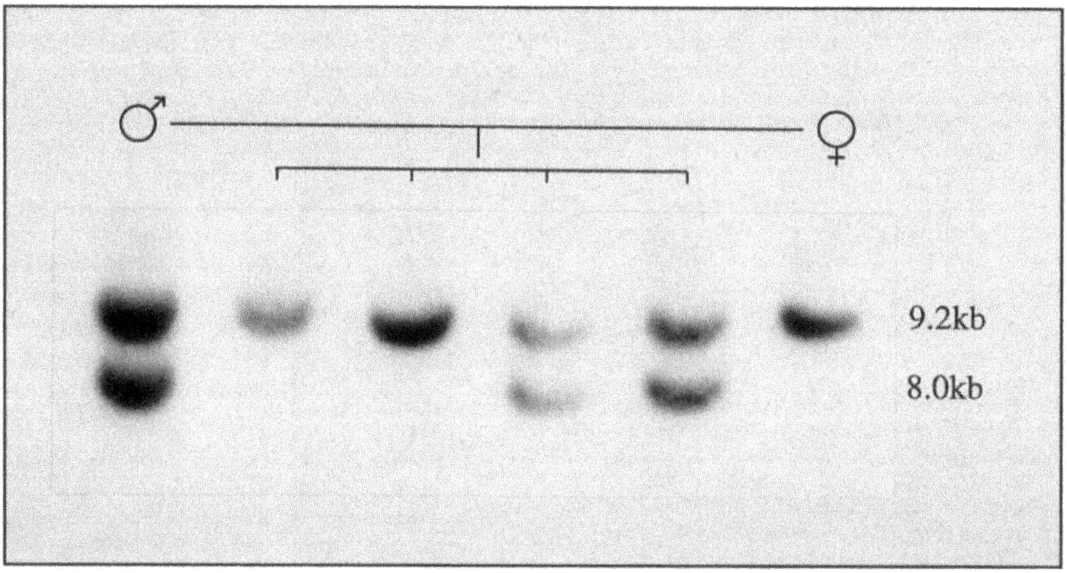

Fig. 5.6. Detection of variation in DNA fragment size in a sire (left lane), a dam (right lane) and their four offspring (middle lanes), using a technique known as Southern blotting. The fragments of different sizes are created by the use of a restriction enzyme; these are then separated by gel electrophoresis, 'blotted' onto a membrane, and detected using a DNA probe. (Courtesy of Professor Alan Archibald.)

markers in genome mapping and for marker-assisted selection. However, most of the applications of genetic marker technology to livestock breeding are now based on *SNP markers*.

- **Single-nucleotide polymorphism markers.** From the late 1980s, microsatellites were used as markers in various livestock improvement programmes and also to help identify the right parents when pedigree information was missing or recorded incorrectly for some animals. However, limitations of microsatellite markers include that they are laborious and expensive to genotype, they are not amenable to automation, and the markers are often a considerable distance from the loci of genes that control the traits of economic importance. These loci with genes that control traits of economic importance are usually referred to as quantitative trait loci (QTL). Microsatellite markers were not very useful in precisely mapping the position of QTLs on chromosomes in the genome, nor as genetic markers to assist in prediction of breeding values. As a result of the efforts to sequence the human genome, a huge amount of variation at the DNA level resulting from a substitution of a single nucleotide at a specific position in the genome has been discovered. The DNA sequence variation occurring when a single nucleotide (adenine (A), thymine (T), cytosine (C), or guanine (G)) in the genome differs between members of a population of a particular species, or paired chromosomes in an individual, is referred to as a SNP. In other words, a SNP represents a difference in a single DNA building block (nucleotide), in a certain stretch of DNA, between members of a population of a particular species. For example, at a specific base position in an animal genome, the C nucleotide may appear in most individuals but in a minority of individuals the position is occupied by an A. This means that there is a SNP at this specific position, and the two possible nucleotide variations, C or A, are said to be alleles for this position. Usually, SNPs are bi-allelic, that is they have only two alleles, but this is not always the case. A SNP may result from a single nucleotide being changed (substitution), removed (deletion) or added (insertion) during meiosis. SNPs are the most common types of genetic variation at the DNA level. They occur almost once in every 1000 nucleotides on average (depending on the species and population), which means there are roughly 4 to 5 million SNPs in a typical farm animal genome. The abundance of SNPs and the plausibility of genotyping SNPs in very large numbers makes them very useful as biological markers, helping scientists locate QTL that are associated with disease or traits of economic importance in animals, and more recently to improve accuracy of estimating breeding values. The livestock breeding industry has made a great use of SNPs as the major marker of choice (see Vignal *et al.* (2002) for a review of marker development, and Georges *et al.* (2018) for a recent review of their application).
- **Using SNP markers.** The value of SNP markers is that two versions of the SNP may be in LD with other variations in DNA sequence that affect traits of interest. In other words, the different versions of the SNP may be on haplotypes which contain interesting variations of a gene, or other key DNA features, which affect the trait of interest differently. Advantages of SNP markers include: (i) they are found throughout the genome, for example in exons, introns, promoters, enhancers, etc.; (ii) SNPs generally are more stable than other forms of polymorphism, meaning they are less likely to be affected by mutations between generations or populations than microsatellites (Schork, *et al.*, 2000); and (iii) given their simple structure as base changes, various technologies have been developed to allow the rapid and efficient genotyping of thousands of individuals for thousands of SNPs simultaneously. The measurement of genetic variations in SNPs between members of a species or population is referred to as SNP genotyping, and is described immediately below.
- **SNP marker technology.** Several approaches have been used for SNP genotyping but one of the most popular is the use of SNP *microarrays*. In so-called high-density oligonucleotide SNP arrays, hundreds of thousands of short fragments of DNA (oligonucleotides, also called probes) are placed onto on a small chip, allowing for many SNPs to be genotyped simultaneously (see Fig. 5.7). These probes are copies of known parts of the genome from the species that we are analysing. SNP markers are commonly used in the context of genome-wide studies by selecting suitably evenly spaced SNPs across the genome and making them available as commercial chips. These so-called 'SNP chips' comprise thousands of probes on a chip, each of which contains a short stretch of fluorescently labelled DNA.

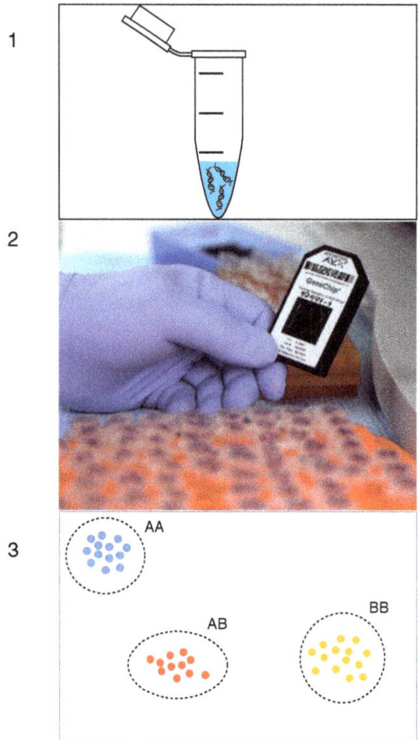

Fig. 5.7. Summary of the steps involved in genotyping animals using SNP markers. Step (1): DNA extracted from blood, semen or hair follicles. The DNA of the animal is converted to fragmented sequences, amplified, and labelled with fluorescent dyes. Step (2): The DNA is genotyped for genome-wide SNP markers using a SNP array. The array contains immobilized allele-specific oligonucleotide probes. The DNA is hybridized to the array and a detection system records and interprets the hybridization signal which varies according to the specific SNP alleles an individual carries. Step (3): The outputs of the SNP array genotyping of individuals is a form of cluster plot that is based on the amount of signal from each allele-specific probe. Specialist software is used to define clusters that correspond to specific genotypes (i.e. AA, AB, BB) and then to call individuals' genotypes based on their position relative to those clusters. (Photo: public domain).

These probes contain the two alternative sequences around a particular SNP and adhere to their appropriate section of DNA from our candidate animals. Because of the fluorescent labelling and some clever technology, it is possible to 'read' the signals from the chip and determine which versions of the SNP, at any given locus, an animal has. Chips commonly contain ~50,000 SNPs (referred to as a 50K chip) but they may range from a few hundred to over 1 million SNPs in size. The chips are typically produced by commercial companies such as Illumina (2019a) or ThermoFisher (2019, a company which purchased another main genotyping provider, Affymetrix, recently) which provide genotyping services for determining the genotypes at genome-wide SNPs of individuals using DNA extracted from tissue samples such as blood or hair.

- **Genotyping-by-sequencing (GBS) methodology.** Genotyping-by-sequencing is a technique based on using high-throughput, short-read (reading between 100 to 600 base pairs at a time) sequencing technology, combined with restriction enzymes, to generate accurate sequence information for a subset of an animal's genome (i.e. the regions flanking restriction enzyme cut sites). There are various techniques based on similar principles, all of which can result in similar SNP data sets comparable to commercial SNP chips. The potential benefits of using GBS on the complete genome have also been investigated in livestock breeding (Gorjanc *et al.*, 2015). It may help in investigating cases where there is so-called ascertainment bias in the generation of the SNP chips. Ascertainment bias can result when the SNPs placed on a SNP chip are most informative in the populations which were sequenced to discover the SNPs, making the SNP chip more suitable for use in some populations and breeds than others. GBS is distinct from whole-genome sequencing, the uses of which will be discussed later in this chapter.

Genome mapping

The main driving force for the production of the human genome map was that it enabled the investigation, and potentially the treatment, of a wide range of human diseases with a genetic component. Comparison of the genome maps produced for different species has provided, and continues to provide, a powerful tool for the study of evolution. Studies so far highlight the similarity between genomes of all species; the closer the species in evolutionary time, the greater the similarity between genomes. Similarly, genome maps can be used to make more informed decisions about which breeds, strains or individuals should receive highest priority in conservation of genetic resources. In farm livestock and crop species, genome maps can be useful in making informed choices of markers for economically important traits to accelerate conventional selection programmes, and for locating genes of potential interest for gene transfer. These applications are discussed in more detail in later sections.

As we have seen in Chapter 2, chromosomes are made up of long double strands of DNA. These strands of DNA are made up of paired bases adenine (A), thymine (T), guanine (G) and cytosine (C). Functional genes are sequences of these bases which form the codes for the production of proteins. However, functional genes are thought to account for less than 3% of the total DNA (the whole genome). The rest of the DNA is either involved in controlling when, and in which tissues, particular genes are switched on, or its function is unknown at present.

The ultimate purpose of a genome (or gene) map is to describe the location of genes, or other sequences of functional DNA, on each of the chromosomes of the species concerned. The enormity of this task will be easier to appreciate from some statistics on the genomes of mammals. The genomes of mammals are estimated to be composed of 3000 million base pairs, and to contain at least 25,000 genes, averaging about 3000 base pairs each. If the complete sequence of base pairs for one of these mammalian species was known and was written in a series of books, it would fill 200 volumes, each of 1000 pages. For comparison, the genomes of fruit flies, yeast and the bacterium *Escherichia coli* would take up 10 books, 1 book and 300 pages, respectively (US Department of Energy, 1992).

A range of methods have been developed over the years to map the genome and a number of different mapping criteria have been developed. These include *physical mapping* methods such as *linkage maps* and cytogenetic maps, but a full description of them are outside the scope of this book. An advanced text such as Russell (2014) provides much useful background material on these techniques. Figure 5.8 illustrates some of the different types of map used and their levels of resolution. With the advent of whole-genome sequencing (WGS) methods it has become possible to locate 'genes' on an animal's chromosomes using the order of bases found in the DNA sequence of each chromosome. This has led to a number of breakthroughs in genetic methodology which have already become applied in practice, many based on publicly available databases of molecular genetic information.

Whole-genome sequencing methods

As indicated earlier, DNA sequencing is the process of determining the order of nucleotides in DNA. It has been widely used in studying human and livestock genomes and led to practical applications in many fields of study. *Sanger sequencing* was the initial widely used method. It is also known as dideoxy or capillary electrophoresis sequencing. It was developed by Frederick Sanger and colleagues in 1977 but was commercialized by Applied Biosystems in the 1980s. It is based on the selective incorporation of chain-terminating dideoxynucleotides by DNA polymerase, a DNA synthesizing enzyme, during *in vitro* DNA replication. In other words, DNA polymerase adds fluorescent nucleotides

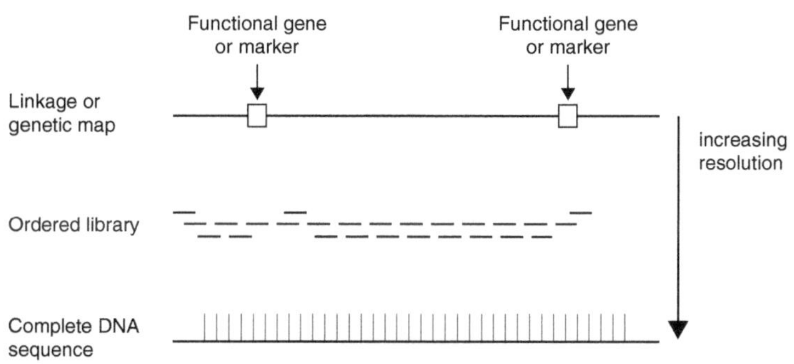

Fig. 5.8. A schematic diagram illustrating some of the different types of map used in human and livestock genome mapping, and their levels of resolution. (After Billings *et al.*, 1991.)

one by one onto a growing DNA template strand, with each incorporated nucleotide identified by its fluorescent tag. The Sanger method only sequences a single DNA fragment at a time. This limits its application to small-scale analysis of specific regions of the genome. The advent of *next-generation* or *second-generation sequencing* (NGS) methods which are highly scalable, has transformed the field of molecular biology, making it possible for the entire genome to be sequenced at once. In general, the concepts behind Sanger sequencing and NGS are similar, but NGS is massively parallel, i.e. it sequences millions of fragments simultaneously per run of a sequencing instrument. NGS involves fragmenting the genome into small pieces, randomly sampling for a fragment, and sequencing it using one of a variety of technologies. Thus, the entire genome can easily be sequenced because many millions of fragments (or reads) are sequenced at once in an automated process. NGS also offers the added advantage of being more sensitive to detecting low-frequency, rare and novel sequences (called variants), and so gives a more comprehensive coverage of the genome. Note that single base-position variants are sometimes referred to as *single-nucleotide variants* (SNVs) in papers dealing with NGS, but SNVs are essentially the same as SNPs but can include insertions and deletions (indels) as well.

Generally, DNA sequencing involves a sequence assembly stage which aligns and merges DNA fragment sequences in order to reconstruct the original sequence. This may involve assembling reads against an existing backbone (called a *reference sequence* or *reference genome*), building a sequence that is similar but not necessarily identical to the backbone sequence. However, in some cases, there is no reference sequence and building the genome sequence is referred to as *de novo sequencing*, i.e. determining the sequence of DNA with no previously known sequence for alignment. The term '*de novo*' is a Latin phrase meaning 'from the beginning'. The process of *de novo* genome sequencing involves the sequencing of small DNA fragments and assembling them into longer sequences (called '*contigs*', short for contiguous sequences) and finally ordering the contigs to obtain the entire genome sequence. The coverage quality of *de novo* sequence data depends on the size and continuity of the contigs, that is, the number of gaps in the data. Gaps in the assembled sequence may be filled by primer walking, which is a sequencing method for sequencing DNA fragments between 1.3 and 7 kilobases (kb) in length. Such fragments are too long to be sequenced in a single sequence read but the method works by dividing the long sequence into several consecutive short ones. For large genomes, *shotgun sequencing* is often used; this is designed for analysis of DNA sequences longer than 1000 base pairs, up to and including entire chromosomes. This requires the target DNA to be broken into random fragments. After sequencing individual fragments, the sequences can be reassembled on the basis of their overlapping regions; however, the assembly is complex, particularly with sequence repeats often causing gaps in the genome assembly. You may see a genome described as having 10× coverage. This means that the sequencing has been carried out ten times on average per section of the genome and we usually expect genomes with higher coverage to be more accurate representations of the sequence.

In more recent years, long-read sequencing technology (also called 'third-generation' sequencing) has begun to supersede short-read sequencing for assembly of reference genomes. The increased capability and reduced cost of third-generation long-read sequencing technology as delivered by Pacific Biosciences and Oxford Nanopore platforms, have allowed the rapid generation of high quality and contiguous reference genome sequences for several livestock species, and the long reads can also be applied to fill gaps in previous reference genome assemblies generated from short reads.

Sequence databases

Generating genome sequences is expensive, so it is efficient to make data available for other researchers, to improve the accuracies of research outcomes and reduce overall cost. This has given rise to databases for various types of sequence. A sequence database is typically a biological database stored on a computer, composed of publicly available nucleic acid or protein sequences. The databases contain both genomic and expressed nucleotide sequences (sequences derived from the genome by transcription and translation) from essentially all organisms for which some sequence data has been determined. They are very valuable to researchers as they enable them to analyse, query and retrieve nucleotide sequences for various scientific purposes, such as investigating a specific gene, or set of genes, related to a trait of interest.

A variety of bioinformatics tools are available to interrogate the sequence databases. One of the most common uses of these tools is searching for sequences similar to a certain gene whose sequence is already known to us, using programs such as BLAST, SAMtools or Clustal. BLAST is an algorithm for comparing primary biological sequence information from the nucleotides of DNA sequences; Clustal is a series of computer programs used for comparing multiple sequences; and SAMtools is a set of utilities for interacting with, and analysing, short DNA sequences.

The sequence databases may be classified on the basis of the sequences they hold. The three most comprehensive nucleotide databases which comprise the 'International Nucleotide Sequence Database Collaboration' and hold sequence data for more than 160,000 species are GenBank (2019), ENA the European Nucleotide Archive (2019) and DDBJ, the DNA DataBank of Japan (2019).

Examples of protein and protein sequence databases include: Entrez Protein, Swiss-Prot, PIR-International: Protein Information Resource and PDB: Protein Data Bank. An example of database on genomes and maps is Entrez Genome.

There are other specialized databases containing information on individual organisms, specific categories/functions of sequences, or data from specific sequencing technologies. Some examples of specific categories or function sequences include TRANSFAC (Transcription Factors and Vector Database) and organism specific sequences include the Mouse Genome Database. Other databases like KEGG (2019) contain a vast array of useful information for following up on individual genes, proteins or biological pathways.

These are just some current examples of useful resources for livestock genomics, but they may change, be updated and new ones added in time.

Current status of livestock genomes

The first draft of the human genome sequence was completed in 2001, but it was several years later that the genomes of most livestock species were delivered. The first sequence of the cow was in 2004 and then those for the chicken, horse, pig, rabbit and sheep followed in 2005, 2007, 2010, 2014 and 2014, respectively. As mentioned earlier, the availability of these genome sequences not only offers researchers the opportunity to study the structure of the genome and genes related to performance traits or diseases, but also provides a useful reference for faster and more accurate assembly of new WGS data from other animals of the same species. An outcome of genome-sequencing projects is the publication of the total size of the genome specific to each species. The size for the chicken genome is 1.2 gigabase pairs (Gbp), 2.5 Gbp for pig and horse, 2.6 Gbp for sheep, 2.7 Gbp for rabbit and cow, and 3 Gbp for Atlantic salmon. The human genome is slightly larger at 3.1 Gbp. See Blasco and Pena (2018) for more details on each of these genomes in terms of the number of protein-coding genes, non-coding genes, gene transcripts and sequence variants.

Details of the genomes of all the farmed species covered in this book can be found at NCBI (2019) by entering the appropriate species name. To increase the usefulness of genome sequences, the various regions of the genome, and the possible function they perform, are usually identified. This process is called *genome annotation* and the next section discusses this in greater detail.

Genome maps of the major livestock species are freely available on websites such as the UCSC *genome browser* (UCSC, 2019) or ENSEMBL (Fig. 5.9; ENSEMBL, 2019). At its basic level, these genome maps comprise a string of bases (A, C, G or T) from the start of each chromosome, for each chromosome in turn. The basis of a genome map for a particular species is what is called a reference genome; often the DNA from a single animal of that species. These are constantly updated and refined and so the version of the reference genome used is critical when describing any results. For example, the notation Chr11:423192 of Btau UMD3.1 refers to a position 423,192 bases from the start on chromosome 11 of the cattle (*Bos taurus*) genome using a variation of the third build of the genome developed by the University of Maryland. By referring to the ENSEMBL website it is possible to see the species and the versions of the genome of all publicly-available sequenced organisms. Since the reference genome is a long string of base letters (A, C, G and T) and is not much use on its own, it clearly needs further explanation and information.

As an aside, you may come across positions on a chromosome expressed in '*morgans*' or *centimorgans* (cM). This refers to an older system of mapping genes implemented before WGS methods were available. This unit of measurement is named after the scientist who first proposed the method, Thomas Morgan. A centimorgan is defined as the distance between two positions on a chromosome with a 1% chance of being separated by a crossing-over

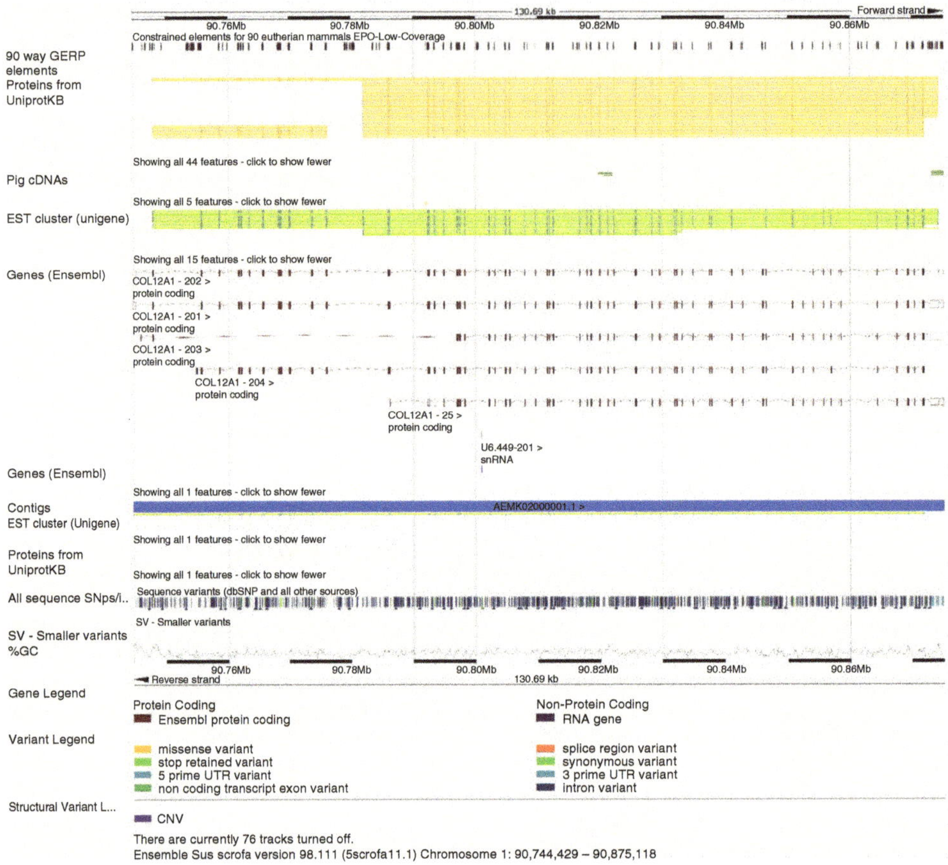

Fig. 5.9. Output from a genome browser (ENSEMBL; https://www.ensembl.org/) showing detailed information for a given region of a livestock genome assembly (in this case *Sus scrofa* (pig)) version 11.1, Chromosome 1, 90,774,429–90,875,118. Predicted genes and proteins are shown, conserved regions across other mammals, genome contigs, polymorphic variants and their potential functional consequences, and putative structural variants. There are also many additional 'tracks' that can be used to highlight other features and data associated with the region.

event in a single generation. This may seem a rather odd definition in the modern era, but it is based on test matings between organisms with known versions of two or more genes and noting how many offspring showed recombination. It is not as precise a method of locating genes on a chromosome as WGS but the two systems clearly have some equivalence.

The reference genome for any given species is just a starting point since each animal may have a different base at any given position. Actually, many base positions show no variation at all for a number of very good reasons. Perhaps the most important of these is that many genes need to be conserved from one generation to the next (and even one species to another) in order to preserve basic biological functions. For example, the genes controlling all aspects of breathing in mammals need to be maintained in a fairly similar form from one generation to the next, in order for the animals to live and thrive. Obviously, several mutations do occur each generation, as discussed in Chapter 2, but the process of evolution ensures that those changes that are detrimental are lost and only changes that confer some advantage to the animal, or are neutral in effect, survive.

Variation from the reference genome at many sites is expected and these variations (the previously described polymorphisms or variants) form the basis of mapping projects to chart such differences found within a species. So, for example, the 1000 Bull Genomes Project (2019) aims to collect WGS sequences from 1000 animals in order to explore the variation that exists at the genome level in cattle. At the time of writing this project has collected data on over 2700 cattle and identified more than 88 million variants, about 3% of the genome. It is these variants that provide the material for improving the traits of interest in our livestock breeding programmes, but we need to know which ones are useful and how best to use the information gathered.

One of the broader results of the molecular genomic revolution has been the burgeoning understanding gained on the various functions of the genome. Clearly the protein-coding sections of the genome (often loosely referred to as genes) play a crucial rôle in the underlying biology of our species of interest. Having a reference genome for a species does not tell us about the function of any part of the genome. Additional resources are required to place the genes of interest at particular points on the genome, and this process is known as genome annotation. Currently, RNA sequencing of selected tissues of an animal, often at different developmental time points, can be used to provide data for a comprehensive annotation of a species' reference genome (discussed in the section immediately below). *Gene mapping* was going on before WGS techniques were available, but the new methodology has provided an added tool to locate genes precisely. QTL databases predate WGS methods and provide a source of information about the approximate position of genes affecting livestock traits. With the advent of WGS methodology it has become possible to identify protein-coding regions (often called CDSs, from *coding sequence*) using bioinformatic methods. It is outside the scope of this book to discuss these methods but websites such as UCSC (2019) or ENSEMBL (2019) contain links to gene information from any chromosome position on the genome. In addition, the NCBI (2019) website contains links to all known genes in many species. This 'gene' information not only includes the CDS regions but also an ever-increasing range of DNA features, as outlined in Chapter 2.

Also, the Animal QTL database (Hu *et al.*, 2019) provides a useful source of reference for the species covered in this book. It provides a number of search options including searching for information on traits, breeds, publications, genes of interest (called *candidate genes*) and tools for data analysis. It also gives access to genome browsers to visually search for chromosome features and provides downloads of sequences for further analysis. No doubt databases like this will evolve over the coming years to provide a more comprehensive set of tools for animal breeders to use.

Genome annotation

After the sequences are established, the next step when building a genome map is to annotate the genetic elements underlying each genome. This annotation step is constantly evolving as new elements are still being discovered. The word annotate means 'to add critical or explanatory notes or comment'. *Genome annotation* therefore involves the process of attaching biological information to sequences to increase their usefulness and enhance practical application. It consists of two main steps of initially identifying elements on the genome, a process called gene prediction and referred to as *structural annotation*, followed by the second step of attaching biological information to these elements, usually referred to as *functional annotation*. Structural annotation involves identification of genomic elements such as coding regions, gene structure, transposons, repeats, location of regulatory motifs (short nucleotide sequences that control the expression of genes), and the identification of open reading frames (ORF) and their locations. ORF are continuous stretches of codons that begin with a start codon (usually ATG) and end at a stop codon (usually TAA, TAG or TGA), codons marking the beginning and end of protein-coding regions. The functional annotation involves allocating biological information such as biochemical, regulatory and biological functions and gene expression to genomic elements. It is aimed at understanding how the individual components of a biological system work together to produce a particular protein or phenotype. RNA sequencing has been widely applied to annotate transcribed regions of reference genomes, and other techniques allow mapping of putative transcription factor binding sites and other genome features, which are key to the regulation of gene expression.

Annotation is usually carried out automatically using sophisticated software packages based on sequence or structure comparisons. At times, the annotation process may involve biological experimentation or gene expression studies. Results from different organizations working in this area are in publicly available databases. Examples include: Encyclopaedia of DNA elements (ENCODE), GENCODE, ENSEMBL, Entrez Gene, Gene Ontology Consortium GeneRIF and RefSeq.

Use of molecular markers in selection

Two main applications of individual molecular markers prior to the availability of genome-wide SNP assays are initially considered in this section before examining methods based on SNP markers. The first is the use of markers to assist in the introduction of a single gene with a favourable effect from one population into another. For example, there may be interest in introducing a single gene controlling polledness or resistance to a disease to a different breed, cross or family. The traditional route for introducing a gene of this sort is to cross the current preferred breed to a breed carrying the gene of interest, and then backcross to the original preferred breed for several generations. Molecular markers may be useful in identifying animals carrying the favoured allele, and so help speed up the 'recovery' of the rest of the original genetic makeup. This type of application is called *marker-assisted introgression (MAI)*. The second application is the use of markers to accelerate selection for a particular trait within a population. In this case, the aim of using markers is simply to boost the improvement made by conventional means, by 'homing in' on genes already present in the breed concerned. This use of markers is called marker-assisted selection (MAS).

In both MAI and MAS, the gene of interest may be either a single gene with a large effect (*major gene*), such as those affecting coat colour, polledness and double muscling, or it may be one of many genes affecting a quantitative trait of interest, such as milk yield and quality, growth rate or wool production. These are QTL as discussed above.

In addition to these two applications, molecular markers can provide a more definitive test of ancestry. For instance, the probability of excluding an incorrect parentage can increase from one in a few thousand using 12 traditional blood type markers, to one in several million by using between 5 and 10 DNA-based markers (Haley *et al.*, 1996). This makes the techniques very powerful for pedigree verification in livestock (and of great value in forensic science). They are also valuable as an alternative to pedigree recording at birth in difficult or very extensive management systems (e.g. in fish breeding or where breeding animals are kept under extensive range conditions). Similarly, the techniques could be used to confirm the breed of animals or their products. This is popular where branding animal products on their breed of origin is critical (e.g. retailers in several countries sell beef specifically labelled as from Aberdeen Angus crosses, or 'traditional' beef breeds, lamb from traditional hill breeds and milk from specified breeds including the Channel Island and Ayrshire breeds).

Molecular markers are also useful in ensuring that breeds or individuals carrying particularly rare or useful genes are included in conservation programmes. A related application of the techniques is in the control of inbreeding in selection or conservation programmes. As we saw in Chapter 4, inbreeding coefficients estimate the average level of inbreeding of offspring from a particular mating. In fact, there will be some variation around this average because, by chance, some offspring receive more and some receive fewer genes than average from the common ancestor. Molecular markers can be used to identify those offspring that receive fewer genes than average from the common ancestor, and so are less inbred than average for that group of sibs (see Moore *et al.* (2019) for an example of using SNP data to investigate relatedness and pedigree).

The choice of markers and methods of establishing a link between a marker and a trait of interest are outlined next, before giving more detailed examples of the use of markers in MAI and MAS.

Choice of markers

The ideal marker for both MAI and MAS would be the causative polymorphism which has a direct effect on the trait of interest, or a shorter sequence of DNA or a SNP very close to this causative polymorphism. Causative polymorphisms may typically occur in a gene, or close to a gene where they may act by regulating expression of that gene. For example, the ideal marker for selecting for polledness would be the mutation/polymorphism coding for polledness itself. This means that selection on the 'marker' always delivers the expected genotype. However, most markers are not the causative polymorphisms themselves but are nearby linked markers in LD with the gene. In these cases, it is important to recognize that the marker and the causative polymorphism will sometimes become separated from each other from one generation to the next, because of recombination. The more closely linked the marker and the causative polymorphism, the less often this will happen, and the more useful the marker is. Using WGS methodology it is possible to find a SNP marker with a very close association between the marker and the causative polymorphism, or the polymorphism itself. For MAI of a favourable allele between two very different breeds, it should be relatively easy to find a close marker which will remain associated with the trait of interest for long enough to be useful, because the two breeds are likely to have different genotypes at many loci. This situation is illustrated in Fig. 5.10. However, within a population the same marker allele may be associated with favourable performance in one family, and unfavourable performance in another. This arises because the two genes have been segregating in the population for many generations, so there have been many opportunities for recombination. Hence, for MAS it is important that markers are identified and used within families. This situation is illustrated in Fig. 5.11.

There are two main approaches to choosing markers to investigate whether or not they are linked to traits of interest:

- **The map-based approach.** If WGS data are available, then this is the best way to locate good markers. This may be too expensive in some circumstances so a suitable SNP chip coupled with *genome-wide association study* (GWAS) methodology, as outlined below, can indicate a suitable marker to use.
- **The candidate gene approach.** In this case a known mapped gene may be chosen because it has a similar function to the gene of interest and may be linked to it. For example, a mapped gene with a major effect on disease resistance in one

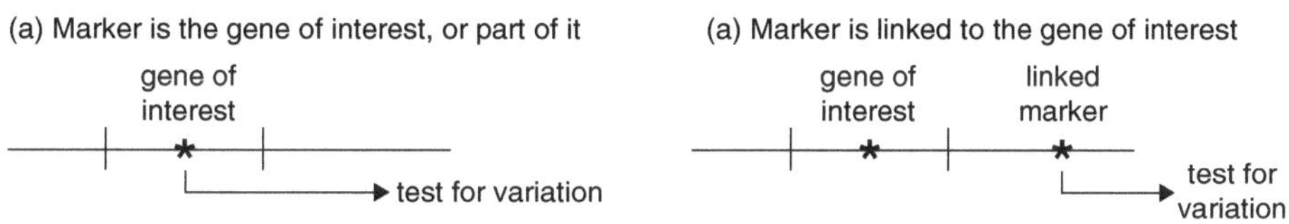

Fig. 5.10. Two possible uses of markers. (a) In the first case a test is available for the gene of interest directly (i.e. the marker is the gene responsible for the trait of interest, or it is a shorter sequence of DNA within this gene). (b) In the second case the marker is not the gene of interest, but it is closely linked to this. In the initial generations of crossing between divergent breeds or lines it should be possible to find markers in which one marker genotype is always associated with favourable performance, since the two breeds are heterozygous at many loci. However, following many generations of selection in offspring from these initial crosses, this linkage will break down because of recombination. The more closely linked the marker and the gene of interest, the longer it will take for this association to break down. (After Womack, 1996.)

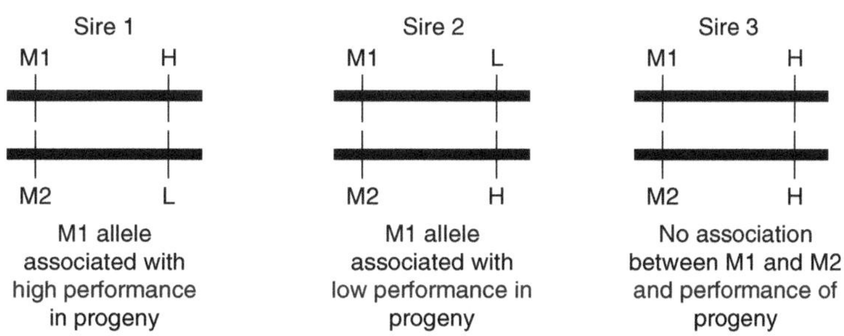

Fig. 5.11. Marker and QTL genotypes for three sires within a breed, and the expected association between marker genotype and performance in progeny of these three sires. One marker allele may be associated with favourable performance in some families, and unfavourable performance in others. This arises because the two alleles have been segregating in the population for many generations, so there have been many opportunities for recombination. Hence for MAS within a breed it is important that markers are identified and used within families. (Source: Haley, 1995.)

species would be an ideal candidate as a marker for a similar disease in another closely related species. Similarly, within a species, a candidate gene may be chosen because it has a known function linked to the trait of interest (e.g. a gene coding for a hormone affecting milk yield may be investigated as a marker for yield).

Establishing a link between a marker and a trait of interest

The linkage-based methods, outlined in the previous version of this book (Simm, 1998), to establish markers for genes and traits of interest have been superseded by the widespread use of genome-wide association studies (see below). Such studies typically use an appropriate SNP chip or SNPs produced from WGS in conjunction with the appropriate physical performance data from the population under study. There are many GWAS studies in the livestock species and a key development is the use of databases of results to highlight genes of interest. The OMIA database and the AnimalQTLdb are two such repositories of information on livestock. It is expected that others will follow.

An example of marker-assisted introgression

The introduction of the polled gene from a polled breed of cattle to a horned breed provides a good example of MAI. In most countries, hornless cattle are preferred to horned cattle, because of the reduced risk of injury to humans and other cattle. However, many popular breeds are horned, so calves need to be dehorned at a young age. This is costly and may compromise the welfare of the calf in the short term, even if it improves it in the long term. In most western breeds of cattle, the polled allele (P) is dominant over the recessive horned allele (p) (Allais-Bonnet *et al.*, 2013). In some breeds both the horned and polled types are present. Also, occasional mutations to the polled type occur within breeds which are normally horned, and animals with this mutation could be useful in programmes to introduce polledness. However, since mutations are rare, polled strains of breeds which are normally horned can be established by crossing to animals from a polled breed followed by backcrossing to the original breed. This could be achieved without the use of markers by the following steps, which are also illustrated in Fig. 5.12:

1. Mate horned cows of the preferred breed A to bulls of a polled breed B. All the resulting calves will be heterozygous polled animals (Pp), with 50% of their genes from breed A and 50% from breed B.
2. Mate the F_1 crossbred females back to bulls of the preferred breed A. This will result in calves of two genotypes with respect to polledness; on average half of the calves will be heterozygous polled animals (Pp), and half homozygous horned animals (pp). The calves will now average 75% breed A genes and 25% breed B genes.
3. Backcross only the polled (Pp) animals to breed A again. About half of the calves will be heterozygous polled and half will be homozygous horned animals, as before. The calves now average 87.5% breed A genes and 12.5% breed B genes.
4. Repeat step 3 until the proportion of genes from the preferred breed is high enough (e.g. overall performance is close to that of pure breed A animals, or the proportion of breed A genes is high enough to allow pedigree registration).
5. Mate graded-up heterozygous polled animals to each other. This will produce three genotypes of calves: 25% PP (homozygous polled - the desired genotype), 50% Pp (heterozygous polled) and 25% pp (horned) on average.
6. Progeny test polled bulls by mating them to horned cows. Those which are homozygous polled will never produce horned calves. On average, heterozygous polled bulls will produce horned calves from 50% of matings to horned cows. About seven polled calves (and no horned calves) would need to be produced from matings to horned cows to be 99% sure of detecting a heterozygous polled bull.
7. Select and breed from homozygous polled bulls only.

Step 6 in the above procedure is very time consuming and expensive but it can be completely abolished by using the widely available SNP markers for polledness to distinguish between homozygous and heterozygous polled animals. Similarly, in breeds with both horned and polled animals present already, markers could be used to identify homozygous polled animals (this would be an example of MAS rather than MAI).

In steps 2 to 5 above it was possible to eliminate 50% or 25% of the animals (the horned ones) from the grading-up programme by visual inspection. MAI could be of even more value if the aim is to introgress genes for a trait which cannot be readily observed in the animals or is expensive or difficult

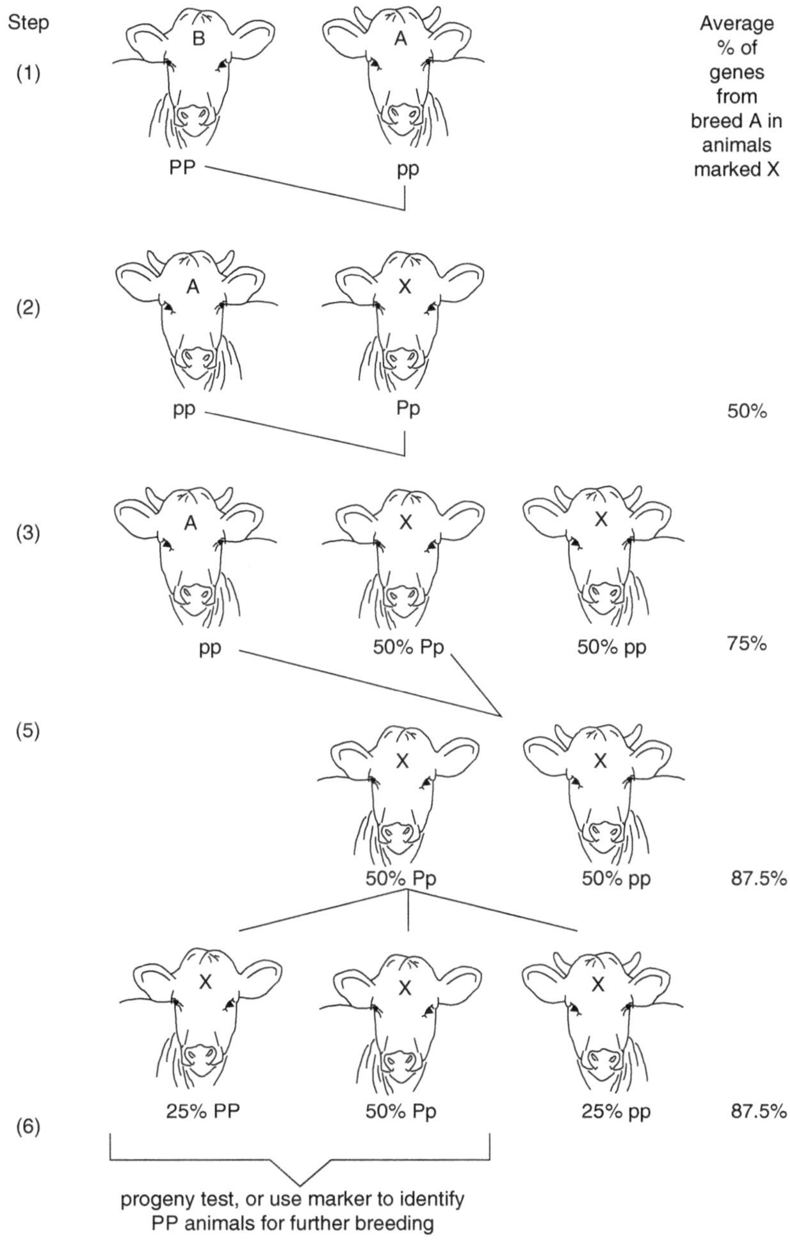

Fig. 5.12. The steps involved in a backcrossing programme to introduce the polled gene from breed B to a horned breed, breed A. The diagram shows only two generations of backcrossing to breed A after the initial cross between breeds A and B. This produces offspring with an average of 87.5% of their genes from breed A, which are then interbred. Further generations of backcrossing could be undertaken if a higher proportion of breed A was required.

to measure. Also, markers in other regions of the genome, apart from the one being introduced, can be used to identify and exclude animals with a high proportion of genes from the least desirable breed in the backcrossing programme.

Disease resistance genes, or genes affecting traits seen in only one sex, or post slaughter, could all be potential candidates for MAI. This approach has been used by some pig breeding companies in crosses between Chinese and European breeds. The aim is to introgress genes conferring high litter size from the Meishan (Chinese) breed while maintaining the higher genetic merit for growth and carcass traits of the European breeds. MAS is most suitable for traits where the genetics is such that a major QTL explains a high proportion of the genetic variation, and otherwise it has largely been superseded by genomic selection.

Although MAI is more efficient than alternative programmes without molecular markers, all grading-up programmes of this sort are time consuming and costly. Also, there is often little scope to select for traits of economic importance, other than the one being introgressed. So, before embarking on a MAI programme, it is important to check whether the economic benefits at the end of the programme are likely to exceed those which could have been obtained by continuing conventional selection (Visscher and Haley, 1995). A good example of this sort of analysis was reported by Gootwine *et al.* (2001) for introgressing the Booroola gene into Israeli dairy sheep breeds.

Gene editing (discussed in more detail below) can provide an alternative to MAI, because theoretically it is possible to directly introduce the favourable allele into the recipient population of interest in a single generation. Furthermore, editing also allows favourable alleles in closely related species to be inserted into target populations in a way that would not be possible with MAI. An example is the creation of genome-edited polled cattle (Carlson *et al.*, 2016) mentioned above.

An example of marker-assisted selection

For the purposes of illustration, a good example of MAS in dairy cattle breeding in the 1990s was in the selection of dairy bulls for progeny testing by some companies in the US. This has now been superseded by the application of genomic methods which are discussed later. The aim was to improve the accuracy of identifying high merit young bulls for progeny testing. This involved the use of markers at the loci controlling the secretion of the milk proteins κ-casein and β-lactoglobulin. There are two alleles segregating at each locus, abbreviated to A and B in both cases. The B allele at the κ-casein locus has favourable effects on milk processing properties, so there may be benefits in direct selection on genotype. However, the genotypes at these loci also serve as linked markers, within sire families, for QTL affecting the milk, fat and protein yields and fat:protein ratios (Cowan, 1994; Gambra *et al.*, 2013).

This is illustrated in Table 5.2, which shows the mean *predicted transmitting ability* (PTA) for sons of three double heterozygous Holstein Friesian bulls (i.e. these grandsires were heterozygous at both the κ-casein and β-lactoglobulin loci). Sons with the genotypes AA for κ-casein and BB for β-lactoglobulin have the poorest PTAs for milk and protein yield, and the highest (i.e. worst in many western milk markets) fat:protein ratio. Conversely, the genotypes BB for κ-casein and AA for β-lactoglobulin had the highest PTAs for protein, and lower (i.e. better) fat:protein ratios. The most favourable combination of genotypes will depend on the current milk pricing policy in the country concerned. However, based on US prices at the time, the sires with the five 'best' genotypes had PTAs which were 108 kg milk and 1.9 kg protein higher than the overall average, and had PTAs for protein 4.0 kg higher than their PTAs for kg fat (Cowan, 1994).

Table 5.2. Mean predicted transmitting abilities (PTAs) for the sons of three Holstein Friesian bulls heterozygous at both the κ-casein and β-lactoglobulin loci. (Source: Cowan, 1994.)

κ-Casein genotype		β-Lactoglobulin genotype		
		AA	AB	BB
AA	No. sons	7	20	11
	PTA milk kg	458.0	592.0	427.0
	PTA protein kg	19.3	18.9	14.0
	PTA fat kg	22.3	23.3	22.3
AB	No. sons	7	19	20
	PTA milk kg	754.0	680.0	601.0
	PTA protein kg	22.3	19.7	18.4
	PTA fat kg	19.1	19.5	23.1
BB	No. sons	6	4	3
	PTA milk kg	732.0	690.0	781.0
	PTA protein kg	26.2	18.2	23.2
	PTA fat kg	18.2	16.0	19.0

A larger study on markers for QTL in dairy cattle involved 14 elite Holstein Friesian sire families in the US, with a total of 1500 progeny tested sons (Georges *et al.*, 1995). This study showed evidence of chromosomal regions associated with effects of up to +8 kg on protein production and +300 kg milk on milk production.

With the advent of genomic selection (see below), the use of MAS at single QTL is now limited to cases where a large proportion of the genetic variation in the trait is explained by a single QTL, for example resistance to the viral disease infectious pancreatic necrosis in salmon (Houston *et al.*, 2008), and subsequent application of MAS to reduce mortalities due to this disease (discussed in more detail in Chapter 13).

Genome-wide association studies

The advent of SNP chips has spawned the development of so-called GWAS to investigate the concordance between known phenotypic differences and differences at particular points on the genome (see Bush and Moore (2012) for a review). GWAS are based on the association between differences in phenotype for a specific trait and the known SNP genotypes at individual loci derived from SNP chip data. At its basic level we may use GWAS to seek to answer a question like 'Is calf mortality associated with one particular genotype at the loci on our SNP chip?' (see Brickell *et al.* (2010) as an example). Each SNP can have two versions (say A and T) so the two chromosomes of a homologous pair can have AA, AT or TT, referred to as genotypes. At each informative SNP (i.e. one where there are differences in genotype in our population under study) we carry out some form of statistical test to see if there is an association between one of the three genotypes and calf mortality, a categorical trait with two values (alive or dead).

There are several types of test that we could apply at each SNP, depending on the trait being analysed. This might be a chi-squared test with a 3×2 table of incidences, as in the case of mortality mentioned above. For quantitative traits we could apply an allele substitution regression at each SNP. This involves fitting a model such as a regression equation substituting one SNP at a time as the independent variable (right-hand side of the regression equation) with the trait of interest as the dependent variable (left-hand side of the regression equation). To ensure that the pedigree relationships in the population being studied do not influence the results, the *genomic relationship matrix* or some other measure of known relationships is included in the form of mixed model analysis. (These concepts are discussed more in Chapters 6 and 7.) The SNPs used in such studies could be derived from SNP chips (e.g. 50K or 800K) or derived from whole-genome sequences or genotyping by sequencing. Normally a probability threshold level (p value) is set to determine which SNP will be considered to have a significant effect on the trait. With one SNP being fitted at a time, multiple tests are carried out on the same data to determine which SNP has a significant effect. This multiple testing using the same data set increases the chance of obtaining false-positive results (called a type I error in statistics). In other words, the probability of identifying at least one significant result due to chance increases as more hypotheses are tested. To reduce the chance of a type 1 error, a *Bonferroni correction* is usually applied (Dunn, 1961). The Bonferroni correction involves testing each individual hypothesis at a significance level of $-\log10(\alpha/n)$, where α is the desired overall significant level (p value) and n is the number of hypotheses or SNPs being tested. For example, if we are testing n = 2000 SNPs, with a desired $\alpha = 0.05$, then the Bonferroni correction would test each individual hypothesis at $-\log10(\alpha/2000)$ = $-\log10(0.05/2000) = 4.602$. Usually the profiles of the p values presented as $-\log10(p$ values) for all SNPs on each chromosome (y-axis) is plotted against each chromosome (x-axis) and is usually called a Manhattan plot. It presents a summary of the GWAS results and indicates which chromosomes harbour SNPs of significant effects. As an example, Fig. 5.13 shows a Manhattan plot for the causal mutation of the Lavender Foal Syndrome (Brooks *et al.*, 2010 as published in the supplementary material of Pollott, 2018). This plot is the result of carrying out a chi-squared test at each of 36,651 SNPs based on a 3×2 table of SNP genotype and disease status.

An alternative to fitting one SNP at a time is fitting models to several adjacent SNPs together to try to account for LD, or to use a genome-wide method such as SSGBLUP (outlined in Chapter 7) which can provide solutions at each SNP. There are several software packages available for GWAS including PLINK (Purcell *et al.*, 2007; Chang *et al.*, 2015), a standalone download; Bioconductor, a set of routines based on open source software in R (R Development Core Team, 2013) and a host of

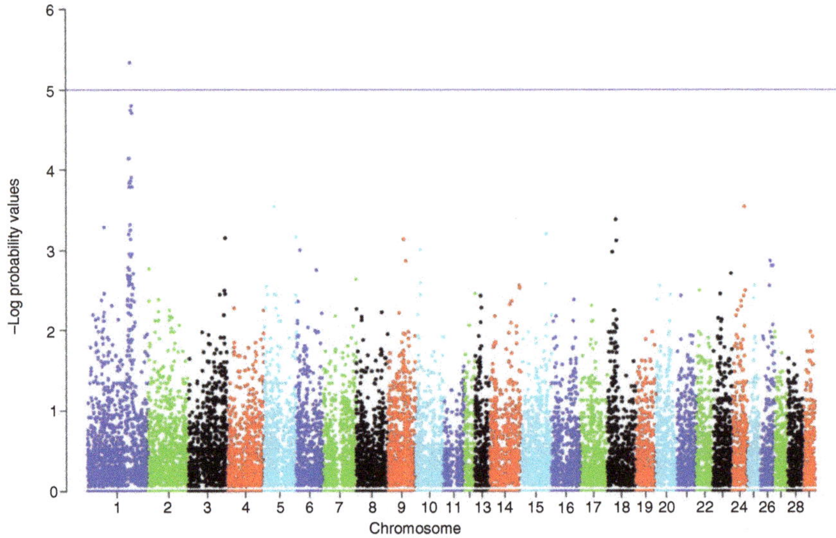

Fig. 5.13. Results of analysing the Lavender Foal Syndrome data set (Brooks *et al.*, 2010) using a genotypic model (3×2) with Fisher's Exact Test. –Log10 probabilities shown for all 36,651 autosomal single-nucleotide polymorphisms with a minor allele frequency > 0.05. Bonferroni correction value p = 5.85 from Pollott (2018). The bottom axis lists all autosomal chromosomes in order from 1 on the left to 29 on the right. Note that the convention for naming chromosomes means that 1 is the largest and 29 the smallest. (Based on the EquCab2.0 build of the horse genome. Reprinted with permission of Cambridge University Press.)

others. In some cases, the results from GWAS are used in functional analysis to identify putative genes and biochemical pathways to help explain the results obtained. This involves using the genomic annotation files for the relevant species, that are publicly available, and various sophisticated software packages as outlined above.

GWAS have provided much information about the cause of genetic variation in animals in recent years. GWAS have been carried out in several livestock species for various traits. For dairy cattle, for example, a number of significant SNPs have been found in *Bos taurus* autosome 14 (BTA14), which hosts *DGAT1*, a gene with a major effect on milk fat content (Grisart *et al.*, 2002) and several other production traits (Nayeri *et al.*, 2016). Other examples are studies on fertility in dairy using GWAS and functional annotation (Cai *et al.*, 2019; Nani *et al.*, 2019). A catalogue of GWAS results can be found at EBI (2019).

Signatures of selection

Detecting *signatures of selection* provides another approach to linking genomic regions and putative genes with traits of interest. Signatures of selection studies involve detecting regions of the genome which are conserved over many generations due to the fact that they confer enhanced fitness or productive ability to individuals in the population. Such conserved regions are thus preferentially kept in the population, with the frequency of favourable alleles, and of particular haplotypes in the region, driven towards fixation. Such regions, called *selective sweeps*, can be detected by reduced haplotype diversity (or increased homozygosity) and a different LD pattern when compared to those of the surrounding background genome. Signatures of selection studies involve characterizing such regions so that inferences on the functionality of these genomic regions, and possibly the effects of specific genes or gene combinations on specific traits, can be made.

There are several approaches for the detection of selective sweeps but one of the simplest is the Wright's F_{ST} statistic, which is a measure of the degree of genetic differentiation between two populations, and is defined as 'the correlation between gametes chosen randomly from within the same sub-population relative to the entire population'. For instance, two populations may be subjected to different selective pressures, with the alternative alleles being favoured in each population at the loci under selection. This will reduce the heterozygosity in the two populations and, hence, increase their genetic differentiation at these loci (high F_{ST}).

Another approach is the selective sweep analysis which has been used in cattle, chickens and pigs (Rubin *et al.*, 2012) and involves using full genome sequence data. This analysis assesses heterozygosity in pre-specified windows along the genome to identify regions with low heterozygosity relative to the entire genome. Given that positive selection usually leads to a reduction in genomic diversity, then regions with high homozygosity are indicative of selective sweeps.

Also, several other approaches based on the concept of *extended haplotype homozygosity* (EHH) have been applied. The EHH at distance x from a core region can be defined as 'the probability that two randomly chosen chromosomes carrying the core haplotype of interest are identical by descent for the entire interval from the core region to the point x' (Sabeti, *et al.*, 2002). This can be detected when positive selection causes a rapid increase in the frequency of a favourable allele in a short time period, giving rise to an unusually long haplotype.

Functional analysis of the identified genome regions from signatures of selection studies can be achieved using various databases for genome annotation with functional annotation tools and software. Signatures of selection studies have been carried out in various livestock species and an interpretive review of selective sweep studies in *Bos taurus* cattle populations, with the aim of identifying unique and shared selection signals across breeds, was carried by Gutiérrez-Gil *et al.* (2015). They examined 21 genomic studies of European *Bos taurus* breeds, compiled a list of 1049 selection sweeps described across 37 cattle breeds (17 beef breeds, 14 dairy breeds, and 6 dual-purpose breeds), and four different beef versus dairy comparisons. Defining *core selective sweep* (CSS) regions as consecutive signals within 1 Mb of each other, they identified a total of 409 CSS across the 29 bovine autosomes, 232 (57%) of which were associated with a single breed. For each CSS, they performed a candidate gene survey that identified 291 genes within the CSS intervals linked to dairy and meat production, stature, and coat colour traits. A complementary functional enrichment analysis of the CSS positional candidates highlighted other genes related to pathways underlying behaviour, immune response and reproductive traits. Bahbahani *et al.* (2015) examined positive signatures of selection in East African Shorthorn Zebu and identified 24 candidate genome regions with positive signatures of selection within 14 autosomes and the X chromosome. A total of 37 candidate genes were identified in these regions and these genes were involved in various biological pathways related to immunity, reproduction, development and heat tolerance.

Genomic selection

The use of MAS as described above has been largely superseded by the use of SNP-based markers. As we have seen, SNPs which are very close to genes of interest in a DNA sequence on a chromosome tend to be inherited together during the process of meiosis and are therefore said to be in linkage. Such SNPs can therefore be used to predict the genetic merit of animals for the performance traits controlled by those genes. The use of such SNPs to predict the breeding value of animals is called genomic prediction and the predicted genetic merit is called the *direct genomic breeding value* (DGV). The use of DGV to select animals of superior genetic merit for breeding is termed genomic selection (Meuwissen *et al.*, 2001). The details, steps and approaches for the implementation of genomic selection are presented in more detail in Chapter 7.

Genomic selection was implemented for dairy cattle in 2008 in the USA, Canada, Denmark, Sweden, Finland and New Zealand with many other countries following in later years. This method has also been implemented subsequently in pigs, sheep, fish, goats and beef cattle. Briefly, it involves an initial step of genotyping a group of animals, called the *reference population*, with phenotypic records for traits of economic importance. A set of equations, similar to the simultaneous equations mentioned in Chapter 2, are then used to compute the relationship between the SNPs and the phenotypic records. This process estimates the effect of the genes associated with each SNP on the trait. Then the accuracy of these SNP estimates is determined in another group of animals, called the *validation set*, by estimating the genetic merit of these animals using only the SNP solutions. These estimates are then correlated with some measure of the genetic merit of these animals that was based on their phenotypic records. The higher the correlation between the estimates of genetic merit from SNP solutions only and those based on phenotypic records, the more reliable are the SNP estimates. Estimates of these correlations vary from trait to trait but may typically be from 0.40 to 0.75. Once the accuracy of the prediction based only on the SNP solutions is satisfactory, they can be used to compute DGVs of very young animals with no phenotypic records. In some species, selection on the basis of DGVs (genomic selection) predicted early in life, can reduce the generation interval, and so accelerate rate of response. In fish breeding (see Chapter 13), genomic selection capitalizes on information from testing of full sibs for traits difficult, or impossible, to measure on selection candidates. Here, it does not result in a reduction of generation interval, but it does significantly improve accuracy of breeding value prediction due to capturing the within-family genetic variation.

More recently, embryo genomic selection (or preimplantation genetic screening) is being used increasingly to select the best embryos within cattle breeding programmes. The steps involve the collection of a few cells (biopsy) from each of the embryos before they are individually cryopreserved. The biopsy samples are then genotyped with a SNP chip, and the genomic estimated breeding value for each embryo is then computed using prediction equations developed from large reference populations of previously genotyped and phenotyped animals. On the basis on the genomic estimated breeding value, a decision is made whether to transfer the embryo or not. The process has become economically feasible due to the availability of cheap, low-density SNP chips with only a few thousand SNPs. Usually, the genotypes from these low-density chips are imputed (see next section) to a 50K SNP chip or high-density chip of about 700–800K before *genomic breeding values* are computed. Thus embryo genomic selection is being used in breeding programmes to accelerate the rate of genetic gain compared to animal-based genomic selection.

Genotype imputation

Genotype *imputation* refers to the process of predicting genotypes that are not directly measured in a sample of individuals genotyped using a low-density SNP chip. The prediction uses data from animals genotyped using a higher density SNP chip. This is usually done to increase the number of genotypes in a sample of animals, to increase the accuracy of genomic prediction and GWAS. The initial SNP chips developed for the application of genomics to livestock in the mid-2000s were the 50K SNP chip for cattle by Illumina (2019b) and the bovine high-density (HD) SNP chips with 700 to 800K SNPs developed by Illumina (2019c) and Affymetrix (2019). These were followed by other 50K SNP and HD chips for sheep, goats and chickens. The use of these chips for the genotyping of individual animals was expensive, thereby limiting the total number of animals that could be genotyped. In an attempt to reduce genotyping cost, several low-density chips with 3–20K SNPs were developed by Illumina and Affymetrix. To increase the accuracy of genomic breeding values when these low-density chips are used in genomic prediction, the genotypes of animals are usually imputed to either that of the 50K or HD chips. The SNPs in the low-density chips are mostly a subset of those in the 50K or HD chips. Therefore imputation is like doing a crossword, with the genotypes of animals in the 50K or HD chips that are missing in the low-density chips filled in using pedigree information (if available) and information on SNPs that are in LD (haplotypes). In the most recent genomic evaluation of UK dairy cattle, information was included from over 37 different types of SNP chips, with 10 of these being responsible for 96% of the information.

There are several algorithms that have been applied in the imputation process (see Marchini and Howie (2010) for a review) but the approach usually involves a set of animals called the reference animals which are genotyped with the target SNP chip. For instance, if we want to impute the genotypes of some animals to the 50K chip, then the reference population will consist of animals genotyped with the 50K chip. The larger the size of the reference population, the higher the accuracy of our imputation. Using the reference population, a group of animals with low-density data are imputed to the target SNP chip using software packages such as Beagle, FImpute, Minimac and Alphaimpute. The accuracy of imputation is computed by masking some of the genotypes of a subset of animals genotyped with the target SNP chip. Then imputation is undertaken with the masked genotypes imputed in this subset of animals. The concordance of imputed genotypes with actual genotypes which were masked in the subset of animals give a measure of accuracy. Imputation accuracies of about 95–99% have been reported for imputing several LD chips to 50K or HD chips in livestock data. In aquaculture, imputation from very LD panels genotyped on offspring to HD panels genotyped on parents has been shown to be highly cost effective, as described in more detail in Chapter 13.

Genetic engineering

Genetic engineering relates to the direct manipulation of an animal's genes using biotechnology. It has been widely researched in farmed livestock. The high level of conservation of DNA between species means that there are prospects for the transfer of genes not only within species, but also between species, and potentially even between different classes of organism. The initial efforts in livestock focused on *transgenesis*, which is the insertion of DNA from another organism into the genome of a target organism (see Figs 5.14 and 5.15). This was initially achieved via direct injection of exogenous DNA into embryos at the one-cell stage. This allowed the insertion of gene constructs but without control of the location and indeed the timing of integration (in terms of embryo development) of the construct into the recipient's genome (Laible *et al.*, 2015).

Genetic engineering approaches have been used to insert or remove genes, or other sections of an animal's genome, and have been widely applied to assess gene function. An animal resulting from genetic engineering is considered to be genetically modified (GM). Genetic engineering has the potential to improve animal production, for example via the insertion of a gene from a different breed or species that has a favourable impact on production or disease resistance traits. Genetically engineered crops with resistance to disease or herbicides have become widely used globally with reported benefits to farmers and processors. However, the technology and its applications are controversial, with strong opposition from certain groups, and a strict regulatory framework governing the use of GM organisms in many countries.

There are four steps involved in conventional gene transfer:

- **Identification and multiplication of a gene with a significant and desirable effect.** This remains a limitation to conventional gene transfer. There are many genes present in the mammalian genome, but for only a fraction of these is the function and exact location in the genome

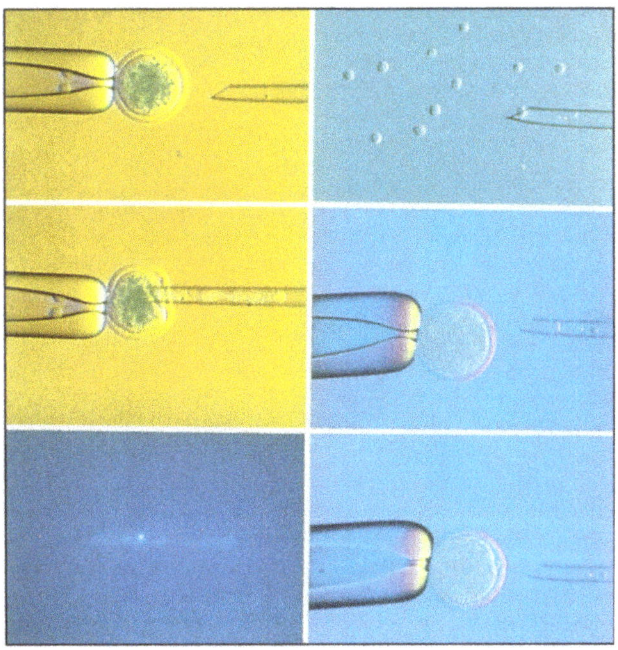

Fig. 5.14. Some of the stages involved in nuclear transfer (anticlockwise from the top left): (i) an oocyte (unfertilized egg) held by suction from a pipette; (ii) a smaller pipette is inserted to remove the chromosomes; (iii) the presence of the chromosomes in the pipette is confirmed under special lighting; a cell to be transplanted is (iv, v) picked up by pipette, inserted into the oocyte, and (vi) the pipette is removed. (Courtesy of Professor Sir Ian Wilmut.)

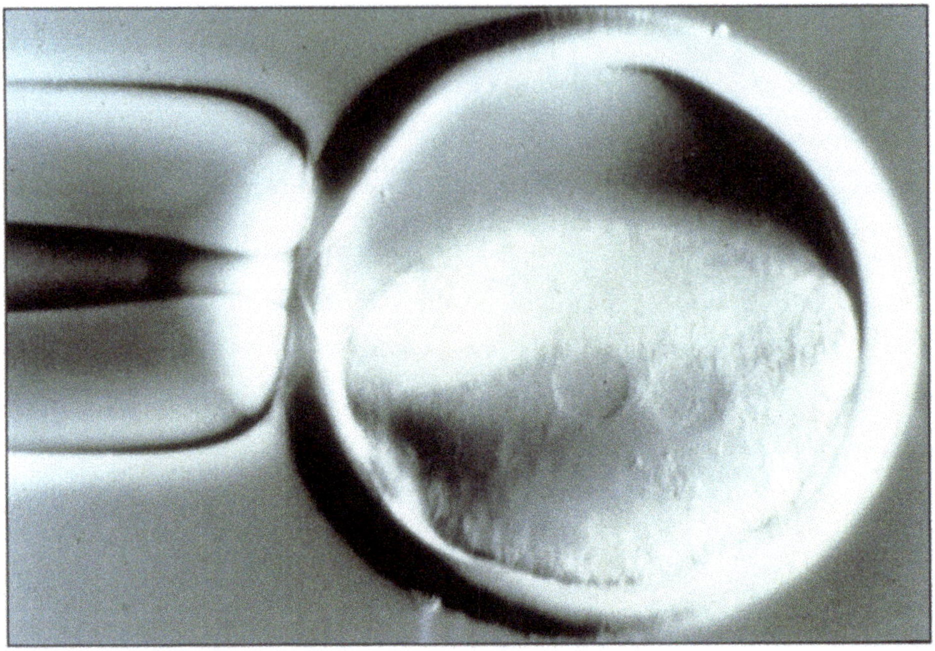

Fig. 5.15. Gene transfer by microinjection of DNA. The plate shows a single-cell embryo which has been treated by centrifugation to allow the pronuclei to be seen clearly (these are the two separate structures containing the chromosomes from the sperm and the egg, which will later form the single nucleus in the cell; they appear as two circles in the centre of the picture). DNA is about to be inserted into one of these pronuclei by micropipette. (Courtesy of Professor Sir Ian Wilmut.)

known at present. When a gene of interest is identified, multiple copies can be produced using one of the techniques outlined earlier.

- **Introducing the DNA coding for the desired gene to the preferred breed or line.** This was achieved experimentally in mammals initially by direct injection of several hundred copies of the foreign DNA sequence into the nucleus of an early stage embryo. This sounds a fairly crude approach, but it appears to work, albeit with low efficiency. For example, in the early applications, less than 1% of manipulated embryos successfully developed into *transgenic* young, though not all transgenic offspring expressed the *transgene* (e.g. Pursel *et al.*, 1989; Wilmut *et al.*, 1990). Alternative methods include the use of vectors, such as retroviruses, which carry copies of the cloned DNA coding for the new gene. This method has been used to create transgenic poultry. Transgenic animals may have different numbers of copies of the foreign gene incorporated into their genome, and they may be incorporated in different places, which can affect the level of expression. The success rate for creating transgenic animals could be improved if these factors could be controlled.
- The developments discussed earlier which have enabled the production of cloned animals from cultured cells have been applied in more recent work on gene transfer. If particular site-specific genetic changes are made to cells in culture, then cloned transgenic animals can be produced. The efficiency of this approach was very low due to the reliance on primary cells (Laible *et al.*, 2015). Both of the drawbacks of these initial approaches have been overcome via the development of genome-editing technology, discussed in detail in the section below.
- **Regulating expression of the introduced gene.** It is clearly vitally important that the right genes get switched on in the right tissues, at the right time. Genes can be coupled to a variety of controlling sequences of DNA which cause the gene to be expressed in response to different hormones.

But understanding of regulation of expression is far from complete. In some experiments, genes with a very specific effect, such as secretion of a human milk protein by sheep, have been transferred successfully. That is, the desired effect was achieved, and there were no apparent undesirable effects (Wright *et al.*, 1991). However, in other early experiments involving transfer of growth hormone genes into pigs and sheep, there were highly undesirable side effects, including serious physiological and anatomical problems such as lameness, arthritis and infertility (Pinkert *et al.*, 1990). These early unintended consequences have probably adversely influenced public opinion on genetic engineering in animals.

- **Confirming transmission of the transferred gene to the next generation of animals.** If the aim of gene transfer is to create improved animals for breeding rather than for the production of modified products themselves, then it is important to confirm that the desired effects are observed in offspring, as well as in the original modified animals. It appears that most transgenic animals produced by early methods, and which actually express the transferred gene, do pass on this new gene to their offspring.

As a result of the low technical efficiency of some of the techniques, public concern over the use of the technologies, including unintended consequences, and tight regulatory controls in many countries (see Chapter 14 for more details) there have been few practical applications of conventional GM technologies in livestock to date (Simm, 1998; Wheeler, 2013; Lotti *et al.*, 2017). The only GM animal product to be approved for human consumption so far is the AquaBounty Atlantic salmon, which shows improved growth rate due to the insertion of a growth hormone (GH) gene from Chinook salmon linked to a promoter from another fish species that drives high GH expression.

The major technical drawbacks of initial GM approaches have been overcome via the development of genome-editing technology, discussed in detail in the section below.

Genome editing

Genome-editing technologies have been developed which allow very precise and targeted changes to genomic DNA at a specific location on the genome using repurposed CRISPR/Cas9 systems (Cong *et al.*, 2013; Mali *et al.*, 2013), which occur naturally as a defence mechanism against pathogens in bacteria. This system functions with the Cas9 enzyme making a double-stranded cut in the genomic DNA at a specific target site, which is enabled by the design of so-called guide RNA. The resulting changes to the genomic DNA arise from one of two major categories of DNA repair mechanisms. *Non-homologous end joining* (NHEJ) will repair the DNA at the cut site in the absence of a homologous template and will result in small insertions or deletions at the cut site. This process is essentially relying on an error occurring in the repair of the DNA and the Cas9 enzyme will continue to cut the DNA until that error occurs. These small insertions or deletions can result in targeted knockout of genes of interest. *Homology-directed repair* (HDR) involves the provision of a DNA template which is similar to the flanking sequence of the cut site (but may contain a user-targeted change in sequence) and the cell uses the template to repair the genomic DNA at the cut site. HDR is more precise than NHEJ but can be less efficient, depending on the cell type and species. CRISPR technologies have major potential to help understand the functional genetic basis of traits of economic importance in livestock but also have potential to improve those traits via incorporation into selective breeding programmes if the regulatory environment permits it.

There are a number of potential applications of genome editing for increasing the understanding of biology and improving traits of importance for animal production and welfare. CRISPR/Cas9 is also likely to be used to test hypotheses relating to causative variants underlying QTLs affecting traits of economic interest in livestock production. In these experiments, HDR approaches could be applied to 'swap' one version of the allele at the candidate variant for the alternate version before assessing the impact on the trait of interest. The field is still in its infancy in terrestrial livestock and aquaculture, but it is still important to consider and, if possible, exclude potential off-target effects (i.e. unwanted genome editing at regions other than the target site). Nonetheless, there are several exciting potential applications of genome editing in livestock breeding programmes (subject to public and regulatory acceptance) which could include: (i) fixing of favourable alleles at QTLs affecting traits of economic interest to speed up genetic gain; (ii) rapid 'introgression' of favourable alleles from other populations, strains or species into a closed breeding population without the negative consequences of traditional introgression (e.g. the time needed to remove the 'unwanted' genomic contribution of the donor breed, see section on MAI above); and (iii) creation of *de novo* alleles based on knowledge of the biology of the trait in question. Simulation of the impact of the first approach demonstrated that integration of genome editing into a genomic selection programme rapidly increases the rate of genetic gain for a target trait (Jenko *et al.*, 2015). An example of the latter approach from livestock is the removal of an exon of the *CD163* gene in pigs, which results in complete resistance to the porcine reproductive and respiratory syndrome virus (PRRSV; Burkard *et al.*, 2017). Likewise, genome editing has been used to produce hornless cattle (Carlson *et al.* 2016). For any of these approaches, it is important to consider how the genome editing could potentially be integrated into a selective breeding programme to improve production.

To perform genome editing in practice, it is generally necessary to access newly fertilized embryos, the feasibility of which varies according to the species (for example, it is straightforward in Atlantic salmon but challenging in chickens). This influences how likely the technology is to be applied commercially. Another major challenge is the identification of target loci for successful genome editing, i.e. selecting a locus or variant that has a causative effect on a trait. This has been notoriously challenging in farm animal genetic research to date and the number of known causative variants for economically important traits is still rather low (Georges *et al.*, 2018).

However, there are new approaches which could help in identifying functional genes and variants. For example, genome-wide gene knockout screening approaches, including the use of the genome-scale CRISPR knockout (GeCKO) technique (Shalem *et al.*, 2014), may facilitate identification of genes involved in traits of importance, particularly traits that can be measured in cell cultures (e.g. resistance to viral disease). GeCKO involves delivery of a library of tens of thousands of unique guide RNAs into cell cultures for genome-wide gene knockout followed by negative or positive selection screening (Shalem *et al.*, 2014), using a lentivirus as the mechanism of delivery. For example, a cell culture could be created with knockouts of different genes in different cells, and this cell culture could be challenged with a pathogenic virus of interest. In theory, the cells that survive the challenge are likely to be edited at genes that are related to resistance to that particular virus. Identification of these genes *in vitro* could then be followed by assessment of the consequences of their perturbation *in vivo*. However, as with all targeted changes to the genome, it is important to assess whether there could be any pleiotropic effects (or side effects) associated with the change. This may be particularly pertinent if the variant that is created by genome editing does not exist elsewhere in nature to the best of our knowledge.

The regulatory and public perception landscape surrounding genome editing must be carefully considered when discussing future applications of genetic engineering and genome editing in livestock production. The methods have the potential to address major production challenges, and in some cases may offer solutions that are not otherwise possible (for example, perhaps, complete resistance to infectious diseases). However, there is still considerable debate about what exactly constitutes GM and whether genome editing should be considered as a separate technology and/or split into different categories according to the nature of the induced change to the genome. Involvement of a wide variety of stakeholders, including in the farming and retail industries, policymakers, consumers and other members of the public is important to reach informed decisions. Although arguments have been presented that gene editing for alleles that occur naturally in agricultural populations should not be considered gene modification even under strict legal frameworks (Custers, 2017), the recent ruling by the European Court of Justice that gene-edited crops should be considered GM organisms presents a potential barrier to adoption in European countries (Callaway, 2018). Furthermore, the potential treatment of genome-edited animal regulation in a similar way to how a new drug would be treated does not bode well for speedy commercial application of genome-edited animals in North America. However, the AquaBounty GM salmon strain has been ruled as fit for human consumption by the US Food and Drug Administration and the Canadian Food Inspection Agency, after a lengthy regulatory process (Waltz, 2017). Research and development relating to genetic modification and genome editing in livestock and aquaculture is developing very rapidly, and it is important that the dialogue surrounding regulation and public acceptability continues in parallel in order to facilitate application of this research in a timely and safe manner.

As an interesting example of the use of gene editing, Mueller *et al.* (2019) described the potential for adding the polled gene to the US dairy population, taking the MAI example used above one stage further. Carlson *et al.* (2016) describe the results of actually adding the polled gene to cattle (see Fig. 5.16) but the regulatory authorities in the USA found that two of the calves produced contained unintended genome alterations, one of which resulted in reduced antibiotic resistance. Debate about the use of the technology is on-going but Carroll *et al.* (2016) argue for the regulation of the products rather than the technology itself.

Modern Data Capture Tools

In order to make progress in selecting for traits of interest in farmed animals, we need to be able to measure these traits, or at least measure proxies related to them. The rise of genomic technologies means that we may not need to measure all candidates for selection, but we do need to measure at least some (i.e. the reference population) in order to establish relationships between genomic markers and traits of interest in the first place. In many cases, it may continue to be cost effective, or operationally efficient, to record all potential candidates for selection for at least some traits of interest. The rate of genetic progress is influenced by the accuracy with which the genetic merit of animals is predicted, and this in turn depends on the accuracy of phenotype measurements. Over the last couple of decades there have been significant developments in sensor, digital, communications and other technologies, that enable more accurate, more widespread, or cheaper recording of existing phenotypes and access to new ones. This is proving especially valuable for measurement of reproductive and health events, feed intake and carcass traits, which have long been recognized as important but are difficult and expensive to measure. A range of new measurement techniques is being investigated that potentially allow selection for reduced environmental impact. The current cost, portability and practicality of new techniques will dictate how widely they are used. However, even relatively expensive techniques may be cost effective when used in nucleus populations, or reference populations to establish genomic predictions. We give some examples below of some of these emerging techniques.

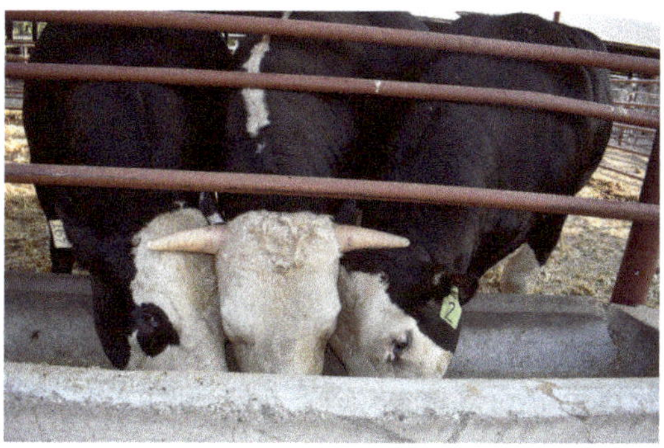

Fig. 5.16. A horned bull flanked by polled progeny of a genome-edited bull. (Courtesy of Dr Alison Van Eenennaam, University of California, Davis.)

Milk mid-infrared spectral data

Mid-infrared (MIR) spectral data from milk samples can be used to determine its chemical composition. This method has been used for many years to predict major milk components such as fat, protein, urea, and lactose content (Luinge *et al.*, 1993). In the last 5 years, there has been an increasing use of milk spectral data as a low-cost and innovative phenotyping strategy for other traits related to health and resilience. Milk contains signals or properties that reflect the physiological status of the cow, her performance and behaviour. Hence, MIR spectra of milk have been used in equations to predict several traits of economic or other importance in dairy cattle. These include individual milk fatty acids, milk coagulation properties and milk mineral content (Soyeurt *et al.*, 2011; Toffanin *et al.*, 2014); cow feed intake and feed efficiency (McParland *et al.*, 2012, 2014); susceptibility to ketosis (De Roos *et al.*, 2007); and methane emissions (Vanlierde *et al.*, 2018). The estimates of correlation coefficient squared (R^2) between various milk fatty acids predicted from MIR and actual measurements in the validation data sets reported by Soyeurt *et al.* (2011) varied from 0.38 to 0.98. Using MIR to predict methane emissions, Vanlierde *et al.* (2018) reported a validation accuracy of 0.57 compared to methane measurements in a respiration chamber. These authors concluded that MIR spectra could be used as a potential proxy to estimate daily methane emissions from dairy cows, cheaply, reliably, rapidly and on a large scale.

Nitrogen in the urine of grazing animals can be an important source of groundwater pollution.

Beatson *et al.* (2019) reported moderately heritable (0.22) measures of milk urea nitrogen (MUN) concentration, based on MIR analyses from NZ dairy cattle, opening up the possibility of selection for lower MUN.

Sensors for health, reproduction and live weight traits

A growing number of sensors has been developed over the past few years, particularly for dairy cattle, to identify health or reproductive events, and the need for associated management interventions, and potentially to reduce labour requirements and labour costs. Many of these techniques also produce data of potential value in breeding programmes. Sensors are devices that measure a physiological or behavioural parameter, e.g. related to the fertility or health of an individual cow, and that enable automated, on-farm detection of changes that warrant a management intervention (Rutten *et al.*, 2013). Sensors can be classified into two categories: attached and non-attached. Attached sensors are either on-animal sensors that are fitted on the outside of the animal's body, or in-animal sensors that are inside the body (e.g. in a rumen bolus or implant). In the case of non-attached sensors, animals may pass by, over or through these for the measurements to be taken. This class of sensors includes in-line sensors that take measurements in a continuous flow of a product (e.g. milk from cows during milking) or on-line sensors that automatically take a sample (e.g. of milk) that is analysed by the sensor.

Several sensors exist for the automated detection of oestrus, usually based on the activity of the cow or on progesterone level in milk. The sensors used to measure cow activity are pedometers, activity meters (sometimes referred to as activometers) and three-dimensional (3D)-accelerometers (Rutten *et al.*, 2013). These are on-cow sensors with the pedometers and 3D-accelerometers usually attached to one of the cow's legs and the activity meters to a neck collar. The level of progesterone is measured in automatically collected milk samples using biosensors and immunostrips, and so can be considered as on-line sensors. These sensor systems provided the farmer with an oestrus alert, some with a probability value to describe the reliability of the alert. Some sensors report the reproductive state such as postpartum anoestrus, oestrus cycling or potentially pregnant.

The electrical conductivity (EC) of milk is employed as a routine in-line test for the diagnosis of sub-clinical mastitis (Milner *et al.*, 1996). Milk EC is determined by measuring the concentration of cations and anions. The concentrations of Na^+ and Cl^- ions are increased while concentrations of lactose and K^+ are decreased in milk during infection. The sensor systems use the statistical relationship between a gold standard measure for mastitis, such as the California Mastitis Test, and the EC measurements, to provide farmers with a mastitis alert, and the reliability of this.

Activity meters have been used to automate the detection of locomotion problems in dairy cows. Sensors such as 3D-accelerometers and/or video cameras have also been used to measure walking behaviour/gait in cattle and poultry. Several off-animal sensors such as four balance-weighing floors, weighing platforms, parallel force plates and force distribution plates have been used to automate locomotion problems by studying the weight distribution among the cow's legs (Rutten, *et al.*, 2013). The animals are required to stand on, or walk over, these sensors. Such systems provide producers with an alert for abnormal locomotive behaviour, with some level of reliability, or analyses of processed sensor data such as weight or walking activity over time.

Automated weighing techniques are used increasingly in several species to monitor growth or to monitor changes in weight that may provide an early indicator of health problems. Typically, animals walk over platforms mounted on weigh cells, with both weights and animal identities being captured using non-attached sensors.

Automated systems for measuring feed intake

Feed constitutes one of the major production costs in most livestock systems, therefore improving efficiency of feed usage has a major impact on farm profitability, and also on the environmental impact of livestock production. However, measuring individual animal feed intake is very difficult and expensive. The older systems to record feed intake required the use of specialized equipment that consisted of an individual bin containing feed. Each animal accessed only one bin through the use of an electronic identification device mounted in a collar. A weighed amount of feed was added to the bin initially and after a certain time interval (24 hours, for instance) the feed remaining in the bin was weighed and discarded. The food consumed by the animal with access to the bin was then calculated as the difference between the two weights. Although this system was cheap, it was labour intensive; feed had to be manually weighed in and out of the bin, and it could also influence the cows' feeding behaviour.

Recent advances have resulted in several automatic systems to measure feed intake by animals (Fig. 5.17). Most of these systems are expensive and tend to be used mostly in research farms or nucleus breeding populations. Examples of these modern techniques for measuring individual feed intake (and in some cases water intake) include the Insentec Roughage Intake Control system (Hokofarm Group, 2019), GrowSafe (GrowSafe Systems, 2019) and the Calan Broadbent Feeding System (American Calan Inc., 2019). These newer systems have feed bins mounted on weigh cells that are constantly monitored. An aerial mounted on the entry to the bin captures the identity of animals accessing it from an electronic identity device on the ear tag or neck collar. As the weight of the feed bin is constantly monitored, the feed intake records are simply the change in weight of the bin during the period a particular animal is registered as present at the feed bin. Animals can feed at any bin and the system offers the additional benefit of being able to capture daily profiles of feed intake per animal, frequency of feeding, meal size and meal duration. Thus, individual animal feeding behaviour can be studied.

In vivo prediction of carcass traits

The ability to accurately measure carcass composition is important for selection of meat-producing animals. Carcass and meat quality traits are expensive and difficult to measure. Obviously, direct measurement can only take place after slaughter, which usually precludes direct measurements on candidates for selection. Breeding programmes in the more prolific species sometimes use carcass measurements on relatives. However, considerable research has gone into finding methods to predict various carcass traits, such as carcass fat and lean weight, or proportion or distribution, using non-invasive techniques on live animals (*in vivo*). For a detailed review on these non-invasive techniques, see Scholz *et al.* (2015).

Generally, non-invasive techniques for predicting body or carcass composition work with electromagnetic or mechanical energy, which is able to pass completely or partially through body or carcass tissues, like muscle, fat and bone. The electromagnetic signal produced by the instrument may originate from mechanical energy such as sound waves (ultrasound – US), 'photon' radiation (X-ray-computed tomography – CT, dual-energy X-ray absorptiometry – DXA) or radio frequency waves (magnetic resonance imaging – MRI) (Scholz *et al.*, 2015). The signal interacts with tissues in the body or carcass at the atomic or molecular level, resulting in secondary signals which are detected by the instruments and processed to measure tissue depths, areas, volumes or

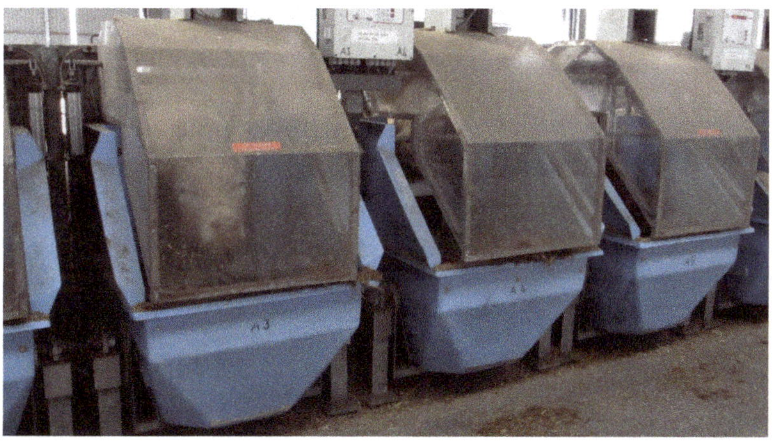

Fig. 5.17. Automated feeder which records feed intake of individual animals. (Courtesy of Scotland's Rural College.)

distributions of fat, muscle and bone or bone mineral (Fig. 5.18). Validation of measurements from these devices usually involves comparison with equivalent measurements obtained directly from the carcass, or with proportions or weights of tissues from carcass dissection. This usually involves regression equations, with the measures from these devices used to predict the measurements from the carcass. The R^2 of the regression analysis gives a measure of the accuracy of the method with high R^2 values indicating high precision of prediction.

Ultrasonic measures have been the most widely used *in vivo* predictors in meat animal breeding, as a result of being relatively cheap, mobile and moderately accurate. CT has been used more recently in livestock breeding programmes, especially meat sheep, and it is considered to be the most accurate of the methods discussed above (see Fig. 10.23). CT scanning has been used in UK terminal sire breeding programmes since 2000 to accurately estimate carcass composition and muscularity (Bunger *et al.*, 2014). The details of the carcass traits measured and their application in sheep breeding programmes is covered in detail in Chapter 10. CT scanning has also been applied to measure intra-muscular fat (IMF) in live lambs and carcass cuts as a measure of meat quality (Lambe *et al.*, 2017, 2018). Using CT measurements, in addition to carcass and loin weights, IMF was predicted with a moderate precision (R^2 = 0.36). Generally, results indicate that the use of CT within a selection index can maintain IMF, for improved eating quality, while increasing lean and decreasing total fat, to improve carcass quality and reduce waste in commercial slaughter lambs.

Video image analysis/computer vision to measure weight, conformation and carcass traits

Video image analysis (VIA)/computer vision techniques are being used to predict live weight and conformation of live animals, and carcass conformation, fatness and meat yield, in a number of livestock species (Rius-Vilarassa *et al.*, 2009; Pabiou *et al.*, 2011; Fernandes *et al.*, 2019). In live animals, repeated images can be captured over time and used to monitor changes in weight and conformation, and predict optimal time of slaughter, based on earlier calibration trials.

Automated VIA carcass grading procedures, utilizing video cameras on the slaughter line and specialist software to classify carcasses, are in use in a growing number of countries. For example, VBS2000 VIA machines (E + V Technology, 2019) are used in several abattoirs in the UK. The procedure involves suspending one side of the carcass on a holding frame while a digital camera on the VIA machine takes a 2D (under normal lighting) and 3D (under striped lighting) image, using a previously calibrated lighting arrangement. These images are analysed to predict weight of individual primal cuts, as well as carcass weight and conformation and fat class (e.g. on the EUROP carcass classification grid

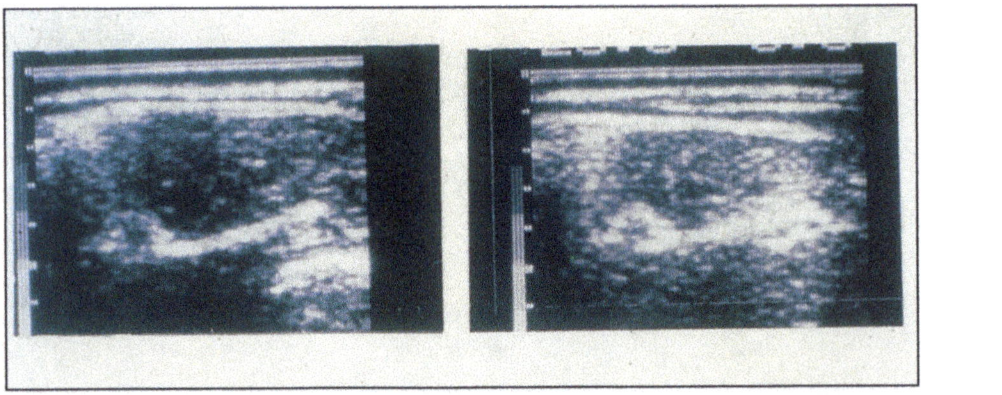

Fig. 5.18. Ultrasonic scans from the loin area of two Suffolk ram lambs. The scan on the right is from an animal with a relatively high fat depth and relatively low muscle depth, that on the left is from an animal with a lower fat depth and a higher muscle depth.

used in the European Union). The prediction of the weights of carcass cuts is based on a multiple-regression method using both the carcass weight and the VIA information. Pabiou *et al.* (2011) reported precision of prediction (R^2) values from 0.65 for predictions of low value cuts (lean trimmings, ribs, flank and brisket) in heifers to 0.93 for predictions of high value cuts (silverside, topside, knuckle, salmon cut) in steers. The automation of this process means that carcass weights and primal cuts can be measured in a large number of animals and genetic evaluations can be carried out for these traits. Moore *et al.* (2017) reported medium to high estimates of heritability of 0.40 to 0.46 for a range of cuts in crossbred beef cattle in the UK. This allows breeding animals to be selected for a higher proportion of high-priced cuts. In addition, the use of these traits in genomic selection (see above and Chapter 7) means that the genetic merit for carcass weight and primal cuts can be predicted, and selection carried out, early in life, thereby reducing the generation interval.

Greenhouse gas emissions

There is growing attention globally on the rôle of agriculture in greenhouse gas emissions. Methane emissions from ruminants are especially important, accounting for around 80% of all livestock emissions, with cattle responsible for the majority of these (Hristov *et al.*, 2013). Methane is produced as a natural part of the digestion process, where microbes in the rumen break down feed and release methane as a by-product, primarily through eructation or belching.

As a first step towards selective breeding to reduce methane (CH_4) emissions from livestock, various approaches have been developed to measure the amount of methane originating from individual animals. The gold standard method is the use of respiration chambers (Fig. 5.19). There are two types: an open-circuit chamber which involves analysing the composition of the in-flowing and out-flowing air, which is then compared. The second type uses a closed-circuit chamber where the increasing concentration of methane is measured (Boadi *et al.*, 2002). Many other proxy methods are being investigated since respiration chambers are expensive to operate and allow only a limited throughput of animals. These include the SF_6 (sulphur hexafluoride) tracer technique, which involves inserting a calibrated source of SF_6 into the rumen of each participating animal. The ratio of CH_4 to SF_6 in the breath of an animal is measured over a 24-hour period, at regular intervals, and corrected with reference to the background methane concentration. Given that the concentration of the tracer is known, the rate of production of CH_4 can be calculated. Repeated 24-hour samples collected over five successive days generally display good day-to-day consistency in daily emissions for each animal. A downside to this technique is that the marker SF_6 is itself a potent greenhouse gas. A hand-held laser methane detector (LMD), or laser gun, has also been used to measure methane outputs from an animal over short periods of time. The LMD is positioned about 1 m distance from the mouth and nostril area of the animal and methane concentrations are recorded at regular short intervals (Chagunda and Yan, 2011). For complete reviews of the methods used to monitor greenhouse gas emissions see Hill *et al.* (2016) and Chapter 3 of National Academies of Sciences, Engineering and Medicine (2018).

Use of mobile apps to capture phenotypic data

To increase accuracy, avoid translation errors and reduce costs, there has been a growth in the application of digital tools and mobile apps to capture livestock performance data for farmers. This has become very important in low- and middle-income countries where the basic infrastructure for elaborate data capture is lacking due to high cost and small, dispersed herds or flocks. Some of the digital tools use The Open Data Kit (ODK) which is formatted to collect performance data and other farm characteristics. The data are automatically relayed to a database for processing and analysis (Gebreyesus *et al.*, 2013; Ojango *et al.*, 2018). One of the limitations of the ODK system in developing countries is the reliance on an internet connection to relay data to the database, as these connections can be intermittent. Various hand-held tools are also employed for data capture and data viewing. One of the milk recording agents in the UK, National Milk Records (NMR), has developed the Pocket Companion, NMR's mobile data service (National Milk Records, 2019). The Cattle Information Service, another milk recording company in the UK, has a mobile app for iPhone or Android called MobileHerd (Cattle Information Service, 2019)

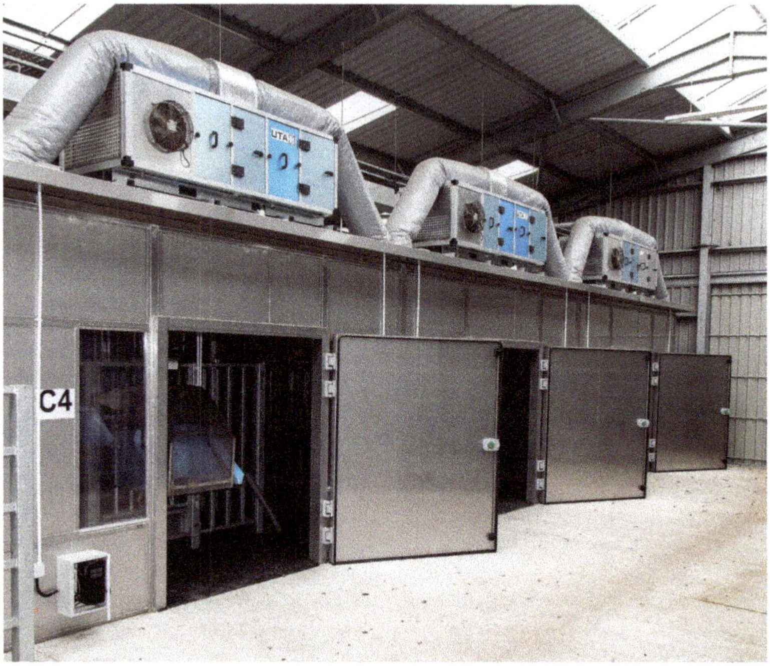

Fig. 5.19. Respiration chamber used to measure greenhouse gas emissions from livestock. (Courtesy of Scotland's Rural College.)

that enables data to be collected and analysed while out and about on the farm. In addition to data collection, the mobile phone has been used for a range of farmer training and advisory applications by sending specific training materials and alerts to improve management, e.g. by the company Green Dreams Tech, operating under the name iCow, in Kenya, Tanzania and Ethiopia (Green Dreams Tech, 2019).

Summary

- New reproductive and molecular genetic technologies could lead to more effective genetic improvement programmes in livestock, or to more rapid dissemination of improved genes from elite to commercial sectors of the livestock industries. While most of these technologies are relevant in all species, some are likely to be of particular value in ruminants.
- Artificial insemination is already widely used in cattle breeding but, largely because of technical difficulties, it is not yet so widely used in sheep breeding. AI can allow higher male selection intensities, shorter male generation intervals and higher accuracy of selection, as well as providing genetic links across herds or flocks. Hence, it is a highly effective method for increasing rates of genetic improvement. It is also an extremely useful method for dissemination.
- Multiple ovulation and embryo transfer (MOET) potentially offers similar benefits in the selection of females to those offered by AI in males. However, in practice the benefits are often smaller. As a result of this and its relatively high cost, the technique is largely confined to specialized breed improvement schemes (often involving elite nucleus populations), to facilitate international trade in genetic material, and to accelerate multiplication of newly introduced breeds.
- *In vitro* production of embryos can dramatically increase embryo yield compared to conventional MOET. This could accelerate rates of improvement in breeding schemes, especially when oocytes are collected from live elite donors (ovum pick up). However, it could also allow more effective

dissemination to the commercial sector, for example when oocytes are collected from slaughtered beef heifers of high performance, for transfer to dairy or suckler cows of lower beef merit.

- While the use of reproductive technologies such as MOET can substantially increase rates of genetic improvement, rates of inbreeding often increase proportionately more. However, much of this gain can often be achieved with minimal increase in inbreeding by modifications to the design of the breeding scheme.
- In most circumstances, sexing of either semen or embryos appears to be of little value in accelerating genetic improvement. However, the development of a cheap, reliable technique for sexing semen in large enough quantities for conventional AI, has led to improvements in the dissemination of genetic improvement and in the efficiency of animal production. Embryo sexing on a smaller scale could still allow more effective dissemination if it is coupled with *in vitro* production of embryos.
- Cloning appears to be of fairly limited value in accelerating genetic improvement, but the potential of the technique to accelerate dissemination of genetic improvement to commercial herds or flocks is clear if the techniques become more cost effective and efficient. Surrogate sire technology, where elite donor germplasm is disseminated via germ-cell ablated surrogate males, also has major potential to achieve similar impacts.
- To date, most selection in livestock has been practised with little or no knowledge of what is happening at the DNA level. Selection has been on the effects of the genes, rather than directly on the genes themselves. However, modern molecular genetic technologies offer the opportunity to improve on these methods. Genome mapping and the use of molecular markers are already having an impact on livestock improvement. Experimental applications of gene editing look promising.
- These molecular technologies are based on advances in molecular and cell biology including: (i) the discovery of restriction enzymes which are capable of 'cutting up' sequences of DNA; (ii) the development of techniques to allow DNA fragments of different lengths to be separated and detected; (iii) the development of techniques to multiply sequences of DNA rapidly; (iv) the development of techniques to determine the sequence of bases on short strands of DNA and whole genomes, including high-throughput short- and long-read sequencing technology; (v) the development of DNA probes and labelling techniques; and (vi) the development of SNP chips and genotyping by sequencing to rapidly genotype genome-wide SNP markers in populations of animals.
- Any identifiable segment of DNA in the genome, which varies between animals, can act as a marker. Hence, markers may be all or part of a 'functional' gene, or they may be a part of the rest of the genome which does not code directly for the production of a protein. Several different types of marker have been developed, based on some of the methods described above, for detecting variation at the DNA level, but SNP markers have become the marker of choice. These markers are of value in genome mapping, marker-assisted selection, parentage verification, genomic selection and product identification.
- The purpose of a genome map is to describe the location of functional genes or other sequences of DNA (e.g. markers) on the chromosomes. There are different types of map which have different levels of resolution. The ultimate level of resolution for a genome map is the full DNA sequence of the genome.
- Livestock genome maps can be useful in making informed choices of markers for economically important traits to accelerate conventional selection programmes, and for locating genes of potential interest for gene editing, introgression or selection. Genome maps are also useful in deciding which breeds, strains or individuals should receive highest priority in conservation programmes.
- Linkage maps have been published for each of the livestock species, but these tend to be superseded by whole-genome sequence maps and their associated tools and databases.
- A sequence database is a typical biological database stored on a computer, composed of publicly available nucleic acid sequences, or protein sequences. The three most comprehensive nucleotide databases which comprise the International Nucleotide Sequence Database Collaboration and hold sequence data for more than 160,000 species are: GenBank, EMBL: European Molecular Biology Laboratory and DDBJ: DNA Data Bank of Japan.
- Molecular markers may speed up introduction of a gene of interest from one breed to another

(marker-assisted introgression). Compared to conventional backcrossing programmes, markers can help by: (i) identifying backcrosses carrying the particular favoured allele from the new breed; and (ii) amongst animals with one or two copies of this allele, identifying those with the least of their genome from the new breed. Genome editing has the potential to achieve introgression of favourable alleles without the negative impacts of linkage drag.

- Markers may also accelerate selection for traits of economic importance within a population (marker-assisted selection). In this case the aim of using markers is simply to boost the improvement made by conventional means, by 'homing in' on genes already present in the breed concerned. The gene of interest may be either a single gene with a large effect, or it may be one of many genes at a locus affecting a quantitative trait (a QTL). Genomic selection has become routine in most advanced livestock breeding sectors and has largely superseded MAS, except where the QTL of interest is of major effect.
- To establish an association between a marker and the trait of interest, genome-wide association studies are carried out using a suitable SNP chip and performance data.
- Signatures of selection studies involve detecting regions of the genome which are conserved over many generations due to the fact that they confer enhanced fitness or productive ability. Such conserved regions are, thus, preferentially kept in the population with the frequency of favourable alleles and haplotypes increasing towards fixation.
- Genomic selection involves selecting animals on the basis of their genetic merit predicted from SNP genotypes. These predictions of genetic merit called direct genomic breeding values. The approach uses the linkage disequilibrium between SNPs and QTLs that control traits of economic importance.
- Gene editing allows the alteration of a single base or a small number of bases, to alter genotypes for traits affecting health or production.
- The rate of genetic progress is influenced by how early in life phenotypes for traits of interest can be recorded, and by the quality and quantity of data available to predict breeding values. Several technologies now exist to allow (automatic or other) recording of hitherto difficult-to-measure performance traits (e.g. traits associated with disease, reproduction, feed intake, carcass composition and greenhouse gas emissions) or enable recording of such traits earlier in life. These include the use of milk mid-infrared spectral data to measure various performance traits in dairy cattle, sensors for measuring disease and fertility-related traits, automated feed intake recording systems, video imaging and a range of scanning techniques for predicting live animal or carcass composition, and several methods for predicting methane production.

References

1000 Bull Genomes Project (2019) Available at: http://www.1000bullgenomes.com/ (accessed 20 November 2019).

Affymetrix (2019) Available at: https://www.affymetrix.com/support/help/genotyping_glossary/index.affx (accessed 21 October 2019).

Alberts, B., Johnson, A. and Lewis, J. (2002) *Molecular Biology of the Cell*, 4th edn. Garland Science, New York.

Allais-Bonnet, A., Grohs, C., Medugorac, I. *et al.* (2013) Novel insights into the bovine polled phenotype and horn ontogenesis in Bovidae. *PLoS ONE* 8, e63512. DOI: 10.1371/journal.pone.0063512.

American Calan Inc. (2019) Available at: http://americancalan.com/code/template.cfm?page=2 (accessed 21 October 2019).

Baguisi, A., Behboodi, E., Melican, D.T. Pollock, J.S., Destrempes, M.M. *et al.* (1999) Production of goats by somatic cell nuclear transfer. *Nature Biotechnology* 17, 456–461. DOI: https://doi.org/10.1038/8632.

Bahbahani, H., Clifford, H.H., Wragg, D., Mbole-Kariuki, M.N., Van Tassell, C. *et al.* (2015) Signatures of positive selection in East African Shorthorn Zebu: A genome-wide single nucleotide polymorphism analysis. *Scientific Reports* 5, 11729. DOI: 10.1038/srep11729.

Baird, N.A., Etter, P.D., Atwood, T.S., Currey, M.C., Shiver, A.L. *et al.* (2008) Rapid SNP discovery and genetic mapping using sequenced RAD markers. *PLoS ONE,* 3, e3376. DOI: 10.1371/journal.pone.0003376.

Beatson, P.R., Meier, S., Cullen, N.G. and Eding, H. (2019) Genetic variation in milk urea nitrogen concentration of dairy cattle and its implications for reducing urinary nitrogen excretion. *Animal* 13, 2164–2171. DOI: 10.1017/S1751731119000235.

Bergstein-Galan, T.G., Weiss, R.R. and Kozicki, L.E. (2019) Effect of semen and donor factors on multiple ovulation and embryo transfer (MOET) in sheep. *Reproduction in Domestic Animals* 54, 401–407. DOI: 10.1111/rda.13381.

Betteridge, K.J., Smith, C., Stubbings, R.B., Xu, K.P. and King, W.A. (1989) Potential genetic improvement of cattle by fertilization of fetal oocytes *in vitro*. *Journal of Reproduction and Fertility, Supplement* 38, 87–98.

Billings, P.R., Smith, C.L. and Cantor, C.R. (1991) New techniques for physical mapping of the human genome. *FASEB Journal* 5, 28–34. DOI: 10.1096/fasebj.5.1.1846833.

Blasco, A. and Pena, R.N. (2018) Current status of genomic maps: genomic selection/GBV. In: Niemann, H. and Wrenzycki, C. (ed.) *Livestock in Animal biotechnologies 2. Emerging Breeding Technologies (eBook)*. Springer, New York, pp. 61–80.

Boadi, D.A, Wittenberg, K.M. and Kennedy, A.D. (2002) Validation of the sulphur hexafluoride (SF_6) tracer gas technique for measurement of methane and carbon dioxide production by cattle. *Canadian Journal of Animal Science* 82, 125–131. DOI: 10.4141/A01-054.

Boni, R. (2012) Ovum pick-up in cattle: a 25 yr retrospective analysis. *Animal Reproduction* 9, 362–369. Available at: https://www.animal-reproduction.org/article/5b5a605af7783717068b46f3 (accessed 31 August 2020).

Brickell, J.S., Pollott, G.E., Clempson, A.M., Otter, N. and Wathes, D.C. (2010) Polymorphisms in the bovine leptin gene associated with perinatal mortality in Holstein-Friesian Heifers. *Journal of Dairy Science* 93, 340–347. DOI: 10.3168/jds.2009-2457.

Brooks, S.A., Gabreski, N., Miller, D., Brisbin, A., Brown, H.E. *et al.* (2010) Whole-genome SNP association in the horse: identification of a deletion in Myosin Va responsible for Lavender Foal Syndrome. *PLOS Genetics* 6, e1000909. DOI: 10.1371/journal.pgen.1000909.

Bünger, L., Moore, K., McLean, K.A., Kongsro, J. and Lambe, N.R. (2014) Integrating computed tomography into commercial sheep breeding in the UK: cost and value. *Proceedings of the 3rd Farm Animal Imaging Conference*, Denmark, Copenhagen. SRUC, Edinburgh, UK. Available at: https://pure.sruc.ac.uk/en/publications/integrating-computed-tomography-ct-into-commercial-sheep-breeding (accessed 4 October 2020).

Burkard, C., Lillico, S.G., Reid, E., Jackson, B., Mileham, A.J. *et al.* (2017) Precision engineering for PRRSV resistance in pigs: macrophages from genome edited pigs lacking CD163 SRCR5 domain are fully resistant to both PRRSV genotypes while maintaining biological function. *PLoS Pathogens* 13, e1006206. DOI: 10.1371/journal.ppat.1006206.

Bush, W.S. and Moore, J.H. (2012) Genome-wide association studies. *PLoS Computational Biology,* 8, e1002822. DOI: 10.1371/journal.pcbi.1002822.

Caballero, A., Santiago, E. and Toro, M.A. (1996) Systems of mating to reduce inbreeding in selected populations. *Animal Science* 62, 431–442. DOI: 10.1017/S1357729800014971.

Cai, Z., Guldbrandtsen, B., Lund M.S. and Sahana G. (2019) Prioritizing candidate genes for fertility in dairy cows using gene-based analysis, functional annotation and differential gene expression. *BMC Genomics,* 20, Article number: 255. DOI: 10.1186/s12864-019-5638-9.

Callaway, E. (2018) CRISPR plants now subject to tough GM laws in European Union. *Nature* 560, 16. Available at: https://www.nature.com/articles/d41586-018-05814-6 (accessed 31 August 2020).

Campbell, K.H.S. and Wilmut, I. (1997) Totipotency or multipotentiality of cultured cells: applications and progress. *Theriogenology* 47, 63–72. DOI: 10.1016/S0093-691X(96)00340-8.

Campbell, K.H.S., McWhir, J., Ritchie, W.A. and Wilmut, I. (1996) Sheep cloned by nuclear transfer from a cultured cell line. *Nature* 380: 64–66. Available at: https://www.nature.com/articles/380064a0 (accessed 30 August 2020).

Carlson, D.F., Lancto, C.A., Zang, B., Kim, E.S., Walton, M. *et al.* (2016) Production of hornless dairy cattle from genome-edited cell lines. *Nature Biotechnology* 34, 479–481. DOI: 10.1038/nbt.3560.

Carroll, D., Van Eenennaam, A.L., Taylor, J.F., Seger, J. and Voytas, D.F. (2016). Regulate genome-edited products, not genome editing itself. *Nature Biotechnology* 34, 477–479. Available at: https://www.nature.com/articles/nbt.3566 (accessed 31 August 2020).

Cattle Information Service (2019) Available at: http://www.thecis.co.uk/services/MobileHerd (accessed 21 October 2019).

Chagunda, M.G.G. and Yan, T. (2011) Do methane measurements from a laser detector and an indirect open-circuit respiration calorimetric chamber agree sufficiently closely? *Animal Feed Science and Technology* 165, 8–14. DOI: 10.1016/j.anifeedsci.2011.02.005.

Chang, C.C., Chow, C.C., Tellier, L.C.A.M., Vattikuti, S., Purcell, S.M. and Lee, J.J. (2015) Second-generation PLINK: rising to the challenge of larger and richer datasets. *GigaScience,* 4, 7.

Ciccarelli, M., Giassetti, M.I., Miao, D., Oatley, M.J., Robbins, C. *et al.* (2020) Donor-derived spermatogenesis following stem cell transplantation in sterile NANOS2 knockout males. *Proceedings of the National Academy of Sciences* 202010102; DOI: 10.1073/pnas.2010102117

Colleau, J.J. (1991) Using embryo sexing within closed mixed multiple ovulation and embryo transfer schemes for selection on dairy cattle. *Journal of Dairy Science* 74, 3973–3984. DOI: 10.3168/jds.S0022-0302(91)78592-5.

Cong, L., Ran, F.A., Cox, D., Shuailiang L., Barretto, R. *et al.* (2013) Multiplex genome engineering using CRISPR/Cas systems. *Science* 339, 819–823. DOI: 10.1126/science.1231143.

Cowan, C.M. (1994) Use of genetic marker technology to select AI bulls. *British Cattle Breeders Club Digest* 49, 45–48.

Cran, D.G. and Johnson, L.A. (1996) The predetermination of embryonic sex using flow cytometrically separated X and Y spermatozoa. *Human Reproduction Update,* 2, 355–363. DOI: 10.1093/humupd/2.4.355.

Custers, R. (2017) The regulatory status of gene-edited agricultural products in the EU and beyond. *Emerging Topics in Life Sciences* 1, 221– 229. DOI: 10.1042/ETLS20170019.

de Boer, I.J.M., Meuwissen, T.H.E. and Van Arendonk, J.A.M. (1994) Combining the genetic and clonal responses in a closed dairy cattle nucleus scheme. *Animal Production* 59, 345–358. DOI: 10.1017/S000335610000787X.

de Graaf, S.P., Leahy, T. and Vishwanath, R. (2014) Biological and practical lessons associated with the use of sexed semen. *Reproduction in Domestic Ruminants* 8, 507–522.

de Roos, A.P.W., van den Bijgaart, H.J.C.M, Hørlyk, J. and De Jong, G. (2007) Screening for subclinical ketosis in dairy cattle by fourier transform infrared spectroscopy. *Journal of Dairy Science* 90, 1761–1766. DOI: 10.3168/jds.2006-203.

Dingwall, W.S. and McKelvey, W.A.C. (1993) Artificial insemination and embryo transfer technology for sheep and goats. *World Agriculture* 1993, 78–81.

DNA Databank of Japan (2019) Available at: https://www.ddbj.nig.ac.jp (accessed 21 October 2019).

Dunn, O.J. (1961) Multiple comparisons among means. *Journal of the American Statistical Association* 56, 52–64. DOI: 10.1080/01621459.1961.10482090.

E + V Technology (2019) Available at: http://www.eplusv.de/start_E.htm (accessed 21 October 2019).

EBI (2019) Available at: https://www.ebi.ac.uk/gwas/docs/faq (accessed 21 October 2019).

ENSEMBL (2019) Available at: https://www.ensembl.org/index.html (accessed 24 September 2019).

European Nucleotide Archive (2019) Available at: https://www.ebi.ac.uk/ena (accessed 21 October 2019).

Evans, K.M. (2010) Interpretation of sex-sorting process and new developments. *Proceedings of the 25th Technical Conference on Artificial Insemination and Reproduction*, Wisconsin, 93–98.

Fernandes, A.F.A., Dórea, J.R.R., Fitzgerald, R., Herring, W. and Rosa, G.J.M. (2019) A novel automated system to acquire biometric and morphological measurements and predict body weight of pigs via 3D computer vision. *Journal of Animal Science* 97, 496–508. DOI: 10.1093/jas/sky418.

Foote, R.H. (2002) The history of artificial insemination: Selected notes and notables. *Journal of Animal Science* 80, 1–10. DOI: 10.2527/animalsci2002.80E-Suppl_21a.

Galli, C., Lagutina, I., Crotti, G., Colleoni, S., Turini, P. *et al.* (2003) Pregnancy: a cloned horse born to its dam twin. *Nature,* 424, 635–635. DOI: 10.1038/424635a.

Gambra, R., Peñagaricano, F., Kropp, J., Khateeb, K., Weigel, K.A. *et al.* (2013) Genomic architecture of bovine κ–casein and β-lactoglobulin. *Journal of Dairy Science,* 96, 5333–5343. DOI: 10.3168/jds.2012-6324.

Gebreyesus, G., Dessie, T., Wamalwa, M., Agaba, M., Benor, S. and Okeyo, A.M. (2013) Harnessing "ODK collect" on smartphones for on-farm data collection in Africa: The ILRI-BecA goat project. Poster prepared for the *ILRI APM 2013*, Addis Ababa, 15-17 May 2013. ILRI, Nairobi. Available at: https://cgspace.cgiar.org/handle/10568/29059 (accessed 21 October 2019).

GenBank (2019) Available at: https://www.ncbi.nlm.nih.gov/genbank/ (accessed 21 October 2019).

Georges, M., Nielsen, D., Mackinnon, M., Mishra, A., Okimoto, R. *et al.* (1995) Mapping genes controlling milk production: towards marker assisted selection in livestock. *Genetics* 139, 907–920.

Georges, M., Charlier, C. and Hayes, B. (2018) Harnessing genomic information for livestock improvement. *Nature Reviews Genetics* 20, 135–156. Available at: https://www.nature.com/articles/s41576-018-0082-2 (accessed 31 August 2020).

Gjedrem, T. and Rye, M. (2018) Selection response in fish and shellfish: a review. *Reviews in Aquaculture* 10, 168–179. DOI: 10.1111/raq.12154.

Gootwine, E., Zenu, A., Bor, A., Yossafi, S., Rosov, A. and Pollott, G. E. (2001) Lamb and milk production in the Afec-Awassi and Afec-Assaf strains carrying the B allele of the FecB fecundity gene. *Livestock Production Science* 71, 49–58. DOI: 10.1016/S0301-6226(01)00240-8.

Gordon, I. (1994) *Laboratory Production of Cattle Embryos.* CAB International, Wallingford, UK.

Gordon, I. (1996) *Controlled Reproduction in Cattle and Buffaloes.* CAB International, Wallingford, UK.

Gordon, I. (1997) *Controlled Reproduction in Sheep and Goats.* CAB International, Wallingford, UK.

Gordon, I. and Lu, K.H. (1990) Production of embryos in vitro and its impact on livestock production. *Theriogenology* 33, 77–87. DOI: 10.1016/0093-691X(90)90599-O.

Gorjanc, G., Cleveland, M.A., Houston, R.D. and Hickey, J.M. (2015) Potential of genotyping-by-sequencing for genomic selection in livestock populations. *Genetics, Selection and Evolution* 47, 12. DOI: 10.1186/s12711-015-0102-z.

Gottardo, P., Gorjanc, G., Battagin, M., Gaynor, R.C., Jenko, J. *et al.* (2019) A strategy to exploit surrogate sire technology in livestock breeding programs. *Genes, Genomes, Genetics* 9, 203–215.

Granleese, T., Clark, S.A., Swan, A.A. and van der Werf, J.H.J. (2015) Increased genetic gains in sheep, beef and dairy breeding programs from using female reproductive technologies combined with optimal contribution selection and genomic breeding values. *Genetics Selection Evolution* 47, 70. DOI: 10.1186/s12711-015-0151-3.

Green Dreams Tech (2019) Available at: http://icow.co.ke/about (accessed 21 October 2019).

Grisart, B., Coppieters, W., Farnir, F., Karim, L., Ford, C., *et al.* (2002) Positional candidate cloning of a QTL in dairy cattle: identification of a missense mutation in the bovine *DGAT1* gene with major effect on milk yield and composition. *Genome Research* 12, 222–231. DOI: 10.1101/gr.224202.

GrowSafe Systems (2019) Available at: https://growsafe.com/our-platform/ (accessed 21 October 2019).

Grundy, B., Caballero, A., Santiago, E. and Hill, W.G. (1994) A note on using biased parameter values and non-random mating to reduce rates of inbreeding in selection programmes. *Animal Production* 59, 465–468. DOI: 10.1017/S0003356100008011.

Gutiérrez-Gil, B., Arranz, J.J. and Wiener, P. (2015) An interpretive review of selective sweep studies in *Bos taurus* cattle populations: identification of unique and shared selection signals across breeds. *Frontiers in Genetics* 6, 167. DOI: 10.3389/fgene.2015.00167.

Haley, C.S. (1995) Livestock QTLs - bringing home the bacon? *Trends in Genetics* 11, 488–492. DOI: 10.1016/S0168-9525(00)89158-1.

Haley, C.S., Willams, J., Woolliams, J. and Visscher, P. (1996) Gene mapping and its place in livestock improvement. *British Cattle Breeders Club Digest* 51, 5–15.

He, L., Martins, P., Huguenin, J., Van, T.-N.-N., Manso, T. *et al.* (2019) Simple, sensitive and robust chicken specific sexing assays, compliant with large scale analysis. *PLoS ONE* 14, e0213033. DOI: 10.1371/journal.pone.0213033.

Hernandez Gifford, J.A. and Gifford, C.A. (2013) Role of reproductive biotechnologies in enhancing food security and sustainability. *Animal Frontiers* 3, 14–19. DOI: 10.2527/af.2013-0019.

Hill, J., McSweeney, C., Wright, A-D.G., Bishop-Hurley, G. and Kalantar-zadeh, K. (2016) Measuring methane production from ruminants. *Trends in Biotechnology* 34, 26–35. DOI: 10.1016/j.tibtech.2015.10.004.

Hokofarm Group (2019) Available at: https://www.hokofarmgroup.com/ric/management-software/ (accessed 21 October 2019).

Houston, R.D., Haley, C.S., Hamilton, A., Guy, D.R., Tinch, A.E. *et al.* (2008) Major quantitative trait loci affect resistance to infectious pancreatic necrosis in Atlantic salmon (*Salmo salar*). *Genetics* 178, 1109–1115. DOI: 10.1534/genetics.107.082974.

Hristov, A.N., Oh, J., Lee, C., Meinen, R., Montes, F. *et al.* (2013) Mitigation of greenhouse gas emissions in livestock production – A review of technical options for non-CO2 emissions. In: Gerber, P.J., Henderson, B. and Makkar, H.P.S. (eds) FAO Animal Production and Health Paper No. 177. FAO, Rome. Available at: http://www.fao.org/3/i3288e/i3288e00.htm (accessed 31 August 2020).

Hu, Z-L., Park, C.A. and Reecy, J.M. (2019) Building a livestock genetic and genomic information knowledgebase through integrative developments of Animal QTLdb and CorrDB. *Nucleic Acids Research* 47, D701–D710. DOI: 10.1093/nar/gky1084.

Illumina. (2019a) Available at: https://www.illumina.com/ (accessed 21 October 2019).

Illumina. (2019b) Available at: https://www.illumina.com/products/by-type/microarray-kits/bovine-snp50.html (accessed 21 October 2019).

Illumina. (2019c) Available at: https://www.illumina.com/products/by-type/microarray-kits/bovinehd.html (accessed 21 October 2019).

Jenko, J., Gorjanc, G., Cleveland, M.A., Varshney, R.K., Whitelaw, C.B.A. *et al.* (2015) Potential of promotion of alleles by genome editing to improve quantitative traits in livestock breeding programs. *Genetics Selection Evolution* 47, Article number: 55. Available at: https://gsejournal.biomedcentral.com/articles/10.1186/s12711-015-0135-3 (accessed 31 August 2020).

Johnson, L.A., Flook, J.P. and Hawk, H.W. (1989) Sex preselection in rabbits: live births from X and Y sperm separated by DNA and cell sorting. *Biology of Reproduction* 41, 199–203. DOI: 10.1095/biolreprod41.2.199.

Kageyama, S. and Hirayama, H. (2012) Sexing of bovine preimplantation embryos using loop-mediated isothermal amplification (LAMP). *Journal of Mammalian Ova Research* 29, 113–118. DOI: 10.1274/jmor.29.113.

Kasinathan, P., Wei, H., Xiang, T., Molina, J. A., Metzger, J. *et al.* (2015). Acceleration of genetic gain in cattle by reduction of generation interval. *Scientific Reports* 5, 8674. DOI: 10.1038/srep08674.

KEGG (2019) Available at: https://www.genome.jp/kegg/ (accessed 21 October 2019).

Kruip, T.A.M. (1994) Oocyte retrieval and embryo production *in vitro* for cattle breeding. *Proceedings of the 5th World Congress on Genetics Applied to Livestock Production,* vol 20, pp. 172–179. Available at: http://www.wcgalp.org/proceedings/1990 (accessed 31 August 2020).

Kruip, T.A.M. and den Daas, J.H.G. (1997) In vitro produced and cloned embryos: effects on pregnancy, parturition and offspring. *Theriogenology* 47, 43–52. DOI: 10.1016/S0093-691X(96)00338-X.

Laible, G., Wei, J. and Wagner, S. (2015) Improving livestock for agriculture — technological progress from random transgenesis to precision genome editing heralds a new era. *Biotechnology Journal* 10, 109–120. DOI: 10.1002/biot.201400193l.

Lambe, N.R., McLean, K.A., Gordon, J., Evans, D., Clelland, N. and Bunger L. (2017) Prediction of intramuscular fat content using CT scanning of packaged lamb cuts and relationships with meat eating quality. *Meat Science* 123, 112–119. DOI: 10.1016/j.meatsci.2016.09.008.

Lambe, N., McLaren, A., Clelland, N., Kaseja, K., Boon, S. and Bunger, L. (2018) Using CT scanning to simultaneously breed UK slaughter lambs for improved carcass and meat quality. *Proceedings of the World Congress on Genetics Applied to Livestock Production*, Auckland, New Zealand, 11, 295. Available at: http://www.wcgalp.org/proceedings/2018 (accessed 12 October 2020).

Land, R.B. and Hill, W.G. (1975) The possible use of superovulation and embryo transfer in cattle to increase response to selection. *Animal Production* 21, 1–12. DOI: 10.1017/S000335610003035X.

Lin, C.Y., Xing, G. and Xing, C. (2012) Measuring linkage disequilibrium by the partial correlation coefficient. *Heredity* 109, 401–402. DOI: 10.1038/hdy.2012.54.

Lohuis, M.M. (1993) Strategies to improve efficiency and genetic response of progeny test programs in dairy cattle. Doctoral thesis, University of Guelph, Canada.

Lotti, S.N., Polkoff, K.M., Rubessa, M. and Wheeler, M.B. (2017) Modification of the genome of domestic animals. *Animal Biotechnology* 28, 198–210. DOI: 10.1080/10495398.2016.1261874.

Luinge, H.J., Hop, E., Lutz, E.T.G, van Hemert, J.A. and de Jong, E.A.M. (1993) Determination of the fat, protein and lactose content of milk using Fourier transform infrared spectrometry. *Anaytica Chimica Acta* 284, 419–433. DOI: 10.1016/0003-2670(93)85328-H.

Luo, Z.W., Woolliams, J.A. and Simm, G. (1994) An assessment of present and future effectiveness of embryological techniques in ruminants. *AgBiotech News and Information* 6, 13N–18N.

Mali, P., Yang, L., Esvelt, K.M., Aach, J., Guell, M. *et al.* (2013) RNA-guided human genome engineering via Cas9. *Science* 339, 823–826. DOI: 10.1126/science.1232033.

Marchini, J. and Howie, B. (2010) Genotype imputation for genome-wide association studies. *Nature Genetics Review* 11, 499–511. Available at: https://www.nature.com/articles/nrg2796 (accessed 31 August 2020).

McParland S., Banos, G., McCarthy, B., Lewis, E., Coffey, M.P. *et al.* (2012) Validation of mid-infrared spectrometry in milk for predicting body energy status in Holstein-Friesian cows. *Journal of Dairy Science* 95, 7225–7235. DOI: 10.3168/jds.2012-5406.

McParland S., Lewis, E., Kennedy, E., Moore, S.G., McCarthy, B. *et al.* (2014) Mid-infrared spectrometry of milk as a predictor of energy intake and efficiency in lactating dairy cows. *Journal of Dairy Science* 97, 5863–5871. DOI: 10.3168/jds.2014-8214.

Meuwissen, T.H.E. (1997) Maximizing the response of selection with a predefined rate of inbreeding. *Journal of Animal Science* 75, 934–940. DOI: 10.2527/1997.754934x.

Meuwissen, T.H., Hayes, B.J. and Goddard, M.E. (2001) Prediction of total genetic value using genome-wide dense marker maps. *Genetics* 157, 1819–1829. Available at: https://www.genetics.org/content/157/4/1819 (accessed 31 August 2020).

Milner, P.K.L., Page, A.W. and Hillerton, J.E. (1996) Detection of clinical mastitis by changes in electrical conductivity of fore milk before visible changes in milk. *Journal of Dairy Science* 79, 83–86. 10.3168/jds.S0022-0302(96)76337-3.

Moore, K.L., Mrode, R. and Coffey, M.P. (2017) Genetic parameters of Visual Image Analysis primal cut carcass traits of commercial prime beef slaughter animals. *Animal* 11,1653–1659. Available at: https://doi.org/10.1017/S1751731117000489 (accessed 31 August 2020).

Moore, K.L., Vilela, C., Kaseja, K., Mrode, R. and Coffey, M. (2019) Forensic use of the genomic relationship matrix to validate and discover livestock pedigrees. *Journal of Animal Science* 97, 35–42. DOI: 10.1093/jas/sky407.

Mueller, M.L., Cole, J.B., Sonstegard, T.S. and Van Eenennaam, A.L. (2019) Comparison of gene editing versus conventional breeding to introgress the POLLED allele into the US dairy cattle population. *Journal of Dairy Science* 102, 4215–4226. DOI: 10.3168/jds.2018-15892.

Nani J.P., Rezende, F.M. and Peñagaricano, F. (2019) Predicting male fertility in dairy cattle using markers with large effect and functional annotation data. *BMC Genomics* 20, Article number: 258. DOI: 10.1186/s12864-019-5644-y.

National Academies of Sciences, Engineering, and Medicine (2018) *Improving Characterization of Anthropogenic Methane Emissions in the United States*. The National Academies Press, Washington. DOI: 10.17226/24987.

National Milk Records (2019) Available at: https://www.nmr.co.uk/software/pocket-companion (accessed 21 October 2019).

Nayeri, S., Sargolzaei, M., Abo-Ismail, M.K., May, N., Miller, S.P. *et al.* (2016) Genome-wide association for milk production and female fertility traits in Canadian dairy Holstein cattle. *BMC Genetics* 17, Article No. 75. DOI: 10.1186/s12863-016-0386-1.

NCBI (2019) Available at: https://www.ncbi.nlm.nih.gov/ (accessed 24 September 2019).

Nicholas, F.W. (1980) The genetic implications of multiple ovulation and embryo transfer in small dairy herds. *Annales de Génétique et de Sélection Animale* 12, 114. DOI: 10.1186/1297-9686-12-1-114B.

Nicholas, F.W. (1996). Genetic improvement through reproductive technology. *Animal Reproduction Science* 42, 205–214. DOI: 10.1016/0378-4320(96)01511-4.

Nicholas, F.W. and Smith, C. (1983) Increased rates of genetic change in dairy cattle by embryo transfer and splitting. *Animal Production* 36, 341-353. DOI: 10.1017/S0003356100010382.

Niemann, H. and Wrenzycki, C. (Eds) (2018) *Animal Biotechnology 2. Emerging Breeding Technologies* (eBook). Springer, New York. DOI: 10.1007/978-3-319-92348-2.

Oatley, J.M. (2017) Recent advances for spermatogonial stem cell transplantation in livestock. *Reproduction,*

Fertility and Development 30, 44-49. DOI: 10.1071/RD17418.

Ojango, J.M.K., Audho, J., Mogaka, D. and Oyieng, E. (2018) ADGG-ODK-1. Installing ODK & Update Tools. Available at: https://africadgg.files.wordpress.com/2018/04/adgg-odk-tool-installation-20180402.pdf (accessed 21 October 2019).

Pabiou, T., Fikse, W.F., Cromie, R., Keane, M.G., Näsholm, A. and Berry, D.P. (2011) Use of digital images to predict carcass cut yields in cattle. *Livestock Science* 137, 130–140. DOI: 10.1016/j.livsci.2010.10.012.

Pinkert, C.H., Dyer, T.J., Kooyman, D.L. and Kiehm, D.J. (1990) Characterization of transgenic livestock production. *Domestic Animal Endocrinology* 7, 1–18. DOI: 10.1016/0739-7240(90)90049-6.

Polejaeva, I.A., Chen, S.-H., Vaught, T.D., Page, R.L., Mullins, J. *et al.* (2000) Cloned pigs produced by nuclear transfer from adult somatic cells. *Nature* 407, 86–90. Available at: https://www.nature.com/articles/35024082 (accessed 31 August 2020).

Pollott, G.E. (2018) Invited review: Bioinformatic methods to discover the likely causal variant of a new autosomal recessive genetic condition using genome-wide data. *Animal* 12, 2221–2234. DOI: 10.1017/S1751731118001970.

Pryce, J.E. and Daetwyler, H.D. (2012) Designing dairy cattle breeding schemes under genomic selection: a review of international research. *Animal Production Science* 52, 107–114. DOI: 10.1071/AN11098.

Public Private Partnership for AI Delivery (2019) Available at: https://www.landolakesventure37.org/Where-We-Work/50 (accessed 20 August 2019).

Purcell, S., Neale, B., Todd-Brown, K., Thomas, L., Ferreira, M.A.R. *et al.* (2007) PLINK: a toolset for whole-genome association and population-based linkage analysis. *American Journal of Human Genetics* 81: 559–575. DOI: 10.1086/519795.

Pursel, V.G., Pinkert, C.A., Miller, K.F., Bolt, D.J., Campbell, R.G. *et al.* (1989) Genetic engineering of livestock. *Science* 244, 1281–1288. DOI: 10.1126/science.2499927.

R Development Core Team (2013) *R: A Language and Environment for Statistical Computing*. R Foundation for Statistical Computing, Vienna. Available at: http://www.R-project.org/ (accessed 19 October 2019).

Rius-Vilarrasa, E., Bünger, L., Maltin, C., Matthews, K. R. and Roehe, R. (2009) Evaluation of Video Image Analysis (VIA) carcasses on-line under UK abattoir conditions. *Meat Science* 82, 94–100. DOI: 10.1016/j.meatsci.2008.12.009.

Roberts, R.J. (2005) How restriction enzymes became the workhorses of molecular biology. *PNAS* 102, 5905–5908. DOI: 10.1073/pnas.0500923102.

Robinson, J.J. and McEvoy, T.G. (1993) Biotechnology - the possibilities. *Animal Production* 57, 335–352. DOI: 10.1017/S1357729800042661.

Rubin, C.-J., Megens, H.-J., Barrio, A.M., Maqbool, K., Sayyab, S. *et al.* (2012) Signatures of selection in the pig genome. *Proceedings of the National Academy of Sciences* 109, 19529–19536. DOI: 10.1073/pnas.1217149109.

Russell, P.J. (2014) *iGenetics: A Molecular Approach*. 3rd edition. Pearson, San Francisco, CA.

Rutten, C.J., Velthuis, A.G.J., Steeneveld, W. and Hogeveen, H. (2013) Invited review: Sensors to support health management on dairy farms. *Journal of Dairy Science*, 96, 1928–1952. DOI: 10.3168/jds.2012-6107.

Sabeti, P.C., Reich, D.E., Higgins, J.M., Levine, H.Z.P., Richter, D.J. *et al.* (2002). Detecting recent positive selection in the human genome from haplotype structure. *Nature* 419, 832–837. Available at: https://www.nature.com/articles/nature01140 (accessed 31 August 2020).

Scholz, A.M., Bünger, L., Kongsro, J., Baulain, U. and Mitchell, A.D. (2015) Non-invasive methods for the determination of body and carcass composition in livestock: dual-energy X-ray absorptiometry, computed tomography, magnetic resonance imaging and ultrasound: invited review. *Animal* 9, 1250–1264. DOI: 10.1017/S1751731115000336.

Schork, N.J., Fallin, D. and Lanchbury S. (2000) Single nucleotide polymorphisms and the future of genetic epidemiology. *Clinical Genetics* 58, 250–264. DOI: 10.1034/j.1399-0004.2000.580402.x.

Seidel, G.E. Jr. (2012) Sexing mammalian sperm – where do we go from here? Review. *Journal of Reproduction and Development* 58, 505–509. Available at: https://www.jstage.jst.go.jp/article/jrd/58/5/58_2012-077/_pdf (accessed 31 August 2020).

Seidel, G.E. Jr. and Garner, D.L. (2002) Current status of sexing mammalian spermatozoa. *Reproduction* 124, 733–743. DOI: 10.1530/rep.0.1240733.

Shalem, O., Sanjana, N. E., Hartenian, E., Shi, X., Scott, D. A. *et al.* (2014). Genome-scale CRISPR-Cas9 knockout screening in human cells. *Science* 343, 84–87. DOI: 10.1126/science.1247005.

Sharpe, J.C. and Evans, K.M. (2009) Advances in flow cytometry for sperm sexing. *Theriogenology* 71, 4–10. DOI: 10.1016/j.theriogenology.2008.09.021.

Simm, G. (1998) *Genetic Improvement of Cattle and Sheep*. CAB International, Wallingford, UK.

Smith, C. (1984) Rates of genetic change in farm livestock. *Research and Development in Agriculture* 1, 79–85.

Smith, C. (1986) Use of embryo transfer in genetic improvement of sheep. *Animal Production* 42, 81–88. DOI: 10.1017/S000335610001775X.

Soyeurt, H., Dehareng, F., Gengler, N., McParland, S., Wall, E. *et al.* (2011) Mid-infrared prediction of bovine milk fatty acids across multiple breeds, production systems, and countries. *Journal of Dairy Science* 84, 1657–1667. DOI: 10.3168/jds.2010-3408.

Taylor, St.C.S., Moore, A.J., Thiessen, R.B. and Bailey, C.M. (1985) Efficiency of food utilization in traditional and sex-controlled systems of beef production. *Animal Production* 40, 401–440. DOI: 10.1017/S0003356100040125.

ThermoFisher. (2019) Available at: https://www.thermofisher.com/uk/en/home.html (accessed 21 October 2019).

Thibier, M., and Wagner, H.G. (2002) World statistics for artificial insemination in cattle. *Livestock Production Science* 74, 203–212. 10.1016/S0301-6226(01)00291-3.

Toffanin, V., De Marchi, M., Lopez-Villalobos, N. and Cassandro, M. (2014) Effectiveness of mid-infrared spectroscopy for prediction of the contents of calcium and phosphorus, and titratable acidity of milk and their relationship with milk quality and coagulation properties. *International Dairy Journal* 41, 68–73. DOI: 10.1016/j.idairyj.2014.10.002.

Toro, M.A., Silio, L., Rodrigañez, J. and Dobao, M.T. (1988) Inbreeding and family index selection for prolificacy in pigs. *Animal Production* 46, 79–85. DOI: 10.1017/S0003356100003135.

UCSC (2019) Available at: https://genome.ucsc.edu/ (accessed 24 September 2019).

US Department of Energy (1992) *DOE Human Genome Program. Primer on Molecular Genetics*. US Department of Energy, Office of Energy Research, Office of Health and Environmental Research, Washington. Available at: https://web.ornl.gov/sci/techresources/Human_Genome/publicat/primer2001/primer.pdf (accessed 19 October 2019).

Vanlierde, H., Soyeurt, N., Gengler, F.G., Colinet, E., Froidmont, M. *et al.* (2018) Short communication: Development of an equation for estimating methane emissions of dairy cows from milk Fourier transform mid-infrared spectra by using reference data obtained exclusively from respiration chambers. *Journal of Dairy Science* 101, 7618–7624. DOI: 10.3168/jds.2018-14472.

van Vliet, R.A., Verrinder Gibbins, A.M. and Walton, J.S. (1989) Livestock embryo sexing: A review of current methods, with emphasis on Y-specific DNA probes. *Theriogenology* 32, 421–438. DOI: 10.1016/0093-691X(89)90008-3.

Vignal, A., Milan, D., Sancristobal, M. and Eggen, A. (2002) A review on SNP and other types of molecular markers and their use in animal genetics. *Genetics, Selection and Evolution* 34, 275–305. DOI: 10.1186/1297-9686-34-3-275.

Villanueva, B. and Simm, G. (1994) The use and value of embryo manipulation techniques in animal breeding. *Proceedings of the 5th World Congress on Genetics Applied to Livestock Production* 20, 200–207. Available at: http://www.wcgalp.org/proceedings/1994 (accessed 16 June 2020).

Villanueva, B., Simm, G. and Woolliams, J.A. (1995) Genetic progress and inbreeding for alternative nucleus breeding schemes for beef cattle. *Animal Science* 61, 231–239. DOI: 10.1017/S1357729800013758.

Vishwanath, R. and Moreno, J.F. (2018) Review: Semen sexing – current state of the art with emphasis on bovine species. *Animal* 12, S1, s85–s96. DOI: 10.1017/S1751731118000496.

Visscher, P.M. and Haley, C.S. (1995) Utilizing genetic markers in pig breeding programmes. *Animal Breeding Abstracts* 63, 1–8.

Waltz, E. (2017) First genetically engineered salmon sold in Canada. *Nature* 548, 148. DOI: 10.1038/nature.2017.22116.

Watson, M. (2018) Commercial applications of SCNT in livestock. In: Niemann, H. and Wrenzycki, C. (eds). *Livestock in Animal Biotechnologies 2. Emerging Breeding Technologies* (eBook). Springer, New York, pp. 21–36.

Wells, D.N., Misica, P.M. and Tervit, R.H. (1999) Production of cloned calves following nuclear transfer with cultured adult mural granulosa cells. *Biology of Reproduction* 60, 996–1005. DOI: 10.1095/biolreprod60.4.996.

Wheeler, M.B. (2013) Transgenic animals in agriculture. *Nature Education Knowledge* 4, 1. Available at: https://www.nature.com/scitable/knowledge/library/transgenic-animals-in-agriculture-105646080/ (accessed 31 August 2020).

White, K.L. (1989) Embryo and gamete sex selection. In: Babiuk, L.A. and Phillips, J.P. (eds). *Animal Biotechnology: Comprehensive Biotechnology, First Supplement*, Pergamon Press, Oxford.

Wilmut, I., Archibald, A.L., Harris, S., McClenaghan, M., Simons, J.P. *et al.* (1990) Methods of gene transfer and their potential use to modify milk composition. *Theriogenology* 33, 113–123. DOI: 10.1016/0093-691X(90)90602-P.

Wilmut, I., Haley, C.S. and Woolliams, J.A. (1992) Impact of biotechnology on animal breeding. *Animal Reproduction Science* 28, 149–162. DOI: 10.1016/0378-4320(92)90101-I.

Wilmut, I., Schnieke, A.E., McWhir, J., Kind, A.J. and Campbell, K.H.S. (1997) Viable offspring derived from fetal and adult mammalian cells. *Nature* 385, 810–813.

Womack, J.E. (1996) The bovine gene map. In: Phillips, C.J.C. (ed.). *Progress in Dairy Science*, CAB International, Wallingford, UK, pp. 89–103.

Woolliams, J.A. (1989) Modifications to MOET nucleus breeding schemes to improve rates of genetic progress and decrease rates of inbreeding in dairy cattle. *Animal Production* 49, 1–14. DOI: 10.1017/S0003356100004190.

Woolliams, J.A. and Wilmut, I. (1989) Embryo manipulation in cattle breeding and production. *Animal Production* 48, 3–30. DOI: 10.1017/S0003356100003743.

Wray, N.R. and Goddard, M.E. (1994a) Increasing long-term response to selection. *Genetics Selection Evolution* 26, 431–451. Available at: https://gsejournal.biomedcentral.com/track/pdf/10.1186/1297-9686-26-5-431 (accessed 31 August 2020).

Wray, N.R. and Goddard, M.E. (1994b) MOET breeding schemes for wool sheep. 1. Design alternatives. *Animal Production* 59, 71–86. DOI: 10.1017/S0003356100007522.

Wright, G., Carver, A., Cottam, D., Reeves, D., Scott, A. *et al.* (1991) High level expression of active human alpha-1-antitrypsin in the milk of transgenic sheep. *Biotechnology* 9, 830–834. DOI: 10.1038/nbt0991-830.

Zoheira, K.M.A. and Allam, A.A. (2010) A rapid method for sexing the bovine embryo. *Animal Reproduction Science* 119, 92–96. DOI: 10.1016/j.anireprosci.2009.12.013.

Recommended Reading

Amer, P., Allain, D., Avendano, S., Baselga, M., Boettcher, P. *et al.* (2015). Breeding strategies and programmes. *Animal Science White Papers, Technical Reports & Fact Sheets. 6.* Available at: https://lib.dr.iastate.edu/ans_whitepapers/6 (accessed 19 October 2019).

Animal Genetics (Journal of the International Society for Animal Genetics).

Mammalian Genome (Journal of the International Mammalian Genome Society).

Nicholas, F.W. (2010) *Introduction to Veterinary Genetics*, 3rd edn, Wiley-Blackwell, UK.

Niemann, H. and Wrenzycki, C. (eds) (2018) *Animal Biotechnologies 2. Emerging Breeding Technologies.* Springer, New York. DOI: 10.1007/978-3-319-92348-2.

Proceedings of the World Congresses on Genetics Applied to Livestock Production. Available at: http://www.wcgalp.org/proceedings (accessed 16 June 2020).

Theriogenology (Journal of the International Embryo Transfer Society).

Trends in Genetics.

6 Analysing Genetic Variation in Farm Animals

Introduction

In Chapter 2, we saw how genes act in different ways to influence the characteristics of animals. In this chapter, we consider how to quantify the extent to which genes affect measured traits and how to use this information in breeding programmes. Because it is practically impossible to discover the exact impact of the many individual genes affecting most traits of interest, we usually consider their collective action on the characteristics of importance to breeders. Some examples of quantitative traits affected by many genes are how much milk a cow produces a day, or how many eggs a hen will lay in a year. One of the key features in developing breeding programmes for many production traits is looking for similarities between animals within families, and differences between animals across families, to assess the genetic variation in such traits. In order to do this, we need to consider how we use the information available on each animal – its pedigree, production data and any available molecular genetic information – and then examine how this information can be combined to indicate the level of genetic control associated with the traits of interest.

Estimating Heritability

Additive variance

It may have seemed a bit theoretical at the time, but the discussion in Chapter 2 on variances has a very important place in the genetic improvement of farmed animals. As we have seen in the preceding chapters, one of the key genetic characteristics of any trait we wish to improve in a breeding programme within a population is its heritability. This is a measure which tells us how much of the variation that we see in our trait is due to the additive effects of the genes that the animals are carrying (additive genetic variance or VAR_A; see Chapter 2) and how much is due to the other factors influencing the performance of our animals, previously called the environmental factors (management, health, nutrition, etc.). The ratio of the additive variance to phenotypic variance for any trait (VAR_A/VAR_P) is called the heritability. Values for heritability lie between 0 and 1 because the additive variance is always a part of the phenotypic variance. A heritability of 0 indicates that there is no genetic variation in the trait concerned, but this is a very rare occurrence in animal populations, as most traits are controlled by genes to some extent. A heritability of 1 is also rare in the polygenic traits found in animal populations and the usual range is between about 0.05 and 0.75 with typical values for a trait like body weight around 0.35.

Note that if we are interested in, say, five traits in our breeding programme then we need to know the heritability of all five traits, and these will probably differ from each other. So, each trait has its own heritability value in any given population. It is also worth noting that the same trait measured in different populations may have a similar heritability value, but it may also vary considerably, depending on the environmental factors coming into play in the different populations, and differences in the genetic makeup of different populations, even within the same breed.

We saw the importance of heritabilities in breeding programmes in Chapters 3 and 4 but we did not address the key question of how to calculate the heritability of a trait. Several genetic principles rely on comparing the phenotypes of related individuals. We instinctively think that offspring tend to look like their parents; not exactly, but they share some of their parents' features. After all, each offspring receives half its genes from each parent. It is no different with quantitative traits, except that in many cases it is harder to see the similarities just by looking. However, by comparing measured values of offspring and parents, or measured values

Genetic Improvement of Farmed Animals (G. Simm *et al.*)
DOI: 10.1079/9781789241723.0006

between families, we can 'see' similarities and differences in the same way. So, heritability measures the resemblance between relatives (and the differences between non-related individuals) and this gives us a clue as to how to calculate heritability.

Actually, there are several ways to estimate heritability. One of the conceptually simplest ways is to calculate the regression of offspring value on parent average (sometimes called the mid-parent value) for a specific trait. We might expect heavier lambs to be born from larger parents and this regression coefficient is a crude way to estimate the heritability of body weight. However, it gives us a clue about how to estimate heritability more generally. When we have pedigree relationships between a group of animals, then related animals should be more similar and unrelated animals less so.

The graph in Fig. 6.1 shows that the weight of offspring is related to the weight of their parents; heavier parents gave birth to heavier offspring. In this case, the heritability of mature weight in sheep would equal the slope of the regression line (the regression coefficient), which is 0.27. While this is a crude example of calculating heritability, it nevertheless demonstrates the principal quite nicely.

Observational and causal variances

So far (in Chapter 2) we have considered the phenotypic (measured) variance of a trait, VAR_P, to be comprised of VAR_A and VAR_E plus one or two other effects. These VAR values are called the *causal components of variance* because they refer directly to the biological origins of the differences between animals. Apart from VAR_P, they are impossible to measure directly in our population so we have to use other features of the population to help us estimate them. Not surprisingly, the key features that we use are the family structure and the relationships between animals in our population, usually in the form of a pedigree. These can be used to calculate what are called *observational components of variance*. The reason that this is important is because the impossible-to-measure causal components of variance need to be estimated in order to calculate measures like the heritability of a trait.

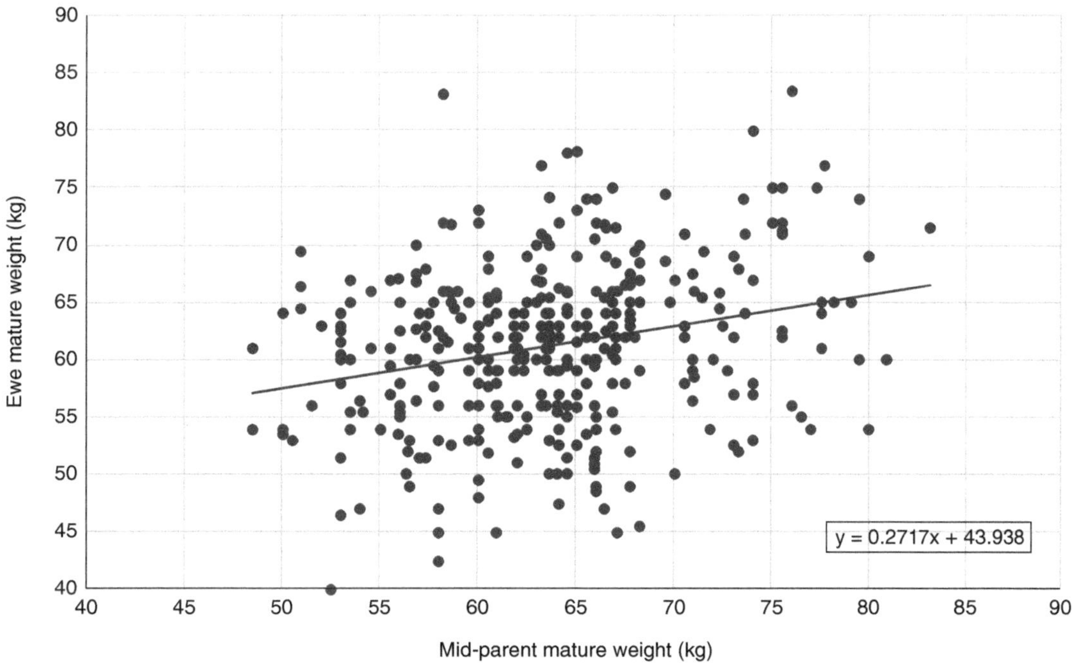

Fig. 6.1. The regression of offspring value on mid-parent value. These data are taken from a flock of sheep in the UK and show the mature weight of 359 ewes at their fourth mating. The fitted regression line is $y = 0.27x + 43.9$; hence the regression coefficient is 0.27 and the heritability of mature weight in this population is 0.27.

Because we can often find an equivalent value from the observational components of variance we can equate them to the causal components of variance, usually in a fairly straightforward manner, and calculate the required causal components from the relevant observational components. By convention we use the Greek letter sigma (σ) to refer to an observational component of variance; technically, sigma refers to the standard deviation so we use σ^2 to indicate the variance (remember in Chapter 2 we saw that the standard deviation of a set of measurements was the square-root of their variance). Also, remember from Chapter 2 that if we are considering two traits then the equivalent of the variance of a single trait is called the covariance, when we want to know how two traits vary together. If we are interested in estimating, say, the genetic correlation between two traits then we will need the covariances of them at both the genetic and phenotypic levels. Sometimes you will see these observational components of *covariance* referred to as cov_{XY} (or cov(X,Y)), where X and Y are the two traits, or as σ_{XY}; they are all equivalent.

The example mentioned in the previous section using a mid-parent/offspring regression (the 'observational component of variance') to estimate heritability (i.e. VAR_A and VAR_P) may not, at first glance, seem to fit this idea of equating two types of variance to find the heritability of the trait. In fact, the covariance between mid-parent and offspring values estimates half the additive variance of the trait. This is because offspring inherit half the genes from each parent or any two offspring from the same parents have half their genes in common (on average). This factor of a half is said to be the additive genetic relationship (A) between the two groups of animals, parents and offspring.

Now remember (from Chapter 2) that:

$$\text{regression of trait 2 on trait 1} = \frac{\text{covariance between traits 1 and 2}}{\text{variance of trait 1}}$$

So, in our present example:

$$\text{Regression of offspring on mid-parent value} = \frac{\text{covariance between the values}}{\text{variance of mid-parent value}}$$

$$\text{Heritability} = \text{regression coefficient}$$

$$\text{Heritability also} = \frac{VAR_A}{VAR_P}$$

Stating this in terms of the casual and observational components of variance (covariance), since the covariance between mid-parent value and offspring value (cov_{XY}) = $0.5 \times VAR_A$ and the variance of mid-parent (σ^2_{MP}) = $0.5 \times VAR_P$ it is straightforward to see that the regression coefficient equals the heritability, since 0.5 cancels out on the top and bottom of the equation (Falconer and Mackay, 1996).

In the case of using a single parent value, rather than the mean of two parents, the covariance between one parental value and offspring value is still = $0.5 \times VAR_A$, the variance of the single parent value = VAR_P. Hence, the heritability is twice the regression coefficient when only using a single parental value.

You can use the data in Spreadsheet 6.1 (see online resources) to rerun the calculations for Fig. 6.1 and calculate the variance and covariances described above. You will need a spreadsheet programme which contains statistical functions to do this. For example, Microsoft Excel currently has these features if you use the 'add-in' called Analysis ToolPak loaded from the 'Options' menu of the 'File' tab. Of course, this may change over time. Read the data into a suitable spreadsheet and use the spreadsheet's built-in regression function to calculate the variances and covariances. Your spreadsheet may also contain a graph plotting function which you can use to plot the data to reproduce Fig. 6.1.

Sire-based methods

One of the earliest methods of estimating heritability in farmed animals was to use the fact that sires produce many gametes and are therefore often used to produce large offspring cohorts (often by artificial insemination). The variance within and between sire cohorts was used to estimate heritability, often done in an *analysis of variance* (ANOVA) and called a *sire model* method of analysis. An analysis of variance is a general statistical method used to analyse data when several different factors affect our data and we wish to ascribe a certain amount of the variance in our measured population to these factors. We do this using a mathematical equation which relates the phenotypic measurements to the different factors we are using to describe them. This equation is commonly called a mathematical 'model' because it tries to reflect the real-world situation in a series of mathematical terms. Because we are interested in the genetic effects of the sires in this case, we include 'sire' as one of the terms in the model and the method is described as using a 'sire model'. Clearly, in order to do this, we need some performance data from the offspring of all sires in our analysis and some idea of the parentage of the offspring (in this case, just the sire).

The analysis of variance is used to calculate the variation ascribed to the differences between sires, as well as the other factors that we may include in the model. In this case the 'between sires' component of variance estimates a quarter of the additive genetic variance (the additive genetic relationship, A, between half sibs) and the measured variance equals VAR_P. Note in the following explanation that the value 4 used to multiply the between-sire component of variance to get the additive genetic variance is the same as 1/0.25, dividing by the additive genetic relationship. So:

$$\text{Heritability} = \frac{(4 \times \text{'between-sire' component of variance})}{VAR_P}$$

There is an example in Spreadsheet 6.2 (see online resources) which you can use to try out a sire model calculation. Read this dataset into a suitable spreadsheet program and use the one-way ANOVA to produce the results. Currently, in Excel, this is found under the 'Data Analysis' tab using the 'ANOVA: single factor' option. The between-sire component is calculated from the 'Between groups' Mean Square (MS) by subtracting from it the 'Within-Groups' MS and dividing by 4.6946 (abbreviated to 4.96 in Table 6.1). This last value is the (weighted) average number of offspring per sire in our dataset and, of course, will differ for any new dataset that you use. Table 6.1 shows the results of doing this set of calculations.

If you are proficient in using the software packages in R (R Core Team, 2013) then we have included a suitable script called R Script 6.1 in the online resources. Note that you will have to edit this script to give it the correct path to the CSV file of data.

We have now seen two examples of how to calculate heritability and a general picture is emerging. We equate the causal and observed components of variance, adjust with the additive genetic relationship and calculate heritability from the estimated additive genetic and phenotypic variances. We can use any relationship group to estimate heritability using the additive relationship between them. Not surprisingly, doing these calculations with real data is slightly more complicated than has been implied so far but the basic principles still apply.

You may have been thinking, hold on a minute, some lambs grow faster than others because they are singles not twins, or because their mother was a mature ewe not a ewe lamb. These 'environmental' factors will affect some lambs 'unfairly' so we may not get a true picture of the genetics of these lambs. Most modern methods of estimating heritability can take such environmental influences into account (if they are recorded) as well as including the maternal contribution to the performance of an animal in the calculations, where appropriate. This is commonly referred to as using a *mixed animal model* and is the method of choice for estimating heritabilities these days.

Table 6.1. The analysis of variance (ANOVA) table produced from analysing the ewe weights (kg) in spreadsheet 6.2 plus the calculation of the heritability from a sire model.

Source of variation from ANOVA table	Sum of squares	Degrees of freedom	Mean square
Between groups	15,093	167	90.38
Within groups	29,265	616	47.51

Steps in calculation	Value	Calculation
Weighted mean sire-group size	4.69	See text
Between-sire component of variance	9.13	(90.38 – 47.51) / 4.69
Additive genetic variance (VAR_A)	36.52	4 × 9.13 (see text)
Phenotypic variance (VAR_P)	56.64	Variance of ewe weight
Heritability	0.64	36.52 / 56.64

Animal model

In the late 1940s and early 1950s, Charles Henderson, a pioneer of modern quantitative genetics, outlined how to estimate the genetic merit of animals, taking into account the known environmental influences which may also affect a trait. This methodology was called *best linear unbiased prediction* (BLUP) and has been the basis for much work to estimate the breeding values of animals. It is interesting to note that at that time there was no way that the BLUP method could be implemented on even a moderate-sized dataset, due to the small size/power of computers available then. The first real-life implementation of BLUP probably occurred in the late 1960s.

Although the initial aim of BLUP methodology was to estimate the genetic merit of animals, the approach was extended to estimate causal components of variance, notably by Patterson and Thompson in 1971. They first described the *restricted maximum likelihood* (REML) approach that has since become the method of choice for estimating the genetic parameters of traits in a population. The method uses a function called the log likelihood function, which looks at the likelihood of the genetic parameters being correct given the characteristics of the data after firstly correcting observations for any environmental effects. The equations to be solved using this function are very complex and so scientists have looked for ways to make solving them easier and less time consuming. The software used to calculate these *variance components* takes in large volumes of pedigree and performance data and stores them as a two-way table, referred to as a matrix in mathematics. Making these calculations easier to compute involves avoiding a complicated mathematical process called inverting a matrix, referred to as *derivative free REML* (DFREML; Smith and Graser, 1986). There are several methods available to average the matrices with the information needed to compute the variance and genetic parameters (*average information REML*; Gilmour *et al.*, 1995).

Several software packages are available for animal breeders to use to estimate heritability using this REML approach (see later section on software solutions). Usually these packages take a computer file of pedigree information from our recorded animals, extending back as far as possible into breed history, plus a file of the recorded traits and environmental effects on the recorded animals. The pedigree information can also be replaced or complemented by genomic information, as described later. The packages then use these files, plus a suitably constructed list of effects to be fitted in the animal model, and produce estimates of how each environmental effect influences our traits and also the additive genetic and phenotypic variances of those traits. These can then be used to compute the heritability. You will often see this method referred to as the mixed animal model; this is because there is a mixture of what are called *fixed* and *random effects* in the model. This is a statistical distinction between different types of model terms used. The environmental effects are commonly fitted as categorical data (males or females; singles, twins or triplets) or may be covariates (e.g. age at weighing when analysing weight data); these are called fixed effects because they have a 'fixed' or limited number of categories. The random effects are considered to have an unlimited number of levels and we are just using a 'random' sample of them in our analysis. These random effects include estimates of VAR_A, and others which we shall learn about in the next section, as well as an estimate of the variance that we cannot account for with any 'known' factors in the model. This is referred to as the *residual variance* or *error variance* and is used in every mixed model that we fit.

You may think that this method sounds complicated and does not fit with our idea of equating causal and observed components of variance, modified by the additive genetic relationship, to estimate heritability. In fact, it does, but in a more comprehensive manner. The 'basic genetic group' is now the animal itself and the additive genetic relationship used is *all* relationships in the pedigree file, right back to when the pedigree started. The mixed animal model methodology effectively computes the relationships between all animals in the pedigree file and applies them to all pairs of relationships in the data. You will see this referred to as the *additive genetic relationship matrix,* often abbreviated to the *relationship matrix* in papers describing variance component estimates.

The animal model is a much more complex calculation than the ones we have attempted so far and the details of achieving it are outside the scope of this book. If you are competent in R (R Core Team, 2013) and would like to try an example we suggest you look at Gorjanc (2019) which provides a simple example of using the animal model. Also consult Mrode (2014) for a straightforward account of the details, and the paper by Thomson *et al.* (2018) for a good summary of using animal models.

Alternative models

If you can grasp the concepts of using an animal model or a sire model with *normally-distributed traits* then you will be able to appreciate most of the work carried out to analyse the traits of interest in animal breeding. However, there are other models, and other types of trait, which you may need to be aware of, and which we introduce here.

Most of the alternative models were used before the animal model became the method of choice. The most common was the *sire–maternal grandsire model*. As its name suggests, it concentrates on the relationships within the dataset used, based on the sires and maternal grandsires of the measured animals. This is because in populations using artificial insemination (AI) these links are the most influential.

Not all traits fit the normal distribution or bell-shaped curve. As mentioned earlier, some of these may be transformed using a particular mathematical function to make them normally distributed. The most suitable transformation will depend on the distribution of the phenotypic values. As an example of this, Pollott and Greeff (2004) used a cube-root transformation of faecal egg count data when investigating parasite resistance in sheep. When analysing such data, it is best to consult a statistician first to see what type of transformation is most appropriate for your data.

Some traits have a limited number of alternative values, despite having an underlying polygenic basis. These often have two phenotypic states such as resistant/susceptible in relation to a particular disease or live/dead at a particular age. In this case, it is possible to use a special type of animal model, a so-called threshold model, to analyse these data which assumes an underlying normal distribution to the limited number of states. In other words, the *liability* of being in one state or another is normally distributed, even though there are few final states. You can read a good account of using this approach with dairy cattle data in Kadarmideen *et al.* (2000).

Additional causal components of variance

So far, we have used the terms VAR_A and VAR_P to indicate two causal components of variance seen in our population for any given trait. There are a number of useful additional components of variance that we can estimate from particular types of data. For example, when analysing pre-weaning traits in mammals there are additional factors which may influence performance of our animals. If a breeding female is a good mother, she will tend to rear heavier offspring than a poor mother. We can estimate the effect of the mother in our animal model if she has had several litters, i.e. repeated lambings,

Table 6.2. Causal components of variance used in animal breeding with a description and some example references.

Variance component	Symbol	Description and reference where it has been estimated
Additive genetic	VAR_A	Variance of breeding values for a trait – Maniatis and Pollott (2002c)
Total genetic	VAR_G	All genetic influences on a trait combined – Maniatis and Pollott (2002c)
Environmental	VAR_E	All non-genetic influences on a trait combined – Maniatis and Pollott (2002c)
Common environment	VAR_{Ec}	Variance due to animals being kept together in specific groups
Permanent environment	VAR_{Ep}	Variance due to common effects across litters or lactations. See VAR_{ME} below
Phenotypic	VAR_P	Variance of measured values of a trait – Maniatis and Pollott (2002c)
Maternal (permanent) environmental	VAR_{ME}	Effect of the mother on a trait of her offspring which is common to all the litters she produces – Maniatis and Pollott (2002c)
Maternal additive genetic	VAR_{AM}	The effect of the mother's genes on the rearing of her offspring as expressed by the offspring's trait – Maniatis and Pollott (2002c)
Dominance	VAR_D	Collective effect of all the dominant genes influencing a trait – Sun *et al.* (2014)
Litter	VAR_{Litter}	Variance in offspring trait due to being born and reared in the same litter – Maniatis and Pollott (2002a)
Associative effect genetic variance	VAR_{SBV}	Variance due to associative effect of individuals on group members – Bijma *et al.* (2007)
Sire by environment (G × E)	VAR_{SE}	The variation in a trait due to a sire's genotype having a different effect in each environment where its offspring are found – Maniatis and Pollott (2002a)
Mitochondrial	VAR_M	Variation only inherited through the maternal line due to differences in the mitochondrial DNA, found outside the cell nuclei but in the cytoplasm – Maniatis and Pollott (2002b)

calvings, farrowings, etc. (referred to as VAR_{Ep} in Chapter 4). This maternal variance component may be further split into a genetic part and a non-genetic (environmental) part, called VAR_{AM} and VAR_{ME}.

A number of other variance components can be estimated using the animal model with REML methodology. These are listed in Table 6.2, along with some references that estimate the variance component concerned and provide more details. Interestingly, maternal components of variance have been found in chickens, which presumably measures the effects of egg size or weight on the performance of the offspring (Koerhuis and Thompson, 1997) since in modern poultry systems hens and eggs are separated soon after laying.

You may ask why it is necessary to complicate further what is already a quite complex set of ideas. Our basic aim in animal breeding is to identify the best animals, genetically speaking, so that we can breed future generations of improved animals from them. If we can identify non-genetic factors which may reduce the accuracy of identifying the best animals and 'remove' their effects from our genetic evaluations, then we should identify more accurately those animals with the highest genetic merit, and so make faster genetic progress. Most of the variance components listed in Table 6.2, other than the phenotypic, additive and total genetic variances, fall into this category of important influences that may add 'noise' to the system, which need to be removed. An exception to this is the maternal additive genetic variance, which may be useful in selection schemes to identify animals who are genetically better mothers. Also, the permanent environmental effect is commonly used to measure the repeatability of a trait (see Chapter 4).

Once we have identified important sources of variation which may reduce the efficacy of our breeding programme, we may choose to account for this in the genetic evaluation procedures outlined in Chapter 7. Fitting these terms in the genetic evaluation model, usually a mixed animal model these days, should make our genetic improvement programme more accurate and therefore lead to faster genetic gains. The articles listed in Table 6.2 give examples of where some of these additional components of variance have been calculated and the size of their effect. There are few current examples of genetic evaluation systems using these additional components, but these are likely to be more common in the future. The dominance variance mentioned in Table 6.2 and its impact on the performance of animals is briefly discussed below.

Estimating Non-Additive Parameters, Correlations and Genotype-by-Environment Interactions

Non-additive components of variance

By definition, the additive genetic variance is the component of most interest in animal breeding because it is the major predictable effect that is passed on from one generation to the next. However, dominance effects and heterosis are also well-known genetic phenomena and estimating their effects has become more tractable in recent years, particularly with the use of molecular genetic information. A good example of this is discussed by Sun *et al.* (2014) who looked at dominance effects of genes in dairy cattle.

We have already mentioned dominance in Chapter 2 when discussing Mendelian gene action. For qualitative traits (i.e. traits that we can observe directly), when there is dominant gene action, we can see the effect of one allele overriding the effect of another in heterozygous individuals (e.g. coat colour in some breeds). When genes act additively on quantitative or measured traits, we expect a smooth, linear progression in performance when comparing animals with 0, 1 or 2 copies of a particular allele. With dominant gene action, we do not see this smooth progression. Dominance results in a different phenotype for heterozygotes than that expected from just the additive effects of the different alleles at a particular locus. Hence, dominance is called a non-additive genetic effect. This effect is not passed on predictably from an individual to its offspring because the offspring inherit only one of the alleles at this locus from each parent, i.e. it is individual alleles, not genotypes, that pass from parents to offspring. With dominant gene action, we need to know which alleles an offspring inherited from *each* parent in order to predict the effect of this genotype on its performance. Quantitative traits are usually controlled by many genes, and it is likely that dominance is occurring at some loci. We cannot observe what is going on at each individual locus using current methods. However, in a population, we can estimate the overall effect of deviations from additive gene action at many different loci for a particular trait. This is called the dominance variance.

Genetic correlations

As mentioned in Chapter 2, we commonly record more than one trait on our populations and breed for genetic improvement in a range of traits. In order to do this, we need to know the relationships between the traits in our population. We measure this using the correlation coefficient described in Chapter 2. There we drew a parallel between calculating a variance and a covariance, from which the correlation is calculated. It should be no surprise to learn that all the variances mentioned in Table 6.2 can have corresponding correlations. The most commonly used correlations are the genetic correlation (strictly speaking the correlation between additive genetic effects) and the phenotypic correlation.

We can estimate these, and any other correlations equivalent to the variances shown in Table 6.2, using REML methodology with a suitable animal model as described above. Technically, we use a *multi-trait animal model* to do this. In practice, as the number of variance components to estimate becomes greater, many of them become inestimable due to the lack of good data structure. An example of this can been seen in Maniatis and Pollott (2003) who discuss the effect that various data structures had on estimating maternal genetic components of variance in pre-weaning lamb traits. You will see examples of the use of multi-trait models in the species chapters of this book (Chapters 8 to 13) when genetic parameters are discussed.

Genotype-by-environment interactions

It is well recognized that a given genotype may perform differently in different environments. This was described in Chapter 3 as a genotype-by-environment interaction (G × E). In its simplest form it can be recognized as the effect of two very contrasting environments on two different breeds. The most noticeable examples of this are when a temperate breed is used in a tropical environment. Technically the performance of the tropical breed should also be measured in a temperate environment too, but this rarely happens. However, in Australia and the US where a range of breeds and environments can be found in the same country it is possible to test this more accurately.

Frisch and Verco (1979) give a nice example of this where growth rate was measured in three types of cattle in three environments. Their data are shown in Fig. 6.2. The Brahman is an improved tropical breed of cattle while the Hereford × Shorthorn is representative of a temperate cross breed. The three environments in this case were different levels of stress relating to various combinations of housing, feeding and parasite treatment. The key point to note is that the three genotypes rank differently in the three environments and the often-assumed superiority of temperate breeds over tropical breeds only holds true in the low stress

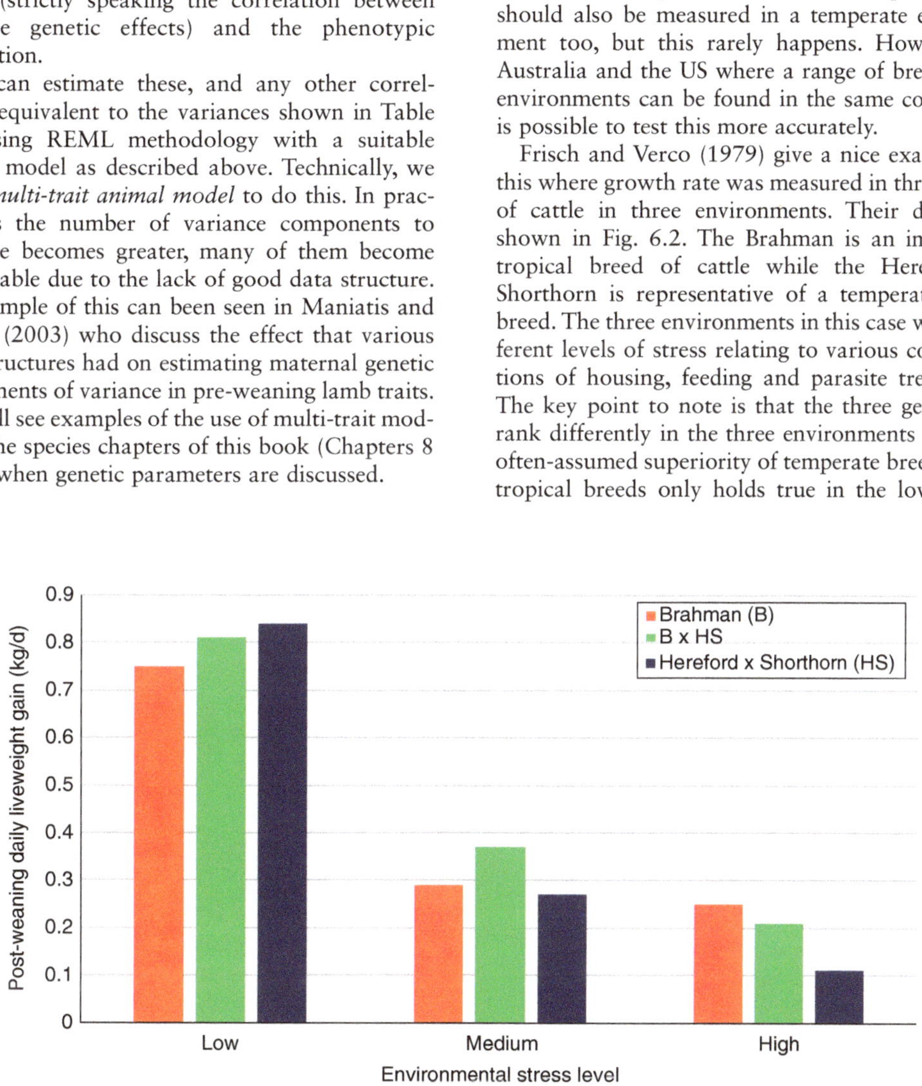

Fig. 6.2. Genotype-by-environment interaction at the breed level for post-weaning daily live weight gain (kg/d) in temperate and tropical breeds of cattle. (After Frisch and Vercoe, 1979.)

environment, and even then its superiority is not that great.

This idea has been extended to look at how multiple genotypes respond in many environments, often using a measure of the environment as an independent variable. These G × E methods have been reviewed by Strandberg (2013) and Hayes *et al.* (2016). One approach is to consider a given trait in two different countries as separate traits, and then to calculate the genetic correlation between them. For instance, Ojango and Pollott (2002) looked at the ranking of Holstein bulls for milk production in the UK and Kenya and found a genetic correlation of 0.49 between them. Clearly, bulls did not rank the same in both countries, although there was some similarity. This idea has been extended to look at how a sire's genetic merit changes as some measure of the environment changes too, using data from AI sires used in a variety of different farming systems within a country. This can be achieved using *random regression* methods for sires across farms and estimated using REML methodology in an extension of the animal model approach. When merit changes with environment, this is referred to as the trait showing *plasticity* and the method used is commonly referred to as a *reaction norm* approach, often used in environmental genetics. Maniatis and Pollott (2002a) found that G × E effects in lambs accounted for about 3% of the variation in scanning weight, fat and muscle depth in a UK sire-referencing scheme. Using random regression methods, Pollott and Greeff (2004) demonstrated that for Merino wool traits and faecal egg count (FEC), an indicator of parasite resistance/susceptibility, the level of G × E was also low (<4% of phenotypic variance) but certain sires were very susceptible to different environments. This paper gives an interesting discussion of using reaction norm models with production traits and is worth reading for a more complete discussion than is possible here.

Random regression

In the previous section, we introduced the topic of random regression. This statistical method is used when a trait varies across a known range of an environmental variable. We may want to fit a line across this range of the environmental variable and use the characteristics of the line to explain how the trait varies with the changing environment. In animal production this is most commonly used when considering how milk yield of dairy animals changes as the lactation progresses, called the lactation curve. If we want to investigate the genetics of different stages in lactation, for example, we could break the lactation data up into different sections and analyse each section as a different trait. A more elegant solution is to model individual lactations using random regression methods and consider specific days of lactation as points to study. In animal breeding we may be interested in how breeding value or heritability changes across the lactation. This method is often used when it is difficult to characterize a trait which changes over time in a simple manner, without losing some of the information in our analysis. There is a good example of this for milk yield in dairy cows in Olori *et al.* (1999) and a review of other studies in Druet *et al.* (2003). Growth curves are another example of when random regression methods are often used. Both growth curves and lactation curves are difficult to characterize individually. The random regression approach has some appeal because it fits an overall shape to the data but there is genetic variation among animals in deviations from this overall curve, which can be analysed and translated into breeding values.

In the previous section we saw a different use of random regression where Merino traits were modelled across different farm environments. In this case it is important to find some variable which can describe the farm environment succinctly so that it can be used as the independent variable (*x* or horizontal axis) in our analysis. Pollott and Greeff (2004) used the mean performance of the trait on each farm as a way to characterize its environment for the production of that trait and showed how the heritability of FEC varied across the range of environments found. This is conceptually simple but is not ideal since we would prefer an independent measure of the environment not already used in the analysis.

McLaren *et al.* (2015) applied a reaction norm model using linear random regressions by sire for a range of traits in Texel sheep. They conducted a survey of the farms in their study and asked for information on a range of flock factors including concentrate feed use and flock size. They used a statistical procedure called canonical correlation analysis to develop a numerical scale for each farm. This scale was then used as the independent variable in their analyses. They found a somewhat higher G × E effect (~10%) than that reported by Pollott and Greeff (2004).

Software solutions

As we have seen, the estimation of variances, covariances, heritabilities and correlations is based on measuring the degree of similarity in performance between relatives. In the past, these parameters were usually estimated from designed experiments involving particular classes of relatives (e.g. parents and offspring; half sibs). The modern methods described above account for the similarity in performance between many different classes of relatives, and they separate genetic and environmental influences on performance in the best possible way, simultaneously. As a result, they can be used to estimate genetic parameters from field records, as well as from designed experiments. (Field records usually contain data from many different types of relatives, often spread unevenly across many herds or flocks, seasons, etc., which complicates analysis.) For more details on parameter estimation, and some of the computer packages available to do this, see Hill and Mackay (1989), Cameron (1997), Mrode (2014) and the *Proceedings of the World Congresses on Genetics Applied to Livestock Production*, particularly Druet and Ducrocq (2006).

It should be noted at this point that there are two basic statistical approaches to estimating genetic parameters: 'Bayesian' and 'frequentist' methods. A detailed discussion of these methods is outside the scope of this book, but you may see papers that refer to these different approaches. There is much discussion amongst statisticians about which approach is best. Both provide parameter estimates that animal breeders require and can use, but each method has some benefits over the other. The DFREML approach we described earlier is a frequentist approach. For a discussion of Bayesian methods see the review by Ben Zaabza *et al.* (2017).

Molecular Genetics and Trait Variation

Early in this chapter we considered how the traits that we are interested in vary between animals. This was measured in terms of trait variance and the 'level of measurement' was the animal (i.e. the records used are the animals' growth rates, milk yields, etc.). With the advent of molecular methods, we are now able to analyse variation in our traits of interest at a much finer level – the gene, single nucleotide polymorphisms (SNPs) or region of the genome. Now we are able to think in terms of a specific change in the genome at one base position having an effect on the traits that we see. This is easier to comprehend when talking about Mendelian traits. In this case a single base change at one position can cause dramatic differences at the phenotypic level. Two good examples of this are the *DGAT1* gene mutation in dairy cattle (see Grisart *et al.*, 2004) and the Booroola gene in sheep (see Wilson *et al.*, 2001). In both cases, a single base change at the DNA level results in a noticeable change in phenotype in milk production and litter size, respectively. When considering quantitative traits, such dramatic changes are exceptional. Our model for gene action with quantitative traits is that these traits are influenced by many genes, each having a small effect on the phenotype. Genetic improvement occurs by selecting the versions of these many genes which, when combined together, have a positive effect on the trait under consideration. These combined effects may be small from one generation to the next, but they accumulate over time to create bigger changes. Ideally, we would like to know the individual effects of all versions (polymorphisms) of all genes on all traits in our breeding programme. At present, this is not feasible, but current genomic selection methodology can utilize these polymorphisms to predict breeding values without knowledge of the specific variants that have causative effects.

The advent of cheap and high-throughput DNA sequencing technologies has made discovery of genome-wide polymorphisms a relatively easy task in farmed animal species. To achieve this, we see how the genomes of a group of animals, often of the same breed, differ at the individual DNA-base level. A useful precursor for this is the availability of reference genome sequences, which are detailed maps of the genomes of our target species. As described in Chapter 5, these are available for all major farmed animal species. Following the reference genome assemblies, research communities have focused on surveying population-level variation, including initiatives such as the *hapmap* project and '1000-genomes' project (1000 Bull Genomes Project, 2019; Hayes and Daetwyler, 2019; International Sheep Genomics Consortium, 2019).

Such work demonstrates some very interesting aspects of livestock genomes which can help us understand how variation at the phenotypic level can arise, be selected for, and be managed. Firstly, as we have always suspected, animals within a particular breed are not identical at the genome level. The cattle genome comprises about 3 Gb (3 billion (1000 million) bases) of DNA sequence. In an experiment using 32 Holstein-Friesian cattle, Szyda *et al.* (2015) found that only 1.5% of these 3 billion base positions showed any polymorphisms. Thus, over 98% of these cattle genomes were identical. Secondly the cattle genome, for example, comprises about 25,000 genes (i.e. recognized protein-coding regions) which comprise less than 2% of the genome (BGSAC, 2009).

These two aspects of cattle genomes allow us to concentrate on the base positions which vary within genes as the source of the genetic variation in our selected populations. Currently, we use a short-cut method to try to evaluate animals at the genomic level. This uses evenly-spaced SNP markers along the genome as the source of information about how the genomes vary in our population under selection. Each SNP is then assessed to see how much variation in the trait is associated with it, based on the linkage disequilibrium between markers and genes. So, if we were using, say, 1 million SNPs in an analysis, only a proportion of them capture some variance for any given trait, and a different proportion will be relevant for different traits. Modern genomic evaluation methods attempt to give a value for each SNP haplotype for each trait and the sum of these is the genetic merit of the animal. Details of this genomic selection methodology are given in Chapter 7.

Currently, this approach has not changed the basic way we think about variance components and the genetic parameters derived from them. However, by using evenly spaced SNPs across the genome it is possible to look at the heritability of regions across the genome. This helps to identify regions of the genome which have a noticeable effect on a trait of interest. In Chapter 5, we outlined another method for investigating the parts of the genome which have a particular significance for a trait, probably where a gene influencing that trait may be found, called a genome-wide association study (GWAS). In an interesting study, Riggio *et al.* (2013) compared the two methods when investigating nematode parasite resistance in sheep. They concluded that the regional heritability approach (whereby the contribution of a 'window' of SNPs to the genetic variance in the trait is assessed) was able to find more regions of the genome influencing the trait that was found by single SNP GWAS. Both types of analysis can be the first step in a process to investigate the genes associated with particular traits by looking at points on the genome where known genetic differences (the SNPs) can be shown to be associated with differences in performance. There are many instances of this in the literature and the Animal QTLdb website (https://www.animalgenome.org/cgi-bin/QTLdb/BT/index) contains many examples of regions associated with quantitative trait differences in livestock.

Not surprisingly, the molecular genetic approach has led to the concept of *genomic heritability* (de los Campos *et al.*, 2015). This idea uses all the SNPs in a particular study and attempts to combine all their effects on a trait to compute the heritability of that trait. Two major advantages of this approach are: (i) the genomic data capture the genetic differences between full sibs, i.e. the Mendelian sampling component of variation; and (ii) genomic data can be used to capture 'hidden' relationships between animals, for example, where pedigree records do not exist or are incomplete. This method appears to provide a similar answer to traditional methods of calculating heritability only when all the SNPs associated with a trait are used in the analysis.

In Chapter 7 we discuss the various extensions to BLUP methodology made possible by the use of different genomic relationship matrices. These methodologies also have a role in variance component estimation. Hence the *single-step method* of Misztal *et al.* (2010) and Legarra *et al.* (2014) can be used to estimate variance components in a similar manner to that described for *genomic breeding values* in Chapter 7. Interestingly, this methodology can also be used for GWAS analyses as well.

Calculating inbreeding using SNP markers

In Chapter 4 we outlined the traditional approach used to estimate the inbreeding coefficient through the pedigree, tracing the ancestry of animals back to a common ancestor. Ultimately, we could trace back to what is termed the *base population* – essentially the animals that originally formed the breed. The inbreeding coefficient (F) is the probability that two randomly chosen alleles at a homologous locus within an individual are identical by descent (IBD), i.e. the alleles are identical because they are passed down from a common ancestor, compared with the base population in which all alleles are said to be independent. Note that segments of the genome may be IBD if the animal is the result of the mating of closely related individuals; these are often described as being *autozygous* segments.

The estimate of F is usually obtained from the pedigree using what is called the path coefficient method (see Table 4.10). With this approach, the inbreeding coefficient for an animal equals half of the relationship between its parents. For example, a male animal (X) will have half of his genes in common with his female offspring (Y). If X is mated with Y to produce Z, then the inbreeding coefficient for the animal Z is half of the relationship between X and Y. In this case, it will be 0.5 × 0.5 and this equals 0.25. Estimating F from pedigrees is based on the expected proportion of the genome that is IBD given the *average* genetic relationships among animals. We know that, because of Mendelian sampling, the actual proportion of the genome that is IBD can vary from the expected average proportion for the given class of relatives.

Using SNP markers, the realized proportion of the genome that is IBD can be estimated for each individual. However, identifying the proportion of the genome which is IBD due to common ancestors requires the allele frequencies of base animals, which is often not very feasible. However, using the genomic relationship matrix derived from SNPs, several studies have estimated F (Bjelland *et al.*, 2013). The results from simulation have shown that when base population allele frequencies are known, F estimated from the genomic relationship matrix is very close to the true value. However, using estimated base allele frequencies results in less accurate estimates of F. Some studies have suggested that using intermediate allele frequencies of 0.5 was more beneficial than attempting to estimate them in the base population (Forutan *et al.*, 2018). However, the availability of SNPs makes it possible to directly measure homozygosity in the genome. More accurate estimates of F can be obtained using such an approach, and it is not dependent on obtaining estimates of base population allele frequencies. Several studies have shown that characterizing inbreeding based on long stretches of consecutive homozygous genotypes (*runs of homozygosity*; ROH) provides a better measure of individual autozygosity than estimating overall inbreeding based on pedigree information or the genomic relationship matrix. Estimates of F_{roh} based on the proportion of the genome that is in runs of homozygosity (of a specified length but variable length) can be derived (Keller *et al.*, 2011) as the total length of the genome in a ROH divided the by the overall length of the genome. Defining different minimum lengths of ROH is similar to changing the depth of pedigree or base population in pedigree inbreeding. The shorter ROH reveal more ancient inbreeding, while longer ROH show more recent inbreeding. Usually, software such as PLINK or BCTtools are used for estimating F_{roh}. The studies of Keller *et al.* (2011) and Forutan *et al.* (2018) demonstrated that estimates of inbreeding by ROH were better than those from the pedigree-based approach and other genomic methods. These newer methods do not require a knowledge of the base population, as is the case with the pedigree method, but rather base their inbreeding calculations in relation to the current generation and relate all other animals back from it. This removes the inherent difficulty of never really knowing which animals were in the base population, often because there was no herd or flock book at that time.

Summary

- Estimating the genetic parameters of traits in livestock populations is a key requirement for genetic improvement programmes. These parameters include the heritabilities of all traits of interest as well as the genetic and phenotypic correlations among them.
- The heritability is calculated from recorded livestock performance data and the pedigree relationships in the population. The basic approach is to equate the phenotypic variance measured in certain family groups with the expected relationships between them, using what are called causal and observational components of variance.
- Modern methods of parameter estimation use the animal model which uses all relationships between an animal and the other recorded individuals in the population, using a genetic relationship matrix (A).
- There are several additional variance components that can be estimated from such data using the animal model. These include maternal effects for pre-weaning traits in mammals, genotype-by-environment interactions, which measure how the same genotype differs in performance in different environments, and several environmental effects accounting for additional and systematic influences on animal performance.
- The calculation of genetic correlations between traits in our population follows a similar methodology to that used for calculating heritabilities. The multi-trait animal model is the current method of choice.

- Random regression methods look at how a trait varies across a measurable range of factors. Commonly, growth curves or lactation curves are analysed in this way, but genotype-by-environment interactions can also be assessed by this methodology. This approach may be useful, for example, when a sire's offspring are recorded in a range of environments (different farms) and there is a measurable difference between the farms, e.g. in climate, levels of husbandry.
- Advances in molecular genetics are allowing us to investigate traits of interest at the genome level, rather than solely at the whole animal level. The availability of SNP chips allows genome-wide studies of the main livestock traits to identify which regions of the genome are associated with differences between animals in performance traits. There are databases available which catalogue the known links between genes and performance.
- The concepts of regional heritability and genomic heritability have expanded our vision of how molecular genetic variation in animals is linked to performance.

References

1000 Bull Genomes Project (2019) *1000 Bull Genomes Project* Available at: http://www.1000bullgenomes.com/ (accessed 20 November 2019).

Ben Zaabza, H., Ben Gara, A. and Rekik, B. (2017) *Bayesian Modelling in Genetics and Genomics.* DOI: 10.5772/intechopen.70167.

BGSAC (2009) The genome sequence of taurine cattle: A window to ruminant biology and evolution. *Science* 324, 522–528. DOI: 10.1126/science.1169588.

Bijma, P., Muir, W.M. and Van Arendonk, J.A.M. (2007) Multilevel selection 1: quantitative genetics of inheritance and response to selection. *Genetics* 175, 277–288. DOI: 10.1534/genetics.106.062711.

Bjelland, D.W., Weigel, K.A., Vukasinovic, N. and Nkrumah, J.D. (2013) Evaluation of inbreeding depression in Holstein cattle using whole-genome SNP markers and alternative measures of genomic inbreeding. *Journal of Dairy Science* 96, 4697–4706. DOI: 10.3168/jds.2012-6435.

Cameron, N.D. (1997) *Selection Indices and Prediction of Genetic Merit in Animal Breeding*. CAB International, Wallingford, UK.

de los Campos, G., Sorensen, D. and Gianola, D. (2015) Genomic heritability: what is it? PLoS *Genetics* 11, e1005048.

Druet, T. and Ducrocq, V. (2006). Innovations in software packages in quantitative genetics. *Proceedings of the 8th World Congress on Genetics Applied to Livestock Production.* Available at: http://www.wcgalp.org/proceedings/2006 (accessed 16 June 2020).

Druet, T., Jaffrézic, F., Boichard, D. and Ducrocq, V. (2003) Modeling lactation curves and estimation of genetic parameters for first lactation test-day records of French Holstein cows. *Journal of Dairy Science* 86, 2480–2490. DOI: 10.3168/jds.S0022-0302(03)73842-9.

Falconer, D.S. and Mackay, T.F.C. (1996) *Introduction to Quantitative Genetics*, 4th edn. Longman, Harlow, UK.

Forutan, M., Mahyari, S.A., Baes, C., Melzer, N., Schenkel, F.S. and Sargolzaei, M. (2018) Inbreeding and runs of homozygosity before and after genomic selection in North American Holstein cattle. *BMC Genomics* 19, 98. DOI: 10.1186/s12864-018-4453-z.

Frisch, J.E. and Vercoe, J.E. (1979) Adaptive and productive features of cattle growth in the tropics: their relevance to buffalo production. *Tropical Animal Production* 4, 214–222.

Gilmour, A.R., Thompson, R. and Cullis, B.R. (1995) Average information REML: An efficient algorithm for variance parameter estimation in linear mixed models. *Biometrics* 51, 1440–1450. DOI: 10.2307/2533274.

Gorjanc, G. (2019) Quantitative genetic (animal) model example in R. Available at: https://www.bioconductor.org/packages/release/bioc/vignettes/GeneticsPed/inst/doc/quanGenAnimalModel.pdf (accessed 21 October 2019).

Grisart, B., Farnir F., Karim, L., Cambisano, N., Kim, J-J. *et al.* (2004). Genetic and functional confirmation of the causality of the DGAT1 K232A quantitative trait nucleotide in affecting milk yield and composition. *Proceedings of the National Academy of Sciences* 101, 2398–2403. DOI: 10.1073/pnas.0308518100.

Hayes, B.J. and Daetwyler, H.D. (2019) 1000 Bull Genomes Project to map simple and complex genetic traits in cattle: Applications and outcomes. *Annual Review of Animal Biosciences* 7, 89–102. DOI: 10.1146/annurev-animal-020518-115024.

Hayes, B.J., Daetwyler, H.D. and Goddard, M.E. (2016) Models for genome x environment interaction: examples in livestock. *Crop Science* 56, 1–9.

Hill, W.G. and Mackay, T.F.C. (Eds) (1989) *Evolution and Animal Breeding: Reviews on Molecular and Quantitative Approaches in Honour of Alan Robertson*. CAB International, Wallingford, UK.

International Sheep Genomics Consortium (2019). Available at: https://www.sheephapmap.org/hapmap.php (accessed 21 October 2019).

Kadarmideen, H.N., Thompson, R. and Simm, G. (2000) Linear and threshold model genetic parameters for disease, fertility and milk production in dairy cattle. *Animal Science* 71, 411–419. DOI: 10.1017/S1357729800055338.

Keller, M.C, Visscher, P.M. and Goddard, M.E. (2011) Quantification of inbreeding due to distant ancestors and its detection using dense single nucleotide polymorphism data. *Genetics* 189, 237–249. DOI: 10.1534/genetics.111.130922.

Koerhuis, A.N.M. and Thompson, R. (1997) Models to estimate maternal effects for juvenile body weight in broiler chickens. *Genetics, Selection and Evolution* 29, 225–249. DOI: 10.1186/1297-9686-29-2-225.

Legarra, A., Christensen, O.F., Aguilar, I. and Misztal, I. (2014) Single step, a general approach for genomic selection. *Livestock Science* 166, 54–65. DOI: 10.1016/j.livsci.2014.04.029.

Maniatis, N. and Pollott, G.E. (2002a) Genotype-by-environment interactions in lamb weight and composition traits. *Animal Science* 75, 3–14. DOI: 10.1017/S1357729800052772.

Maniatis, N. and Pollott, G.E. (2002b) Nuclear, cytoplasmic and environmental effects on growth, fat and muscle traits in Suffolk lambs from a sire referencing scheme. *Journal of Animal Science* 80, 57–67. DOI: 10.2527/2002.80157x.

Maniatis, N. and Pollott, G.E. (2002c) Maternal effects on weight and ultrasonically measured traits of lambs in a small closed Suffolk flock. *Small Ruminant Research* 45, 235–246. DOI: 10.1016/S0921-4488(02)00114-1.

Maniatis, N. and Pollott, G.E. (2003) The impact of data structure on genetic (co)variance components of early growth in sheep, estimated using an animal model with maternal effects. *Journal of Animal Science* 81, 101–108. DOI: 10.2527/2003.811101x.

McLaren, A., Brotherstone, S., Lambe, N.R., Conington, J., Mrode, R. and Bünger, L. (2015) The effects of different farm environments on the performance of Texel sheep. *Animal* 9, 1624–1634. DOI: 10.1017/S1751731115001123.

Misztal, I., Aquilar, I, Legarra, A., Tsuruta, S. , Johnson, D.L. and Lawlor, T,.J. (2010) A unified approach to ultilise phenotypic, full pedigree and genomic information for genetic evaluation. *Proceedings of the 9th World Congress Applied To Livestock Production.* Available at: http://www.wcgalp.org/proceedings/2010 (accessed 16 June 2020).

Mrode, R. (2014) *Linear Models for the Prediction of Animal Breeding Values*, 3rd edn. CAB International, Wallingford, UK.

Ojango, J.M.K. and Pollott, G.E. (2002) The relationship between Holstein bull breeding values for milk yield derived in both the UK and Kenya. *Livestock Production Science* 74, 1–12. DOI: 10.1016/S0301-6226(01)00282-2.

Olori, V.E., Hill, W.G., McGuirk, B.J. and Brotherstone, S. (1999) Estimating variance components for test day milk records by restricted maximum likelihood with a random regression animal model. *Livestock Production Science* 61, 53–63. DOI: 10.1016/S0301-6226(99)00052-4.

Patterson, H. D. and Thompson, R. (1971) Recovery of inter-block information when block sizes are unequal. *Biometrika* 58, 545–554.

Pollott, G.E. and Greeff, J.C. (2004) Genotype by environment interactions and genetic parameters for fecal egg count and production traits of Merino sheep. *Journal of Animal Science* 82, 2840–2851. DOI: 10.2527/2004.82102840x.

R Core Team (2013) R: A Language and Environment for Statistical Computing. R Foundation for Statistical Computing, Vienna. Available at: http://www.R-project.org/ (accessed 01 September 2020).

Riggio, V., Matika, O., Pong-Wong, R., Stear, M.J. and Bishop, S.C. (2013) Genome-wide association and regional heritability mapping to identify loci underlying variation in nematode resistance and body weight in Scottish Blackface lambs. *Heredity* 110, 420–429. DOI: 10.1038/hdy.2012.90.

Smith, S.P., and Graser, H.-U. (1986) Estimating variance components in a class of mixed models by restricted maximum likelihood. *Journal of Dairy Science* 69, 1156–1165. DOI: 10.3168/jds.S0022-0302(86)80516-1.

Strandberg, E. (2013) Animal genetic in environment interaction. In: *Encyclopedia of Sustainability Science and Technology*. Springer-Verlag, Berlin.

Sun, C., VanRaden, P.M., Cole, J.B. and O'Connell, J.R. (2014) Improvement of prediction ability for genomic selection of dairy cattle by including dominance effects. *PLoS ONE* 9, e103934. DOI: 10.1371/journal.pone.0103934.

Szyda , J., Fraszczak, M., Mielczarek, M., Giannico, R., Minozzi, G. *et al.* (2015) The assessment of inter-individual variation of whole-genome DNA sequence in 32 cows. *Mammalian Genome* 26, 658–665. DOI: 10.1007/s00335-015-9606-7.

Thomson, C.E., Winney, I.S., Salles, O.C. and Pujol, B. (2018) A guide to using a multiple-matrix animal model to disentangle genetic and nongenetic causes of phenotypic variance. *PLoS ONE* 13, e0197720. DOI: 10.1371/journal.pone.0197720.

Wilson, T., Wu, X.Y., Juengel, J.L., Ross, I.K., Lumsden, J.M. *et al.* (2001) Highly prolific Booroola sheep have a mutation in the intracellular kinase domain of bone morphogenetic protein IB receptor (ALK-6) that is expressed in both oocytes and granulosa cells. *Biology of Reproduction* 64, 1225–1235. DOI: 10.1095/biolreprod64.4.1225.

Recommended Reading

Cameron, N.D. (1997) *Selection Indices and Prediction of Genetic Merit in Animal Breeding*. CAB International, Wallingford, UK.

Falconer, D.S. and Mackay, T.F.C. (1996) *Introduction to Quantitative Genetics*, 4th edn. Longman, Harlow, UK.

Hill, W.G. and Mackay, T.F.C. (Eds) (1989) *Evolution and Animal Breeding: Reviews on Molecular and Quantitative Approaches in Honour of Alan Robertson*. CAB International, Wallingford, UK.

Lynch, M. and Walsh, B. (1998) *Genetics and Analysis of Quantitative Traits*. Sinauer Associates, Sunderland, Massachusetts.

Mrode, R. (2014) *Linear Models for the Prediction of Animal Breeding Values*, 3rd edn. CAB International, Wallingford, UK.

Nicholas, F.W. (2010) *Introduction to Veterinary Genetics*, 3rd edn. Wiley-Blackwell, Chichester, UK.

Proceedings of the World Congresses on Genetics Applied to Livestock Production. Available at: http://www.wcgalp.org/ (accessed 16 June 2020).

Russell, P.J. (2014) *iGenetics: A Molecular Approach*, 3rd edn. Pearson, San Francisco, California.

7 Predicting Breeding Values

Introduction

In Chapter 4 we concentrated on how to *predict* responses to selection in simple breeding programmes. This is useful for comparing alternative breeding programmes, and helping to make sensible investment decisions. When it comes to actually implementing selection there are a number of steps that can be taken to improve the chances of *achieving* the responses predicted. In this chapter, we will outline the steps that are required to obtain the most appropriate breeding values for any species, and discuss the issues involved. This process of predicting breeding values is often termed *genetic evaluation*.

Figure 7.1 shows the typical steps involved in producing breeding values in modern breeding schemes. We discuss each of these steps in the following sections. However, it will be easier to understand how modern schemes work if we first examine some of the principles, and the earlier approaches, on which modern schemes are founded. Of course, the country, species and type of organization involved will all influence how these steps are implemented in practice. In this chapter we focus on the principles and generic approach, and in the later chapters we highlight the particular issues relevant to each species.

Performance Data and Pedigrees

All genetic evaluation requires performance data of some type. These will either be direct measurements of the traits of interest in the selection programme or correlated, or proxy, traits which can be used as selection criteria. These data will need to be recorded on the animals in the breeding programme and their relatives, along with any appropriate details which will be used later to build the most appropriate model for analysis. For instance, the ages at weighing and the sexes of the lambs are two such factors if we are considering predicting the genetic merit of a population of sheep for body weight. Obviously, performance records should be as accurate as possible since any inaccuracies in data will increase the phenotypic variation of the trait (strictly speaking, the environmental component of this) and make it harder to predict the 'true' breeding values.

For the various methods of evaluation, it is essential to collect complete and accurate pedigrees. This seems obvious too, but is not always easy, partly due to human error. For instance, the availability of genomic data has identified fairly high levels of incorrect parentage recording (typically 10–12% errors). Hence, it is important to have a proper database for the storage of pedigree data, and their validation at collection. When genomic data are available for a population, these can also be used to validate and correct pedigree records. Genomic data also offer another option for populations where pedigree data are not available, or are difficult to collect. Some genomic methods do not require pedigree data but the relationships among animals is computed from the genomic data. This means that genetic evaluation can be implemented without the requirement for pedigrees. This is discussed later in greater detail.

In cattle, sheep and goats, collation and checking of performance and pedigree records tends to be carried by a recording agency. These recording agencies could be commercial companies that offer a charged service to farmers or breed associations. However, for fish, pigs and poultry, the recording operations are carried out mostly within breeding companies. For cattle, sheep and goats, the prediction of breeding values tends to be carried out at a national level, providing estimates of the genetic merit for all animals in the country, or at least those that have their pedigrees recorded. Usually, a national body is responsible for the genetic evaluation and the data are usually transferred from the recording agencies to the evaluation centre. Examples of national evaluation centres for dairy cattle include

Genetic Improvement of Farmed Animals (G. Simm *et al.*)
DOI: 10.1079/9781789241723.0007

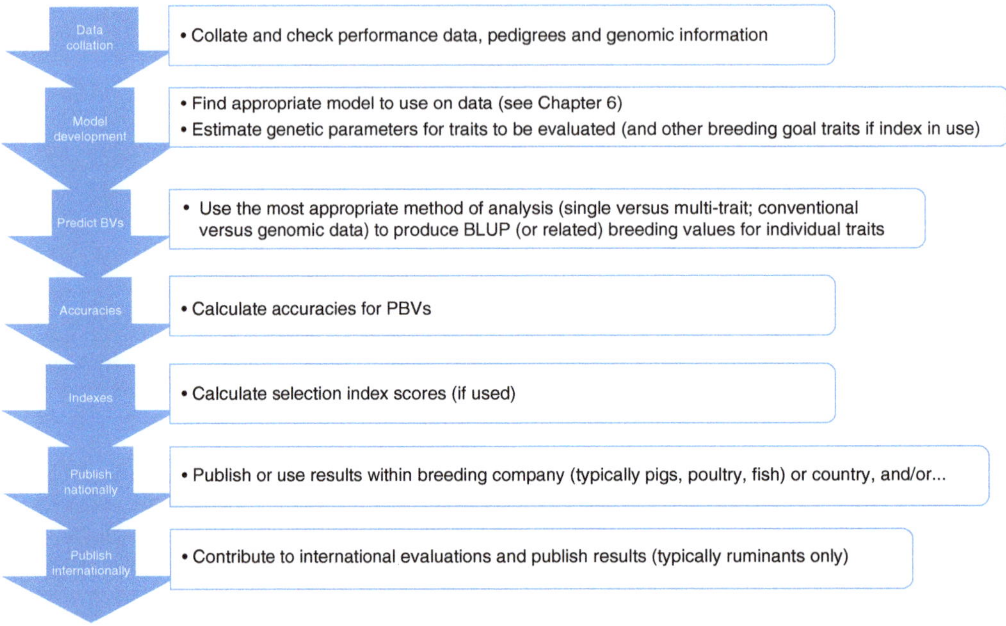

Fig. 7.1. A flow diagram of a typical pathway to producing predicted breeding values.

Edinburgh Genetic Evaluation Services (EGENES) 2019 in the UK, the Canadian Dairy Network (CDN), 2019 in Canada and the Council on Dairy Cattle Breeding in the USA (CDCB), 2019. Examples for sheep and goats include France Génétique Elevage (2019) in France, Sheep Improvement Limited (SIL), 2019 in New Zealand, Sheep Genetics-LambPlan (2019) and KidPlan (2019) in Australia. Evaluations are usually carried out separately for each breed, although across-breed evaluations are becoming more common, especially when records from crossbred animals are available. National systems for genetic evaluations often include a large amount of historical and current performance data and require deep pedigrees, usually spanning many generations. Pig, fish and poultry companies typically perform their genetic evaluations in house.

Management of Candidates for Selection

In most breeding programmes we attempt to disentangle the effects of genes and the environment, in order to select animals that have high genetic merit, and not those that perform well simply because they are well fed and managed. As far as possible, animals that are going to be compared should be managed to give them equal opportunity to express their genetic merit. For example, comparisons of post-weaning growth of animals will be fairest if they are all weaned at the same age and have equal access to feed.

The environmental factors that obscure true genetic merit can be divided into two types: those that are difficult to attribute to individual animals, and those that we can identify as affecting particular animals and can do something about. An example of the first type would be a subclinical disease affecting the performance of some animals in a herd or flock, but not others. In general, we know that this sort of thing happens, but it is difficult to identify with certainty all of the animals that have been affected. Probably the best that we can do in this situation (unless selecting for resilience to disease) is to discard the performance records from animals that we believe have been affected.

The second type of environmental influences are those that we can attempt to adjust for. These include factors such as age of dam, birth rank (single, twin, triplet, etc.) or litter size, lactation number, season or date of birth or age at measurement. Although we can never know the *exact* effect that any of these factors has on an individual animal's performance, we can estimate the *average* effect that any of these factors has on a group of animals. Adjusting for this is usually better than doing nothing about it. Methods of adjusting records for this type of environmental effect are discussed in the following section.

In species such as cattle, sheep and goats, the performance records of animals are collected from several farms which may be spread across the country. Therefore, accurate recording is very important for the identification of all environmental influences. In general, the adjustment for these environmental influences is more of a challenge compared to pigs and poultry, which are usually reared in more controlled environments by breeding companies.

It is the environmental effects of the first type, and those of the second type which we may not have completely corrected for in our analysis, that contribute to the environmental and hence phenotypic sources of variation in animal performance which were described in earlier chapters.

Objective methods of genetic improvement rest heavily on comparisons of the performance of animals which have been treated in a similar way, e.g. born over a relatively short period of time, on the same farm, and fed and managed similarly. These animals are often called contemporaries, and the groups they belong to are called *contemporary groups*. The accuracy of selection will be improved by ensuring that animals in a contemporary group get as similar treatment as possible. Ideally, contemporary groups should be as large as possible, to allow the best possible separation of genetic and environmental effects on performance. In practice, a compromise has to be reached between making the groups large, but including animals which are not really contemporaries, and accepting smaller groups of animals which really do share a similar environment. For instance, in pedigree beef herds there is often quite a wide spread in calving date. When records from these herds are analysed, the size of contemporary groups can be increased by expanding the range of birth dates over which calves are eligible to join a group. But at some stage this defeats the object, as ignoring the increasing seasonal effects on calf performance outweighs any advantage from making the contemporary groups larger. There are various statistical methods of deciding on the optimal group size in these situations, and references to some of these are listed at the end of the chapter.

Adjusting Records of Performance

There are a number of methods of adjusting records of performance that have been used historically to help to deal with the second type of environmental influence described above. They are outlined only briefly here, since modern methods of estimating predicted breeding values (PBVs) simultaneously adjust records and predict breeding values, rather than doing this stepwise. (For more details on the earlier approaches see Simm, 1998.) However, adjusted records are often used as input variables in predictions of breeding values using genomic information, and so are still relevant in this context.

Additive correction factors

The simplest approach is to use *additive correction factors*, so called because they involve adding amounts to (or subtracting amounts from) the performance records of animals which belong to particular classes, like singles or twins. For example, we could weigh lambs at weaning and note which animals were born and reared as singles or twins. If we averaged the weights for the singles and twins separately, we might find that singles were 3 kg heavier than twins, on average. If we wanted to select for growth rate alone, regardless of litter size, the simplest way to compare animals fairly would be to add 3 kg to the weaning weight of all twin lambs (or subtract 3 kg from the weight of all single lambs) to create a set of adjusted records. Then all the lambs could be compared as a single group and those with the heaviest adjusted weights selected for breeding. An example is given in Table 7.1.

Multiplicative correction factors

Multiplicative correction factors are similar to additive factors but, as the name suggests, the records of performance are adjusted by multiplying by the correction factors, rather than adding the correction factors. For example, rather than expressing the correction factor for 20-week weight of triplet-born lambs as +2.51 kg, as in Table 7.1, we could also express this in terms of triplets being 4% lighter than twins, and so multiply all weights from triplets by 1.04 to bring them to the level expected for twins. Multiplicative correction factors are more appropriate when the scale of the correction depends on the mean level of performance in the herd or flock.

Table 7.1. Additive correction factors used to adjust live weights, ultrasonic fat and muscle depths in Suffolk ram lambs, prior to calculating index scores. Lambs were involved in a selection experiment at SAC. A separate set of correction factors was used for ewe lambs. The values shown were subtracted from or added to the records from the class of lambs shown, to make them equivalent to records from twin born lambs from ewes of 3 years of age and older. The values shown for age at scanning were subtracted for each day of age in excess of 150 days at scanning or added for each day of age under 150 days on the day of scanning.

	Correction factors for:						
	Birth rank			Dam age (years)		Age at scanning (days)	
Trait	Single	Twin	Triplet	2	3 and over	under 150	over 150
Live weight	−4.25 kg	0	+2.51 kg	+1.75 kg	0	–	–
Fat depth	−0.52 mm	0	+0.21 mm	–	0	+0.07 mm/day	−0.07 mm/day
Muscle depth	−0.69 mm	0	+0.63 mm	–	0	+0.10 mm/day	−0.10 mm/day

Standardizing to adjust records

A third method of adjusting records involves assigning records from animals born in a specified time period to a contemporary group, based on the factors to be adjusted for. Within each of these groups each record is then expressed as a deviation from the mean of the group, in standard deviation units. For example, records from lambs born over a period of a few weeks (a 'season') could be assigned to four groups: single reared from 2-year-old dams, single reared from older dams, multiple-reared from 2-year-old dams and multiple reared from older dams. The mean and standard deviation (s.d.) of the trait concerned are then calculated separately for each of the four groups. Finally, the performance record of each animal is expressed as a deviation from the mean of its own group, and then divided by the s.d. for that group. This gives records expressed in s.d. units (i.e. typically ranging from about −3 to about +3), rather than the units in which the trait was measured – though they can easily be converted to units of measurement again. These standardized measurements can be compared directly across contemporary groups within a flock or herd.

Principles of Breeding Values and Indexes

Clues to an animal's breeding value

In most modern breeding programmes, we attempt to rank potential candidates for selection on their additive genetic merit or breeding value. We never know the *true breeding value* of an animal, though we can come close to this by recording very large numbers of offspring. Usually this is impractical and very expensive, and so we have to rely on predicted or *estimated breeding values* (EBVs) of the candidates for selection.

The clues we can use to predict breeding values have already been mentioned. They include records of performance, and increasingly genomic information, from:

- the animal itself;
- the animal's ancestors;
- the animal's full or half sibs;
- the animal's progeny;
- any other relatives of the animal; and
- combinations of the classes of relatives listed above.

Predicting an animal's breeding value is a bit like completing a large, complicated jigsaw puzzle, where each piece of the puzzle is a record of performance from the animal itself or one of its relatives. The more pieces of the puzzle we have, the easier it is to see the true picture. However, some pieces of the puzzle are more informative than others. Generally, the higher the proportion of genes in common between the animal and a given relative, the more useful the record of performance from that relative. But, as we saw in Chapter 4, records from progeny are of most value. As the number of records on progeny increases, the correlation between predicted and true breeding values (the accuracy of selection) approaches 1. So widespread progeny tests produce predicted breeding values which are very close to true breeding values. With other classes of relatives, the accuracy of prediction never reaches 1, and for all classes of relatives there are diminishing returns in accuracy as the number of records increases.

Calculating PBVs

The general principle underlying the calculation of PBVs is that the phenotypic performance is a product of two components: environmental and genetic effects. Therefore, the calculation of PBVs always involves 'correcting' for the environmental effects and computation of the PBV from the corrected records, whether this is done as a two-stage process or simultaneously.

Using the animal's own performance

In the simplest case, when we have a single record of performance on the animal itself, the predicted or estimated breeding value is the deviation in performance from contemporaries, multiplied by the heritability of the trait concerned. The deviation in performance is calculated after adjusting the performance records for the type of environmental effects discussed in the last section:

$$\text{PBV or EBV} = h^2 \times \text{deviation in performance from contemporaries}$$

This is equivalent to the formula used at the beginning of Chapter 4 to predict response to selection, except that the PBV refers to a single animal, whereas the response refers to the average performance of the progeny born from selected parents. Table 7.2 illustrates how PBVs are calculated for two groups of animals in separate herds, when each animal has a single record of performance. When PBVs are calculated in this way, the animals rank in exactly the same order within a herd as they rank on their performance record, or on their deviation from the mean of contemporaries. However, the PBV predicts how much of the superiority or inferiority in the animal's performance is due to its (additive) genes – half of which will be passed on to its progeny. The table also illustrates several other features of PBVs:

- They can have positive or negative values or be equal to zero.
- The sign indicates whether they are expected to be genetically above (+) or below (–) the mean (average) of the group of animals on which the calculations were performed, or some other defined group of animals whose PBVs are set to average zero, e.g. those animals born in a particular year. It is important to know which these animals are. The group of animals from which deviations in breeding value are expressed is often called the *genetic base*.
- They span a narrower range than the deviations in performance – this regression or 'shrinking' reflects the fact that part of the variation in performance is environmental (as shown in Fig. 2.24). For an animal with a single record of performance, the regression coefficient, which determines the extent of this shrinking, is simply the heritability of the trait concerned. The higher the heritability, the lower the proportion of environmental variation, and so the less severe the shrinking.
- They are expressed (at least initially) in the same units as the record of performance (e.g. kg of live weight, litres of milk, mm of fat).
- In the example in Table 7.2 we have no way of knowing whether the 20 kg difference in the average weight of animals in the two herds is due to breeding or to feeding and management, or a combination of these. In this case, the best we can do is to calculate and use the PBV within herd only.

As outlined in Chapter 4, using repeated records of performance from the same animals can increase the response to selection. Similarly, the use of repeated records of performance can increase the accuracy of predicting breeding values for individual animals. In this case:

$$\text{PBV} = b \times \text{average deviation of individual's performance records from mean of contemporaries}$$

where b is a regression coefficient which depends on the number of repeated records, and on the heritability and repeatability of the trait concerned (see Van Vleck *et al.* (1987) and Mrode (2014) for details of the calculation of this regression coefficient).

Using information from relatives

Calculating PBV from the performance of relatives can be a bit more difficult. The simplest case is

Table 7.2. An example of the calculation of PBVs for 400-day weight in beef cattle when each animal has a single record of performance. There are groups of ten contemporary animals in each of two herds. The performance records have been adjusted for the type of environmental effects discussed in the last section, e.g. age of dam. The heritability of 400-day weight is assumed to be 0.4. In this example we have no way of knowing whether the 20 kg difference in the average weight of animals in the two herds is due to breeding, feeding and management, or a combination of these. So, the best we can do is to calculate and use the PBVs within herd only.

Herd 1				Herd 2			
Animal	Adjusted 400-day weight (kg)	Deviation from mean (kg)	PBV (kg)	Animal	Adjusted 400-day weight (kg)	Deviation from mean (kg)	PBV (kg)
1	450	−70	−28	11	470	−70	−28
2	600	+80	+32	12	530	−10	−4
3	440	−80	−32	13	550	+10	+4
4	480	−40	−16	14	490	−50	−20
5	530	+10	+4	15	640	+100	+40
6	570	+50	+20	16	480	−60	−24
7	500	−20	−8	17	520	−20	-8
8	520	0	0	18	570	+30	+12
9	550	+30	+12	19	610	+70	+28
10	560	+40	+16	20	540	0	0
Mean	520	0	0	**Mean**	540	0	0

when the only records available are from the parents. If we first calculate PBVs for each parent, then the PBV of their offspring is simply:

PBV of offspring = ½PBV of sire + ½PBV of dam

So, if we mated a bull with a PBV for 400-day weight of +30 kg to a cow with a PBV of +10 kg, the PBV of the offspring for 400-day weight would be +20 kg. This is illustrated in Fig. 7.2(a). This formula should come as no surprise, because we have already seen that offspring get exactly half of their genes from each parent. If we only have a PBV for one parent, then the best we can do is to assume that the other parent is of average genetic merit. If PBVs are expressed relative to the average merit of animals born in the recent past, then a parent of unknown PBV is usually given a PBV of zero. So, for example, if we mated the bull mentioned above with a PBV of +30 kg for 400-day weight to a cow of unknown PBV, the PBV of the offspring would be +15 kg ([30+0]/2; see Fig. 7.2(b)). Or more directly, when the PBV of one parent is unknown, we simply halve the PBV of the other parent to get the offspring's PBV.

In some cases, we have a PBV for the sire and for the dam's sire, but not for the dam herself. We can still get a PBV for offspring in two steps. Firstly, we get a PBV for the dam by halving her sire's PBV. Then we average the sire's and the dam's PBV as before. For example, if we stick with the bull mentioned above, but mate him to a cow of unknown PBV, whose sire has a PBV of +8 kg, then our prediction of the cow's BV is +4 kg (8/2) and so the offspring PBV is +17 kg ([30 + 4]/2; see Fig. 7.2(c)). Alternatively, and more directly, we can add half of the sire's PBV to one quarter of the maternal grandsire's PBV. PBVs calculated in this way from ancestor's PBVs are known as *pedigree indexes*. They are very valuable in providing an early prediction of an animal's genetic merit before it has performance records of its own or records from collateral relatives. (Increasingly, the availability of genomic information is allowing more accurate PBVs for animals without performance records themselves.)

Similarly, if we only had a PBV *based on a single record of performance* from any relative, our best prediction of the BV of a related animal would be:

PBV = proportion of genes in common with the relative × PBV of the relative

So, for example, if we had a PBV of a full or a half sib based on a single measurement of their own performance we would multiply their PBV by 0.5 or 0.25, respectively, to get a PBV for the unrecorded relative. (See Fig. 4.6 for the proportions

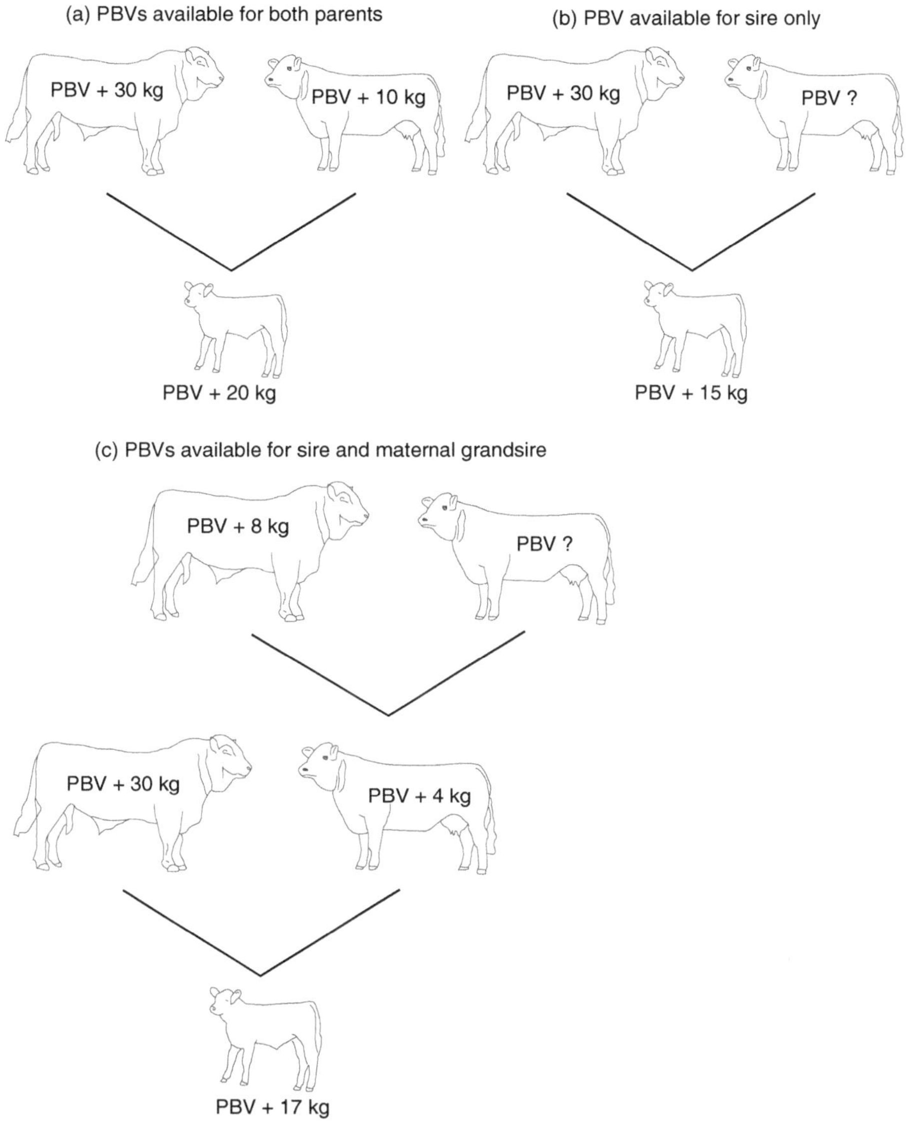

Fig. 7.2. Calculating the expected genetic merit of offspring (a) when both parents have PBVs, (b) when only the sire has a PBV and (c) when the sire and maternal grandsire have PBVs. In this example the PBVs are for 400-day weight.

of genes in common between an animal of interest and some other relatives.)

We saw earlier that if we have PBVs for both parents we can average these to get the PBVs for offspring. This is because the two parents contribute independent samples of genes to their offspring (unless the parents are related). However, if we have more than one of any other type of relative we cannot simply average their PBVs, because progeny or sibs, for example, have genes in common with each other as well as the animal whose PBV is being derived, and so there is 'overlap' in the information they provide – this was illustrated in Chapter 4 by the diminishing returns in accuracy with increasing numbers of relatives.

As an example, let us consider the prediction of a bull's BV from single records on his progeny, which are not related to each other except through him. In this case:

PBV = b × deviation of progeny records from overall mean

where b is a regression coefficient which depends on the number of progeny (n), and on the heritability (h^2) of the trait concerned (after Van Vleck *et al.*, 1987):

$$b = \frac{2n}{n + (4 - h^2)/h^2}$$

This may look complicated, but all we need to note here is that: (i) the higher the number of progeny, the greater the value of b, and (ii) the higher the heritability, the higher the value of b. Table 7.3 shows the values of b for traits with different heritabilities, and for sires with different numbers of progeny. The values in the table show that b approaches a maximum value of 2 when there are records on many progeny. In other words, with many progeny, a bull's PBV is simply the superiority or inferiority of his progeny multiplied by 2. Again, this value of 2 should come as no surprise – progeny have half of their genes in common with each parent, so the progeny performance is a measure of half the bull's breeding value.

To illustrate this further, let us consider two dairy bulls, one whose daughters yield 500 kg more milk than average, and one whose daughters yield 500 kg of milk less than average. The PBVs of the two bulls depend on the number of daughters on which these yield deviations are based. Table 7.4 shows PBVs for the two bulls, assuming that these daughter yield deviations are produced from 1, 5, 10, 100, 1000 or 10,000 daughters of each bull. The heritability of milk yield is about 0.35, so with 1 to 10,000 daughters we get values of b between 0.175 and 1.998, as shown in Table 7.3. With a record from only a single daughter of each bull, we have very little information to base our prediction on. This is reflected by the fact that the value of b is low, and so the PBV are severely 'shrunk' compared to those derived from the same daughter yield deviation based on large numbers of daughters.

The table also shows results for a third bull, Bull C, which has an average daughter yield deviation of +300 kg milk. Comparing results for this bull with those for Bull A illustrates that, even though the average daughter yield deviation is lower, the PBV of Bull C may be higher than that for Bull A when Bull C has more daughters recorded than Bull A (e.g. compare the PBV for Bull A with 10 daughters with that for Bull C with 100 daughters).

Combining information from different types of relatives can become complex. The most common method used, prior to the widespread use of BLUP, was to produce an index that weights the contributions from different types of relatives according to the class of relative, and the number of records

Table 7.3. Values of the multiplier or regression coefficient (b in the formula presented in the text) used to derive PBVs from progeny records for traits with different heritabilities, and for sires with different numbers of progeny.

No. of progeny	Value of 'b'			
	$h^2 = 0.1$	$h^2 = 0.25$	$h^2 = 0.35$	$h^2 = 0.5$
1	0.050	0.125	0.175	0.250
5	0.227	0.500	0.648	0.833
10	0.408	0.800	0.979	1.176
100	1.439	1.739	1.811	1.869
1,000	1.925	1.970	1.979	1.986
10,000	1.992	1.997	1.998	1.999

Table 7.4. PBVs of three bulls with average daughter yield deviations of +500 kg, −500 kg and +300 kg milk, assuming that these deviations are produced from 1, 5, 10, 100, 1000 or 10,000 daughters of each bull, and that the heritability of milk yield is 0.35.

	Bull A	Bull B	Bull C
Average daughter yield deviation (kg milk):	+500	−500	+300
PBV (in kg milk) if yield deviation is based on single records from the following number of daughters:			
1	+87.5	−87.5	+52.5
5	+324.0	−324.0	+194.4
10	+489.5	−489.5	+293.7
100	+905.5	−905.5	+543.3
1,000	+989.5	−989.5	+593.7
10,000	+999.0	−999.0	+599.4

available from each class. This approach is described in the next section.

Selection indexes

Historically, selection indexes were used to combine adjusted records of performance in: (i) *a single trait* measured on the animal itself, and one or more classes of relatives; (ii) *several traits* measured on the animal itself; or (iii) *several traits* measured on the animal itself and on one or more classes of relatives. Index selection on more than one trait is termed *multi-trait* index selection. Today, selection indexes are typically based on PBVs, but we will return to that later.

Combining information from relatives on a single trait

In the first case listed above, the object is to produce a single score for selecting animals, based on information from different types of relative. In this case, we can define the index as:

$$I = b_1P_1 + b_2P_2 + b_3P_3 \ldots$$

where

I = the index score for an individual animal

b_1, b_2, b_3 = the weighting factors or *index coefficients* by which the phenotypic measurements P_1, P_2, and P_3 are multiplied. (These are equivalent to the regression coefficients used earlier to calculate PBVs from records of performance from an individual or averages from groups of progeny.)

P_1, P_2, P_3 = the phenotypic measurement on the animal itself, or the average measurement from different groups of relatives, for the single trait under selection, after adjustment for known environmental effects. For example, if we were selecting for weaning weight in sheep, and had a flock with 100 breeding females, and 5 sires used per annum, we would have three main sources of information: a record of weaning weight for each of the candidates for selection which we call P_1, plus an average weaning weight of the two parents which we call P_2, and an average weaning weight of around 20 paternal half sibs which we call P_3. In this example there are 3 sources of information, but in practice there may be more or less than this.

The problem is then to derive a set of index coefficients which give appropriate emphasis to each of the three sources of information, to get the highest possible correlation between the index score for weaning weight (which is a prediction of breeding value) and the animal's true breeding value for weaning weight. The problem can be solved using algebra, but we will not go into that here. The relative size of the resulting index coefficients, and thus the emphasis on the different sources of information, depends mainly on: (i) the heritability of the trait under selection – the higher the heritability, the greater the emphasis which goes on the animal's own record of performance, and the lower the emphasis on records from relatives; (ii) the class of relatives concerned – the closer the relationship, the more emphasis that these records receive; as mentioned before, progeny records are of most value; the value of other records is proportional to the expected proportion of genes in common with the animal being scored; and (iii) the number of records available for each class of relative – the more records, the greater the emphasis which is put on the average measurement from this group. Table 7.5 shows some examples of the relative importance of different sources of information when indexes are derived for traits with different heritabilities.

Although this type of index makes optimal use of information from different classes of relatives, it does have drawbacks. The main one is that it does not deal adequately with records from animals reared in different environments. Also, in practice, the animals being evaluated have records available from different combinations of relatives, and they have different numbers of relatives of each type. This means that many different index coefficients have to be calculated and used. More modern (BLUP) methods, which overcome these problems, are discussed in a later section.

Combining information on different traits

In most livestock production systems, profitability depends on several different animal characteristics rather than on any single trait. It is important to reflect this in genetic improvement programmes, and animals are usually selected (whether objectively or subjectively) on a combination of traits. This can be achieved in a number of ways, as described in Chapter 3. However, multi-trait index selection is widely agreed to be the most efficient method of improving several traits at once. In this context, an *economic selection index* is often used; this is an extension of the type of index already discussed.

Table 7.5. Some examples of the approximate emphasis given to different sources of information on an animal and its relatives by selection indexes for a trait with (a) low heritability ($h^2 = 0.1$), and (b) high heritability ($h^2 = 0.5$). Accuracies of the resulting PBVs are also shown – see later sections in this chapter for definition and discussion of accuracy. The emphasis shown for half sibs and progeny is the total emphasis on records from this source – the emphasis on each record from a half sib or a progeny can be obtained by dividing this total emphasis by the number of animals of the type concerned. The percentage emphasis in each row does not always add up to 100 because of rounding. (Dr R E Crump, personal communication; after Johansson and Rendel, 1968.)

(a) Low heritability ($h^2 = 0.1$)

No. of records of performance on the animal itself	No. of paternal half sibs with a performance record	No. of progeny with a performance record	% emphasis on record from animal's sire	% emphasis on record from animal's dam	% emphasis on record from animal itself	% emphasis on record from half sibs	% emphasis on record from progeny	Accuracy of PBV
0	0	0	50.00	50.00	0	0	0	0.22
1	0	0	24.32	24.32	51.35	0	0	0.38
1	5	0	14.88	16.60	34.18	34.34	0	0.40
1	10	0	10.72	13.19	26.61	49.47	0	0.42
1	50	0	3.31	7.13	13.15	76.41	0	0.49
1	10	5	5.67	3.14	7.89	32.54	50.76	0.64
1	10	10	4.79	2.66	6.68	27.53	58.34	0.67
1	10	50	2.15	1.19	2.99	12.33	81.34	0.81
1	10	100	1.27	0.70	1.77	7.30	88.96	0.87
1	10	500	0.30	0.17	0.41	1.71	97.41	0.97

(b) High heritability ($h^2 = 0.5$)

No. of records of performance on the animal itself	No. of paternal half sibs with a performance record	No. of progeny with a performance record	% emphasis on record from animal's sire	% emphasis on record from animal's dam	% emphasis on record from animal itself	% emphasis on record from half sibs	% emphasis on record from progeny	Accuracy of PBV
0	0	0	50.00	50.00	0	0	0	0.50
1	0	0	20.00	20.00	60.00	0	0	0.76
1	5	0	13.02	17.67	50.70	18.60	0	0.76
1	10	0	9.66	16.55	46.21	27.59	0	0.77
1	50	0	3.15	14.38	37.53	44.94	0	0.78
1	10	5	5.27	3.69	11.85	31.13	48.06	0.88
1	10	10	4.51	3.15	10.14	26.63	55.58	0.90
1	10	50	2.09	1.46	4.70	12.34	79.42	0.95
1	10	100	1.25	0.87	2.81	7.38	87.68	0.97
1	10	500	0.30	0.21	0.67	1.75	97.08	0.99

As well as combining information on different traits, this type of index still allows records from the animal itself and from different classes of relatives to be combined into a single score. To derive an economic selection index, we need to know:

- Which traits we want to improve, collectively called the *breeding goal, breeding objective* or *selection objective*.
- The economic values of each of the traits in the breeding goal. The economic value of a trait is often defined as the *marginal profit* resulting from a genetic change of one unit in that trait. That is, for example, the increase or decrease in profit resulting from a change of 1 kg in live weight, 1 litre of milk, or 1 mm of backfat, compared to the current average value in the herd or flock, with no change in other traits in the breeding goal. Economic values can be calculated from several different perspectives; for example, with the aim of maximizing the profitability of an enterprise for an individual producer or with the aim of improving the efficiency of a national livestock industry. Often there are arguments over which method is most appropriate. (See Amer (1994) and Weller (1994) who discuss the pros and cons of the different approaches, and the attempts to unify them.) Despite these differences of approach, economic values are usually fairly robust. Also, in practice, it is the *relative* economic values of goal traits (i.e. the value of each goal trait relative to the others), rather than their *absolute* values, which affects response most. Relative economic values tend to be particularly robust.
- The set of traits for which measurements will be available for all candidates for selection – called the *index measurements* or selection criteria. These may be the same as the traits in the breeding goal (e.g. if the goal traits can all be measured in both sexes, and on the live animal) or they may be different from the goal traits (e.g. if they are only available on one sex, or are measured after slaughter, in which case measurements from relatives or indirect measurements will often be used).
- The additive genetic and phenotypic variances for traits in the breeding goal and the index measurements, and the additive genetic and phenotypic covariances among them.

With this information it is possible to calculate a set of weighting factors, or index coefficients which, when used in selection, will maximize genetic progress in overall economic merit. These index coefficients are applied to the measurements from candidate animals, or their relatives, in order to calculate a single index score for each candidate.

The aim of multi-trait index selection is to maximize the change in breeding value for total economic merit. The breeding value for total economic merit can be expressed as the sum of the breeding values for all of the traits in the breeding goal, each weighted by its economic value:

$$BV_{TEM} = v_1BV_1 + v_2BV_2 + v_3BV_3 \ldots$$

where:

BV_{TEM} = true breeding value for total economic merit (TEM)

v_1, v_2, v_3 = economic values for breeding goal traits 1, 2 and 3

BV_1, BV_2, BV_3 = true breeding values for breeding-goal traits 1, 2 and 3 – there are only 3 goal traits in this case, e.g. carcass weight, carcass fat class and carcass conformation class, but there may be many more in comprehensive indexes.

In theory, the breeding goal for total economic merit should include all heritable characters which influence profitability. In practice, there is often insufficient information on the genetic and phenotypic variances and covariances of all of these to do so, and so only the main characters are included.

The index on which selection is based, is the sum of the phenotypic measurements on index traits from the animal itself, or the average measurements from groups of relatives, each weighted by the appropriate index coefficient:

$$I = b_1P_1 + b_2P_2 + b_3P_3 + b_4P_4 + b_5P_5 + b_6P_6 \ldots$$

where

I = the index score for an individual animal – unless the index has been rescaled, the index scores are the predicted breeding values for total economic merit, expressed in £, €, $ or whatever currency the economic values were measured in. However, indexes are often rescaled to make the numbers more manageable, or to make the mean index score equal in different flocks or herds - this reduces the temptation to compare absolute values across flocks, if the indexes were not calculated in a way which makes this valid.

b_1 to b_6 = the index coefficients which are applied to the phenotypic measurements P_1 to P_6, respectively. These are calculated to make maximum genetic gain in the breeding value for total economic merit, as defined in the equation for BV_{TEM}. (This equation defining the breeding goal is used solely to allow optimum b values to be calculated.)

P_1 to P_6 = the phenotypic measurements on the animal itself, or groups of relatives, for the index traits or selection criteria, adjusted for known environmental effects. In this case there are six different criteria which contribute to the overall index score e.g. the animal's own live weight (P_1), ultrasonic fat depth (P_2) and ultrasonic muscle depth (P_3), and the average weight (P_4), fat depth (P_5) and muscle depth (P_6) of its half sibs. There may be more or fewer measurements than this in practice.

As before, the problem in constructing a multi-trait selection index is to find the values of b_1, b_2, b_3, and so on, which will maximize the change in breeding value for total economic merit. The mathematical solution to the problem is to set up a series of simultaneous equations and solve them to get the values of the index coefficients. (These equations contain the economic values and the genetic and phenotypic variances and covariances mentioned above.) If there are only a few goal traits and a few index measurements, it is feasible to calculate the b values with a calculator or spreadsheet. Examples of the type of calculations involved can be found in the references listed at the end of this chapter. However, with more traits it becomes cumbersome to do the calculations this way, and it is easiest to solve the large number of equations using a mathematical technique called matrix algebra, on a computer. Matrix algebra is like the algebra we learnt at school but using blocks of numbers in place of single numbers in our calculations. This can be done using software packages such as Mathcad, Matlab, Genstat or SAS or software like SelAction (2019) (Rutten *et al.*, 2002) purposely written for calculation of selection indexes. Although calculating index coefficients may be difficult, the principles of index selection, actually using the index coefficients, and understanding the outcome are all much more straightforward.

A practical example

A practical example of the steps involved in deriving a multi-trait index, and the results obtained, may be useful. The example involves an index derived at Lincoln College, New Zealand, to help select for leaner sheep (Simm *et al.*, 1987). (It was used both in an experimental flock and in the New Zealand industry, in this or modified forms, for many years afterwards.)

- The first step was to decide on the breeding goal. It was decided that two traits would be included: carcass lean weight and carcass fat weight, both measured at a constant age. The aim was for selection on the index to increase carcass lean weight at this age and to reduce carcass fat weight, or at least limit any further increase in it. (The fairly strong positive genetic correlation between carcass lean and fat weights makes it difficult to increase lean weight without also increasing fat weight at a constant age. However, if lean weight is increasing faster than fat weight, the proportion of fat in the carcass can still be reduced.)
- The next step was to calculate economic values for carcass lean and fat weights. At the time, payment for lamb carcasses destined for export from New Zealand was based on carcass weight and the tissue depth (mainly fat) over the 12th rib, at a point 11 cm from the midline (the so-called 'GR' site). Payments on this scale were first converted to payments per kg lean and per kg fat, by using published information on the carcass lean and fat weights of carcasses of different weight and GR depth. The marginal costs of production of lean and fat, which were mainly feed costs, were then estimated and subtracted from the respective marginal returns. This gave marginal profits of NZ$ +5.65 per kg carcass lean, and NZ$ –4.12 per kg fat. In other words, increasing carcass lean weight by 1 kg, compared to the current average, at the same fat weight, was worth NZ$5.65. The minus sign on the marginal profit from increasing fat weight indicates that there is a marginal *loss* from increasing fat weight. Hence, increasing carcass fat weight by 1 kg, compared to the current average and with lean weight remaining the same, would incur a penalty of NZ$4.12. These marginal profits were used as the economic values in the index. So, we can write down the breeding goal as:

$$BV_{TEM} = [5.65 \times BV_{lean\ wt}] + [-4.12 \times BV_{fat\ wt}]$$

- The third step was to decide on index measurements. Since neither of the traits in the breeding goal could be measured directly on the live animal, three index measurements were used as indirect predictors of carcass merit. These were live weight (LW), ultrasonic fat depth (UFD) and ultrasonic muscle depth (UMD), all measured on candidate animals for selection, at a constant age. So, the index to be constructed can be written:

$$I = b_1LW + b_2UFD + b_3UMD$$

- The next task was to find appropriate values for b_1, b_2 and b_3 to maximize change in the breeding value for total economic merit. As described above, this requires values of the phenotypic and genetic variances and covariances, as well as the economic values. In this example, average values of phenotypic variances, heritabilities, phenotypic and genetic correlations for traits in the breeding goal and index were obtained from a comprehensive review of the scientific literature, and the variances and covariances required for the index calculations were derived from these. Ideally, the variances and covariances should be estimated from the population of animals in which the index will be used. However, in many circumstances this is too expensive and time consuming, and so existing literature values have to be used initially. Once sufficient data have been collected on the animals under selection, it makes sense to estimate the required genetic parameters, and to update the index if the new parameters differ from the ones used originally. In this case, the index coefficients calculated to maximize response were +0.10 per kg LW, −0.45 per mm UFD and +0.30 per mm UMD, so we can write the formula to calculate each animal's own index score as:

$$I = [+0.10 \times LW] + [-0.45 \times UFD] + [+0.30 \times UMD]$$

Although we have not gone through the calculations in detail here, intuitively the signs on the index coefficients look sensible. We would expect to favour heavier animals and those with larger muscle depths if we want to increase lean weight, so positive weightings for LW and UMD look reasonable. Conversely, we would expect to penalize animals with high fat depths, so the negative weighting on UFD also looks sensible. If there are more traits than this in an index, especially with complex associations among them, it is not always this easy to check that the size and direction of index weights make sense.

Table 7.6 shows the index scores calculated from this formula for several animals with different live weight and ultrasonic measurements. The table illustrates that animals with the more favourable combinations of measurements get the highest index scores. It also illustrates that animals which have poor performance in one trait can still get comparatively high index scores if they have excellent performance in other traits. In this particular index, there is a lot of emphasis on reducing fat, so it is harder for animals to compensate for high fat than it is to compensate for low weight or muscle depth. The fact that animals can still get a high score without excelling in all components of the index makes it difficult for some breeders to accept index selection, as they are looking for *individual animals* which excel in all characteristics. However, index selection is still the most efficient method to genetically improve total economic merit *of the whole herd or flock*.

Table 7.6. Index measurements and index scores for eight sheep. Index scores were calculated using the coefficients of +0.10 per kg LW, −0.45 per mm UFD and +0.30 per mm UMD, as described in the text.

Animal	Live weight (kg)	Ultrasonic fat depth (mm)	Ultrasonic muscle depth (mm)	Index score (NZ$)
1	55	4	25	11.20
2	60	4	25	11.70
3	65	4	25	12.20
4	65	3	25	12.65
5	65	5	25	11.75
6	65	4	20	10.70
7	65	4	30	13.70
8	65	5	30	13.25

Further calculations for this particular index showed that including measurements from groups of 10, 20 or 30 half sibs in the index was expected to improve the accuracy of selection by 11.5%, 17.3% and 20.8%, respectively, compared to selection on an index with measurements from the individual only. Hence, selection on indexes with these numbers of half sibs should lead to corresponding increases in response in total economic merit, compared to that from selection on the original index. Other examples of selection indexes are given in Chapters 8 to 13.

Predicting Breeding Values Using Best Linear Unbiased Prediction

Some shortcomings of the traditional methods of adjusting records of performance and predicting breeding values have been mentioned already. These include:

- PBVs can only be compared fairly for animals which are managed and fed similarly e.g. within herds or flocks.
- The results from some of the methods for adjusting performance are specific to the herds or flocks for which they were derived, and it may be unwise to apply them more generally.
- Most of the methods of adjusting records run the risk of removing some true genetic differences (e.g. between the progeny of dams of different ages).
- Several methods of adjusting performance assume that animals in different contemporary groups are of equal genetic merit.
- Although conventional indexes combine information from relatives in an appropriate way, they are not very flexible to use; for example, different weighting factors are needed whenever there are different numbers of records from a particular class of relatives. With large numbers of animals and relatives, the task of calculating all of the index coefficients becomes very difficult or impossible.

Much of the impetus to produce better methods of evaluating animals arose following the commercial uptake of artificial insemination (AI) in dairy cattle. For example, in Britain the first cattle AI station was opened at Cambridge in 1942, following research on the technique by Sir John Hammond and his colleagues in the then Cambridge School of Agriculture. Although the introduction of AI was intended initially to reduce the spread of venereal diseases in cattle, and reduce the risks from handling bulls on farms, its potential for assisting the genetic evaluation of dairy bulls and accelerating genetic improvement was soon recognized.

Progeny testing schemes for dairy bulls were introduced in the 1950s, and bulls were evaluated by a method known as the *contemporary comparison* (CC). Much of the work on statistics and methodology was undertaken by Professor Alan Robertson and his co-workers at the then Institute of Animal Genetics in Edinburgh. The CC system involved comparing the average production of the first lactation daughters of a bull undergoing progeny testing with the average production of the other heifers milked in the same herd, in the same year and in the same season (Robertson, *et al.*, 1956). Deviations in production for daughters of the bull being tested were then combined across herds, after weighting to take into account the number of daughters of the bull undergoing the test, and the number of contemporaries against which these were compared. Comparing cows on a within-herd basis recognized the fact that milk production is not only affected by genetic merit but also by management and feeding (the 'environment'). However, CCs were based on the assumption that all herds were of equal genetic merit and that, apart from sires and their daughters, other animals were unrelated – two assumptions which were increasingly violated by the wide uptake of AI.

Much of the research to overcome these problems and produce a fairer system of predicting breeding values was initiated by Dr C.R. Henderson at Iowa State and Cornell Universities in the United States (Henderson, 1973, 1975). He first proposed a statistical procedure known as *best linear unbiased prediction*, or BLUP, in 1949. Although the workings are complex, and are not described in detail here, BLUP is basically a statistical technique which disentangles genetics from management and feeding in the best possible way, and so produces more accurate predictions of breeding value. It achieves this by:

- Estimating environmental effects (like dam age, season of calving, birth rank) and predicting breeding values simultaneously.
- 'Recognizing' that some performance records are from related animals, and so they are expected to be more alike than those from unrelated animals. Related animals in different contemporary groups provide genetic links between the groups (see Fig. 7.3). These links are necessary in order for BLUP to estimate environmental effects and predict breeding values simultaneously.

BLUP is essentially an extension of the methods used in selection indexes. However, there are several steps involved in conventional index selection – deriving index coefficients, adjusting the records of performance for environmental effects, and then applying the index coefficients to the adjusted records to get PBVs for individual animals. BLUP can achieve these simultaneously, and so it produces PBVs in one step.

How BLUP works

We have already seen that one of the main tasks in deriving a selection index is to calculate the weightings

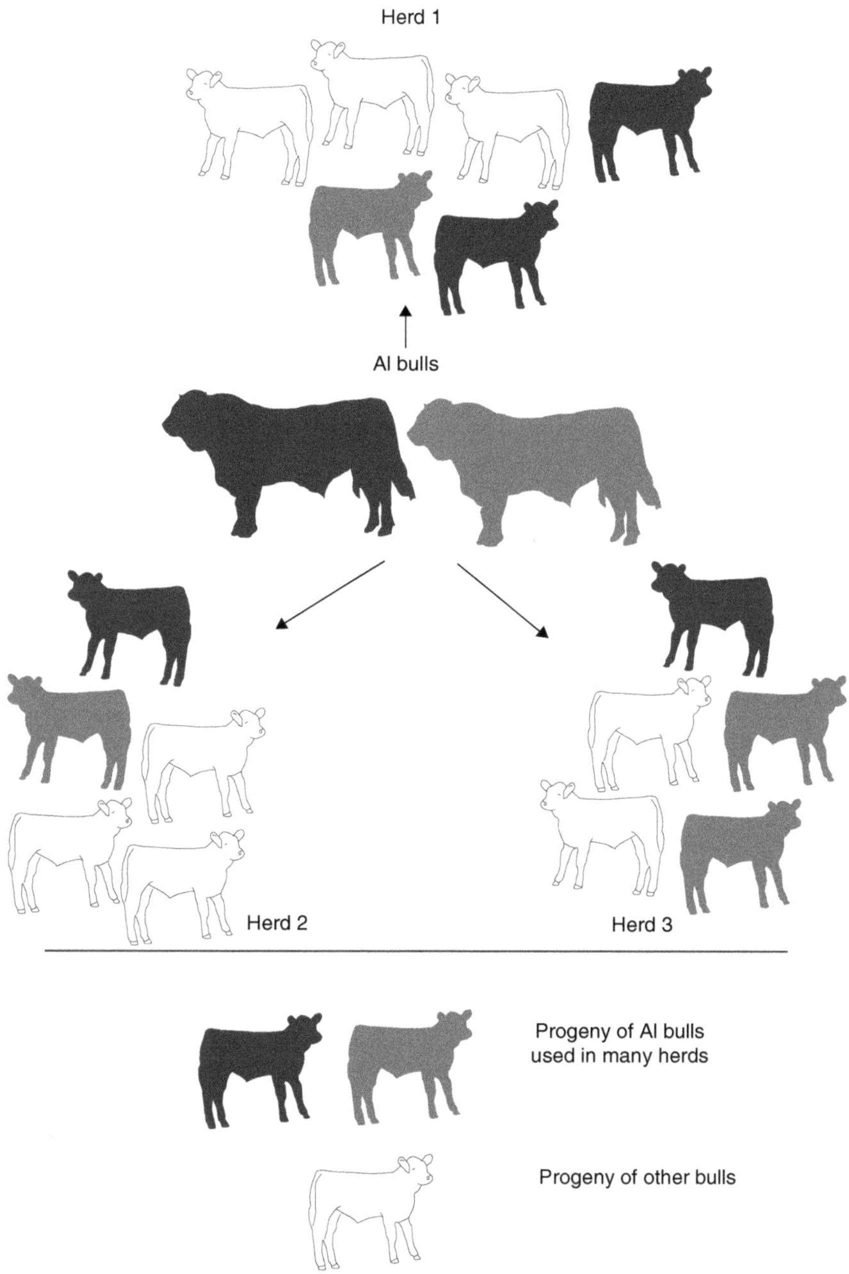

Fig. 7.3. Genetic links between contemporary groups are necessary for BLUP to estimate environmental effects and predict breeding values simultaneously. In cattle these links occur most commonly through the use of AI bulls in many different herds (Wray and Simm, 1991).

to apply to performance records from different classes of relatives, or to records on different traits. With BLUP there are similar problems in calculating the emphasis that ought to be given to different sources of information when predicting animals' breeding values and in estimating environmental effects.

In both selection indexes and BLUP (as well as in many other applications of statistics), the problem of finding the appropriate emphasis to give to different pieces of information is solved by setting up a series of simultaneous equations. This may appear complicated at first, but most of us have solved simultaneous equations at one time or another. If it was at school, then it was probably finding the price of two commodities, given the total price of different quantities of each. For example, if we bought ten apples and five oranges on day one for a total cost of £3.00, we can write this as:

10 apples + 5 oranges = £3.00 [Equation 7.1]

If, on the following day, we bought 5 apples and 15 oranges for £5.25, we can write this as:

5 apples + 15 oranges = £5.25 [Equation 7.2]

One way to find the price of apples and oranges is to multiply both sides of Equation 7.2 by 2, so that it has the same number of apples as Equation 7.1:

10 apples + 30 oranges = £10.50 [Equation 7.2 multiplied by 2]

We can then subtract Equation 7.1 from the new equation, to get a price for oranges alone:

(10 apples + 30 oranges) – (10 apples + 5 oranges) = £10.50 – £3.00

so:

25 oranges = £7.50

and:

1 orange = £0.30

We can then substitute the price of oranges in one of the original equations to get the price of apples. For example, in Equation 7.1 we now know that the 5 oranges cost £1.50, and so:

10 apples = £3.00 – £1.50 = £1.50

and therefore

1 apple = £0.15

In this simple example we were able to solve the equations easily just by rearranging them. However, it is possible to solve this sort of equation directly using matrix algebra. In BLUP, the equations to be solved link the performance records to the environmental effects, and to the animals whose BVs we are predicting. Instead of calculating prices for apples and oranges from a total amount of money spent, we are estimating environmental effects (e.g. herd, dam age, birth rank) and predicting breeding values from a total amount of live weight or milk produced. For example, Table 7.7 summarizes the milk production records from the first lactation daughters of two unrelated dairy bulls. Each bull has some daughters in two different herds, but within each herd the heifers are managed as a single group.

The BLUP equations to solve in order get PBVs for the two sires would be as follows. The abbreviations S1 and S2 are used for sires 1 and 2, and H1 and H2 are used for herds 1 and 2:

$$15H1 + 0H2 + 5S1 + 10S2 = 85{,}500$$

$$0H1 + 18H2 + 12S1 + 6S2 = 113{,}400$$

$$5H1 + 12H2 + (17 + w)S1 + 0S2 = 101{,}900$$

$$10H1 + 6H2 + 0S1 + (16 + w)S2 = 97{,}000$$

Just as the earlier equations explained the total amount of money spent in terms of the number of apples and oranges bought, these BLUP equations explain the total amount of milk produced in terms

Table 7.7. Summary of milk production records available from the daughters of two bulls, milked in two different herds.

(a) Numbers of daughters in each herd

	Sire 1	Sire 2	Total
Herd 1	5	10	15
Herd 2	12	6	18
Total	17	16	33

(b) Total and average milk production for each herd and each sire

	Number of heifers	Total milk production (kg)	Average milk production (kg)
Herd 1	15	85,500	5,700
Herd 2	18	113,400	6,300
Sire 1	17	101,900	5,994
Sire 2	16	97,000	6,063

of the numbers of daughters' lactations recorded in each herd and from each sire. It is the addition of the term **w** in the last two equations which distinguishes them from the equations in the 'fruit' example. BLUP requires a slightly modified approach to solve equations, since we are interested in getting predictions of breeding values and not just fixed prices of commodities as in the fruit example. The term **w** is a weighting factor which accounts for the heritability of the trait concerned and for the relationship between the animals who produced the records and those whose BVs are being predicted. In this case, the records are single lactation records from daughters of two unrelated sires, and the weighting factor is $(4 - h^2)/h^2$. Note that this term also appeared in the formula earlier in this chapter for predicting the breeding value of a sire based on progeny records. (See Van Vleck *et al.* (1987) and Mrode (2014) for the equivalent weighting factors for records from other relatives.) The heritability of milk production is about 0.35, and so the weighting factor in this case becomes approximately 10.43.

Solving these four equations looks like hard work, compared to those in the fruit example. However, modern powerful computers can solve vast numbers of these equations very rapidly indeed. Solving these equations and scaling the results appropriately (see later section on scale of presentation) gives predicted breeding values for the two bulls of:

S1 = −175.3 kg milk

and

S2 = +175.3 kg milk

In this example, the two sires were unrelated and you will notice that the sum of their PBVs is zero. This is explained in the next paragraph. However, in practice the animals being evaluated are often related to each other. These relationships are accounted for in BLUP evaluations by creating what is known as a relationship matrix – essentially a table showing the expected proportion of genes in common between all the animals being evaluated. A simple example is shown in Table 7.8. In this case, there are four bulls being evaluated A, B, C and D. Bulls A and B are full brothers, so they are expected to have 0.5 of their genes in common, but they are unrelated to the other two bulls. Bulls C and D are half-brothers, so they are expected to have 0.25 of their genes in common. These relationships were easy to calculate because we are dealing with only four bulls and their relationships were very straightforward. However, when dealing with data from lots of animals, these relationships can be complicated to work out by hand. There are several computer software packages that can be used in such cases (for example, RelaX2 (2019) and Pedigree Viewer (2019)). In general, the matrix describing the relationship among animals is called the *numerator relationship matrix* (**A** matrix). The numerator relationship matrix is used to derive the appropriate weightings to use in the BLUP equations – these weightings are equivalent to the value of **w** used in the example above when the sires were unrelated. The relationship matrix can also be modified to account for inbreeding – related inbred animals have more genes in common than related outbred animals. (See Nicholas (1987), Van Vleck *et al.* (1987) and Mrode (2014) for more details on the mechanics of BLUP.)

Table 7.8. An example of a simple relationship matrix, showing the degree of relationship between four bulls. An animal's relationship to itself is 1.0 (i.e. it has all of its genes in common with itself), the relationship between full sibs (bulls A and B) is 0.5, and that between half sibs (bulls C and D) is 0.25. (In this example, none of the animals is inbred.)

Bull	A	B	C	D
A	1.0	0.5	0	0
B	0.5	1.0	0	0
C	0	0	1.0	0.25
D	0	0	0.25	1.0

BLUP models

As discussed earlier, a model is an equation that outlines the possible fixed effects (e.g. environment, management, farm) that influence the performance of animals in the trait of interest, and also the random (animal) effects. Random effects usually include the animals whose PBVs we want to calculate. In the use of BLUP, the random effect in the model determines the name given to the model and how the analysis is carried out. For example, when sires are in the random effect part of the model, then it is called a BLUP sire model. If individual animals are in the random effect part of the model, it called a BLUP animal model. Hence, the name of the model indicates the animals for which BVs are being predicted, and the relationships used to predict them. So, sire models predict BVs for sires from their progeny records, sire-maternal grandsire models predict BVs for sires using records from both their progeny and maternal grand-progeny, and individual animal models predict BVs for all animals included in the evaluation, using all relationships among them. In general, the most common BLUP models are: (i) sire models, (ii) sire-maternal grandsire models, and (iii) individual animal models, just as we discussed for genetic parameter estimation in Chapter 6.

The more sophisticated BLUP models recognize more relationships between animals, and hence predict BVs more accurately. So, animal models predict PBVs more accurately than sire-maternal grandsire models, which in turn predict PBVs more accurately than sire models. However, there is a higher computing cost as more effects are included in the analysis and the dataset gets larger. An equation has to be solved for each animal which gets a PBV. In national genetic evaluations there may be hundreds or thousands of sires, and so there are hundreds or thousands of equations to solve in a sire model BLUP evaluation. But there may be millions of individual animals, and so millions of equations to solve, in an individual animal model BLUP evaluation. As a result, one of the main factors governing the uptake of more sophisticated models has been the cost and availability of computing power. However, recent advances in computing technologies have alleviated this limitation, so animal model BLUP evaluations can now be implemented for large data sets. For example, at the time of writing, UK national dairy cattle evaluations for milk yield include more than 9 million cows.

As mentioned above, the impetus for new methods of evaluation came primarily from dairy cattle breeding. Sire model BLUP evaluations were first used in dairy cattle in the USA in the early 1970s, and several other countries soon afterwards. Advances in computing allowed sire-maternal grandsire models to be used in the same decade. This improved the accuracy of evaluations, compared to those from sire model BLUP, by recognizing that not all cows to which test bulls were mated were of equal merit. However, the sire-maternal grandsire model only accounted for differences in the merit of cows via their sire (the maternal grandsire of heifers whose records were being evaluated, hence the name of this model). The emphasis was still on predicting BVs for sires, and indexes for cows were produced by combining their sire's and maternal grandsire's PBVs with their own production records. These difficulties were overcome with the introduction of individual animal model BLUP evaluations in many countries during the late 1980s and early 1990s.

Although BLUP evaluations were first used in dairy cattle, the benefits are also relevant to other species. Over the last few decades BLUP methods have become the methods of choice for evaluating most farm livestock species. Because performance-recorded populations of beef cattle and sheep are usually smaller than those of dairy cattle, and because BLUP methods have been adopted later in these sectors, it has often been possible to skip several generations of BLUP models and adopt animal model evaluations from the start. For example, in Britain BLUP evaluations were used in some sheep-breeding schemes for the first time in 1990, and they were used in beef cattle for the first time in 1991. In both cases individual animal models were used from the start. More details are given in the following chapters.

Direct and maternal genetic effects

There are some traits of interest in livestock breeding where the performance of offspring is affected not only by their own genes and environment, but also by their mothers' genes and the (nurturing) environment the mother provides. For example, the weaning weight of a suckled beef calf is affected not only by the genes for growth which the calf inherits, and the environment it gets, but also by its mother's genes for maternal characteristics such as uterine capacity and milk production, and the environmental influences on her performance in these traits (see Fig. 7.4). So, it is often useful to think of *direct breeding value* and *maternal breeding value* for traits such as weaning weight which are influenced by both direct and maternal genetic merit. Both males and females carry genes for milk production and other aspects of maternal performance, but only females get the chance to express them. However, with sufficient data, BLUP can predict both direct and maternal breeding values for males and females, from the relationships between animals with performance records (e.g. cows with calf weaning weights) and those without (e.g. bulls).

The concept of separating direct and maternal genetic effects appears rather complicated at first

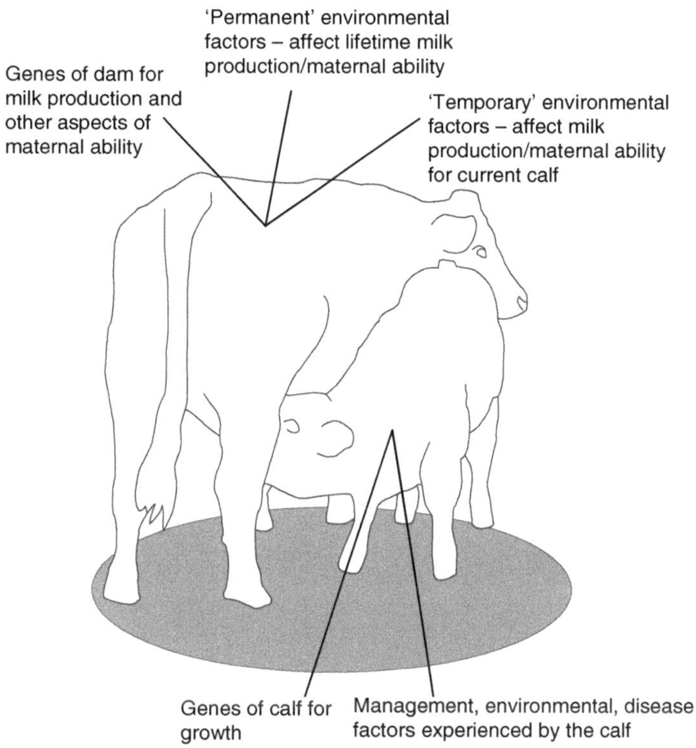

Fig. 7.4. Some of the genetic and environmental factors which influence calf weaning weights, either directly or via the dam. (After Wray *et al.*, 1991.)

sight, but it is really just an extension of the principles we have already considered and discussed in Chapter 6. We can predict the breeding value of dairy bulls for milk traits based on their daughters' milk production records. But, because we cannot easily record the milk yield of lactating pigs, beef cows or non-dairy sheep, and because we are interested in other aspects of maternal performance as well as milk yield, we have to rely on the early growth or weaning weights of offspring to assess maternal genetic merit. Many different types of relative can provide clues to an animal's genes for maternal performance, but the principle is easiest to understand by considering the performance of grand-offspring of a bull, produced by his daughters, as a means to assess his maternal genetic merit. These calves get a quarter of their genes for growth, on average, directly from their grandsire. But their performance is also influenced by the fact that their dams received half of the grandsire's genes for milk production and maternal performance. In contrast, calves sired by sons of the bull we are interested in are only influenced by the genes they inherited for growth (again, a quarter of their genes on average come from their grandsire). If, on average, grand-offspring from daughters of the original bull have heavier weaning weights than grand-offspring from sons of the original bull, then this is likely to be a consequence of that bull carrying genes for high maternal performance. Conversely, if grand-offspring from daughters of the original bull have lower weaning weights than grand-offspring from his sons, then this is likely to be a result of that bull carrying genes for low maternal performance. This is illustrated in Fig. 7.5. By comparing these two types of descendants of a sire – those which were influenced by the maternal performance of his female relatives, and those which were not – BLUP can predict breeding values for both direct and maternal components of weaning weight or other traits influenced by both direct and maternal genetic merit.

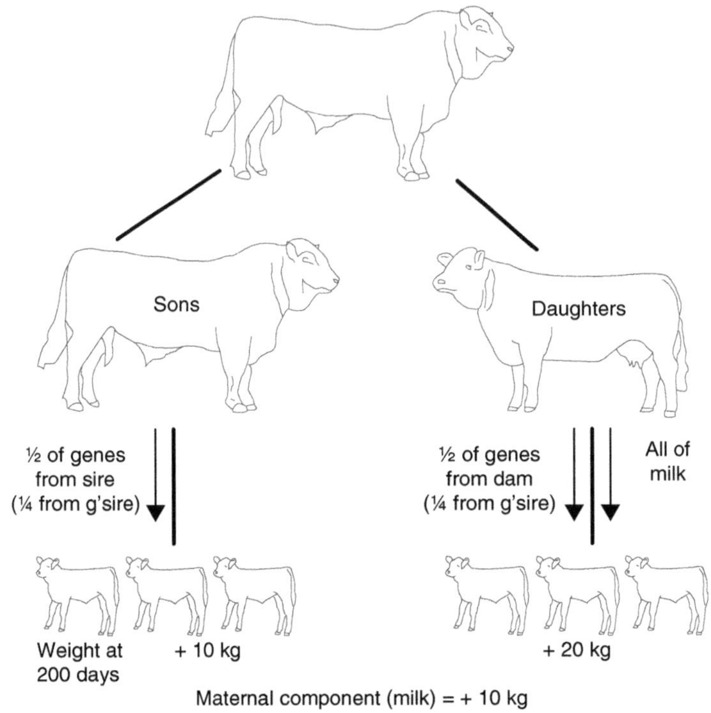

Fig. 7.5. How records of weaning weight from the grand-offspring of a bull can provide clues to his genetic merit for milk production and other aspects of maternal performance.

Single and multi-trait BLUP

Initially, most BLUP evaluations were for one trait at a time (*single-trait* evaluations). However, as mentioned earlier in this chapter, when there is a correlation between two or more different traits, a record of performance in one trait can help to predict an animal's breeding value in other traits and this generally increases the accuracy of the PBVs. The simultaneous evaluation of traits in *multi-trait* BLUP also means that prior selection on correlated traits can be accounted for. For example, a breeder may cull animals that do not achieve a particular weaning weight. If we analyse the animals with yearling weight only with a single-trait BLUP, then our analysis is biased as we have not accounted for the fact that only animals with good weaning weight contributed yearling weight records. A multi-trait BLUP on weaning and yearling weights is the best way to analyse these data. In such multi-trait BLUP, the records for yearling weight for animals sold off at weaning will be coded as missing and BLUP will correct for this culling bias. Multi-trait BLUP evaluations have become widely used both to increase accuracy and to correct for culling or selection bias. As well as the usual information on relationships between animals and estimates of the heritabilities (or variances) of the traits to be evaluated, multi-trait BLUP evaluations require estimates of the correlations (or covariances) between all of the traits included. Modern advances in computing facilities and strategies have made this feasible for a large number of traits and many animals.

Random regression models

In Chapter 6, we introduced the topic of random regression. This statistical method is used when a trait is measured successively on an animal over a range of ages or time periods. Examples include body weight measured at several ages from birth until market weight in beef cattle or pigs, or milk yield measured on different 'days in milk' (test days) throughout the lactation. Repeated observations such as milk test-day yields, or body weight measured over time, are usually referred to as longitudinal data. The heritabilities of measurements made at different stages (e.g. of growth or lactation) can vary. For instance, several studies mentioned in Chapter 6 reported that the heritability of daily milk yields varied with the number of days in milk. Repeated measurements also have different means, and different covariances between them, which change gradually over the time period of measurement. For example, genetic correlations between repeated milk yield measurements tend to decrease as the time between them increases (Pander *et al.*, 1992).

One of the earlier methods used to analyse traits with repeated measurements ignored these differences in the mean and variances at different ages. The repeated records were regarded as the same trait with the same mean and variance over different ages. This model is called the repeatability model. For traits with a high repeatability this model gave very good results. However, a better approach is to analyse such data by fitting a curve that accounts for the different means and variances of the repeated records at the different ages. (Often the change in a trait over time is non-linear, i.e. best described by a curve rather than a straight line.) For example, daily milk yield in dairy cows usually increases steeply from the beginning of the lactation, reaches a peak about 6 weeks later, and then declines gradually until the end of lactation. The curve for the average milk yield per day over the lactation period for a group of first-lactation UK cows is shown in Fig. 7.6. The so-called Wilmink curve or function is used commonly to model test-day milk yields (Wilmink, 1987). It is popular because plotting the lactation curve with this function requires only three parameters to be estimated. These account for the level of production, the increase in production towards peak yield, and the decrease in production after peak yield. In addition, it is easy to solve the Wilmink function as a linear function after log-transformation.

Models that use curves to account for the changes in the mean and variance of repeated records over time for each animal are called random regression models. In these models a curve (referred to generally as the fixed curve) is used to account for the overall shape of the repeated records over time for all animals in the data, or within sub-groups of animals which have similar

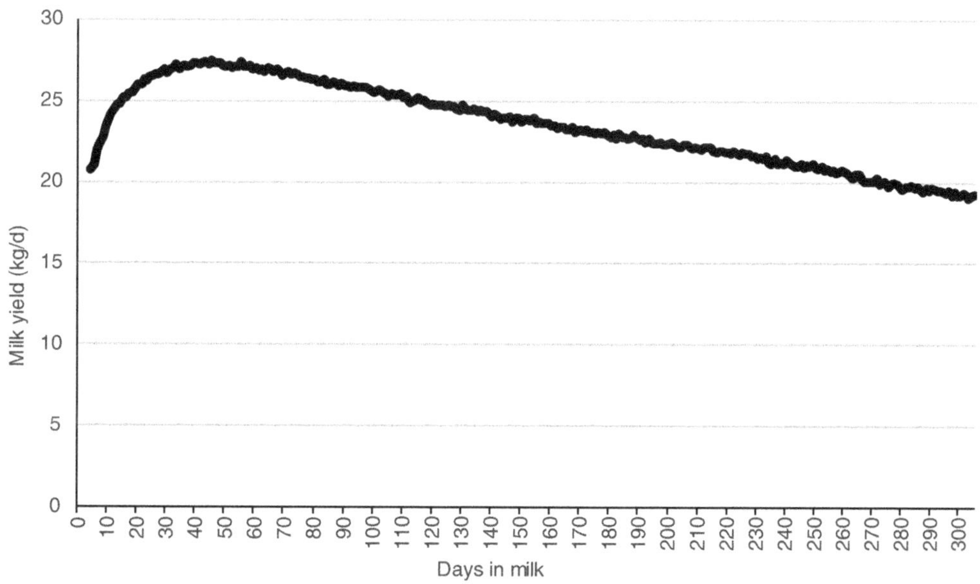

Fig. 7.6. A lactation curve for the average milk yield per day over the lactation period for a group of cows with first lactations in the UK. (Generated from data at EGENES, 2019.)

characteristics, such as those born in the same year and season. Then, another curve (referred to generally as the random regression curve) is fitted to describe the shape of the repeated records over time for each individual animal, relative to the fixed curve. The advantage of the random regression model is that it estimates the regression coefficients of the curve fitted for each animal rather than a single PBV. Using these estimated regression coefficients, we can calculate PBVs for each animal at any age or time interval represented in the data. Similarly, heritabilities for the different time intervals or ages can also be computed, as can the genetic correlations among PBVs at different ages. The equations for the random regression model are formulated using the BLUP approach. The model is used by many countries such as the UK, Canada and Germany to calculate PBVs for test-day milk traits such as daily milk, fat and protein yields. The random regression model has been employed also for the analysis of growth data in pigs (Andersen and Pedersen, 1996) and beef cattle (Meyer, 1999), as well as the estimation of genotype-by-environment interaction effects (Pollott and Greeff, 2004) as mentioned in Chapter 6.

Social interaction model

In a group of animals reared together, social interactions among them can affect the expression of some performance traits (Bijma *et al.*, 2007). For example, the growth rate of some piglets may be reduced by competition for feed within their group. Selection based on individual growth rates in such group settings may mean selecting for the most competitive animals and not just those with the genetic ability to grow fast. Thus, when a group of animals depends on a limiting resource, such as feed, to achieve a desirable trait, such as rapid growth rate, the observed phenotype of an individual is due to the direct genetic effect for growth of the individual and the phenotypic ability to compete for feed with other members of the group. This phenotypic ability to compete for resources, which is termed the *social interaction effect*, has a genetic component (the genes carried by the individual and by others in the group affect how individuals compete) and an environmental component (e.g. the size of the pen, or the number of animals in the group). The genetic component is generally referred to as an indirect genetic effect (IGE; Moore *et al.*, 1997), or an *associative effect*. For traits affected by an associative effect, the selection of animals for breeding is ideally based on the sum of their PBVs for the trait (direct genetic effects) and the IGE. If the IGE is not accounted for, the rate of genetic change may be lower than expected or even in the wrong direction. The inclusion of social interactions among individuals may increase the total heritable variance in a trait by 7–20%. Genetic evaluations for this sort of trait involve using BLUP equations such that PBV effects due to the direct effects of the genes of the individual and IGEs due to the associative effect are estimated simultaneously. Such a model is termed a *social interaction model*. For practical examples and more detailed information see Bergsma, *et al.* (2008) and Mrode (2014).

Estimates of Heritabilities and Correlations for PBV Calculations

The use of the various models described in the preceding section requires estimates of heritabilities and correlations (or the variances and covariances they are derived from) to set up the various equations to estimate PBVs. These estimates of heritabilities (or genetic and phenotypic variances) of the traits being evaluated, and the phenotypic and genetic correlations among traits – are usually referred to as genetic parameters. The procedures for estimating these genetic parameters were covered in Chapter 6. It is particularly important that accurate and relevant estimates of these parameters are used in calculating PBVs, so that emphasis is apportioned properly among the various sources of information contribution to the PBVs of animals, such as the performance record of the animal itself, those from various classes of relatives and for other traits. Accurate estimates of heritabilities and correlations are also important if the estimates of *genetic trends* (annual rates of change in the genetic merit of traits of interest) are to be correctly computed.

Ideally, the genetic parameters should be estimated at each round of genetic evaluation. However, as the genetic parameters tend to be stable over several BLUP runs, it is not usually cost effective to do so. The models and parameters used should be checked periodically though, to ensure that they are still appropriate.

Genomic Prediction of Breeding Values

Genomic markers in the form of single nucleotide polymorphisms (SNPs) were described in Chapter 5.

The use of SNPs to predict the breeding value of animals is called genomic prediction and the predicted genetic merit is called a direct genomic breeding value (DGV). The use of DGV to select animals with superior genetic merit for breeding is termed genomic selection (Meuwissen *et al.*, 2001).

The first step in using SNPs to calculate DGVs is to find out the relationship between these markers (the SNPs) and the performance of a representative group of animals. This group of animals should have genotypes, i.e. SNP information, as well as performance records for the traits of interest. The performance records are usually adjusted, or precorrected, for known environmental and management factors affecting these traits. Variation in the adjusted performance records is then primarily due to the influence of genes on the trait. However, when using bulls for genomic prediction for sex-limited traits such as milk yield, the *de-regressed* PBVs of the bulls are used. The de-regressed PBV approximates the mean of the bulls' daughters' performance and can be calculated as:

$$\text{de-regressed PBV}_{\text{bull}} = \text{PA}_{\text{bull}} + \frac{(\text{PBV}_{\text{bull}} - \text{PA}_{\text{bull}})}{\text{Rel}_{\text{dau}}}$$

where PA_{bull} is the parent average PBV for the bull, PBV_{bull} is the bull's PBV and Rel_{dau} is the bull reliability from daughters with parent information removed.

This de-regression process essentially reverses the 'shrinking' that goes on to account for accuracy in calculating PBVs in order to get back to average daughter performance corrected for environmental effects.

The relationship between the SNPs and the trait of interest is worked out using equations, similar to multiple regression or BLUP calculations, to compute solutions for the SNPs. These solutions are also called the *SNP key* for the trait of interest. The group of animals used to compute the SNP solutions is called the reference population. The larger the size of the group of reference animals, the more accurate the SNP key will be (VanRaden, 2008). As an illustration, Goddard (2009) showed that for a trait with a heritability of 0.4, the required number of animals with both phenotypes and genotypes in the reference population to achieve an accuracy of 0.70 was about 10,000, and to achieve an accuracy of 0.5 it was about 4000 animals. The corresponding numbers of animals for a trait with a heritability of 0.1 were 38,000 and 12,500. In general, the lower the heritability, the larger the size of the reference population needed to achieve a given accuracy of genomic prediction.

The second step is to test how accurate the SNP key is. This is done in another set of animals called the *validation* or *selection animals*. Using the SNP key calculated in the reference population, and only the genotypes of the validation animals, the DGV for the validation animals are predicted. Then the correlation between the DGVs of these animals and their adjusted performance records is calculated to assess how accurately the SNP key is predicting the adjusted records (which, as we said before, vary primarily due to the effects of genes). The higher the correlation, the better the SNP key. Usually we expect this correlation, which is called the accuracy of prediction, to be higher than estimates of accuracy calculated from only the parent average PBV of the animals. The difference between the prediction accuracy in the validation animals and the average accuracy for these animals calculated from only the parent average PBV is called the gain in accuracy due to using genotypes or genomics. In dairy cattle in the USA, VanRaden *et al.* (2009) reported gains in accuracy of 0.20, 0.38 and 0.30, respectively, for milk yield, fat percentage and protein percentage by using this approach. For the UK dairy cattle sector, Mrode *et al.* (2011) reported similar gains of 0.22 for milk yield. These gains are high as a result of having extremely large and informative reference populations; such large reference populations are not always available.

The prediction accuracy from validation animals informs us of the ability to use the SNP key to predict the breeding values for newborn or young animals, or even embryos, using only their genotypes. This is very important as it means that at birth, we can decide which animals have high predicted genetic merit and should be retained for use as parents. In dairy cattle, this has substantially reduced the generation interval and so speeded up the rate of genetic progress. This is because, with conventional progeny testing, it takes about 5 years from the birth of dairy bulls before the records of daughters are available to predict sire breeding values. This 5-year interval can now be cut down to about 2–3 years, as the young bulls of higher genetic merit can be identified at birth and used for breeding as soon as they are sexually mature. For example, the mean sire age for Holstein male progeny born in 2012 in the USA was 2.7 years younger than for males born in 2006; there was a corresponding reduction of 1.3 years for females (Hutchison *et al.*, 2014). This has resulted from the wide usage of young bulls chosen for breeding on the basis of their genomic breeding values. The percentage of US Holstein sons sired by young bulls was 10% in 2008 compared with 59% in 2012, due to the uptake of genomic evaluations. For the Jersey breed, the equivalent figures were 11% in 2008 and 57% in 2012 (Hutchison *et al.*, 2014).

Models for genomic prediction and selection

GBLUP

The models for calculating DBVs are based on the BLUP models described earlier. You will remember that in the BLUP equations, the relationships between all pairs of animals are included in the simultaneous equations to calculate the breeding values. The relationship between animals is calculated using the simple rule that a parent passes exactly half of its genes to its offspring. So, two offspring from the same parent have half of their genes in common, on average. However, parents do not pass on exactly the same half of their genes to each offspring, unless they are identical twins. The relationship matrix (**A**) described earlier is based on the *expected* proportion of genes that animals have in common. Using the genotypes or SNPs we can work out the *observed* or *actual* relationships among all the animals (see VanRaden (2008) for formulae and Mrode (2014) for examples). This is called the *genomic relationship matrix* (**G**). The **G** matrix therefore describes the observed relationships among animals from the genotypes and is more accurate as it is based on the actual genes passed from parent to offspring. When we use **G** in the BLUP equations instead of the **A** matrix calculated from the pedigree, the model is called GBLUP. So GBLUP is similar to BLUP in other respects, but we use observed relationships (**G**) instead of the expected relationships from the pedigree (**A**). GBLUP produces the DGVs which can be used for selection of animals for breeding.

SNP-BLUP

Remember that with animal model BLUP, the equations are set up for each animal. Solving the BLUP equations gives us the PBVs for each animal. The idea is rather different for the SNP-BLUP model, as the equations are set up for the SNP genotypes observed in each animal that also has performance records. You may recall that SNPs are bi-allelic such that the SNP genotype of an individual is AA if it has both dominant alleles, Aa if it has one dominant and one recessive allele, or aa if it has both recessive alleles. Let us code these SNP genotypes, AA, Aa and aa as 2, 1 and 0, respectively. Note that this coding is equivalent to counting the number of dominant alleles that an individual has for this SNP. Thus an individual with the SNP genotype aa is coded 0 as it has no copy of the dominant allele A. See Table 7.9 for an illustration of the coding of the genotypes of six animals with five SNPs. SNP-BLUP involves setting up the BLUP equations using the coded genotypes of 2, 1 and 0 for each SNP. Solving the SNP-BLUP equations gives the solution for each SNP. The DGV for each animal is then obtained by multiplying the solution for each SNP by the genotypes observed for that SNP in the animal and this is summed over all the SNPs used in the analysis. Given that equations are set up for each SNP rather than each animal, this is called the SNP-BLUP model (VanRaden, 2008). This model can be advantageous if there are millions of animals for which we want to calculate DGVs, as the number of SNPs is usually fewer – about 50,000 in most cases – therefore the number of equations to be solved is also fewer.

In practice, it is usually only a proportion of animals in an evaluation that are genotyped, due to cost, or DNA samples not being available for older animals. This means that the parents of some of the younger genotyped animals may not have any SNP information. Therefore, the DGVs calculated for these younger animals from GBLUP or SNP-BLUP models do not contain any information about the

Table 7.9. The coding of SNP genotypes for a sample of animals.

	Actual SNPs					Coded SNPs				
Animal	1	2	3	4	5	1	2	3	4	5
1	aa	AA	Aa	aa	Aa	0	2	1	0	1
2	AA	Aa	Aa	Aa	aa	2	1	1	1	0
3	Aa	AA	aa	AA	Aa	1	2	0	2	1
4	AA	Aa	AA	aa	AA	2	1	2	0	2
5	aa	Aa	aa	AA	Aa	0	1	0	2	1
6	Aa	Aa	AA	Aa	aa	1	1	2	1	0

parents. To include the information from parents there are two steps involved. Firstly, conventional BLUP is carried out for all animals in the population with performance records and pedigree records. Secondly, the DGVs of the younger animals from GBLUP or SNP-BLUP are combined with the parent average from the conventional BLUP evaluations (VanRaden *et al.*, 2009) using their reliabilities as weights to estimate what are termed *genomic breeding values* (GEBVs). The selection of young animals for breeding is usually based on the GEBVs. Due to the two steps involved in calculating GEBV with GBLUP or SNP-BLUP, this is termed the *two-step procedure* in contrast to the *single-step procedure* described in the next session.

Single-step procedure

As mentioned above, data sets can contain a mixture of animals with different combinations of pedigree, phenotypic and genotypic records. For example, in most dairy cattle populations in developed countries, genotyping of bulls and cows started in the late 2000s. This means that cows born before this time will only have phenotypes and/or pedigree information available. Using the phenotypic and pedigree information available for all the cows and bulls in combination with the genotypes of the cows and bulls born more recently, a procedure called *single step* (Misztal *et al.*, 2010) can be used to estimate GEBVs directly for all cows and bulls in the population. The procedure can be used for any species (see Christensen, *et al.* (2012) for an application in pigs and Lourenco *et al.* (2015) for an application in beef cattle). The procedure involves setting up equations for all the animals, as in BLUP. GEBVs for all animals are estimated in one step, as parent information for genotyped animals is included in their GEBVs through the pedigree. Hence the name single step compared to GBLUP or SNP-BLUP. The method also means that genomic information can flow from the younger animals with genotypes to the older animals in the pedigree without genotypes. The single-step procedure involves calculating the relationships among all animals combining both the **A** matrix from pedigree information and the **G** matrix from the SNPs for the genotyped animals. This combined relationship matrix is called *the **H** matrix*. The inverse of the **H** matrix is then used in the usual BLUP equations to produce the GEBVs for the animals.

Benefits of BLUP

As mentioned earlier, there must be genetic links between contemporary groups for BLUP to estimate environmental effects and predict breeding values simultaneously. Providing these links exist:

- The effects of environment and breeding will be separated more effectively by BLUP than with traditional methods, which first adjusted records of performance for environmental effects, and then predicted breeding values. With traditional methods genetic merit and environment can easily be confounded, for example, corrections for age of dam may ignore the fact that genetic improvement is being made. As a result, younger animals of higher merit may be 'undervalued'. Similarly, the use of sires of different genetic merit in different contemporary groups would be overlooked with traditional methods. Also, the use of sires of different merit at different times during the mating season could result in some true genetic differences being treated inadvertently as seasonal effects. In BLUP evaluations, the more relationships between animals that are recognized, the greater the chance of overcoming these problems.
- The resulting PBVs can be compared directly across different contemporary groups. This means that PBVs can be compared across age groups, so allowing more accurate sequential selection or culling, and removing the need to decide in advance on the optimum age structure in the herd or flock.
- PBVs can be compared across herds and flocks, as long as these are genetically linked via related animals. This has a major effect on the selection intensities which can be applied. The benefits of selection across herds or flocks are particularly high when AI is used, as in most dairy cattle industries, because very high male selection intensities can be achieved. However, across-herd or across-flock evaluations are still valuable in industries with less widespread use of AI. This is particularly true in countries like Britain where pedigree herds and flocks are often small, and so within-herd or within-flock selection intensities are typically low.
- PBVs can be compared across years, as long as there are genetic links between years, i.e. related animals which are recorded in successive years (e.g. progeny from the same sires or dams). Plots of PBVs across time show the estimated genetic trend which is occurring in a particular

herd, flock or national population, for the traits evaluated. These trends allow breeders to monitor the success of their breeding programmes, and they allow commercial buyers of breeding stock to select from companies, breeders, breeds or breeding schemes which are making most genetic progress. Several examples of estimated genetic trends are given in the following chapters.

The relationships between some animals have to be identified and included in BLUP evaluations using the **A** matrix, in order to achieve the benefits above. However, increasingly BLUP evaluations involve all relationships, i.e. they are animal model evaluations. There are additional benefits here:

- Including performance information for all relatives in predicting breeding values increases the accuracy of selection, and hence response to selection. An example of this is shown in Table 7.10. This particular example is from pigs, and the benefits vary from one species to the next, depending on the typical numbers of relatives of different classes with performance records. However, these results give an indication of the increase in accuracy which can be obtained. Note that this example shows only the benefits of including information from all relatives with BLUP. These benefits could also be achieved by using a very comprehensive selection index, incorporating information from many different classes of relatives, but it is more practical to incorporate this information using BLUP. Further benefits, not measured here, would result from the better separation of genetic and environmental effects which BLUP achieves.
- When all relationships between animals are included, and all of the traits under selection are being evaluated, BLUP can account for the fact that selection reduces the amount of variation in a trait. It can also account for culling bias and non-random matings. For example, depending on the perceived merit of a young sire, he may be mated to females of lower or higher than average merit in a herd or flock, which will clearly influence the performance of his progeny compared to those of sires mated to average females. Animal model BLUP can account for this, and so produce unbiased PBVs.

Table 7.10. Predicted rates of genetic improvement with various sources of information and methods of predicting breeding values. Rates of improvement are expressed in percentage units relative to that expected from selection on a record of performance on individual animals, for a trait with a heritability of 0.1 (= 100). Accuracies of selection are shown in brackets. The results are from a simulated pig breeding scheme with 10 males and 100 females, with records from three offspring of each sex per annum, and a generation interval of one year. (From Wray (1991) and Dr N R Wray, personal communication.)

Information used, and method of predicting breeding value	Heritability			
	0.1	0.2	0.4	0.6
Record from individual only	100 (0.30)	192 (0.43)	356 (0.59)	511 (0.72)
Records from individual and full brothers and sisters in optimum index	113 (0.35)	208 (0.47)	365 (0.62)	517 (0.73)
Records from individual and all relatives in BLUP	158 (0.50)	244 (0.56)	390 (0.60)	526 (0.75)

The benefits of conventional BLUP listed above are augmented by the use of genomic information, as a result of this allowing more accurate estimates of the actual (rather than expected) proportion of genes in common between related animals, and providing further information about likely genetic merit in traits of interest.

Using Economic Values with BLUP

Both multi-trait selection indexes and multi-trait BLUP use information on the associations between traits to produce more accurate predictions of breeding value. Multi-trait economic selection indexes then go one stage further, to combine the PBVs for breeding-goal traits into a single score based on their economic values. We have already seen that BLUP has several advantages over conventional indexes in predicting breeding values. How do we capitalize on these, and yet still get a PBV for total economic merit? There are basically two approaches, both based on multi-trait selection index methods outlined earlier. In the first case, if we have multi-trait BLUP PBVs for all of the breeding-goal traits we are interested in, we can simply multiply these by their economic values and add them together to get a PBV for total economic merit (Schneeberger *et al.*, 1992):

$$PBV_{TEM} = v_1PBV_1 + v_2PBV_2 + v_3PBV_3 \ldots$$

This formula is very similar to that presented earlier in this chapter for deriving the breeding goal for multi-trait indexes. If we do not have multi-trait BLUP PBVs for the breeding-goal traits (e.g. carcass traits), but we do have them for other correlated traits (e.g. ultrasonic measurements), then an intermediate step is required. This involves deriving PBVs for goal traits from the PBVs for indicator traits, using the genetic correlation between the two traits. The newly calculated PBVs for breeding-goal traits can then be weighted by their economic values as above.

Scale of Presentation of Genetic Merit

In all of the examples discussed so far, the PBV referred to the genetic merit of the animals being evaluated. The beef cattle and sheep genetic evaluation schemes in many countries express genetic merit on this scale. This can cause confusion among bull or ram buyers, because when they breed from the sire they buy, they can expect to see only half of the PBV in terms of extra progeny performance, as only half of the genes of the progeny come from the sire. The same scale of presentation is used for pigs, poultry and fish with genetic merit published as PBVs. However, dairy cattle producers are used to thinking about the merit of a bull in terms of the extra milk produced by his daughters, i.e. genetic merit expressed in terms of the merit of offspring, rather than the merit of the animal (parent) being evaluated. This difference in the way genetic merit is visualized is understandable, as dairy bulls do not produce milk themselves, whereas many of the traits of interest in other animals can be recorded on both sexes. Hence, the results of dairy cattle evaluations in some countries (and sheep and beef evaluations in a few) are expressed as *predicted* or *estimated transmitting abilities* (PTAs or ETAs) or *expected progeny differences* (EPDs). These three terms mean exactly the same thing, but the preferred name varies between countries. PTAs, ETAs or EPDs are simply one half of the PBVs (or EBVs) for the trait concerned, reflecting the fact that offspring receive half of their genes from each parent. So, it is easy to move from one scale to the other, but it is very important to know which scale you are working on! (Unless they are rescaled, the results of sire model BLUP evaluations are expressed as PTAs, while those from animal model evaluations are expressed as PBVs. Hence, the solutions to the equations in the earlier example of the two dairy sires used into two herds were multiplied by 2 to put them on to the PBV scale.)

To summarize:

PTA (or ETA, or EPD) = ½PBV (or ½EBV)

The expected genetic merit of offspring can be calculated from the PTAs or ETAs of parents in exactly the same way as it can from PBVs or EBVs, as shown in Fig. 7.2. That is:

PTA of offspring = ½PTA of sire + ½PTA of dam

However, there is a very important difference in the way the two scales of measuring genetic merit are used to predict the expected difference in *performance* of offspring, as opposed to the *genetic merit* of offspring. If genetic merit is expressed on the BV scale, the expected difference in performance of offspring, compared to using parents of average merit (i.e. PBV of 0) is:

Expected difference in performance of offspring
= ½PBV of sire + ½PBV of dam

If the PBV of the dam is unknown, for example, when a bull or ram is being used on crossbred commercial females, the dams are assumed to be of average genetic merit, and so have a PBV of 0. Since half of 0 is 0, the contribution from the dam is ignored and:

Expected difference in performance of offspring
= ½PBV of sire

For example, if a bull with a PBV of +30 kg for 400-day weight is used across a herd of commercial suckler cows, his calves are expected to weigh 15 kg more at 400 days than those sired by an average bull, i.e. a bull with a PBV of 0 kg (see Fig. 7.7(a)).

In contrast, if genetic merit is expressed on the transmitting ability scale, the merit of parents is already expressed in terms of the expected difference in performance of offspring, and so there is no need to halve the PTA of parents:

Expected difference in performance of offspring
= PTA of sire + PTA of dam

If PTAs are only available for the sire (the most common case) then the dams are assumed to have PTAs of zero, and so:

Expected difference in performance of offspring
= PTA of sire

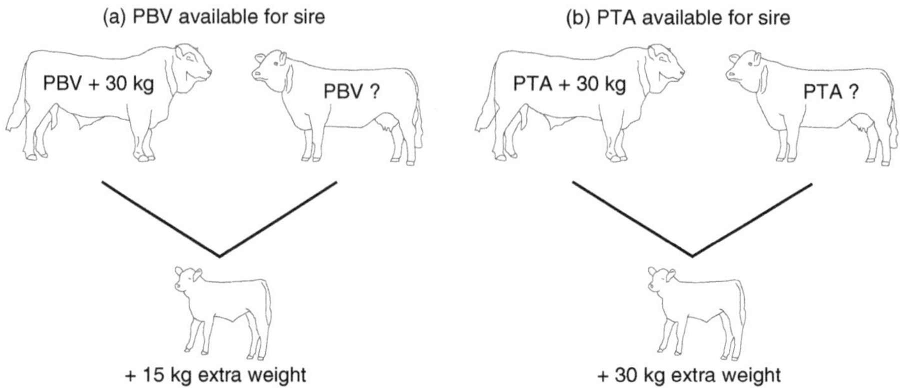

Fig. 7.7. (a) Calculating the expected difference in offspring performance when PBVs (or EBVs) are available on sires. (b) Calculating the expected difference in offspring performance when PTAs (or ETAs or EPDs) are available on sires. In this example the PBVs or PTAs are for 400-day weight, and the difference in weight of offspring is recorded at 400 days of age.

This is illustrated in Fig. 7.7(b). Similarly, if semen from a dairy bull with a PTA of +20 kg protein is used in a herd of cows without PTAs, our best guess is that his daughters will yield 20 kg more protein per lactation than daughters of a bull with a PTA of 0 kg protein.

Accuracies and Reliabilities

Whatever method of genetic evaluation is used, it is useful to know just how accurate individual PBVs are. In statistical terms, accuracies are correlations between predicted and true breeding values, and they range from 0 to 1. However, they are often expressed as percentages by multiplying the correlation by 100. Recall that we never know the true breeding values and always have to predict them in some way. High accuracies indicate that the PBVs are expected to be close to the true BVs, lower accuracies indicate that the association between PBVs and true BVs is weaker. Accuracies are often presented alongside PBVs from beef cattle and sheep evaluations. However, most dairy cattle PBVs or PTAs are accompanied by *reliabilities*. Reliabilities of PBVs or PTAs are simply squared accuracies. In other words, a PBV with an accuracy of 0.5 would have a reliability of 0.25 (0.5 × 0.5), and a PBV with an accuracy of 0.9 would have a reliability of 0.81 (0.9 × 0.9). The relationship between accuracy and reliability is shown in Fig. 7.8.

The fact that two different measures are used with the same aim is a bit confusing, and it is difficult to say with certainty why these different conventions have been adopted. Because of the widespread use of AI and progeny testing in dairy cattle, most bulls end up with very accurate PBVs or PTAs. The risk of a PBV changing is identical for a bull with an accuracy of 0.9 or a reliability of 0.81, and identical for another bull with an accuracy of 0.6 or a reliability of 0.36. But the fact that reliabilities give lower numbers than accuracies may deter people from using all but the most reliably-tested animals. So, the convention of using reliabilities for dairy cattle evaluations probably arose to give particular emphasis to widely proven bulls, and to reduce the emphasis on young bulls and other bulls with a limited proof. Generally, beef cattle and sheep evaluations are based on fewer performance records, and so they are less accurate than those for dairy bulls. Adopting reliabilities, rather than accuracies, could well be self-defeating, as beef and sheep breeders may be deterred from using the majority of animals. Also, accuracies make it a bit easier to discriminate among animals when they all have relatively little information available, simply because the scale of accuracies is wider than the scale of reliabilities 'at the bottom end' of the distribution (i.e. when animals' PBVs are based on relatively little information).

There are several factors that affect the accuracies of PBVs or reliabilities of PTAs:

- The heritability of the trait concerned – the higher the heritability of the trait, the higher the accuracy.

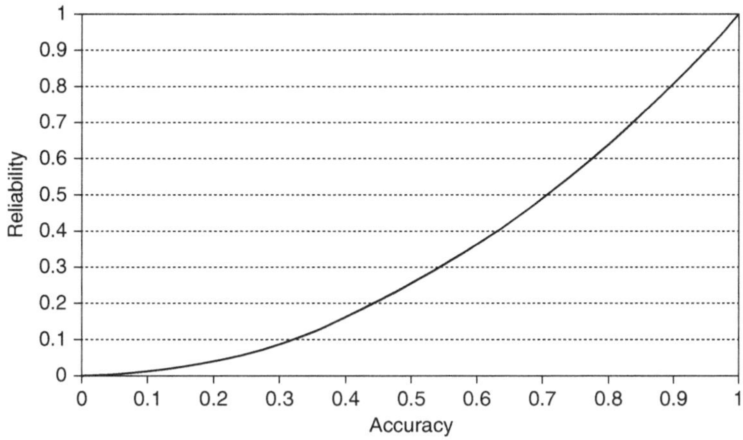

Fig. 7.8. The relationship between accuracy and reliability.

- The amount of performance information on the trait concerned from the animal itself – the more information, the higher the accuracy.
- The amount of performance information on the trait concerned from relatives of the animal – the more information, and the more useful the class of relative in predicting breeding values, the higher the accuracy (as before, progeny are the most valuable class of relatives; others contribute in proportion to the fraction of genes they have in common with the animal concerned).
- If it is a multi-trait evaluation, the amount of information on related traits from the animal itself and its relatives; the more information, and the higher the correlation with the trait of interest, the higher the accuracy.
- The number of contemporaries recorded – the more contemporaries recorded, the higher the accuracy.
- In the case of genomic evaluations, the size of the reference population – the larger the reference population the higher the accuracy.
- In the case of genomic evaluations, the density of the SNP chip. High density chips usually give higher accuracy resulting from a higher linkage disequilibrium between SNP markers and QTLs. If genotypes are imputed from lower-density chips, then the accuracy of imputation will also affect the accuracy of genomic prediction.
- For young animals (selection candidates) with BVs predicted using only genotype information, the higher the degree of genetic relationship between the reference animals and the selection candidates, the higher the accuracy.

Generally, the accuracies of PBVs based on performance and pedigree information alone for an individual animal start off quite low when the animal is young. For example, the PBV of a young dairy bull or maiden heifer might be based exclusively on its parents' PBVs and the accuracy is one quarter of the sum of the reliability of the sire and dam. Young pigs, beef calves or lambs might have an additional measure themselves, e.g. a birth weight, but their PBV would still be based mainly on ancestors' performance. The accuracies increase as records of performance from the animal itself and from its collateral relatives are included in the evaluation. For instance, milk records from sisters contribute to the PBVs of young dairy bulls; heifers have information from their sisters plus their own milk record. Likewise, pigs, poultry, beef cattle and sheep have records of their own plus those from sibs. Accuracies increase further once performance records are available from progeny and other descendants. This increase of accuracy with age is illustrated in Fig. 7.9 using 20-week live weight in lambs as an example.

However, as indicated earlier, historically there has been a trade-off between accuracy and generation interval. In most cases, waiting for many progeny to be recorded in order to get very accurate PBVs increases the generation interval, and so can reduce annual responses to selection. The situation is changing now with the use of genetic markers

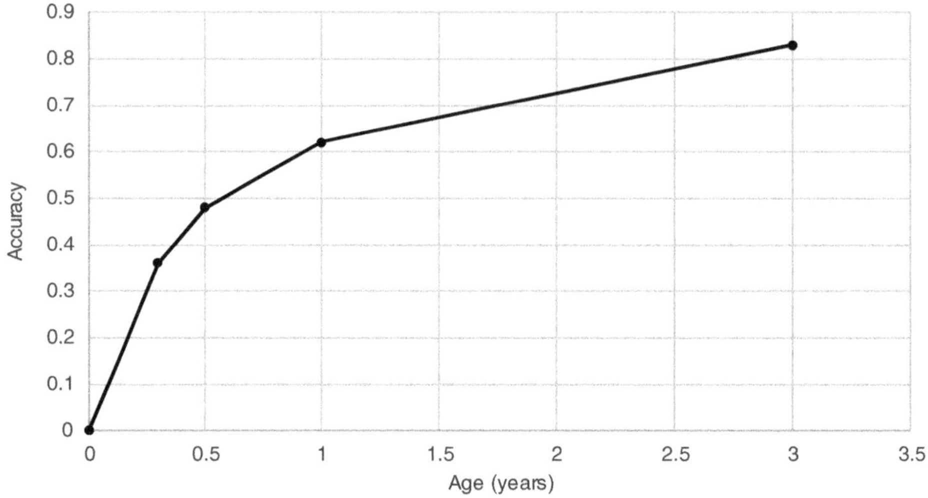

Fig. 7.9. The relationship between accuracy of evaluation and age using lamb early growth as an example (heritability = 0.25). At birth, no information is available (except parental values which are not usually computed at this stage) but parental performance and EBVs are used at, say, 6 months of age. The animal's own performance is added at about 1 year of age and then over the next few years performance from the animal's offspring is available.

linked to the genes affecting performance traits and used in the prediction of genomic breeding values (see section above on genomic predictions and genomic selection). Using these genetic markers across the genome means PBVs are predicted with more information and therefore higher accuracies at younger ages. The accuracy of predicting GEBVs for young dairy animals with no records for production traits (e.g. milk, fat and protein yields) ranges from 0.50–0.85 (Moser *et al.*, 2010; Wiggans *et al.*, 2017). These accuracies can be up to 30–50% higher than those obtained from the parent average PBVs based on performance and pedigree information alone.

The principle behind genetic evaluation in general, and multi-trait animal model BLUP evaluation in particular, is to use all available information on the animal and its relatives to give the most accurate prediction of breeding value possible at that time. Repeating genetic evaluations quite frequently allows new performance information to be included, producing more accurate PBVs. Accuracies also give an indication of the chance that future PBVs will differ from current ones. Low accuracies indicate that there is a high chance that the PBV will change, e.g. when extra performance records become available on the animal itself or its relatives. High accuracies indicate that the PBV is already based on a substantial amount of performance information, and that new information is unlikely to lead to big changes in PBVs. This is illustrated in Fig. 7.10 which shows the possible range of true BVs for animals with PBVs of different accuracies. Typical levels of accuracy achieved in evaluations for different species are given in Chapters 8 to 13.

An important feature of BLUP PBVs is that they are already scaled to account for the amount of performance information on which they are based. PBVs based on very little information get adjusted or 'shrunk' back (regressed) towards the mean PBV. This shrinking applies both to high and low PBVs. In other words, it is difficult to get either a very high or a very low PBV on the basis of little information. The more information available on an animal and its relatives, the less the PBVs are shrunk, and the easier it is to get very high or very low PBVs. This is illustrated in Fig. 7.11 which shows the relationship between accuracy and EBV for 8-week weight in lambs. At low accuracies, there is very little information on the animal, so EBVs are low and similar. As more information becomes available on the animal, as shown by increased accuracy, then the EBVs spread out towards their 'true' values. This feature of BLUP is a very valuable way of accounting for the risk

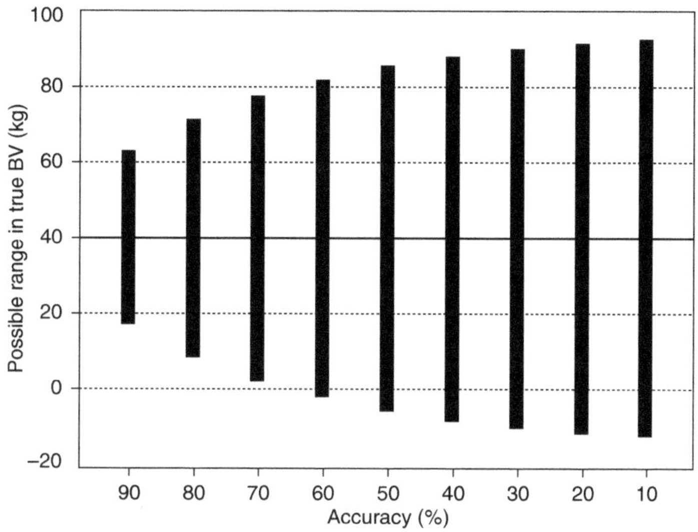

Fig. 7.10. Possible range of true breeding values for a bull with a PBV for 400-day weight of +40 kg with various levels of accuracy. In this example, there is a 90% chance that the true breeding value lies in the range shown. (Dr R.E. Crump, personal communication; see Van Vleck *et al.* (1987) for more details on methodology.)

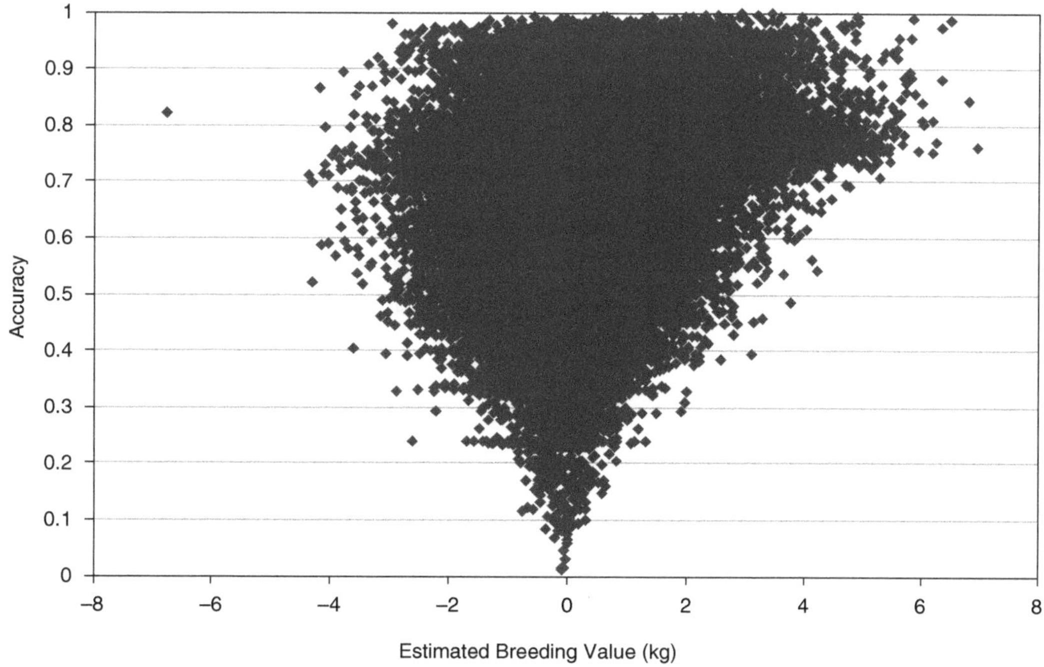

Fig. 7.11. A plot of EBV against accuracy for lamb 8-week weight (kg) showing the conservative nature of using BLUP to compute EBVs. Lambs with little information (low accuracy) have EBVs at average levels (0 on the EBV scale). As more information becomes available (moving up the left-hand axis) then EBVs spread out allowing the identification of better and poorer animals. Really good (or poor) animals can only be found with certainty at high accuracies.

involved in breeding decisions. It helps to avoid selecting animals which initially appear to have high genetic merit on the basis of flimsy evidence, and which might turn out later to be much poorer than expected. The chance of an individual animal's BLUP PBV going down is exactly the same as the chance of it going up, but obviously breeders are more concerned about selecting an animal which turns out to be worse than expected than about selecting an animal which turns out to be better than expected.

Because BLUP PBVs already account for accuracy, many scientists argue that it is irrelevant to look at the accuracy any further; rates of genetic progress in the trait concerned will be highest if selection is based solely on BLUP PBVs. These PBVs have already been adjusted to balance the risk versus the potential gain in order to identify animals which are the 'best bet' overall. Breeders who take any further account of accuracies may reduce the risk but, on average, would also reduce the genetic gain. While this is true, accuracies are still valuable in allowing breeders to assess the risk involved in the purchase of individual animals, and in interpreting changes in an individual animal's PBV over time.

Publishing Results

Depending on the circumstances of the PBV estimation there may be a range of options for publishing the results of the evaluations. In the case of pigs, poultry and fish, where most breeding programmes are run by private breeding companies, typically very limited information is made publicly available. However, for dairy and beef cattle, sheep and goats, with genetic evaluations typically carried out by a national centre or a breed association, results are usually published on their websites and in breed show and sale catalogues. (For examples, see AHDB, 2019; Breedplan, 2019; British Limousin Cattle Society, 2019; CDN, 2019; CDCB, 2019; Sheep Improvement Limited, 2019; Signet, 2019.)

Genetic bases

In the section on calculating PBVs, we mentioned that PBVs are usually expressed as a deviation from the mean PBV of a group of animals, called the genetic base. However, the genetic base has to be appropriately defined. If PBVs are expressed relative to the merit of distant ancestors and genetic progress is being made in the population, the average genetic merit of base population animals could be a lot lower than that of the current breeding population. This may make the current animals appear a lot better than they really are. There are two main solutions to this. One is to express PBVs relative to a more recent group of animals, e.g. those born in a recent year, and to set their average merit in that year equal to zero. This is called a *fixed base* if the definition of base animals remains unchanged for a few years. Fixed bases are usually updated every few years, as they too can become outdated if genetic progress is high. An out-of-date fixed base can be quite misleading because many animals which have positive PBVs are, in fact, well below the average genetic merit of the current breeding population. Fixed bases are used in beef, sheep and dairy cattle evaluations in many countries. The other alternative is a *rolling base*. With a rolling base the predicted transmitting values are expressed relative to the merit of the current population, and so they change with each new evaluation. Rolling bases are used, for example, in dairy cattle evaluations in Canada and France (http://www.interbull.org/ib/geforms).

There are pros and cons to each type of base. For example, it is easier to compare the results of successive evaluations with a fixed base than with a rolling base. But a fixed base can give a false impression of progress if animals are selected on the basis of the sign of their PBV alone. If the population is improving rapidly some animals with positive PBVs compared to a base chosen a few years earlier will be worse than the current breed average. A rolling base avoids the problem of highlighting animals of low merit, but the frequent changes in absolute values of PBVs can lead to confusion. A frequently updated fixed base is a common compromise.

International Evaluations and Conversions

Livestock breeding has become an increasingly international business over the past few decades. In the pig and poultry industries a few international companies are responsible for production of a high proportion of the world's breeding stock, and hence a high proportion of the genes in commercial livestock. In these industries much of the business of comparing breeds and strains internationally has been undertaken 'in house' by breeding companies, via designed trials. However, in the ruminant livestock industries ownership of breeding stock remains much more dispersed, involving many individual breeders and some breeding companies. The international spread of many cattle and sheep breeds has been aided by the development of techniques for AI and semen freezing and, more recently, by the development of equivalent procedures for embryos. Hence, methods are needed to allow fair comparisons of imported strains when they or their offspring appear in national performance recording schemes. This is particularly true in dairy cattle breeding, and much effort has gone into developing procedures to allow breeders in one country to make use of genetic evaluations of bulls in other countries. More recently, a similar system for international comparisons of the genetic merit of beef cattle has been developed. Much of the groundwork in this area has been under the guidance of an organization called INTERBULL – a subcommittee of the International Committee for Animal Recording, based at the Swedish University of Agricultural Sciences in Uppsala.

Where there is an active international trade in genetic material, it is logical to consider comparing evaluations across national boundaries. In the past, this has usually been achieved by deriving formulae to convert PBVs or PTAs calculated in the exporting country to equivalent PBVs or PTAs in the importing country. However, with advances in methodologies, this now involves combining records from several countries in a single international evaluation using a method called *multi-trait across country evaluation* (MACE).

International evaluations

The multi-trait across country evaluation used for international evaluations, especially in dairy cattle, is based on the multi-trait BLUP method described earlier (Schaeffer, 1994). MACE regards records on the same trait from different countries as different traits. This allows MACE to account for differences among countries in the heritability of the trait and differences in scale, or the way the trait is measured, in different countries. MACE estimates the genetic correlations among the countries for the traits of interest, and this is used in the calculation of PBVs. In the case of dairy cattle, MACE uses average daughter yield deviations from sires in different countries (these can be derived approximately, by the process of de-regression mentioned earlier, using the sires' local PTAs, the numbers of daughters contributing to these PTAs and the heritability used locally), rather than individual daughter records, to reduce the computing demands. In addition, this ensures that the records coming from different countries have been adjusted for the non-genetic effects known to be important in those countries. Evaluations are produced for each sire on the scale of the different countries. The different sources of information that contribute to the reliability of the MACE evaluation of any sire in any participating country include the heritability of the trait, the number of daughters the bull has in each of the participating countries, and the correlation between the trait being evaluated in the local country and other countries in which he has daughters.

MACE requires that there are good genetic links among the participating countries. These genetic links make it possible to estimate genetic correlations among the countries for the trait being evaluated. Examples of some genetic correlations between production traits in the UK and some other countries are shown in Table 7.11. The correlations are all high. However, the fact that there are particularly high correlations between the production traits in the UK and the corresponding traits in Ireland, Netherlands, France and Denmark shows that daughter information on bulls among these countries are similar, reflecting the similar production systems in these countries. Conversely, the correlations between production traits in the UK and the corresponding traits in New Zealand and Australia are the lowest, reflecting differences in climate and production systems.

There are several potential benefits from the use of MACE. Firstly, it produces separate PTAs for sires for each country involved in the evaluation, and these are expressed on the local scale and are ready to use. Secondly, because they use information from daughters in all of the countries in which they are present, MACE evaluations are more accurate than the conversions they replace (see next section on conversions). Thirdly, because MACE allows different values for genetic correlations between a trait in different countries, the rankings of sires evaluated can differ among countries. This is particularly useful where there is a genotype-by-environment interaction, e.g. for the same milk production trait in countries with very different management systems. (The correlations in Table 7.11 indicate that the greatest likelihood of re-ranking of sire proofs between the UK and the other countries shown will be

Table 7.11. Estimates of the genetic correlations between milk, fat and protein production in the UK and the same traits in several other countries. These estimates were produced by INTERBULL for the August 2019 MACE evaluations. (INTERBULL; EGENES)

	Genetic correlation with corresponding trait in UK for Holstein/Friesian Breed		
Country	Milk (kg)	Fat (kg)	Protein (kg)
Australia	0.74	0.71	0.70
Belgium	0.81	0.81	0.81
Canada	0.87	0.86	0.85
Czechia	0.80	0.81	0.80
DFS[a]	0.86	0.88	0.86
France	0.87	0.89	0.86
Germany[b]	0.83	0.86	0.82
Ireland	0.82	0.80	0.78
Italy	0.82	0.83	0.81
Netherlands	0.87	0.87	0.86
New Zealand	0.70	0.70	0.69
Spain	0.84	0.84	0.84
Switzerland	0.89	0.90	0.87
USA	0.85	0.87	0.84

[a]Joint Denmark, Finland and Sweden evaluations.
[b]Joint Austria and Germany evaluations.

with New Zealand.) The possibility for different rankings among countries is also useful where the traits being recorded in different countries are similar, but not identical. These benefits are also seen in cows, when MACE evaluations on male relatives are used in calculating cow PBVs.

The INTERBULL Centre produces MACE evaluations routinely for milk, fat and protein yields, udder health (somatic cell count and mastitis), conformation, fertility, and calving traits (calving ease and stillbirth) for dairy cattle. At the time of writing, evaluations are based on data from 35 countries and are carried out three times per year. Evaluations are produced for Ayrshire, Brown Swiss, Guernsey, Holstein and Jersey sires. Some of the countries involved use the INTERBULL international evaluations in place of domestic evaluations or combine them with domestic evaluations for foreign bulls with few daughters in the country. Others use them until a sire has a reliable local proof.

Countries submit PBVs to the INTERBULL centre to be used as input variables for the dairy MACE evaluations. As mentioned above, these PBVs are then de-regressed before they are used in MACE. The INTERBULL centre returns PBVs to each country expressed on their own national scale. However, as a result of the much smaller data sets for beef cattle compared to dairy cattle, and increasing computer power, INTERBULL has developed an international evaluation for beef cattle based on performance records from individual animals rather than PBVs. Otherwise, the approach is similar to the dairy cattle system, i.e. a MACE evaluation is used, with the genetic correlations among the countries incorporated. The beef genetic evaluation system is called INTERBEEF (2019), and the traits evaluated are calving ease, birth weight and weaning weight, for the Limousin and Charolais breeds. These international evaluations started in 2015 and two evaluations are carried out per year.

Additionally, INTERBULL now performs genomic multi-trait across-country evaluations (GMACE), based on the same principles as MACE. GMACE is, however, restricted to young dairy bulls (not more than 7 years old) with only genomic breeding values (i.e. no contribution of daughter information or performance to their genetic merit). The genomic breeding values of young bulls for a particular trait such as milk yield from the different countries are treated as separate traits. Using the same estimates of genetic correlations among the countries used in MACE, the GMACE procedure predicts genomic evaluations for the young bulls for all countries participating in INTERBULL, expressed on their own national scale (Sullivan, 2016). Currently there are 32 countries participating in GMACE for milk production traits. (At the time of writing GMACE is not available for beef cattle.)

International conversions

In the early stages of international trade in dairy cattle semen, and prior to the introduction of MACE, *international conversions* provided the means by which PBVs from one country could be expressed on the scale of another. International conversion formulae were established using the regression methods outlined in Chapter 2. This essentially involved plotting the PBVs or PTAs of a group of bulls, derived from progeny tests in the exporting country, against their PBVs or PTAs derived from progeny tests in the importing country. The slope of the line passing through these points on the graph, and the point at which the line crosses an axis (the intercept) were then used to derive converted PBVs or PTAs for other bulls from the exporting country which had yet to get a progeny test in the importing country. The method had the disadvantage that the countries involved must have a reasonably large number of progeny-tested bulls in common to obtain a reliable conversion formula. In addition, some countries expressed genetic merit on different units (e.g. kg, lb or standardized units) or on different scales (PTA or PBV), which needed to be accounted for. Also, different countries used different models in their evaluation systems making the process of computing conversion equations rather cumbersome. However, with the introduction of MACE for bulls, these limitations have been resolved.

The introduction of MACE meant that there is no need for international conversions for bulls. This is because once a bull has a PBV in one country, MACE produces a PBV for that bull in all other countries in the international evaluation. However, international trade in dairy cattle is not restricted to use of semen from AI bulls only but also occurs via sale of embryos, heifers or cows. So, international conversions are still useful for the conversion of cow PBVs from one country to the scale of another. The procedure for calculating conversion equations is still based on a regression approach but with different sets of rules for selecting the bulls to be used (INTERBULL, 2019). Conversion equations are now calculated based on the international predicted genetic merit (PGM) of bulls with the following requirements for the exporting country: (i) bulls are progeny tested in only one country, the country of origin; (ii) only bulls born since YYYY-15, where YYYY is the current year for the MACE evaluations, are included; (iii) national PGM is based on daughters in at least 20 herds; (iv) national reliability is at least 75%; and (v) a minimum of 20 bulls are required for computation. (In countries where there are not enough bulls that meet the above rules, conversion equations are based on a standard formula.)

Summary

- There are a number of steps involved in the selection of animals to maximize the response achieved. These include: (i) managing the animals as equally as possible to make it easier to disentangle genetics and environment; (ii) adjusting records of performance for known environmental effects, and then (iii) predicting the breeding values of individual animals by the most appropriate method. Modern (BLUP) methods of genetic evaluation achieve the second and third of these steps simultaneously.
- Records of performance may be adjusted using additive or multiplicative correction factors, or by standardizing. Additive and multiplicative correction factors are the simplest to use, but both have to be derived from prior analysis of large data sets. Standardizing records is more complex, but requires no prior information. Using multiplicative correction factors or standardizing records may be most appropriate when the size of the effect being adjusted for is related to the level of performance of animals either within or between herds or flocks. Each of the methods can separate genetic and environmental effects poorly in some circumstances, e.g. when sires have been used unequally across different groups of animals. This type of problem can be reduced or overcome by simultaneous estimation of environmental effects and prediction of breeding values using BLUP methods.
- Predicting an animal's breeding value is a bit like completing a large, complicated jigsaw puzzle, where each piece of the puzzle is a record of performance from the animal itself or one of its relatives. More recently, the genomic information on the animal adds a further piece of the puzzle. Generally, the higher the proportion of genes in common between the animal and a given relative, the more useful the record of performance from that relative. But, records from progeny are of most value. As the number of records on progeny increases, the correlation between predicted and true breeding values approaches one. With other classes of relatives the accuracy of prediction never reaches one, and for all classes of relatives there are diminishing returns in accuracy as the number of records increases.
- PBVs may be expressed relative to a base. If the definition of base animals remains unchanged for a few years, it is called a fixed base. Fixed bases are usually updated every few years, as they can become outdated if genetic progress is high. The other alternative is a rolling base. With a rolling base the PBVs are expressed relative to the merit of the current population, and so they change with each new evaluation.

- PBVs can have positive or negative values or be equal to zero. The sign indicates whether they are expected to be genetically above (+) or below (–) the average of the group of animals on which the calculations were performed, or some other defined group of animals whose PBVs are set to average zero (the base). PBVs are expressed (at least initially) in the same units as the record of performance (e.g. kg of live weight, litres of milk, mm of fat). The PBVs of animals can only be compared within contemporary groups, herds or flocks unless there are genetic links between these groups, and the PBVs were from across-herd or across-flock BLUP evaluations.
- In the simplest case, when we have a single record of performance on the animal itself, the predicted or estimated breeding value (PBV or EBV) is the deviation in performance from contemporaries, multiplied by the heritability of the trait concerned. The deviation in performance is calculated after adjusting the performance records for environmental effects. PBVs calculated from a single record of performance span a narrower range than the deviations in performance; the higher the heritability, the lower the proportion of non-genetic variation, and so the less severe the shrinking.
- Calculating PBVs from the performance of relatives is more difficult. The simplest case is when the only records available are from the parents. If we first calculate PBVs for each parent, then the PBV of their offspring is calculated simply by adding half the PBV of the sire to half the PBV of the dam. PBVs calculated from ancestors' PBVs are known as pedigree indexes. They are very valuable in providing an early prediction of an animal's genetic merit.
- PBVs can be derived from a single record of performance on any relative, by multiplying the PBV of the relative by the expected proportion of genes in common with the animal without a PBV.
- If we have more than one of any other type of relative apart from parents, we cannot simply average their PBVs, because progeny or sibs, for example, have genes in common with each other as well as the animal whose PBV is being derived, and so there is 'overlap' in the information they provide. In these cases PBVs are calculated from the average deviation in performance of the progeny or sibs from their contemporaries, multiplied by a factor which depends on the class of relative concerned, the number of records available, and the heritability of the trait concerned.
- Combining information from different types of relatives is more complex. The most common method is to produce an index which, again, weights the contributions from different types of relatives according to the class of relative, the number of records available from each class, and the heritability of the trait concerned.
- In most livestock production systems profitability depends on several different animal characteristics rather than on any single trait. Index selection is also used to combine adjusted records of performance in several traits measured on the animal itself, or several traits measured on the animal itself and on one or more classes of relatives.
- To derive a multi-trait economic selection index we need to know: which traits we want to improve (the breeding goal or selection objective); the economic values of each of the traits in the breeding goal; the set of traits for which measurements will be available for all candidates for selection (the index measurements or selection criteria); the additive genetic and phenotypic variances for traits in the breeding goal and the index measurements and the additive genetic and phenotypic covariances among them. With this information it is possible to calculate a set of index coefficients which, when used in selection, will maximize genetic progress in overall economic merit.
- Adjusting records of performance and then predicting breeding values in two separate stages has several shortcomings: (i) PBVs can only be compared fairly for animals which are managed and fed similarly, e.g. within herds or flocks; (ii) the results from some of the methods for adjusting performance are specific to the herds or flocks for which they were derived; (iii) most of the methods run the risk of removing some true genetic differences; (iv) several methods of adjusting performance make the assumption that animals in different contemporary groups are of equal genetic merit; and (v) although conventional indexes combine information from relatives in an appropriate way, they are not very flexible to use, e.g. different weighting factors are needed whenever there are different numbers of records from a particular class of relatives.
- BLUP is a statistical technique which disentangles genetics from management and feeding in

the best possible way, and so produces more accurate predictions of breeding value. It achieves this by estimating environmental effects and predicting breeding values simultaneously. BLUP 'recognizes' that some performance records are from related animals. Related animals in different contemporary groups provide genetic links between the groups. These links are necessary in order for BLUP to estimate environmental effects and predict breeding values simultaneously.

- With both selection indexes and BLUP, the problem of finding the appropriate emphasis to give to different pieces of information is solved by setting up a series of simultaneous equations. In BLUP, the equations to be solved link the performance records to the environmental effects, and to the animals whose BVs we are predicting. BLUP equations also include weighting factors which account for the heritability of the trait concerned and for the relationship between the animals who produced the records and those whose BVs are being predicted.
- BLUP can be applied under different sets of assumptions – called models – which differ in sophistication. The most common BLUP models are: (i) sire models; (ii) sire-maternal grandsire models; and (iii) individual animal models. The name of the model indicates the animals for which BVs are predicted, and the relationships used to predict them. The more sophisticated BLUP models recognize more relationships between animals, and hence predict BVs more accurately. An equation has to be solved for each animal which gets a PBV. As a result, one of the main factors governing the uptake of more sophisticated models has been the cost and availability of computing power.
- It is often useful to think of direct and maternal breeding values for traits such as weaning weight, which are influenced by both direct and maternal genetic merit. Both males and females carry genes for milk production and other aspects of maternal performance, but only females get the chance to express them. However, with sufficient data, BLUP can predict both direct and maternal breeding values for males and females, from the relationships between animals with performance records (e.g. cows with calf weaning weights) and those without (e.g. bulls).
- BLUP evaluations can be performed for one trait (single-trait evaluations) or several traits (multi-trait evaluations) at a time. When traits are correlated, multi-trait evaluations produce more accurate PBVs than single-trait evaluations. However, multi-trait evaluations are more demanding on computing resources than single-trait BLUP, and require accurate estimates of covariances among traits.
- There are several benefits from using BLUP. As long as there are genetic links among contemporary groups in different herds or flocks, and across years, BLUP separates genetic and environmental effects more effectively than traditional methods, and the resulting PBVs can be compared directly across different contemporary groups, and hence age groups, herds, flocks or years. Plots of average PBVs across time show the estimated genetic trend which is occurring. The relationships between some animals have to be identified and included in BLUP evaluations in order to achieve these benefits. However, when BLUP evaluations involve all relationships there are additional benefits. Including performance information for all relatives in predicting breeding values increases the accuracy of selection, and, when all of the traits under selection are being evaluated, BLUP can account for the fact that selection reduces the amount of variation in a trait, and it can also account for non-random matings.
- If we have multi-trait-BLUP PBVs for all of the breeding-goal traits we are interested in, we can simply multiply these by their economic values and add them together to get a PBV for total economic merit. If we only have PBVs for other correlated (indicator) traits, we have to derive PBVs for goal traits from the PBVs for indicator traits, using the genetic correlations between the two sets of traits.
- The genetic merit of animals can also be predicted using SNPs, which are DNA markers that are closely linked with genes that control traits of interest. The initial step involves estimating the SNP effects in a reference population that has both SNPs and phenotypic records for the trait of interest. The SNP effects, also referred to as the SNP key, can then be used to estimate DGVs for young animals which are related to the reference population. The DGVs are usually combined with parent averages from BLUP for these young animals to estimate GEBVs. The accuracy of GEBVs for young animals tends to be 30–50 % higher than that from the parent average for traits of high to

medium heritability. The selection of animals as parents on the basis of GEBVs is called genomic selection.

- Models used for genomic prediction include: (i) GBLUP, which is similar to BLUP but the genomic relationship matrix (**G**) is used in the usual BLUP equations instead of the numerator relationship matrix (**A**); (ii) SNP-BLUP, which sets up equations for each SNP genotype, and so produces solutions for each SNP; the genomic breeding values are then obtained by multiplying each SNP solution by the corresponding genotype observed in the animal and summing over SNPs; and (iii) single step, which predicts PBVs combining both the A matrix from the pedigree for non-genotyped animals and the G matrix for genotyped animals, to produce the H matrix.
- The predicted genetic merit of animals is expressed on one of two scales. PBVs refer to the genetic merit of the animals being evaluated. But predicted or estimated transmitting abilities (PTAs or ETAs) or expected progeny differences (EPDs) express genetic merit in terms of the expected superiority or inferiority in the performance of progeny. PTAs, ETAs or EPDs are one half of the PBVs (or EBVs) for the trait concerned. The predicted genetic merit of offspring is simply the average of the PBVs or PTAs of parents. However, the method of predicting differences in offspring performance varies depending on the scale on which genetic merit is expressed. If parents' genetic merit is expressed as PBVs, we average these to get the expected difference in offspring performance, but if parents, genetic merit is expressed as PTAs we *sum* these to get the expected difference in offspring performance.
- The PBVs for dairy and beef cattle, sheep and goats are usually calculated at a national centre or within a breed association and the results tend to be published on their websites and in various sale catalogues. In the case of pigs, poultry and fish, with most breeding programmes run by private breeding companies, typically very limited information is made publicly available.
- Accuracies are correlations between predicted and true breeding values; we never know true BVs. High accuracies indicate that the PBVs are expected to be close to the true BVs, low accuracies indicate that the association between PBVs and true BVs is weaker. The accuracies of PBVs depend on the heritability of the trait concerned, the amount of information on the trait concerned on the animal itself and its relatives, the amount of information on related traits on the animal itself and its relatives (if it is a multi-trait evaluation), and the number of contemporaries recorded. Accuracies also give an indication of the chance that future PBVs will differ from current ones. Low accuracies indicate that there is a high chance that the PBV will change when new information becomes available, and *vice versa*. Reliabilities of PBVs or PTAs are squared accuracies.
- International trade in genetic material has created much interest in comparing evaluations across national boundaries. In the past this was usually achieved by deriving formulae to convert PBVs or PTAs calculated in the foreign country to equivalent PBVs or PTAs in the importing country. There are several disadvantages to this approach, including the fact that conversion formulae have to be derived separately for each foreign country of interest. To surmount these problems and make better use of the international information available on sires, a procedure has been developed to allow international evaluations. This is called multi-trait across country evaluation (MACE). MACE treats records on the same trait from different countries as if they were different traits. This allows for differences among countries in the heritability of the trait of interest and allows for different genetic correlations between this trait recorded in different countries.
- MACE has several potential advantages: (i) it produces separate PTAs for sires for each country involved in the evaluation, and these are expressed on the local scale; (ii) because they use information from daughters in all of the countries in which they are present, MACE evaluations are more accurate than conversions; and (iii) because MACE allows different values for genetic correlations between a trait in different countries, the rankings of sires evaluated can differ among countries (this is particularly useful where there is a genotype-by-environment interaction, or where the traits being recorded in different countries are not identical).
- While the use of conversion equations for bulls has been superseded by MACE, these are still useful for converting the PTAs of imported cows to the local scale. International conversions are now based on a set of at least 20 young bulls with international genetic merit estimated in two countries.

References

AHDB (2019) Breeding and genetics. Available at: https://dairy.ahdb.org.uk/technical-information/breeding-genetics/#.XWsbQigzZPZ (accessed 21 October 2019).

Amer, P.R. (1994) Economic theory and breeding objectives. *Proceedings of the 5th World Congress on Genetics Applied to Livestock Production*, 18, 197–204. Available at: http://www.wcgalp.org/proceedings/1994 (accessed 16 June 2020).

Andersen, S. and Pedersen, B. (1996) Growth and food intake curves for group-housed gilts and castrated male pigs. *Animal Science* 63, 457–464. DOI: 10.1017/S1357729800015356.

Bergsma, R., Kanis, E., Knol, E.F. and Bijma, P. (2008) The contribution of social effects to heritable variation in finishing traits of domesticated pigs (*Sus scrofa*). *Genetics* 178, 1559–1570. DOI: 10.1534/genetics.107.084236.

Bijma, P., Muir, W.M. and Van Arendonk, J.A.M. (2007) Multilevel selection 1: quantitative genetics of inheritance and response to selection. *Genetics* 175, 277–288. DOI: 10.1534/genetics.106.062711.

Breedplan (2019) Available at: https://breedplan.une.edu.au/ (accessed 10 August 2019).

British Limousin Cattle Society (2019) Performance Programmes. Available at: https://limousin.co.uk/performance-programmes/ (accessed 10 August 2019).

Canadian Dairy Network (CDN) (2019) Available at: https://www.cdn.ca/home.php (accessed 21 October 2019).

Christensen, O.F., Madsen, P., Nielsen, B., Ostersen, T. and Su, G. (2012) Single-step methods for genomic evaluation in pigs. *Animal* 6, 1565–1571. DOI: 10.1017/S1751731112000742.

Council on Dairy Cattle Breeding (CDCB) (2019) Available at: https://www.uscdcb.com/ (accessed 21 October 2019).

Edinburgh Genetic Evaluation Services (EGENES) (2019) Available at: https://www.sruc.ac.uk/info/120275/egenes (accessed 21 October 2019).

France Génétique Elevage (2019) Available at: http://en.france-genetique-elevage.org (accessed 21 October 2019).

Goddard, M.E. (2009) Genomic selection: prediction of accuracy and maximisation of long term response. *Genetica* 136, 245–252. DOI: 10.1007/s10709-008-9308-0.

Henderson, C.R. (1973) Sire evaluation and genetic trends. In: *Proceedings of the Animal Breeding and Genetics Symposium in Honor of J.L. Lush.* American Society for Animal Science, Champaign, Illinois, pp. 10–41.

Henderson, C.R. (1975) Best linear unbiased estimation and prediction under a selection model. *Biometrics* 31, 423-447. DOI: 10.2307/2529430.

Hutchison, J.L., Cole, J.B. and Bickhart, D.M. (2014) Short communication: use of young bulls in the United States. *Journal of Dairy Science* 97, 3213–3220. DOI: 10.3168/jds.2013-7525.

INTERBEEF (2019) Available at: https://www.icar.org/index.php/technical-bodies/working-groups/interbeef-working-group/ (accessed 21 June 2020).

INTERBULL (1990) *Recommended Procedures for International Use of Sire Proofs*. INTERBULL Bulletin No. 4, International Bull Evaluation Service, Department of Animal Breeding and Genetics, Uppsala, Sweden.

INTERBULL (2019) Interbull centre document on August Routine Evaluation 2019. Estimated Conversion Coefficients. (Interbull Centre, Unpublished document).

Johansson, I. and Rendel, J. (1968) *Genetics and Animal Breeding*. Oliver and Boyd, Edinburgh, UK.

KidPlan (2019) Available at: http://www.sheepgenetics.org.au/Breeding-services/KIDPLAN-Home (accessed 21 October 2019).

Lourenco, D.A.L., Tsurutai, S., Fragomeni, B.O., Masuda, Y., Aguilar, I. *et al.* (2015) Genetic evaluation using single-step genomic best linear unbiased predictor in American Angus. *Journal of Animal Science* 93, 2653–2662. DOI: 10.2527/jas.2014-8836.

Meuwissen, T.H, Hayes, B. and Goddard, M.E. (2001) Prediction of total genetic values using genome-wide dense marker maps. *Genetics* 157, 1819–1829.

Meyer, K. (1999) Estimates of genetic and phenotypic covariance functions for postweaning growth and mature weight of beef cows. *Journal of Animal Breeding and Genetics* 116, 181–205. DOI: 10.1016/S0301-6226(96)01414-5.

Misztal, I., Aquilar, I., Legarra, A., Tsuruta, S., Johnson, D.L. and Lawlor, T.J. (2010) A unified approach to ultilise phenotypic, full pedigree and genomic information for genetic evaluation. *The 9th World Congress Applied To Livestock Production.* Available at: http://www.wcgalp.org/proceedings/2010 (accessed 16 June 2020).

Moore, A.J., Brodie Jr, E.D. and Wolf, J.B. (1997) Interacting phenotypes and the evolutionary process. I. Direct and indirect genetic effects of social interactions. *Evolution* 51, 1352–1362. DOI: 10.1111/j.1558-5646.1997.tb01458.x.

Moser, G., Khatkar, M.S., Hayes, B.J. and Raadsma, H.W. (2010) Accuracy of direct genomic values in Holstein bulls and cows using subsets of SNP markers. *Genetics, Selection and Evolution* 42, 37. DOI: 10.1186/1297-9686-42-37.

Mrode, R.A. (2014) *Linear Models for the Prediction of Animal Breeding Values*, 3rd edn. CAB International, Wallingford, UK.

Mrode, R., Krzyzelewski, T., Moore, K., Winters, W. and Coffey, M.P. (2011) The implementation of genomic evaluations in the UK. *Interbull Bulletin* 44, 173–175.

Nicholas, F.W. (1987) *Veterinary Genetics*. Oxford University Press, Oxford.

Pander, B.L., Hill, W.G. and Thompson, R. (1992) Genetic parameters of test day records of British Holstein heifers. *Animal Production* 55, 11–21. DOI: 10.1017/S0003356100037211.

Pedigree Viewer (2019) Available at: https://bkinghor.une.edu.au/pedigree.htm (accessed 21 October 2019).

Pollott, G.E. and Greeff, J.C. (2004) Genotype by environment interactions and genetic parameters for fecal egg count and production traits of Merino sheep. *Journal of Animal Science* 82, 2840–2851. DOI: 10.2527/2004.82102840x.

RelaX2 (2019) Available at: https://www.researchgate.net/publication/332144513_RelaX2_program_for_pedigree_analysis_User's_guide_for_version_165 (accessed 21 October 2019).

Robertson, A., Stewart, A. and Ashton., E.D. (1956) The progeny assessment of dairy sires for milk: The use of contemporary comparison. *Proceedings of the British Society of Animal Production* 1956, 43–50. DOI: 10.1017/S0369852100001688.

Rutten, M.J.M., Bijma, P., Woolliams, J.A. and van Arendonk, J.A.M. (2002) SelAction: Software to predict selection response and rate of inbreeding in livestock breeding programs. *Journal of Heredity* 93, 456–458. DOI: 10.1093/jhered/93.6.456.

Schaeffer, L.R. (1994) Multiple-country comparison of dairy sires. *Journal of Dairy Science* 77, 2671–2678. DOI: 10.3168/jds.S0022-0302(94)77209-X.

Schneeberger, M., Barwick, S.A., Crow, G.H. and Hammond, K. (1992) Economic indices using breeding values predicted by BLUP. *Journal of Animal Breeding and Genetics* 109, 180–187. DOI: 10.1111/j.1439-0388.1992.tb00395.x.

SelAction (2019) Available at: https://www.wur.nl/en/Research-Results/Chair-groups/Animal-Sciences/Animal-Breeding-and-Genomics-Group/Research/Software.htm (accessed 21 October 2019).

Sheep Genetics-LambPlan (2019) Available at: http://www.sheepgenetics.org.au/Breeding-services/LAMBPLAN-Home (accessed 21 October 2019).

Sheep Improvement Limited (2019) Available at: https://www.sil.co.nz/ (accessed 21 October 2019).

Signet (2019) Signet Breeding Services. Available at: http://www.signetfbc.co.uk/ (accessed 10 August 2019).

Simm, G. (1998) *Genetic Improvement of Cattle and Sheep*. CAB International, Wallingford, UK.

Simm, G., Young, M.J. and Beatson, P.R. (1987) An economic selection index for lean meat production in New Zealand sheep. *Animal Production* 45, 465–475. DOI: 10.1017/S0003356100002956.

Sullivan, P.G. (2016) Defining a Parameter Space for GMACE. *Interbull Bulletin* 50, 85–93.

VanRaden, P.M. (2008) Efficient methods to compute genomic predictions. *Journal of Dairy Science* 91, 4414–4423. DOI: 10.3168/jds.2007-0980.

VanRaden, P.M., Van Tassell, C.P., Wiggans, G.R.., Sonstegart, T.S, Schnabel, R.D. *et al.* (2009) Invited Review. Reliability of genomic predictions for north American Holstein bulls. *Journal of Dairy Science* 92, 16–24. DOI: 10.3168/jds.2008-1514.

Van Vleck, L.D., Pollak, E.J. and Oltenacu, E.A.B. (1987) *Genetics for the Animal Sciences*. W.H. Freeman and Company, New York.

Weller, J.I. (1994) *Economic Aspects of Animal Breeding*. Chapman and Hall, London.

Wiggans, G.R., Cole, J.B., Hubbard, S.M. and Sonstegard, T.S. (2017) Genomic selection in dairy cattle: The USDA experience. *Annual Review of Animal Biosciences* 5, 309–322. DOI: https://doi.org/10.1146/annurev-animal-021815-111422.

Wilmink, J.B.M. (1987) Adjustment of test day milk, fat and protein yield for age, season and stage of lactation. *Livestock Production Science* 16, 335–348. DOI: 10.1016/0301-6226(87)90003-0.

Wray, N.R. (1991) The estimation of genetic merit. Summaries of papers, British Society of Animal Production, Winter Meeting, March 1991, paper no. 32.

Wray, N.R. and Simm, G. (1991) *BLUP for Pedigree Beef and Sheep Breeders*. SAC Technical Note T265. The Scottish Agricultural College, Perth, UK.

Wray, N.R., Simm, G., Thompson, R. and Bryan, J. (1991) Application of BLUP in beef breeding programmes. *British Cattle Breeders' Club Digest* 46, 29–39.

Recommended Reading

Banos, G. (1994) International genetic evaluation of dairy cattle. *Proceedings of the 5th World Congress on Genetics Applied to Livestock Production* 17, pp. 3–10. Available at: http://www.wcgalp.org/proceedings/1994 (accessed 16 June 2020).

Cameron, N.D. (1997) *Selection Indices and Prediction of Genetic Merit in Animal Breeding*. CAB International, Wallingford, UK.

Falconer, D.S. and Mackay, T.F.C. (1996) *Introduction to Quantitative Genetics*, 4th edn. Longman, Harlow, UK.

Harris, D.L. and Newman, S. (1994) Breeding for profit: synergism between genetic improvement and livestock production (a review). *Journal of Animal Science* 72, 2178–2200. DOI: 10.2527/1994.7282178x.

Hazel, L.N. (1943) The genetic basis for constructing selection indexes. *Genetics* 28, 476–490. Available at: https://www.genetics.org/content/28/6/476 (accessed 3 September 2020).

Hill, W.G. and Mackay, T.F.C. (Eds). (1989) *Evolution and Animal Breeding. Reviews on Molecular and Quantitative Approaches in Honour of Alan Robertson*. CAB International, Wallingford, UK.

INTERBULL Bulletins. International Bull Evaluation Service, Department of Animal Breeding and Genetics, Uppsala, Sweden.

Mrode, R.A. (2014) *Linear Models for the Prediction of Animal Breeding Values*, 3rd edn. CAB International, Wallingford, UK.

Nicholas, F.W. (1987) *Veterinary Genetics*. Oxford University Press, Oxford.
Nicholas, F.W. (2010) *Introduction to Veterinary Genetics*, 3rd edn, Wiley-Blackwell, UK.
Proceedings of the World Congresses on Genetics Applied to Livestock Production. (Especially volumes covering prediction of breeding values, estimation of genetic parameters, computing strategies and software. Available at: http://www.wcgalp.org/ (accessed 16 June 2020).
VanRaden, P.M. and Wiggans, G.R. (1991) Derivation, calculation and use of national animal model information. *Journal of Dairy Science* 74, 2737–2746. Available at: https://www.journalofdairyscience.org/article/S0022-0302(91)78453-1/pdf (accessed 3 September 2020).
Van Vleck, L.D., Pollak, E.J. and Oltenacu, E.A.B. (1987) *Genetics for the Animal Sciences*. W.H. Freeman and Company, New York.
Weller, J.I. (1994) *Economic Aspects of Animal Breeding*. Chapman and Hall, London.

8 Dairy Cattle Breeding

Introduction

The first seven chapters in this book concentrated on the scientific principles of genetic improvement. The aim of the next six chapters is to give some more details of the current and possible future applications of these principles in practical cattle, sheep, goat, poultry, pig and fish breeding. Chapters 8 to 12 follow a similar format. (Chapter 13 has a slightly modified format because of the wide range of species involved in aquaculture.) They begin by examining breeding goals in a general way, to identify animal characteristics likely to be important in genetic improvement programmes. Next, they examine breeds and crosses in widespread use, and methods of selection within breeds, including systems of testing, traits recorded and methods of genetic evaluation. Finally, each chapter has a section on the evidence for genetic improvement and its value, and a list of practical guidelines on selection. We start with dairy cattle breeding as there is probably more information in the public domain about dairy cattle breeding than about any other farmed species, so this is a good starting point to illustrate the principles of genetic improvement in practice.

Most of the examples of dairy cattle breeding discussed in this chapter are from the UK, elsewhere in Europe, New Zealand, Canada and the USA. However, they are intended to illustrate issues of wide relevance in dairy cattle breeding, at least in temperate areas. To show the context into which production in these countries fits, Fig. 8.1 shows the world production of cow milk by continent in 2016. Europe had the highest production, accounting for about 33% of global milk production. Figure 8.2 shows the amount of milk produced in 2016 by the 15 highest-producing countries in the world. The US was by far the largest producer, but The Russian Federation, India, several European countries, New Zealand and Australia featured in the top 15.

Breeding Goals

In broad terms, the breeding goal of most livestock producers is to increase the profitability of their animals. Many breeders and producers would add that this should be achieved without detriment to the animals' health and welfare, or the environment. While there may be broad agreement on this aim, there is often less agreement on what the main animal characteristics affecting profitability are in particular systems, and how to improve them most effectively. Milk production traits have obviously been the focus of attention in dairy cattle since organized breeding programmes began around a century ago. Indicators of health and welfare have received much attention over the past few decades, and indicators of environmental impact are now being studied intensively. Figure 8.3 shows the main sources of returns and the main variable costs in relatively high input and relatively low-input dairying systems in Britain (SRUC, 2018). While these figures do not tell the whole story as far as profitability is concerned, they do highlight some of the key animal characteristics that influence it. Also, although the absolute values of the different inputs and outputs shown varies between countries, there is greater similarity in their relative importance. For example, both milk prices and production costs will be substantially lower in countries such as New Zealand selling at world market prices, and with predominantly pastoral production (see Fig. 8.4). The results show that:

- returns from milk production are by far the most important returns, and are of similar relative importance in both high- and low-input systems;
- returns from the sale of calves and cull cows are relatively low in both systems, but slightly more important in low- than in high-input systems;

Genetic Improvement of Farmed Animals (G. Simm *et al.*)
DOI: 10.1079/9781789241723.0008

- feed costs are by far the most important variable costs in both high- and low-input systems, although the relative importance of concentrate versus forage costs differs substantially between systems; and
- veterinary costs account for a relatively low proportion of the variable costs, although there are other hidden associated costs, such as lost production due to disease itself, or due to milk withdrawal, e.g. following antibiotic treatment.

For most of the last few decades, yield of milk has been the main objective criterion for selecting between and within dairy breeds in most temperate countries. Figure 8.5 shows the approximate change in yield per cow in Britain over the last 70 years or so. By the 1920s and 1930s, yield per cow was about double that produced by a beef cow suckling a calf. The current average yield is over eightfold higher than this. These changes have been brought about by a combination of selection, both between and within breeds, and improved feeding, health and management. Separating the contributions of breeding and management to changes in

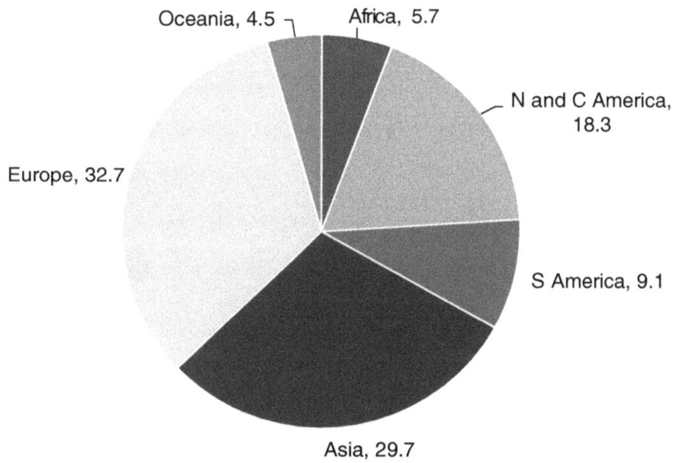

Fig. 8.1. Proportion of world cow milk production by continent in 2016 (%). (After FAO, 2019.)

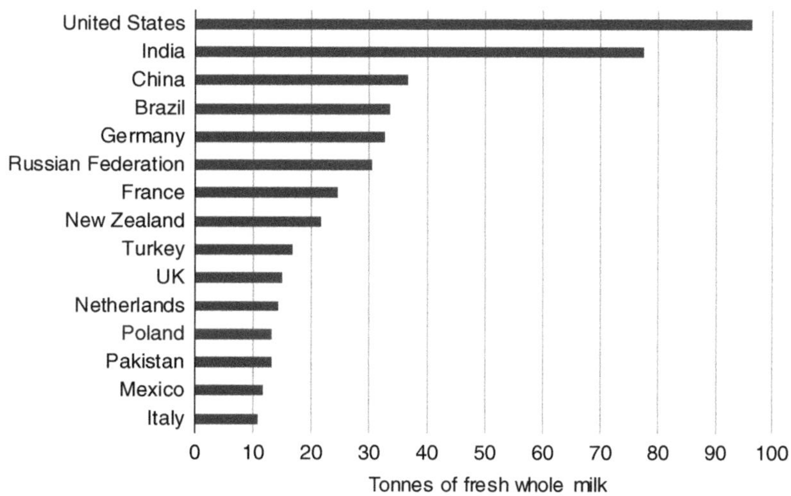

Fig. 8.2. Production of cow milk by the 15 highest-producing countries in the world in 2016. (After FAO, 2019.)

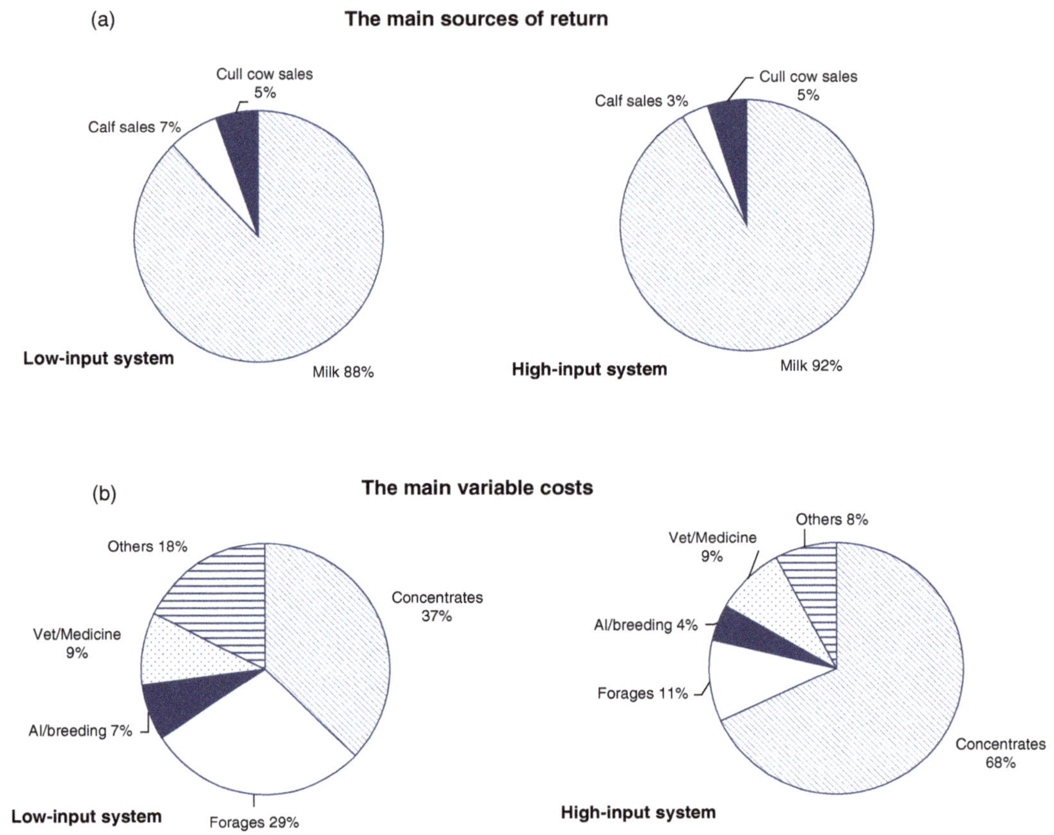

Fig. 8.3. The main sources of return in relatively low-input and relatively high-input dairy systems in Britain. The (a) returns and (b) costs are based on a low-input system with spring calving, an average yield of 5000 litres of milk per cow per annum and 750 kg of concentrates fed per cow per annum, and a higher-input system with an average yield of 10,000 litres milk per cow per annum and 4000 kg concentrates fed per cow per annum. An annual share of heifer replacement costs (about £153 for the low-input system and £459 for the high-input systems) would normally be deducted from the returns (SRUC, 2018).

production is difficult, especially over this time span. Some examples of attempts to do so over shorter periods of time are given later in the chapter.

Although milk yield is clearly a major component of profitability, the emphasis it has received is also due to the ease of measurement compared to some of the other components of profitability. In the 1980s, questions began to be raised over the relevance of continued selection for higher yields, on at least three counts. The first was the increased emphasis in payment schemes in many countries on the composition of the milk. The second was the introduction of milk quotas in some countries as a means of controlling national production, and hence limiting the cost of support. (For example, quotas were introduced throughout the European Union (EU) in 1984 but were abolished in 2015.) The third was the actual or perceived deleterious effect of selection for yield on the health, fertility and welfare of cows. These factors, in addition to other technological developments, began to influence the emphasis on milk yield relative to milk components, and traits related to health, fertility and welfare, in the subsequent decades. The details of these developments are discussed later in the chapter.

The trend for payment schemes to attach more value to milk composition began with schemes which paid premia for high milk fat or total milk solids content, or deducted penalties for low fat or solids content. Later, premia and penalties were

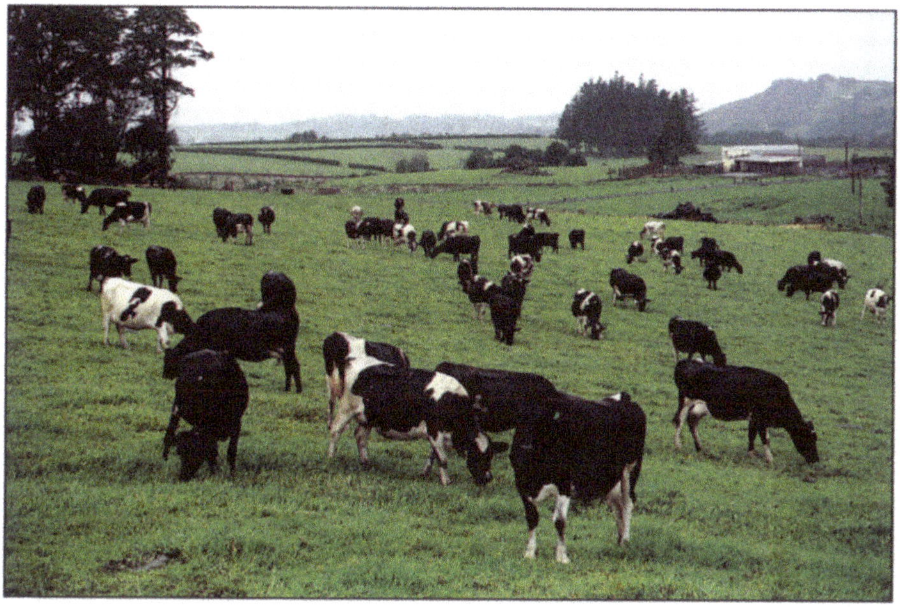

Fig. 8.4. Holstein Friesian cows grazing in Northland, New Zealand. The NZ climate allows low-cost production of milk – entirely from grass in the majority of herds, until recently.

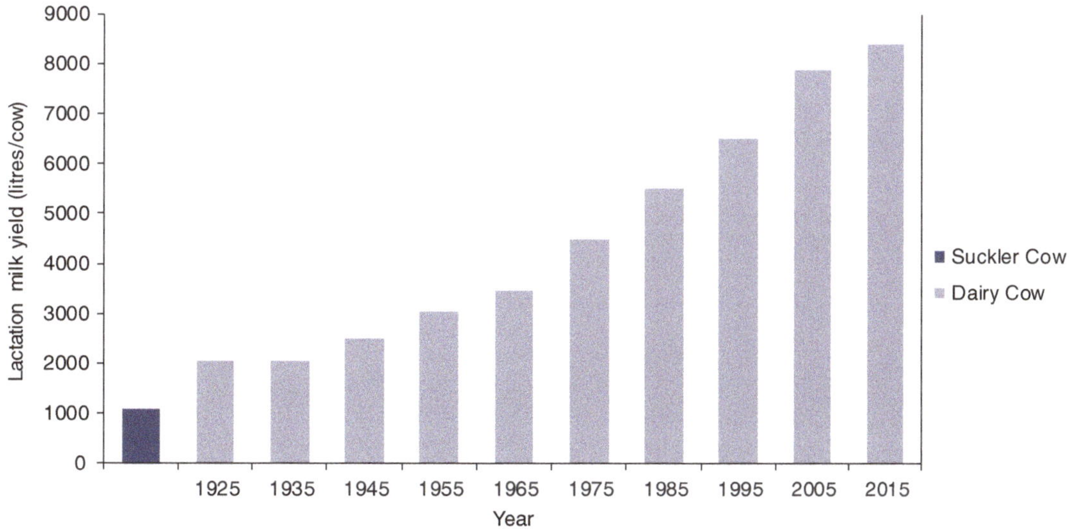

Fig. 8.5. Changes in approximate average yield per cow in Britain since the 1920s, compared to the estimated yield of a beef cow suckling a calf. These changes have been brought about by a combination of selection, both between and within breeds, and improved feeding, health and management (after Simm, 1998; Edinburgh Genetic Evaluation Services (EGENES), Scotland's Rural College).

attached to solids-not-fat (SNF) content, and then directly to protein content. More recently there has been a steady increase in the importance of milk protein relative to milk fat in most countries, due to stronger market demand, and its effect on milk processing properties (Miglior *et al.* 2017). For instance, the relative weight on protein to fat in the national selection index in the UK (Profitable Lifetime Index or £PLI) was 1.5:1 in 1985 but it is 2:1 at the time of writing.

The progressive increase in emphasis on milk solids, especially protein, in milk payment schemes since the 1990s has fuelled the debate on the merits of selection for breeds and individuals with high yields of milk. There is still, however, a huge market for liquid milk (as opposed to milk destined for processing into butter, cheese, milk powder and other dairy products) in many European countries. In 2014/2015 about 48.2% of the raw milk produced in the UK went into the liquid milk market. In a review of 28 major dairy production countries at a similar time, liquid milk accounted for 56.1% of dairy milk production (AHDB, 2015). In general, buyers specializing in liquid milk sales tended to put less emphasis on milk composition than those specializing in processed dairy products. Theoretically it may be argued that this sort of divergence in payment schemes may justify separate breeding goals for producers selling into different markets. However, in practice, the strong genetic association between total milk yield and yield of protein or fat has made separate goals unnecessary, as evidenced by the national breeding objectives of most countries.

In spite of the changes in the selection indexes of many countries, there is still a substantial emphasis placed on milk production traits. One of the reasons is that several studies have shown that the highest-yielding breeds and individuals are generally the most efficient converters of feed energy to milk energy (Bryant *et al.*, 1985; Simm, *et al.*, 1994). More recently, Ledinek *et al.* (2019) evaluated several breeds for the relationship between different efficiency traits, production traits and body condition score. The results from their study are presented in Table 8.1. They concluded that high-yielding breeds (e.g. Holstein Friesian) did not only have higher feed intake but were more efficient in partitioning nutrients to milk production than to body reserves, resulting in the loss of body weight and condition score. However, some earlier studies have indicated that the Jersey breed appears to be an exception to this rule, having a higher efficiency than expected for its yield – this may be due to a higher yield and intake per unit of body size than in other breeds (Oldenbroek, 1986).

Traditionally, the sale of calves for beef production has been seen as an important by-product from many European dairy industries. In several European countries dairy bulls entering progeny tests for milk production are performance tested first for beef characteristics. In Britain, Ireland and a few other countries, there is a further integration of the dairy and beef industries because of the

Table 8.1. Least squares means for milk production data, predicted dry-matter intake, energy balance and efficiency parameters for different breeds in Austria over a period of one year (Ledinek *et al.*, 2019)

	Breed			
Trait	Fleckvieh	Fleckvieh × Red Holstein (25%)	Holstein Friesian	Brown Swiss
Number of performance records	9,942	2,365	6,172	9,286
Milk (kg/day)	26.30[c]	27.00[b]	29.50[a]	26.40[bc]
Fat (%)	4.21[b]	4.28[ab]	4.09[d]	4.13[cd]
Protein (%)	3.53[b]	3.55[ab]	3.35[d]	3.49[bc]
Body condition score (1–5)	3.42[a]	3.24[b]	2.61[c]	2.88[d]
Dry matter (DM) intake (kg DM/day)	19.72[c]	20.24[b]	20.86[a]	19.84[c]
Energy intake (MJ NEL/day)	129.10[c]	132.60[b]	137.40[a]	130.30[bc]
Energy requirement (MJ NEL/day)	130.40[b]	133.80[a]	135.50[a]	126.30[c]
Feed efficiency (kg ECM/kg DMI)	1.333[bc]	1.349[b]	1.381[a]	1.319[c]
Energy efficiency (MJ LE/MJ NEL)	0.654[bc]	0.661[b]	0.674[a]	0.645[c]

[a–d]Least squares means within a row with different superscripts differ significantly ($P < 0.05$)

NEL, net energy for lactation; ECM, energy corrected milk; DMI, dry matter intake; LE, energy in milk.

widespread use of beef × dairy suckler cows. This has led to much debate on the merits of breeding for dual purpose versus more specialized dairy cows. This debate intensified following the influx of specialized North American Holstein strains of black-and-white cattle, with comparatively poor beef characteristics, to most European countries in the 1970s and 80s. The results in Table 8.1 and those from experimental studies comparing the profitability of dual purpose versus specialized dairy strains of black-and-white cattle show that, in most circumstances, specialized dairy strains are the most profitable. Consequently, most European and other temperate dairy industries are generally following a path of increased specialization. In this case, the returns from surplus calves will usually be maximized by mating those cows not required to breed replacements to beef bulls. Good fertility and, where appropriate, a compact calving period both help to maximize the number of cows available for mating to a beef bull, and so help to maximize returns from the sale of beef-cross calves. The growing use of sexed semen in many temperate countries is resulting in fewer matings being required to breed replacement dairy heifers. Advances in these techniques, and in cost effective methods of sexing and transferring embryos, could result in additional opportunities to increase returns from sale of beef-cross calves, or pure beef calves. Similarly, the choice of beef breed for mating to surplus dairy cows, and the choice of sire within beef breeds, both have an important influence on profitability. These issues, together with selection for beef traits in dairy or dual-purpose breeds, are discussed further in Chapter 9.

Figure 8.3(b) shows the importance of feed costs, or at least feed costs relative to milk value, in determining profitability. Because of the difficulty of measuring intake, and the evidence that higher-yielding breeds and individuals are more efficient converters of feed energy to milk energy, most dairy cattle breeding schemes have not considered feed intake or efficiency directly as part of the breeding goal until recently. Also, philosophical (but important) arguments over whether yield 'drives' intake, or intake drives yield, and on the importance of maintaining the capacity for high roughage intake in ruminants, make it difficult to know whether breeding programmes should aim to increase or decrease feed intake. Some of these issues are beginning to be addressed in dairy cattle breeding programmes and are discussed in greater detail later in this chapter.

Direct health costs appear to be relatively minor components of profitability from Fig. 8.3(b). However, the indirect costs through lost production, and the fact that there are animal welfare implications of disease, suggest that genetically improving health deserves greater emphasis than a superficial economic analysis might suggest. Similarly, the direct costs associated with reproduction appear relatively low, but there are indirect costs here too. There is evidence of a genetic decline in some aspects of health and reproduction as a result of selection for yield (Philipsson, 1981; Emanuelson, 1988). This has prompted work to reduce or redress changes in health and reproductive performance as a result of selecting for yield in many dairying countries. This has resulted in the development of broader national selection indexes that include performance and other traits related to health and reproduction. This is discussed further later in the chapter. While the evidence of the higher gross efficiency of higher-yielding breeds and higher-yielding animals within breeds is strong, the need to develop more comprehensive breeding goals for dairy cattle has become even more apparent in the last few decades. Most of the animal characteristics discussed above now feature, either directly or indirectly, in many dairy cattle breeding programmes in temperate countries.

Table 8.2, adapted from Miglior *et al.* (2017), presents the timeline for research and incorporation of these various traits in the breeding goals for dairy cattle. Some of the approaches involved, such as the introduction of national genetic evaluations for a wider range of traits and the development of multi-trait selection indexes for dairy cattle, are discussed in more detail later in this chapter.

Breeds and Crosses Used in Dairying

Figure 8.6 shows the proportion of different breeds and crosses which make up the national dairy cattle populations in several major dairying countries. These charts illustrate that: (i) black-and-white strains predominate; and (ii) there is little use of systematic crossbreeding in most temperate systems, except in New Zealand and to a lesser extent in Australia (see Fig. 8.7). However, compared with equivalent figures in Simm (1998), there is an increasing trend towards cross breeding, partly to address reduced fertility due to intensive selection for milk yield in the Holstein Friesian.

Designed breed comparisons in many countries, together with the results of commercial semen

Table 8.2. Major milestones in the study of traits and introduction of indexes in genetic selection of dairy cattle. (Adapted from Miglior *et al.*, 2017.)

Date	Milestone	Reference
1920	Breeding decisions are mainly based on milk and fat yields from milk testing programmes along with consideration of conformation	Copeland (1927)
1930	Classification programmes are instituted by breed associations	Copeland (1937)
1943	Selection index approach is used for simultaneous selection of multiple traits	Hazel (1943)
1950	Interest increases in the SNF portion of milk due to proposed changes to milk pricing strategies	Johnson (1957)
1970	Fertility and health traits are evaluated in Nordic countries	Philipsson and Lindhé (2003)
1970	Calving traits are introduced	Pollak and Freeman (1976)
1970	Milk protein contents measured in milk-recording programmes and genetic evaluations are available	Shook (2006)
1980	Somatic cell counts are used in selection for udder health indices	Coffey *et al.* (1986)
1990	Workability and longevity traits are added to national genetic evaluations	Meyer and Burnside (1987)
2000	Fertility traits are considered by many non-Nordic countries	Miglior *et al.* (2005)
2010s	Health trait evaluations using producer-recorded health data and their indicators are initiated in several non-Nordic countries	Pryce *et al.* (2016)
	Novel traits (including feed efficiency, milk coagulation properties, milk fatty acid contents, hoof health, and automatic milking systems) are implemented by different countries	Malchiodi *et al.* (2017)

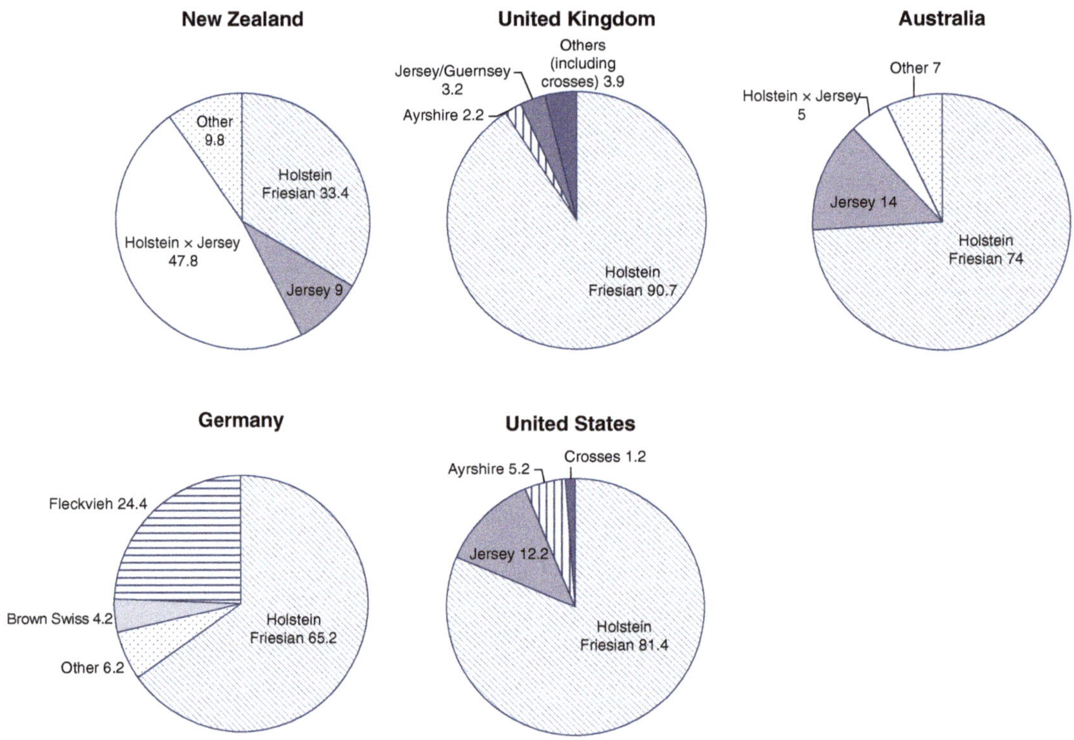

Fig. 8.6. The proportion of different breeds and crosses which make up the dairy cattle populations of some major dairying countries. (After Bundesverband Rind und Schwein, 2018; Datagene, 2018; New Zealand Dairy Statistics, 2018; EGENES, 2019; Guinan *et al.*, 2019).

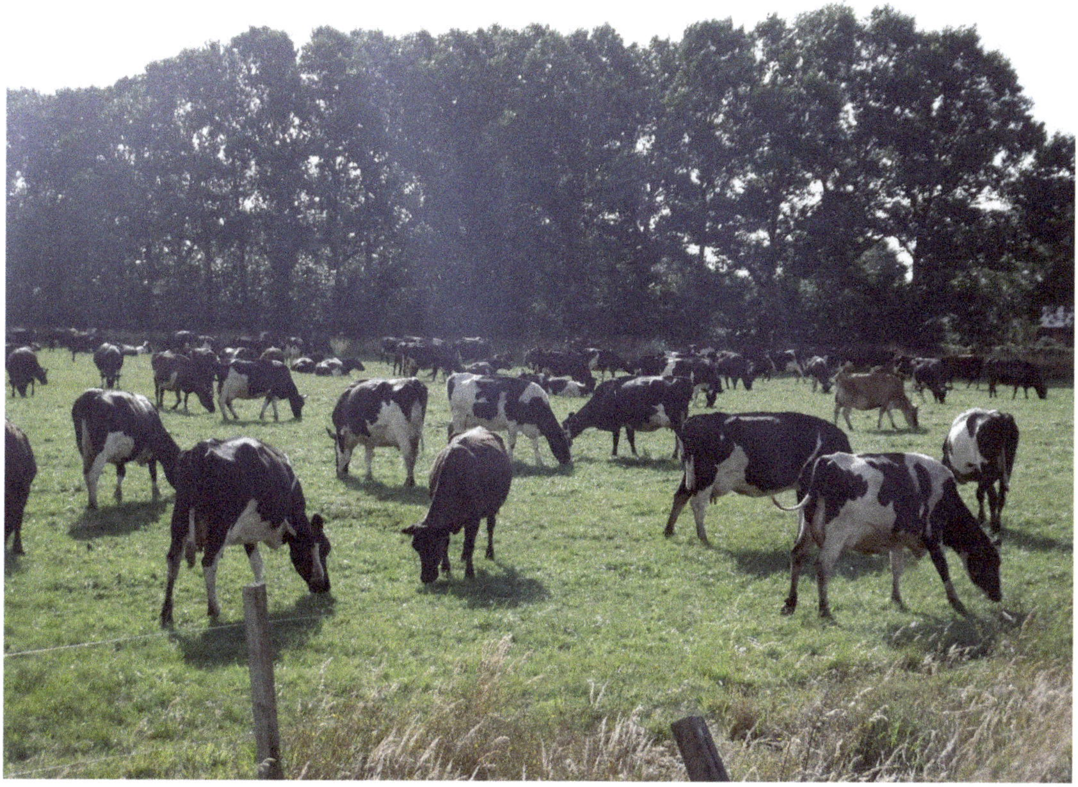

Fig. 8.7. Holstein Friesian, Jersey and crossbred cows in Waikato, New Zealand. The New Zealand dairy industry is one of the few in temperate areas to make use of systematic crossbreeding. (Courtesy of Marie Haskell.)

importations, have demonstrated the higher total yield of milk and milk solids from North American black-and-white strains, compared to local black-and-white strains or other breeds (Jasiorowski *et al.*, 1983; Kakwaya and Peterson, 1991; Ledinek *et al.*, 2019). The average milk yields of different breeds from milk-recording schemes in the UK show the same trend (see Table 8.3). Although they do not conform to some of the rules recommended for proper breed comparisons in Chapter 3, such as comparing different breeds in the same environment, results from these recording schemes have the advantages of including more breeds, being based on more animals and being more up to date than most of the designed comparisons. The results in Table 8.3 also show that although Holstein Friesians have higher total milk and milk solids yield, they have lower compositional quality than several other breeds. Some of the tools developed to put appropriate emphasis on solids yield versus content, on protein versus fat, and on other components of profitability, are discussed later.

Table 8.3. Average annual milk yields of cows that calved in 2017 for different breeds in recorded herds in the UK. (Data courtesy of EGENES.)

Breed	Milk yield (kg)	Butterfat (%)	Protein (%)
Holstein Friesian	8394	4.00	3.23
Ayrshire	6011	4.18	3.33
Jersey	5487	5.25	3.77
Guernsey	5079	4.74	3.52
Dairy Shorthorn	5454	4.03	3.32
Brown Swiss	6493	4.12	3.42
Montbéliarde	6612	4.14	3.36
All breeds	6218	4.38	3.32

Figure 8.8 shows the trend in the proportion of Holstein genes over time in the population of

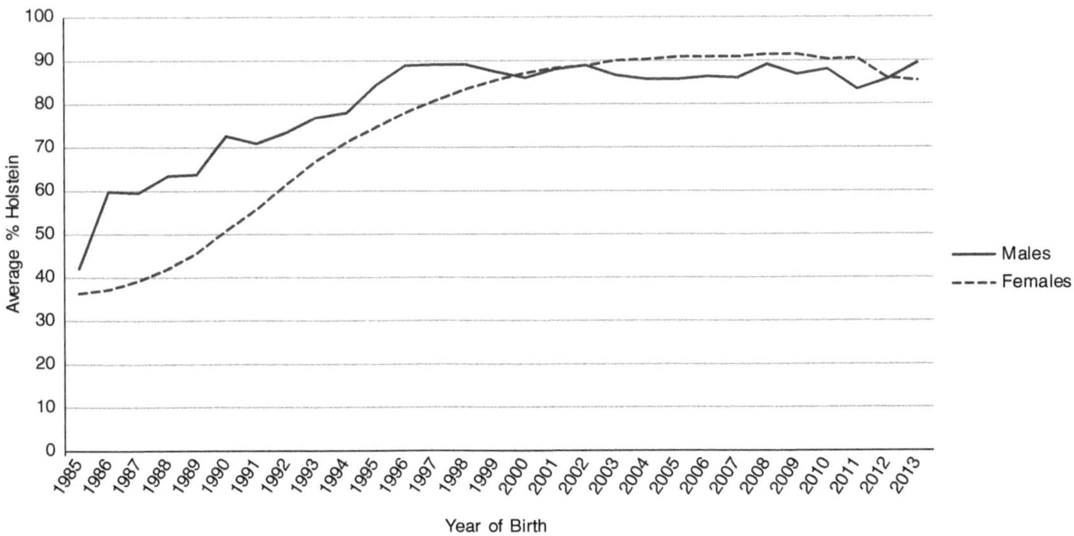

Fig. 8.8. Change in the proportion of Holstein genes in bulls and cows registered by Holstein UK (Holstein UK; EGENES).

black-and-white cows in the dairy national genetic evaluation systems in the UK. The proportion of Holstein genes seems to have stabilized at a high level of about 90% for cows and slightly lower for bulls in the last 10 years or so. The fact that breeding companies, breeders and producers are 'voting with their feet' by continuing to breed, test and select animals with a high proportion of Holstein genes probably provides further evidence of the validity of the results on the profitability of this strain compared to others, at least in relatively high-input, temperate systems. Because of its large global population size, there are more opportunities for selection for 'new' traits in this breed than in many other breeds with smaller populations, even for characteristics where the current mean performance may not be high.

The most appropriate measure of physical and economic performance of dairy herds depends on the most limiting resource in the herd concerned. While production per cow is a major component of profitability in higher-input dairying systems, production per hectare is usually more important in lower-input pastoral systems. The ranking of breeds on production per hectare is less clear than that on production per cow. There is evidence that some strains of Jersey have a higher or equal output per hectare to black-and-white strains, but choosing equivalent stocking rates to make fair comparisons is difficult (see Table 8.4). Table 8.5 shows some results of an early study on the various measures of the physical and economic performance of UK herds comprised of Holstein Friesian or Channel Island breeds recorded by the breeding company Genus. These data do not allow an unbiased comparison of breeds, since some breeds may be more prevalent in some management systems, but they do illustrate how rankings of breeds change, depending on the type of financial margin used to compare them (i.e. margin over purchased feed expressed per litre, per kg fat, per cow or per hectare). More recently, using data from a large farm in California, Kasbergen (2013) indicated that compared with the Holstein, Jersey cows were more economically efficient, generating more income per pound of milk, due to the higher milk components (average SNF % of 9.42% versus 8.78%), higher pregnancy rate, feed efficiency and higher income over feed cost of about 30%. The greater numerical importance of the Jersey breed in countries with mainly pastoral production is probably a result of greater emphasis on production per hectare than on production per cow. For example, in New Zealand, although the proportion of Jersey cows has declined, they still account for about 14% of the dairy cattle population.

Table 8.4. Production of Jersey and Friesian cows grazed at low- or high-stocking rates in New Zealand. (After Bryant, 1993; Holmes, 1995)

Breed	Jersey		Friesian	
Stocking rate (cows/ha)	3.57	4.53	3.02	3.98
Fat plus protein yield				
kg per cow	334	272	372	268
kg per ha	1192	1231	1121	1064
Days in milk	260	223	261	226

Table 8.5. Various measures of economic performance of Genus Milkminder herds in England and Wales, comprised of Holstein Friesian or Channel Island (Jersey and Guernsey) breeds, in 1995/1996. These data do not allow unbiased comparison of these breeds, since some breeds may be more prevalent in some management systems, but they do illustrate how rankings of breeds change, depending on the type of margin used to compare them. (After Genus, 1996)

Breed	Holstein Friesian	Channel Island
Yield per cow (l)	6253	4536
Yield from forage (l per cow)	2497	1442
Milk price (pence per l; ppl)	24.79	29.41
Concentrate used per l (kg)	0.27	0.34
Total concentrate per cow (kg)	1680	1529
Margin over purchased feed (MOPF) per l (ppl)	20.77	23.87
MOPF per kg fat (£)	4.94	4.49
MOPF per cow (£)	1298	1078
MOPF per hectare (£)	2829	2894

There is a similar explanation for the low use of crossbreeding in countries with higher-input systems. In these systems there appear to be no other breeds that consistently produce first crosses (F_1) which have higher yields than pure black-and-white animals. This is partly due to the advantage in additive genetic merit for milk and milk solids yield per cow seen in the black-and-white breeds, and partly due to the typically relatively low level of heterosis for production. In contrast, because of the greater similarity among breeds in production per hectare, crossbred dairy cows do appear to be competitive in pastoral systems. This advantage may be augmented by the fact that heterosis for live weight appears to be lower than that for yield (see Table 3.9). Crossbred cows benefit from higher yield due to heterosis, but show a proportionally lower increase in live weight, and hence in maintenance costs, due to heterosis. The growing awareness of the importance of health and fertility traits in dairy cattle breeding may lead to an increased interest in crossbreeding. Some of the new breeding technologies outlined below and in Chapter 5 may create opportunities for other breeds to compete more effectively with the Holstein Friesian in terms of additive genetic merit.

Crossbreeding is a major strategy for improving productivity in sub-tropical and tropical regions, with crosses between improved exotic taurine breeds and tropically adapted breeds often being particularly valuable (see Fig. 3.3). In Brazil, for example, one of the major dairy cattle breeds is a composite, the Girolando, created by crossing the Holstein and *Bos indicus* Gyr breeds, the latter originally from India. The Girolando was formed with breed contributions of 5/8 Holstein and 3/8 Gyr. The first progeny test was performed in 1997 and at the time of writing, about 13 genetic evaluations have been performed (see Silva *et al.*, 2012, 2017). In Ethiopia and Tanzania, the African Dairy Genetics Gains Project (2019) funded by the Bill and Melinda Gates Foundation supports genomic evaluation of crossbred bulls for use in artificial insemination and natural mating.

Selection Within Breeds

Systems of testing

Progeny testing schemes

One of the fundamental problems in dairy cattle breeding is that most of the traits of interest are expressed only in females. But because fewer males than females are needed in livestock breeding, the scope for genetic improvement is greatest through selection of males, especially when artificial insemination (AI) is used. As outlined in Chapter 5, it was the uptake of AI in the mid-1900s that provided both the stimulus and the means for improved methods of genetic improvement of dairy cattle. The progeny testing schemes which evolved then have been central to the genetic improvement of dairy cattle in most countries for over 50 years. Recent developments in genomic selection have begun to reduce the importance of progeny testing. However, a detailed description of progeny testing is presented below, because of its pivotal historical rôle, before examining the impact of genomic approaches.

HOW PROGENY TESTING WORKS The basis of progeny testing schemes is the comparison of the milk production of the daughters of young bulls being tested with the daughters of other bulls recorded in the same herd, year and season (see Fig. 8.9). Results are then combined across herds, years and seasons and used to predict the genetic merit of the bulls being tested, and of other animals in the recorded population. The procedures involved were introduced in Chapter 7 and they are expanded on later in this section.

Dairy cattle progeny-testing schemes in most countries share the following features, which are illustrated in Fig. 8.10:

- The identification of young bulls of high predicted genetic merit, for progeny testing. Often young bulls are bred specifically for progeny testing by contract matings between the top cows available and the best available AI bulls. These matings are arranged by the breeding organizations (e.g. milk boards, farmer co-operatives and breeding companies) or individual breeders engaged in progeny testing. The increased global trade in semen, embryos and animals, from the 1980s onwards, highlighted differences between countries in the genetic merit of dairy cattle. In particular, this period saw a dramatic influx of semen from black-and-white dairy strains from the US and Canada to many other temperate dairying countries that had made lower genetic gains in milk production traits in the preceding decades. As a result, the importance of contract matings to homebred cows declined in countries which were not near the top of the 'international league table' of genetic merit. In these countries, many of the agencies involved in progeny testing obtained young bulls either by arranging contract matings abroad and importing the resulting embryos or offspring, or they identified high predicted merit young bulls or embryos already available. However, the principle is exactly the same. Prior to the widespread use of genomic selection, pedigree indexes were widely used to identify young bulls of interest, and to monitor their predicted merit at various stages throughout testing. (Following the implementation of genomic selection in most major dairy industries, genomic breeding values are now used for the selection of young bulls at about two years of age. Selected bulls are then used widely via AI at this stage. Genomic breeding values may also be used to pre-select young

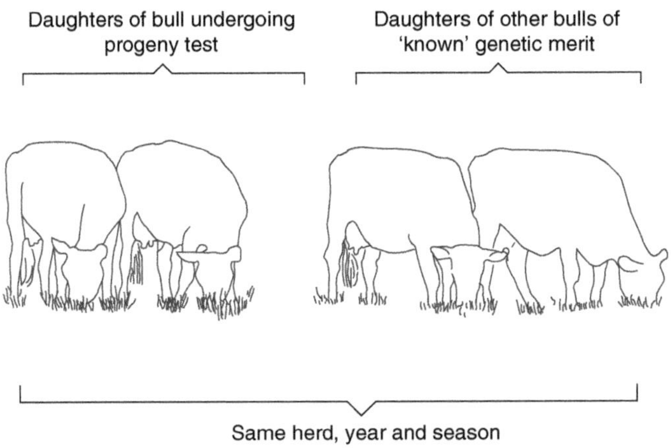

Fig. 8.9. The basis of progeny testing schemes is the comparison of the milk production of the daughters of young bulls being tested, with the daughters of other bulls recorded in the same herd, year and season.

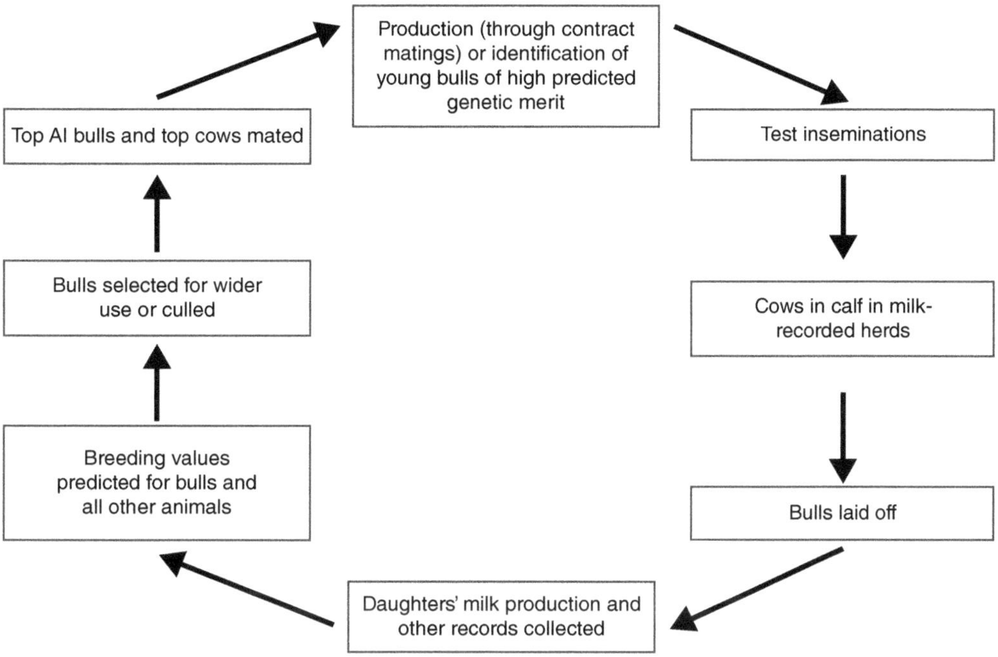

Fig. 8.10. The main features of progeny testing programmes for dairy bulls.

bulls for progeny testing, but this is becoming rarer. A high proportion of bulls used in AI are now young bulls evaluated through genomic prediction. Eventually, these young bulls get progeny test results themselves. The degree of correspondence between the initial genomic predictions and later progeny test results is discussed later.)

- Cows in milk-recorded herds are inseminated with semen from young bulls being progeny tested. The herds used for progeny testing by most of the larger agencies are commercial dairy herds, but they are expected to have high standards of recording, and to treat their animals uniformly. They are contracted to rear, milk and record female calves resulting from these test inseminations alongside the daughters of other bulls used in their herds. One of the criticisms of some smaller progeny testing schemes, or syndicates, was that they are open to bias through the preferential treatment of the daughters of particular bulls. Even with the most modern methods of evaluation, these problems are difficult to overcome, although any initial bias is usually 'diluted' later when records from more daughters in other herds get included in the evaluation of the bull. If the information is available, checking the number of herds in which the bull was tested, and the distribution of his daughters across these herds, helps to identify bulls at risk from this type of problem. (Picking bulls with a high reliability alone does not necessarily guard against this problem. The use of more sophisticated statistical methods in evaluation, described in the section on methods and results of genetic evaluation later, helps to reduce it.)
- At this point the young bulls are 'laid off', or temporarily retired, until their daughters' milk production and other records have been collected and their breeding values have been predicted. (In some countries larger quantities of semen were collected and frozen at the start of testing, and bulls were slaughtered before the results of the progeny test were known.)
- Milk production and other performance records on daughters are collated and the bulls' breeding values are predicted. In most countries breeding values are predicted for kg milk, kg fat, kg protein, % fat and % protein. Additionally, in most countries the appearance, conformation or type of a bull's daughters are scored, spanning a range

of characteristics including body size, the size, shape and placement of udders and teats, and the shape and angle of feet and legs. Type classification is done by either the progeny testing agency itself, or more commonly by a breed society. (Type traits are discussed in more detail in a later section.) Most testing agencies also score additional traits such as the fertility of the bull, the calving ease when his offspring are born, the presence of any genetic abnormalities among calves, and once daughters are milking, their temperament, speed of milking and other 'workability' traits. In some countries the incidence of common diseases is also recorded. Breeding values for production, type and some of the additional characteristics recorded are usually predicted by a national agency established for that purpose (e.g. Edinburgh Genetic Evaluation Services (EGENES, 2019) provides this service in the UK, funded by the Agriculture and Horticulture Development Board (AHDB, 2019a)), or by a breed society, university or government department. Bulls with high predicted breeding values for some combination of these recorded traits are retained for semen production, while those which fail to meet the desired standard are culled. Typically, less than 10% of bulls which enter progeny testing are retained as AI sires for wider use.

The number of bulls born from 2004 to 2007 that were progeny tested annually in some major dairying nations is shown in Table 8.6. Although numbers rose subsequently, the relatively low number of bulls tested annually in the UK in the 1970s and 1980s probably contributed to the low rates of genetic improvement made at that time. Limited initial semen imports in the 1980s and comparatively late access to the US market were also important factors. However, testing more bulls is only helpful if they are of high predicted genetic merit, and there are sufficient recorded cows available to ensure an accurate test. The increasing international trade in dairy cattle, semen and embryos in the 1980s and 1990s stimulated restructuring in many dairy cattle breeding industries worldwide, directed towards improving the merit of bulls entering tests, and increasing the speed and accuracy with which the tests were conducted. In the late 1980s in the UK, for example, this included the revamping of the Genus Sire Improvement Programme, several intranational and international agreements on co-operative progeny testing, and the launch of a new co-operative company, Cogent, which combined the formation of an elite nucleus herd with progeny testing in members' herds. The introduction of international genetic evaluations by INTERBULL meant that the genetic merit of many more bulls progeny tested in other countries could be compared reliably with locally tested bulls. This, followed by semen companies aggressively promoting progeny-tested bulls on the basis of their international evaluation results, resulted in countries with limited resources abandoning their own progeny testing of bulls. The advent of genomic selection has further exacerbated the situation and currently, there is no active progeny testing scheme operating in the UK in any dairy breeds. Figure 8.11 illustrates the increasing usage of genomically evaluated young bulls in the UK. About 70% of inseminations were carried out with semen from young bulls in 2019 compared with only 20% in 2013. Even in countries such as the USA, which progeny-tested large numbers of bulls prior to the genomic era, there has been a gradual drop in the number of inseminations from progeny-tested bulls. Figure 8.12 gives a breakdown of inseminations to various categories of bulls in the USA from 2011 to 2018. In the USA, the first genomic evaluations were published in 2009. Only about 1% of inseminations were from progeny-tested bulls in 2011–2012 and the proportion of inseminations to young genomic bulls rose to 67% by 2018. The pattern in Canada is similar (CDN, 2019). Thus, formal progeny schemes are gradually being phased out with the introduction of genomic selection. However, some breeding companies make a deliberate effort to collect data on low heritability traits such as

Table 8.6. Average number of Holstein Friesian AI bulls progeny tested annually in some major dairying nations. Only domestic bulls born in 2004-2007 with daughters in more than 20 herds are shown. (After V. Palucci, INTERBULL; personal communication.)

Country	Average number of Holstein Friesian AI bulls progeny tested annually
Canada	965
Denmark, Finland and Sweden	477
France	1812
Germany	3285
Italy	1236
Netherlands	245
UK	246
USA	1900

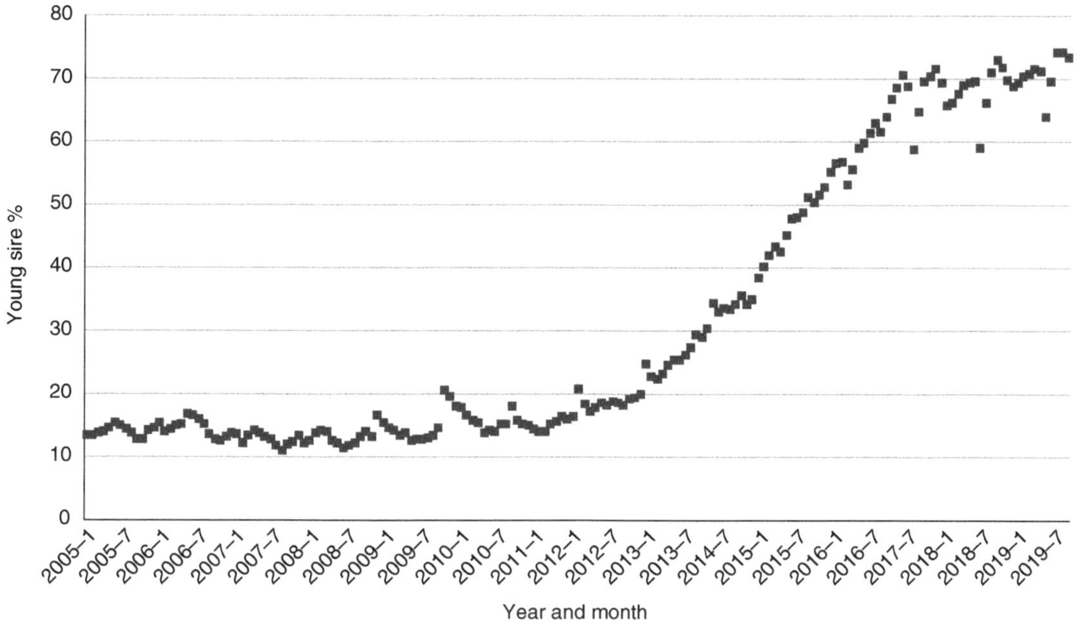

Fig. 8.11. The proportion of young genomically-tested bulls used in inseminations in the UK from 2005 to 2019.

fertility and calving performance on the daughters of the young bulls from the genomic program (Dr George Wiggans, personal communication).

It is worth noting that the number of bulls tested, and their merit, are not the only factors affecting rates of gain in national dairy cattle populations. The level of use of top bulls is another criterion which has a major effect on overall genetic gain. A study in the early 1980s clearly showed that most European countries, except Britain and Ireland, tested a high number of bulls relative to the size of their national dairy herds, but used the best ones on a fairly limited scale. In contrast, in the US and New Zealand proportionally fewer bulls were tested, but the best ones were much more widely used. This gave similar or even higher potential rates of gain than those possible in countries testing more bulls (Cunningham, 1983). The figures in Table 8.6 show a similar pattern to that reported in the early 1990s, in terms of number of bulls tested relative to the size of national dairy herds. However, top bulls are more widely used in Europe now than they were in the 1980s.

PATHWAYS OF GENETIC IMPROVEMENT WITH PROGENY TESTING In dairy cattle populations which depend on progeny testing for genetic improvement, progress can be attributed to four 'pathways' (Rendel and Robertson, 1950; Robertson and Rendel, 1950). These are the selection of: (i) bulls to breed bulls (BB) – that is, the selection of top AI bulls to sire the next generation of young bulls for progeny testing; (ii) cows to breed bulls (CB) – the selection of top cows to breed young bulls for testing; (iii) bulls to breed cows (BC) – the choice of bulls to breed cows in herds which contribute bulls for testing; and (iv) cows to breed cows (CC) – the choice of cows to breed replacement heifers in herds which contribute bulls for testing.

The contributions of these four pathways to overall genetic improvement in a dairy cattle population are potentially about 30%, 39%, 28% and 3%, respectively (Woolliams and Smith, 1988). In other words, about 70% of the progress made in a population is down to the choice of parents to breed the next generation of bulls for testing – decisions which are in the hands of the breeding companies, rather than individual breeders. Of the breeding options available to individual breeders, the choice of AI bull has the greatest impact by far. To allow for losses due to involuntary culling, and to allow for fluctuations in the sex ratio of calves born and

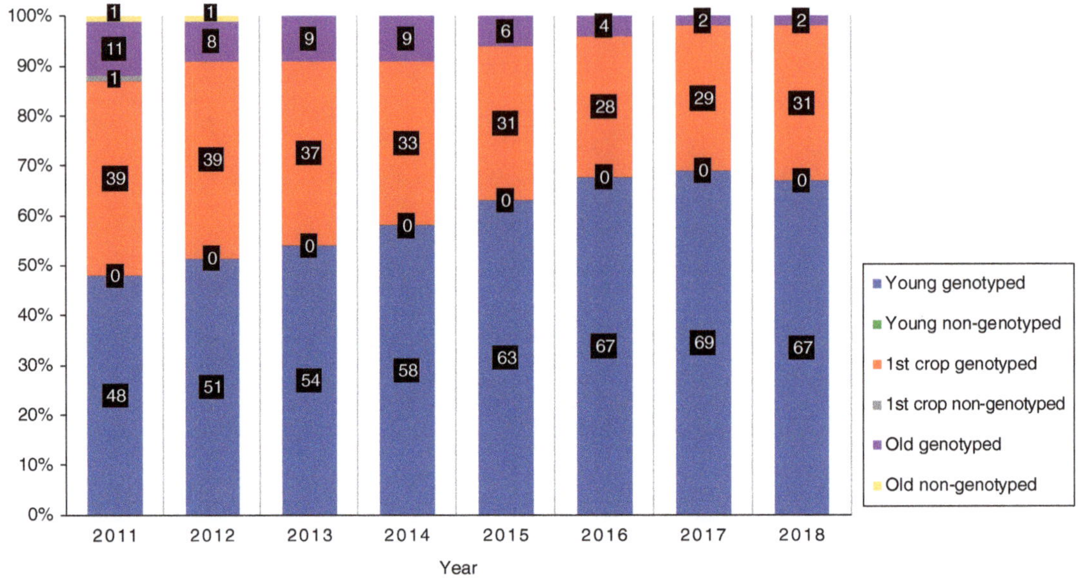

Fig. 8.12. The proportion of inseminations to various categories of bulls in the USA from 2011 to 2018. (After Wiggans, 2019.)

losses during rearing, often 60% of cows, or more, have to be selected as potential dams of replacement heifers, unless sexed semen is used. This gives little scope for selection among them on genetic merit. Prior to the availability of genomic evaluations, one of the few opportunities to practice selection among females arose if extra female calves were reared as potential replacements. In this case it was worth calculating a pedigree index for all female calves prior to selection and retaining those with high index scores. However, it is now possible to apply intense selection on 1-year-old heifers for use as bull dams, on the basis of genomic predicted breeding values. For example, this is practised in the Delta nucleus breeding scheme in the Netherlands (see later section on MOET schemes); 75% of young-bull dams are selected as one-year-old heifers and 25% are first-calved heifers.

García-Ruiz *et al.* (2016) reported the changes in generation interval and selection differential in the four pathways after the introduction of genomic selection in the USA. The generation intervals in the BB, BC, CB, and CC pathways up to 2009, prior to genomic evaluations, were 6.9, 6.9, 3.9 and 3.8 years, respectively. In 2015, 7 years after the introduction of genomic evaluations, the comparable values were 2.4, 5.0, 2.6, and 3.6 years, respectively. This change reflects a 37% reduction in generation interval since the introduction of genomic selection. Selection differentials were relatively stable, with some modest gains recently. The authors noted that Rendel and Robertson's (1950) model assumed a steady-state system where the flow of genetic gain is in equilibrium, and that genomic selection represents a major recent change in gene flow that has not had the opportunity to stabilize. They concluded that with the introduction of genomics the BB pathway appears to be the largest driver of genetic gain, followed by the CB path but with least changes occurring in the BC and CC paths.

Breeding practices in herds which do not contribute bulls for progeny testing (herds in the multiplier or commercial tiers described in Chapter 3) do not affect rates of genetic gain in national breeding schemes. However, widespread use of the top AI bulls in these herds, and efficient selection of replacement heifers, will reduce the genetic lag, or gap in genetic merit, between them and the elite or nucleus tier of herds contributing animals for progeny testing.

PROS AND CONS OF PROGENY TESTING The main advantage of progeny testing is that, providing sufficient daughters are recorded, it produces accurate predictions of a bull's genetic merit. Also, the results are based on the performance of daughters in commercial herds under management systems which are typical for the country concerned, and so they are of direct relevance to many other herds in that country (i.e. the risk of genotype-by-environment interactions is minimized). The disadvantages are that progeny testing schemes are costly to run, and the results take many years to materialize. For instance, most bulls will be about 1½ to 2 years old when the test inseminations are completed, 2½ to 3 years old when their daughters are born, and about 5½ to 6 years old by the time these daughters have completed their first lactations and evaluations have been produced. In many countries, genomic selection is now overcoming this limitation, as already illustrated, and described in greater detail in the next section.

Progeny testing also depends on access to a large population of milk-recorded cows. While most temperate dairying countries have sufficiently large populations of recorded black-and-white cows to run effective progeny testing schemes, it is difficult to sustain these in numerically small breeds. As a result, these breeds often have too few bulls tested, progeny test results of low accuracy, or both of these problems. In numerically small breeds these issues could probably be reduced by greater international co-operation on the identification and testing of young bulls of high predicted merit, if the breed concerned occurs in several countries. The use of alternative breeding schemes such as the nucleus schemes described below, and genomic selection, may also be helpful in these breeds.

Genomic selection

As mentioned above, one of the disadvantages of progeny testing is the long interval of about 5 or 6 years before the genetic merit of bulls can be estimated from their daughters' performance. Using genomic information and the methods described in Chapter 7, young bulls can have daughters at about 2 years of age, resulting in a substantial reduction in the generation interval.

The first step in genomic selection is to identify a group of bulls that have genotypes (single nucleotide polymorphisms, SNPs) as well as very reliable predictions of genetic merit for milk production and all the other traits of interest, as a result of having many performance-recorded daughters. The next step is to construct a set of equations that relate SNP information for this set of bulls with their daughters' average performance. Solving this set of equations provides the solutions for the SNPs which we call the SNP key. The set of bulls used to calculate the SNP key is referred to as the reference population. Their daughters' average performance can be approximated by subtracting from their predicted breeding values (PBVs), the average PBV of their parents and then dividing by the reliability of their PBVs. (This process is called 'de-regression' – essentially reversing the 'shrinking' that goes on to account for accuracy when calculating PBVs, as explained in Chapter 7, in order to get back to average daughter performance corrected for environmental effects.) For traits such as feed intake, which are difficult to measure, genetic evaluations may not be available, or they may have low reliability due to the limited data available. In such cases, the equations for the relationship between SNPs and performance may be calculated using both genotypes and performance records from cows. The performance records for these cows are initially adjusted for known environmental effects before being used to calculate the SNP key.

The next step is to determine the reliability of the SNP key calculated in the reference population when it is used to predict the genetic merit of other animals. This is carried out on data from another set of bulls, called the validation data set, that has both genotypes and PBVs for the trait of interest. Using the SNP key, the genetic merit of the bulls in the validation set is computed from their SNP genotypes. The reliability with which the genetic merit of these bulls in the validation set is calculated is the squared correlation between the computed genetic merit and their daughters' average performance. The higher the squared correlation, the better the reliability; for milk production traits, reliabilities of about 80% are considered adequate.

Once we are satisfied with the accuracy of the SNP key, the final step is using the SNP key to calculate the genetic merit (genomic breeding value) of young bulls or cows based only on their SNP genotype. This can be done as soon as DNA samples are available from animals (or embryos). This means that the generation interval can be shortened, as bulls can be used as soon as they reach sexual maturity. This is illustrated in Fig. 8.13 which shows timelines for conventional progeny testing and typical genomic selection schemes for dairy cattle. This has resulted in more rapid rates of genetic gain especially in dairy cattle in developed countries. In the USA and most other developed temperate dairy countries, the number of genomically evaluated young bulls used as active sires is currently higher than the number of progeny-tested bulls. In the USA, Hutchison *et al.* (2014) reported that young bulls accounted for

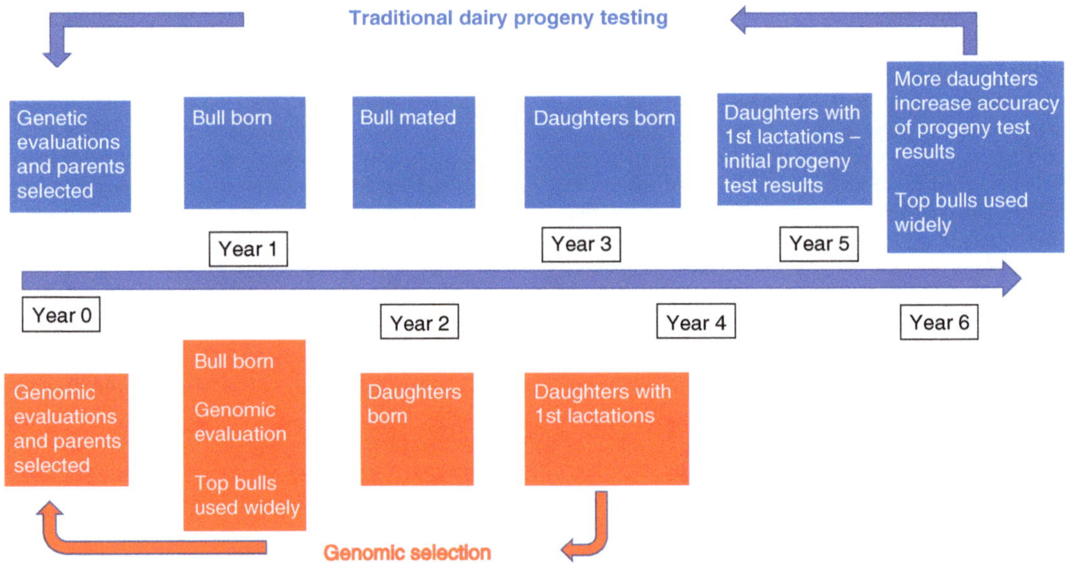

Fig. 8.13. A comparison of the timelines in traditional progeny testing and genomic selection schemes in dairy cattle. The red arrows show the shorter timeline achievable by genotyping bulls soon after birth.

28% and 25% of Holstein and Jersey inseminations in 2007, respectively. These percentages had increased to 51% and 52%, respectively, by 2012 due to the use of genomically evaluated young bulls. As illustrated earlier (see Fig. 8.11), there is increasing usage of genomically evaluated young bulls in the UK, with about 70% of inseminations from young bulls in 2019 compared with 20% in 2013.

In addition to shorter generation intervals, the reliability of genomic breeding values (GEBVs) for young bulls that have not had daughters is higher than that calculated from the parent average PBV. This higher reliability is because the equation for computing GEBVs is based on a large number of bulls with very highly reliable PBVs in most developed countries. This is particularly advantageous for traits of low heritability, such as fertility and calving ease, as high reliabilities can be obtained earlier in life compared to progeny testing.

The disadvantage of genomic selection is the cost of genotyping the animals. This is usually not a limitation to AI companies, as the overall cost of genomic selection is lower than the cost of running a progeny testing scheme. However, the cost of genotyping, which is currently about £50 and £100 per animal for the 50K and HD (600–700K) SNP chip, respectively, limits the widespread usage of genomic selection by individual farmers for the choice of replacement heifers, even in wealthier countries. To overcome this limitation, individual farmers tend to use SNP chips of lower density, varying from 3–20K, which are available at about £10–£20 per animal at the time of writing. For instance, in the UK genomic evaluations systems, about 22% of animals, (bulls and cows) are genotyped with low-density SNP chips of 3–20K. Usually the SNPs in these low-density SNP chips are a subset of those in the 50K or HD chips. Using imputation (see Chapter 5), an equivalent 50K data set can be created for these animals by filling in the missing SNPs using the information from the 50K genotypes, their parents and other relatives. The equivalent 50K genotypes created by imputation are usually about 90–99% as accurate as the genotypes produced by genotyping directly with the 50K chip (Druet *et al.*, 2010).

The reliability of genomic evaluations is influenced by the size of the reference population (see Chapter 7). In numerically small breeds, such as the Ayrshire, Jersey and Guernsey, the difficulty of securing enough animals for the reference population has limited the implementation of genomic selection. Hence, the accuracies or reliabilities reported have been very low. Using 197 genotyped bulls and

1440 genotyped cows, Jenko *et al.* (2016) reported an accuracy of 0.213 ±0.03 for milk yield using only bulls in the reference population, but this increased to 0.376 ±0.02 when cows were included. The accuracy they obtained from BLUP based on pedigree information only was 0.316 ±0.03, indicating very little gain in accuracy from GBLUP. In Canada, de Oliviera *et al.* (2018) reported average reliabilities of 0.46 from Single Step GBLUP (see Chapter 7) compared with 0.42 from BLUP parent average for milk production traits for the Jersey breed. Corresponding estimates for the Ayrshire were 0.57 from genomic prediction and 0.44 from BLUP parent average. To overcome the limitation of the small size of the reference population for the numerically small breeds, the use of multi-breed genomic selection has been investigated. This involves evaluating several small breeds together. However, the gains from this approach have been small and this approach is not implemented routinely yet. The European Brown Swiss Federation has adopted a different approach and initiated genomic selection with data pooled across several countries (Jorjani *et al.*, 2011). The phenotypes used for the genomic predictions are proofs from MACE evaluations for the breed. The project, developed at INTERBULL, called Intergenomics, involves Italy, Germany, Austria, Switzerland, France, Slovenia, USA and Canada. Jorjani *et al.* (2011) reported gains in reliability in the validation data set (young bulls) of 0.43–0.45 for protein yield compared to the average reliabilities calculated from the parent average. However, the gains for fertility were lower at about 0.19–0.32. At the time of writing, INTERBULL carries out three Intergenomics runs per year for the countries involved.

RELATIONSHIP BETWEEN GENOMIC BREEDING VALUES OF YOUNG BULLS AND THEIR SUBSEQUENT PROGENY TEST RESULTS One of the obvious questions arising from the widespread adoption of genomic selection is whether it really works. In other words, how does the GEBVs predicted for young bulls using only genomic information correspond with their genetic merit estimated from daughter records. In the UK, to answer this question, the GEBVs of 7745 young bulls calculated in the August 2014 evaluation run were correlated with their genetic merit calculated in August 2018, when performance data from daughters was included. This analysis was also restricted to a subset of the data consisting of 459 bulls with high reliabilities (average reliability of 0.95) in the August 2018 run, that had an increase of at least 25% in reliability. The correlation between GEBVs from the two runs ranged from 0.85–0.90 for production traits but was slightly lower at 0.80 for lifespan (Table 8.7). For the subset of 459 bulls which had more daughter information in the progeny test, this correlation was 0.80–0.85 for production traits and 0.75 for lifespan (Table 8.7). These results indicate good agreement between initial GEBVs predicted using only genomic data and later

Table 8.7. Changes in, and correlations between, predicted transmitting abilities (PTAs) of young bulls in the UK with genomic information (August 2014) and subsequent PTAs (August 2018) including daughter information. The table shows similar data for a subset of bulls with higher reliabilities. (After Marco Winters, AHDB, personal communication.)

	All bulls (n = 7745)			High reliability bulls (n = 459)		
Reliability and PTA	August 2018 average	Change from August 2014	Correlation	August 2018 average	Change from August 2014	Correlation
Reliability milk traits %	83	15		96	28	
PTA Milk kg	452	30	0.85	425	26	0.83
PTA Fat kg	15.0	−0.6	0.85	16.5	−0.6	0.80
PTA Protein kg	13.7	0.1	0.86	13.6	−0.3	0.81
PTA Fat %	−0.03	−0.02	0.90	0.00	−0.02	0.85
PTA Protein %	−0.01	−0.01	0.87	0.00	−0.01	0.85
Reliability SCC %	83	14		90	20	
PTA SCC	−11	0	0.83	−12	0	0.77
Reliability lifespan %	69	9		79	19	
PTA Lifespan	0.25	−0.01	0.80	0.25	0.00	0.75

progeny test results, demonstrating the accuracy of genomics.

Nucleus breeding schemes

THEORETICAL BENEFITS Before the advent of progeny testing one approach to the genetic improvement of dairy cows was the use of a central cow performance test station (e.g. in Denmark). Comparing the performance of animals under a single management and feeding system has many attractions, and various modifications to this approach have been proposed since. One proposal was the creation of a large nucleus herd for recording the daughters of high predicted merit young bulls (Hinks, 1978). The advantages suggested for this type of scheme, compared to progeny testing in commercial herds, include: (i) greater operational control – for example, it is easier to decide on aims and to control the timing and precision of measurements in a single herd than in a national programme; (ii) removing the risk of preferential treatment; (iii) higher accuracy of recording and selection; (iv) the opportunity to record and select on a wider range of traits than those recorded in progeny testing schemes based on commercial herds; and (v) smaller scale of operation resulting in reduced cost, and opportunities for use in situations where the infrastructure for recording or the population size prevent effective progeny testing schemes in commercial herds (Hinks, 1978; Nicholas and Smith, 1983). Wider interest in this type of scheme was generated by investigations on the use of multiple ovulation and embryo transfer (MOET) in dairy cattle breeding. As outlined in Chapter 5, MOET is a series of reproductive techniques including superovulation of a donor female (hormone treatment leading to higher numbers of ova being shed than usual), mating, recovery of the resulting embryos, and transfer of fresh or frozen embryos to recipient females. This permits elite females to leave many more progeny than they would be able to do by natural means.

In the late 1970s and the early 1980s, Drs Frank Nicholas and Charles Smith proposed a new rôle for MOET in nucleus breeding schemes, as an alternative to progeny testing (Nicholas, 1979; Nicholas and Smith, 1983). Their proposed new schemes used MOET to create families of full sibs, for testing and selecting both young bulls and future embryo donors. In these schemes (referred to from now on as MOET schemes), the selection of males was based primarily on the performance of their sisters rather than the performance of their daughters, as in conventional progeny testing schemes. In other words, breeding companies operating MOET nucleus breeding schemes would market semen from young bulls on the basis of a sib test, rather than a progeny test. Information on sisters is available much sooner than that on offspring, and so these proposed schemes reduced generation intervals substantially compared to those possible in progeny testing, but they also reduced the accuracy of selection on males. However, on balance, the gains from shorter generation intervals outweighed the losses from lower accuracy, and the proposed schemes were predicted to give higher rates of genetic gain.

Nicholas and Smith (1983) examined both 'adult' and 'juvenile' MOET nucleus schemes. In the adult schemes, selection of embryo donors was based on one lactation of the candidate, plus information from other relatives. In the juvenile schemes selection of embryo donors was based solely on performance records from ancestors. The details of the timing of events for these two types of scheme, estimated generation intervals and relative rates of response compared to progeny testing are given in Simm (1998).

Potential problems associated with nucleus schemes include the higher risks from a disease outbreak in the nucleus herd. Also, if management and feeding policy in the nucleus herd is markedly different from those in commercial herds which will use bulls bred in the nucleus, then there is a greater risk of genotype-by-environment interactions with nucleus breeding schemes than with progeny testing in commercial herds. However, steps can be taken to reduce these risks. For instance, different age groups of nucleus animals can be reared in different locations, and frozen embryos can be used as an insurance against disease outbreak. Also, management and feeding policies in the nucleus can be geared towards those in target commercial herds to reduce the risk of interactions.

In the mid-1980s, dairy cattle MOET breeding schemes were established in Britain, Denmark, the Netherlands, Germany, France, Italy, Finland, Poland and Canada, though only a few schemes still operate today, often in a modified form, for example the Delta nucleus herd in the Netherlands and the Nordic open nucleus herd Viken in Sweden. More details on these MOET schemes and mode of operation are given in Medic *et al.* (1999) and Simm (1998).

NUCLEUS SCHEMES IN THE GENOMIC ERA The level of reliability indicated for individual MOET sib-tested bulls with larger full-sib families was about 40-49% for production traits (see Simm, 1998). However, with genomic selection, reliabilities of 65% or more have been reported for the GEBVs of young bulls with no daughters, for various performance traits. This has prompted the incorporation of genomic selection into some nucleus herds. For example, from about 2007, the Delta nucleus scheme in the Netherlands introduced genomic selection within the nucleus breeding unit – initially using about 3000 genetic markers (van der Beek, 2007) – but the number has increased since then. Currently, the selection of young bulls in the scheme is mostly on the basis of genomic prediction. Also, intense selection is applied on one-year-old heifer donors as bull dams on the basis of genomic predicted breeding values. Consequently, the age of bull dams at selection has decrease; 75% of the young-bull dams are 1-year-old heifers and 25% are first-calved heifers. For more details of the current structure of the Delta nucleus scheme and the rôle of genomic selection in it, see Oldenbroek and van der Waaij (2015, Chapter 12).

For difficult-to-measure traits such as feed intake or fertility, nucleus herds are valuable as more detailed recording of such traits can be undertaken in a few herds with a well-defined management structure and a relatively small number of cows. Such nucleus herds could be open or could comprise well-managed herds across a country (a dispersed nucleus). For widespread application of the results of genomic studies from such open or dispersed nucleus herds, it is essential that they are genetically connected with the wider cow population in the country. An example of such an open dispersed nucleus herd is the Genomic Information Nucleus (Ginfo) in Australia (Pryce *et al.*, 2017). This was initiated in an attempt to increase the size of the reference population in the Australian genomic selection system and to allow collection of high-quality data on difficult-to-measure traits. Dairy herds were recruited into Ginfo on the basis of a score which depended on the quality of the records the herds were contributing to the national database. The scoring was based on an index that rewards cows with records on fertility, conformation, survival, workability, somatic cell count and milk yield. More emphasis was given to non-production traits such that complete fertility phenotypes constituted about 10 points out of the maximum score of 25. The highest scoring 103 herds were recruited into Ginfo, proportionately representing the dairy cow population across Australia's main dairy regions. The cows in the Ginfo herds were genotyped and included in the reference population for the genomic selection of the Australian national herd. The average increase in reliability from adding Ginfo to the reference population varied by trait, with gains of between 5% and 7% for Holsteins and between 2% and 3% for Jerseys. For instance, in Holsteins, the reliability for daughter fertility increased from 41%–46%, while the reliability for overall type increased from 42%–49% (Pryce *et al.*, 2017).

The Ginfo herds also offer the opportunity to study four of the most notable groups of health diseases in dairy herds: mastitis, reproductive problems, lameness and metabolic disorders (Abdelsayed *et al.,* 2017). The incidence levels for these four groups of diseases were 16%, 9%, 2% and 1.5%, respectively. Reported heritability estimates from pedigree and genomic analysis ranged from 0.01–0.03 for mastitis, 0.005–0.02 for reproductive disorders, 0.00–0.02 for lameness and 0.00–0.06 for metabolic disorders. Initial genomic prediction with a reference population of 11,458 cows, for bulls with daughters in the reference population, resulted in a comparatively low reliability (<30%), but was more promising for mastitis (about 30%) and a collective disease trait based on all diseases (about 28%).

Traits recorded

Many of the traits recorded and used in dairy cattle breeding programmes have been mentioned already. The purpose of this section is to provide more detail on the manner of recording, on the heritabilities of these traits and the associations among them. An overview of estimates of heritabilities for various categories of traits important in dairy cattle breeding is presented in Fig. 8.14.

Milk recording

National or regional milk-recording schemes have been the main source for capturing milk production traits for progeny testing schemes, and this remains the case even since the introduction of genomics in some temperate countries from the early 2000s. For example, in the UK there are currently two large milk-recording organizations (National Milk

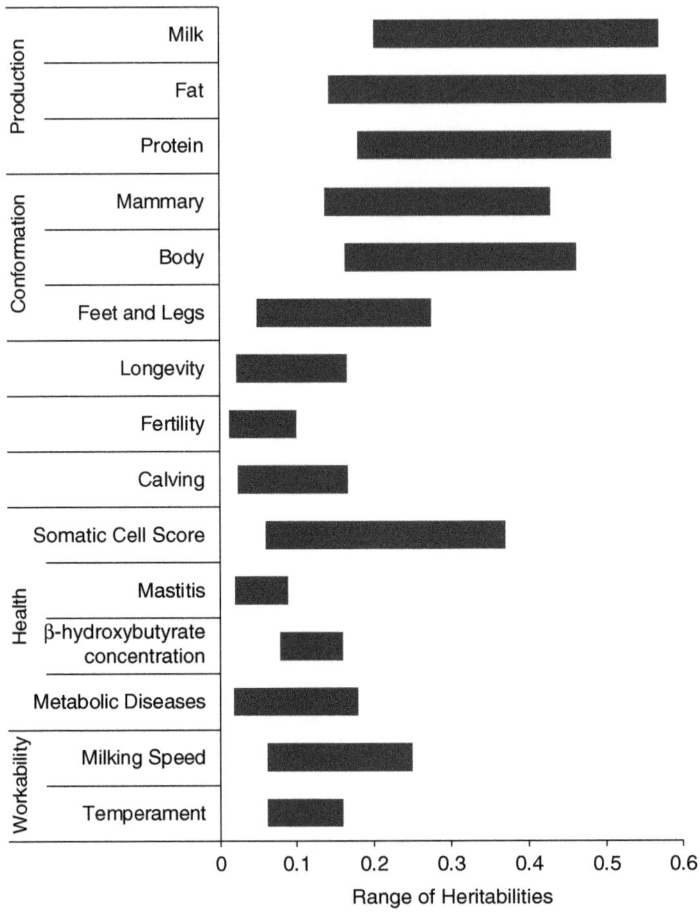

Fig. 8.14. An overview of the ranges of heritabilities for various categories of traits recorded in dairy herds. (After Miglior *et al.*, 2017.)

Records and Cattle Information Services) and both operate across the whole of the UK. More recently, a new milk-recording company, Quality Milk Management Services, began milk-recording activities, primarily in England. About 68% of the dairy cows in the UK are officially milk-recorded, a lower proportion than that in most other major dairying nations in Europe and elsewhere (ICAR, 2019a). In most of these countries, recording services must operate to standards set by the International Committee for Animal Recording (ICAR) before records are used in genetic evaluation.

The basis of most milk-recording schemes in Western countries is that a recorder visits the herd at monthly (or longer) intervals, and records the milk yield of cows at two or three milkings in a 24-hour period. Samples of milk are also obtained from individual cows at each milking for analysis of protein and fat contents. Increasingly, somatic cell counts (SCC) are obtained from these samples too. (High somatic cell counts in milk are usually associated with mastitis. Also, high cell counts in the bulk milk tank result in substantial penalties in milk price in many countries. Thus, individual cow cell counts provide a management tool for culling cows with abnormally high counts, and they provide the basis for genetic evaluations of bulls and cows for resistance to mastitis.) Farmers participating in milk-recording schemes receive reports of yields and other details of their cows at monthly or other regular intervals for management purposes. For the purposes of genetic evaluation, records are collated at regular intervals by the milk-recording organizations and sent to the organization responsible for evaluation.

Historically, milk records of cows were only used for genetic evaluation once lactations were complete. The normal length of lactation for recording purposes in many countries with semi-intensive production systems is 305 days, but some shorter lactations (e.g. those in excess of 200 days, in the UK) are considered to be complete for genetic evaluation purposes if the cow has 'dried off' or been culled. (It is often difficult to achieve 365-day calving intervals in high-yielding herds, so inevitably many lactations are longer than 305 days. There is a view that planning lactations longer than 305 days may be more biologically and economically efficient for high-yielding cows in some non-seasonal production systems.) All of the available milk records (called *test-day records*, as mentioned in Chapter 7) for an individual cow are used to predict that cow's 305-day yield of milk, fat and protein. Typically, there are nine or ten records at monthly intervals. There are strong genetic associations between the yields of milk, fat and protein at successive sampling occasions and the total lactation yield. Therefore the latter can be predicted quite well from a smaller number of test-day records (see Table 8.8). However, the genetic correlation among the test-day records decreases as the days in milk increases between successive milk sampling events. The means and variances of the test-day milk records also vary with days in milk.

To account for this gradual change in the means and variances of test-day records over the days in milk, a method called the random regression model (see Chapter 7 for full details) was developed that involves fitting a curve through the test-day records over the lactation. Such curves account for the fact that milk yield increases from the beginning of the lactation and peaks at about 6 weeks, followed by a gradual decline (e.g. Wilmink, 1987). The use of the random regression model means that cows with at least three test-day records can be included in the genetic evaluation system. The inclusion of cows with a minimum of three test days can reduce substantially the time lag between making test inseminations from a young bull and getting an initial prediction of breeding value, and so it can shorten male generation intervals and improve the efficiency of progeny testing. The random regression model for the genetic evaluation of milk production traits was introduced in the UK in 2005.

Table 8.9 shows estimates of the heritabilities of the most commonly recorded milk traits in the UK, and the correlations among them in the first lactation, using an animal model. More recent estimates of heritability for milk, fat and protein yields in the UK from a random regression model are higher at 0.61, 0.50 and 0.56, respectively (Mrode *et al.*, 2005). These increases in heritability estimates are generally in line with estimates from other countries when test-day models have been used. This has been attributed to the ability of random regression models to better account for the fixed and environmental effects. Yields of milk, fat and protein are all moderate to highly heritable, while fat and protein content are both highly heritable. There are high genetic correlations among milk, fat and protein yields, indicating that selection for any one of these three traits is expected to lead to increases in the other two. However, there are negative genetic correlations between all three yield traits and protein %, and

Table 8.8. Estimates of genetic correlations between individual test-day records for several milk production traits, obtained at approximately monthly intervals throughout lactation, and predicted full lactation records for the same traits. The records were from British Holstein Friesian heifers; all animals had at least eight test-day records, but only a subset had ten test-day records. Except for the first one or two test-day records, most show a high genetic correlation with total lactation production; heritabilities of test-day records follow a similar pattern. (After Pander *et al.*, 1992.)

	Test day (approximately monthly intervals)									
Lactation record	1	2	3	4	5	6	7	8	9	10
Milk yield	0.87	0.89	0.97	0.98	0.99	0.97	0.98	0.97	0.95	0.88
Fat yield	0.77	0.85	0.95	0.97	0.97	0.93	0.97	0.96	0.97	0.98
Protein yield	0.84	0.90	0.97	0.97	0.98	0.95	0.98	0.98	0.95	0.91
Fat %	0.81	0.91	0.98	0.98	0.99	0.98	0.96	0.98	0.94	0.91
Protein %	0.76	0.87	0.95	0.97	0.96	0.98	0.92	0.94	0.89	0.77

between yields of milk or protein and fat %, indicating that selection for yield is likely to lead to a reduction in protein or fat concentration, or both. Table 8.10 shows the correlations between production in successive lactations. The fairly high genetic correlations indicate that there is a reasonably close association between genetic merit for milk production in early and later lactations.

Type traits

As mentioned earlier, assessments of type or conformation are widely used in dairy cattle breeding. Type classification is usually performed by breed society staff, or staff from progeny testing agencies. The records are used both to provide a description of the cow concerned, and to enable predictions of breeding values for cows and bulls. The methods of type classification, and the emphasis that ought to be placed on type versus production, have been a major source of debate between scientists and breeders for decades. Type classification schemes evolved as a method of describing the physical attributes of cows, particularly those thought to be associated with functional fitness, health and longevity, or success in the show ring. However, the early classification systems were based on subjective opinions of individual classifiers, and so they were not very repeatable or easy to interpret. Many breed societies retain classification schemes which include some subjective judgement, but increasingly these schemes are using more objective measurements. In particular, in the late 1970s and early 1980s a new system called linear assessment was developed in North America. This has been adopted since then in most major dairying countries.

Table 8.9. Estimates of the heritabilities of the most commonly recorded milk traits, and the correlations among them, for the first lactation of Holstein Friesian cows. Heritability estimates for yield of milk, fat and protein in later lactations tend to be slightly lower. Those for fat and protein content are similar to the first lactation values. Heritabilities are shown on the diagonal in bold, phenotypic correlations are shown above the diagonal and genetic correlations below the diagonal. (After Visscher and Thompson, 1992.)

Trait	Milk (kg)	Fat (kg)	Protein (kg)	Fat (%)	Protein (%)
Milk (kg)	**0.39**	0.84	0.95	−0.31	−0.42
Fat (kg)	0.75	**0.36**	0.87	0.26	−0.13
Protein (kg)	0.91	0.82	**0.36**	−0.16	−0.10
Fat (%)	−0.42	0.28	−0.20	**0.58**	0.51
Protein (%)	−0.50	−0.09	−0.10	0.60	**0.62**

For most traits, linear assessment still involves visual appraisal of the cow. However, unlike the original classification systems, linear assessment scores the characteristics of the cow in relation to the biological extremes, rather than labelling her as good, bad or indifferent. This means that the results are more repeatable, and more amenable to scientific analysis. Figure 8.15 illustrates the principles of the linear assessment system for some of the traits scored by Holstein UK (HUK). Table 8.11 shows the interpretation of high and low scores for the 15 linear-type traits recorded by HUK and their heritabilities. In addition, HUK allocates scores for five composite traits: dairy capacity, dairy character, rump, legs and feet, and mammary. These scores are assigned subjectively but they are closely related to the relevant linear-type scores. A total score, ranging from 50–97 points, is calculated from the cow's score for these five composite traits, with 10% of total emphasis given to dairy capacity, 10% to dairy character, 10% to rump, 30% to legs and feet, and 40% to mammary. Based on the total score, cows are assigned to final classes of excellent (90–97 points), very good (85–89 points), good plus (80–84 points), good (75–79 points), fair

Table 8.10. Estimates of the phenotypic and genetic correlations among milk production traits recorded in the first, second and third lactations of Holstein Friesian cows. (After Visscher and Thompson, 1992; Mrode *et al.*, 2005.)

	First and second lactation		First and third lactation		Second and third lactation	
Trait	Phenotypic	Genetic	Phenotypic	Genetic	Phenotypic	Genetic
Milk (kg)	0.58	0.87	0.54	0.84	0.60	0.98
Fat (kg)	0.56	0.86	0.51	0.85	0.57	0.97
Protein (kg)	0.58	0.86	0.52	0.82	0.61	0.98
Fat (%)	0.73	0.85	0.71	0.84	0.69	0.74
Protein (%)	0.70	0.78	0.69	0.76	0.71	0.78

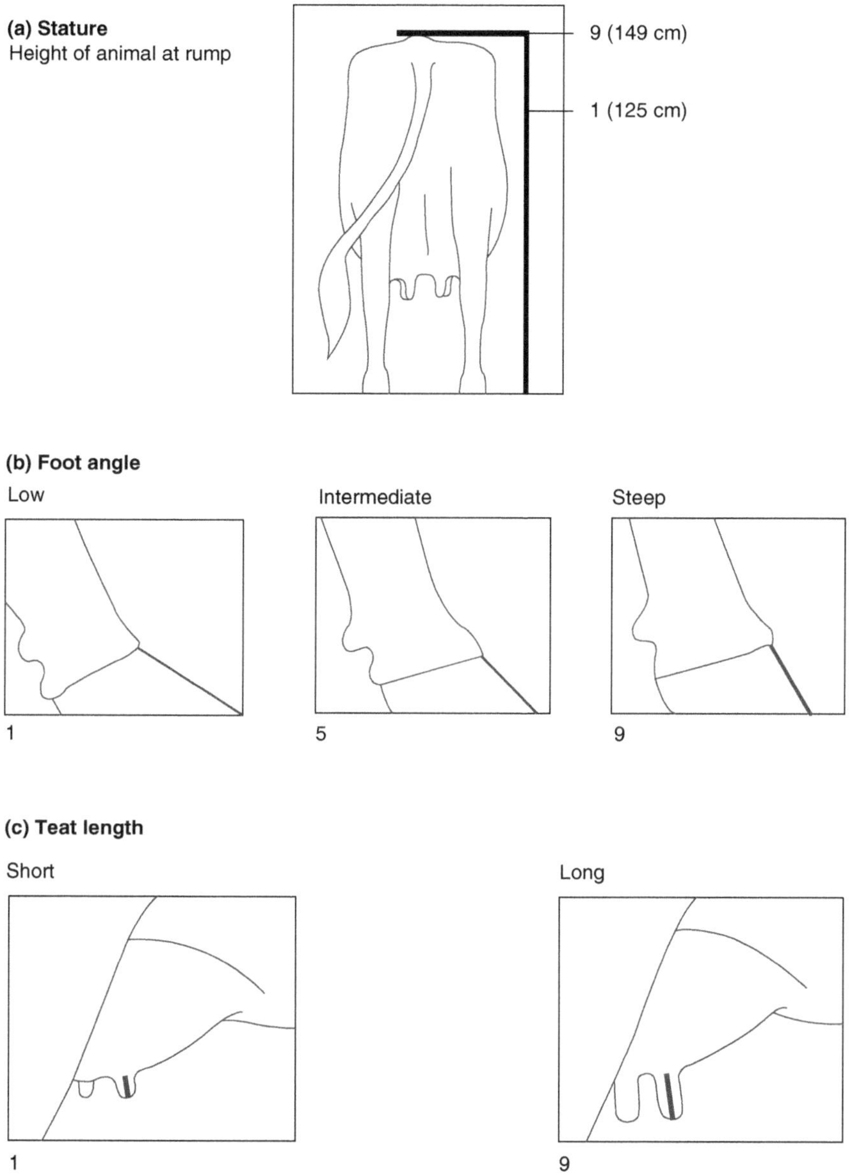

Fig. 8.15. The principles of the linear assessment system for some of the traits scored by Holstein UK. The diagrams illustrate the characteristics of animals with extreme scores (1 and 9) for three traits. (a) Stature; (b) foot angle; (c) teat length. (After Holstein UK, 2019).

(65–74 points) and poor (50–64 points) (Holstein UK, 2019).

The World Holstein–Friesian Federation introduced a type harmonization programme for most countries for the type evaluation of Holstein dairy cows in the early 2000s after a series of workshops. There is now good evidence that trained operators produce linear-type classifications which provide repeatable and heritable descriptions of the appearance of cows. Also, there is growing evidence that some linear-type traits are genetically correlated with economically important traits such as milk production, longevity and disease resistance, live weight and feed intake (see Table 8.12). From the early 1990s, most breeders or commercial producers using type information have based their selection on the animals' scores for individual type traits, or on one of the overall scores of type merit. A number of countries now include these scores along with production traits in indexes of overall

Table 8.11. The interpretation and heritabilities of linear-type traits recorded by the Holstein Friesian Society (now Holstein UK) in Britain and Ireland. (After Brotherstone and Hill, 1991; Holstein Friesian Society of Great Britain and Ireland, 1995; Dr S Brotherstone, personal communication)

	Interpretation of extreme scores		
Trait	1	9	Heritability
Stature	125 cm	149 cm	0.48
Chest width	Narrow	Wide	0.27
Body depth	Shallow	Deep	0.35
Angularity	Thick and coarse	Angular	0.26
Rump angle	High pins	Low pins	0.29
Rump width	Narrow pins	Wide pins	0.22
Rear legs, side view	Straight	Sickled	0.19
Foot angle	Low	Steep	0.27
Fore-udder attachment	Loose	Strong	0.27
Rear udder height	Low	High	0.20
Udder depth	Below hocks	22 cm above hocks	0.39
Central ligament[a]	Flat	Strong	0.16
Front teat placement, rear view	Wide	Close	0.43
Teat placement, side view	Close	Far apart	0.41
Teat length	Short	Long	0.44

[a]Formerly called udder support.

Table 8.12. Genetic correlations between linear-type traits, longevity and milk production traits in UK Holstein Friesians. (After Brotherstone and Hill, 1991; Brotherstone, 1994.)

	Genetic correlation with:			
Linear-type trait	Longevity	Milk yield (kg)	Fat yield (kg)	Protein yield (kg)
Stature	0.00	0.22	0.16	0.25
Chest width	−0.13	−0.14	−0.10	−0.13
Body depth	−0.03	0.24	0.25	0.24
Angularity	0.13	0.44	0.42	0.43
Rump angle	0.03	−0.11	−0.08	−0.11
Rump width	−0.11	−0.01	0.01	0.01
Rear legs, side view	−0.05	0.07	0.06	0.07
Foot angle	0.09	0.02	0.05	0.07
Fore-udder attachment	0.06	−0.29	−0.23	−0.28
Udder depth	0.14	−0.48	−0.40	−0.44
Central ligament[a]	0.02	0.10	0.16	0.15
Front teat placement, rear view	0.03	−0.05	−0.03	−0.01
Teat placement, side view	−0.02	0.38	0.35	0.36
Teat length	−0.19	0.18	0.12	0.17

[a]Formerly called udder support.

merit. For instance, the Canadian Lifetime Performance Index includes composite scores for feet and legs, mammary systems, dairy strength and rump as indirect measures of herd life, and udder depth as an indirect measure of health and fertility. Some of these developments are discussed later in this chapter.

Claw disease traits

Cow foot and leg health has become very important in recent years, due to the fact that lameness has considerable economic cost and is also an indicator of animal welfare. The genetics of foot and leg health and locomotion were reviewed by Boelling and Pollott (1997). Impaired locomotion has been attributed primarily to claw conditions. Some management factors such as the gradual shift from tie stalls to loose house barns in the Nordic countries has led to an increase of infection-related claw diseases such as dermatitis, heel horn erosion and skin proliferation (Johansson *et al.*, 2011). Data on claw traits is usually obtained from professional claw trimmers. In general, trimmings are made twice a year, so that a cow can have several trimming records in each lactation. The claw traits recorded in Germany, Netherlands and several Scandinavian countries include interdigital hyperplasia, laminitis, white line disease, claw ulcers, heel horn erosion, sole haemorrhage, sole ulcer, digital phlegmon and digital dermatitis. These traits may be further classified as infection-related traits (digital and interdigital dermatitis, heel horn erosion, and interdigital hyperplasia); feed-related traits (sole haemorrhage, sole ulcer and white line disease); and malformation traits (corkscrew claws). The wide range of these claw disease traits means that there is a need for clear definitions and harmonization in recording across countries. ICAR has provided such a standardized protocol for recording claw traits (ICAR, 2019b). In addition, a number of countries, including Germany and the Netherlands, are working on adopting a comprehensive and integrative approach to record information on claw conditions using veterinary diagnoses, observations by farmers, regular screening and observations from routine hoof trimming.

The data on claw diseases from professional trimmers are recorded usually as binary (0 = no disorder, 1 = disorder) or as categorical traits with three or four categories depending on the country (e.g. 0 = no disorder; 1 = slight disorder; 2 = moderate disorder; 3 = severe disorder). Sole haemorrhage (SH), digital dermatitis (DD), interdigital dermatitis (ID), wall ulcer (WU), sole ulcer (SU) are scored as categorical traits; interdigital hyperplasia and white line disease are scored as binary traits.

The estimates of heritabilities from several studies are reported in Table 8.13. These are generally low, ranging from 0.01 for wall ulcer to 0.13–0.15 for interdigital hyperplasia.

van der Linde *et al.* (2010) also estimated the genetic correlation between the prevalence of claw disease traits in the first and later parities up to the fifth lactation. The genetic correlations between first and later parities were 0.93, 0.88, 1.00, 0.72, 0.89, 0.83, 0.90 and 0.92 for sole haemorrhage, digital dermatitis, interdigital dermatitis, wall ulcer, sole ulcer, interdigital hyperplasia and white line disease, and combined claw health, respectively. Only the correlations for digital dermatitis, sole ulcer and interdigital hyperplasia were significantly different from one; the other diseases were essentially the same trait across parities.

The genetic correlations among the various claw disease traits tend to be medium to high (0.49 to 0.78), but a few are lower (Johansson *et al.*, 2011). The various claw disease traits are usually used to construct a claw health index for use in selection to improve claw health in breeding programmes. In the Netherlands the claw health index for the Dutch Holstein includes SH, DD, ID, SU, IH and WL (van de Linde *et al.*, 2010). The reliability of

Table 8.13. Prevalence, heritability and repeatability for several claw traits. (After van der Linde *et al.*, 2010; Stock *et al.*, 2017.)

Trait	Prevalence (%)	Heritability	Repeatability
Sole haemorrhage	38	0.06	0.16
Digital dermatitis	22	0.06–0.9	0.31
Interdigital dermatitis	29	0.06–0.11	0.26
Wall ulcer	3	0.01	0.15
Sole ulcer	7	0.08–0.12	0.30
Interdigital hyperplasia	5	0.13–0.15	0.57
White line disease	11	0.03–0.09	0.16
Combined claw health	69	0.07	0.22

this index was 0.59, but including several conformation type traits (feet and legs, rear legs rear view, fore-udder attachment, and locomotion) increased the reliability by an extra 6%. Similar indexes based on claw diseases for Nordic countries and Germany have been reported by Johansson *et al.* (2011) and Stock *et al.* (2017). The correlations between claw disease traits and feet and leg traits are very low in the Norwegian Red cattle (Ødegård *et al.*, 2013); more moderate genetic correlations are found with various type traits. For instance, these authors reported genetic correlations between rear leg rear view and infectious claw disorders and laminitis-related claw disorders of –0.20 and 0.26, respectively, and a correlation between hoof quality and laminitis-related claw disorders of –0.33. They concluded that selection for feet and leg conformation is not an efficient approach to genetically improve claw health in Norwegian Red cattle, and that this should be based on direct selection for these traits.

An alternative approach is to assess the overall effect of feet and leg traits on lameness and locomotion. Boelling and Pollott (1998) reported heritabilities of 0.08–0.11 for locomotion scores of UK Holstein cattle, from heifers up to fourth lactation animals. High correlations were found with some of the type traits. Genetic merit for locomotion and some type traits had declined over the 15-year period studied. The value of locomotion scoring is that it is relatively easy to apply on commercial farms.

Reproduction, health and workability

Most milk-recording agencies collect details of inseminations made, using the information for management purposes or to provide parentage information for the resulting offspring when they produce milk records themselves. More recently, in a large number of dairying countries (e.g. Denmark, the Netherlands, Norway, UK, Germany) these records are also being used to produce routine genetic evaluations of cow (and bull) fertility. This has been enhanced by the introduction of MACE evaluation for cow fertility traits by INTERBULL. Currently, INTERBULL performs MACE evaluations for 21 countries and analyses five female fertility traits: (i) maiden heifer's ability to conceive (e.g. conception rate or number of inseminations); (ii) lactating cow's ability to recycle after calving (e.g. the interval from calving to first insemination); (iii) lactating cow's ability to conceive, expressed as a rate trait (e.g. non-return rate); (iv) lactating cow's ability to conceive, expressed as an interval trait (e.g. interval from first to last insemination); and (v) lactating cow's interval traits (e.g. days open or calving interval).

Several studies have shown an unfavourable genetic correlation between fertility and milk production. For example, an early review in this area showed genetic correlations averaging about 0.35 between fat-corrected milk yield and the interval between calving and first insemination (though this may be influenced by management practices), and about 0.22 between fat-corrected yield and number of inseminations (Philipsson, 1981). A summary of several studies by Pryce et al. (2004) indicated that the estimates of genetic correlations between milk yield and calving interval range from 0.22–0.59, those between milk yield and days open range from 0.16–0.64, and those between milk yield and days to first service range from 0.22–0.44. Consequently, from the early 2000s most major dairying countries commenced prediction of breeding values for cow fertility traits, and their inclusion in national selection indexes, in an attempt to improve fertility. Table 8.14 shows the heritabilities of some measures of fertility. In most cases these are very low, indicating the importance of management, and also the need for large numbers of daughters to be recorded to produce accurate bull proofs for fertility traits in conventional progeny schemes. While heritabilities are low, overall phenotypic variation is high, and hence there is usable genetic variation. Consequently, results have indicated that selection for fertility traits has been effective. For example, in the US, García-Ruiz *et al.* (2016) reported that the decline in daughter pregnancy rate (DPR) stabilized in 2003, the first year after introducing genetic evaluations for DPR. Similar results have been obtained in the UK with the genetic trend for fertility showing improvement from about 2009 following the introduction of genetic evaluations in 2006. With genomic selection, accurate evaluations for fertility traits can be obtained for young bulls at an early age, and therefore faster rates of genetic progress are possible. The rate of change reported in the USA for DPR after the introduction of genomic evaluations was 0.26 per year (2011–2018) compared with 0.02 per year for the period immediately before this (2006–2010).

Calving complications lead to an increase in veterinary and labour costs, a decrease in revenue

Table 8.14. Estimates of the heritability of some measures of fertility, calving difficulty and stillbirth.

Trait	Heritability (s.e.)	Source
Days to first service	0.03–0.04 (0.004)	Hayes *et al.* (1992); Pritchard *et al.* (2013)
Days open	0.05	Hayes *et al.* (1992)
	0.04 (0.02)	Hoekstra *et al.* (1994)
Services per conception	0.03	Hayes *et al.* (1992)
	0.01–0.02 (0.002–0.005)	Swalve *et al.* (1992)
Calving interval	0.03–0.04 (0.02–0.0042)	Hoekstra *et al.* (1994)
Non-return rate at 56 days	0.01 (0.002)	Pritchard *et al.* (2013)
Number of inseminations	0.02 (0.006)	Pritchard *et al.* (2013)
Gestation length (direct)	0.27–0.41(0.02–0.03)	Jamrozik *et al.* (2005); Eaglen *et al.* (2012)
Gestation length (maternal)	0.07–0.09 (0.01–0.02)	Jamrozik *et al.* (2005); Eaglen *et al.* (2012)
Dystocia (calving difficulty)	0.03–0.20[a]	Meijering (1984); Philipsson *et al.* (1979)
	0.05–0.34[b]	Wiggans *et al.* (2003); Jamrozik *et al.* (2005); Eaglen *et al.* (2012)
Stillbirth	0.00–0.06[a]	Meijering (1984); Philipsson *et al.* (1979)
	0.04–0.14[b]	Meijering (1984); Philipsson *et al.* (1979); Jamrozik *et al.* (2005); Cole *et al.* (2007); Eaglen *et al.* (2012)

[a]Heritability on the categorical scale, i.e. measured. The range of heritabilities is similar for both direct and maternal effects on dystocia and stillbirth (i.e. whether they are considered as traits of the calf or as traits of the dam).
[b]Heritability on the underlying continuous scale.

through loss of animals and reduced subsequent performance, and they have implications for animal welfare. Hence the emphasis has shifted from just collecting information on calving difficulty on daughters of bulls undergoing progeny testing in the 1980s, to herd-wide recording of calving data by milk-recording agencies. Most major dairy countries now produce routine genetic evaluations for calving traits.

Calving difficulty is usually recorded on a categorical scale of 1 to 4 or 5, depending on the country or recording organization. Assuming a scale of 4 classes, 1 represents easy and non-assisted calving, 2 is moderate and farmer assisted calving, 3 is difficult and farmer assisted and 4 is difficult and veterinarian assisted. Selection for ease of calving is more complicated than it seems at first sight. Bulls whose progeny are born with little or no calving difficulty generally produce smaller progeny. But, when these small daughters calve themselves, they are more likely to have difficulties than larger cows. Hence, in several countries there are two separate evaluations of calving ease for bulls: firstly a 'direct' evaluation of the bull as a father, and secondly a 'maternal' evaluation of the bull – an evaluation of the bull based on the calving performance of his daughters (see Chapter 7). The typical ranges of heritabilities for calving difficulty and stillbirths are shown in Table 8.15. As with fertility traits, the heritabilities of these traits are usually very low. Given the low heritability of calving traits, some studies have included gestation length in multi-trait analyses of calving traits as an additional source of information in estimating parameters for calving ease. Eaglen *et al.* (2012) reported a genetic correlation of 0.5 ± 0.08 between direct calving ease and gestation length.

Dairy cattle breeding programmes in several countries now include selection for resistance to some common diseases such as mastitis and ketosis. Selection for disease resistance has been practised for many years in the Scandinavian countries. Genetic evaluations there are based on comprehensive national databases of individual cow health events maintained by farmers and veterinary surgeons. In the UK, similar records were collected from the mid-1980s by DAISY (Dairy Information System), a recording service now operated by National Milk Records, but there were relatively few animals involved. However, in recent years recording for disease traits has increased, likely due to the uptake of on-farm software for herd management purposes, the increase in farm assurance schemes, the mandatory recording of veterinary treatments/medicine use in food-producing animals, and contracts with retailers requiring detailed health recording.

As with reproduction traits, there is evidence of unfavourable genetic correlations between milk production and some diseases, and this has stimulated interest in genetic evaluations for resistance to common diseases. Currently INTERBULL undertakes MACE evaluations for direct measures of mastitis for about 10 countries, and 23 other countries provide somatic cell counts as indirect measure of mastitis. While genetic evaluation for ketosis, milk fever and other diseases have been ongoing in Scandinavian countries since the 1980s, other countries have commenced evaluations for these traits more recently. For instance, Canada has started genetic evaluations for metabolic disease resistance based on a combination of three traits: clinical ketosis, subclinical ketosis and displaced abomasum. A displaced abomasum results from the accumulation of gas, which can cause it to move up in the abdomen, generally to the left side of the body. Surgical intervention is often required. Cows with a displaced abomasum have been shown to produce over 300 kg less milk during lactation. The USA introduced genetic evaluations for ketosis, clinical mastitis, retained placenta, metritis, displaced abomasum and milk fever in 2018.

Bovine tuberculosis (bTB) is a chronic bacterial disease of cattle caused by *Mycobacterium bovis* infection, primarily involving the respiratory tract. It is endemic in the UK and other countries and it is regarded as one of the four most important livestock diseases globally. Annual costs of about £175 million are incurred in the UK (Abernethy *et al.*, 2013). Routine genetic evaluation for resistance to bovine tuberculosis was implemented in the UK in January 2016 (Banos *et al.*, 2017). Infected animals are classified as those with a positive skin test or with a positive *post-mortem* examination result. The trait has a low heritability of about 0.09. Predicted transmitting abilities (PTAs) are published as an index called TB Advantage. The index indicates the degree of resistance to bTB that a bull is predicted to pass on to his offspring; it is expressed on a scale which typically runs from −3 to +3. For every +1 point in the index, 1% fewer daughters are expected to become infected during a bTB breakdown.

Table 8.15 shows the heritabilities of some of the diseases mentioned above, and others. The heritabilities of most disease traits are fairly low. For estimates of correlations between some of these disease and milk production traits, see the review by Berry *et al.* (2011).

Although direct evaluations of health traits are being practised in some countries, in many others there is a greater dependence on indicator traits. This is the case for mastitis, as mentioned above, for genetic evaluations at the national level and for MACE evaluations. Thus, somatic cell counts continue to be used as indirect predictors for mastitis in many countries. Somatic cell counts in milk have been shown to be heritable (e.g. heritability of 0.11–0.14 in different dairy breeds in the UK (Mrode *et al.*, 1995; Pritchard *et al.*, 2013)) and genetically associated with the incidence of mastitis (e.g. genetic correlations of 0.4–0.8 with various measures of infection (Coffey *et al.*, 1986; Philipsson *et al.*, 1995; Pritchard *et al.*, 2013)). Selection for reduced somatic cell counts has been shown to decrease the incidence of mastitis. Also, a growing number of milk payment schemes attach direct economic value to somatic cell counts as a measure of the hygienic quality of milk. Currently, all major dairy countries have established genetic evaluations for somatic cell count and INTERBULL carries out MACE evaluations based on cell count for 33 countries, in addition to direct MACE evaluations for mastitis, as mentioned in the last section. Similarly, linear-type traits can be useful indicators of problems of the mammary system or feet and legs (e.g. Groen *et al.*, 1994; Berry *et al.*, 2004). The most useful of these indicator traits are already incorporated into the indexes of overall merit, as explained later.

Table 8.15. Estimates of the heritability of some diseases in dairy cattle.

Trait	Heritability (s.e.)	Source
Mastitis	0.0–0.37	Emanuelson (1988); Pritchard *et al.* (2013)
Ketosis	0.01–0.23	Emanuelson (1988); Vosman *et al.* (2015)
Lameness	0.02–0.10 (0.006)	Berry *et al.* (2011); Pritchard *et al.* (2013)
Claw disorders	0.09–0.31 (0.08–0.10)	Distl *et al.* (1990)
Bovine tuberculosis	0.06–0.18 (0.01–0.04)	Berry *et al.* (2011); Banos *et al.* (2017)
Bovine paratuberculosis	0.05–0.15 (0.02–0.06)	Berry *et al.* (2011)
Hypocalcaemia (milk fever)	0.01–0.13	Berry *et al.* (2011)
Cystic ovaries	0.02–0.22	Berry *et al.* (2011)
Metritis	0.04–0.06	Berry *et al.* (2011)
Retained foetal membrane	0.004–0.08	Berry *et al.* (2011)

Good temperament and ease of milking have long been recognized as important to those at 'the sharp end' of milk production. In the past, most selection pressure on these 'workability' or 'parlour' attributes has been achieved by culling the worst offenders. The importance of milking speed has increased recently, especially in herds with automatic milking systems. Therefore national recording schemes based on farmer's assessment and evaluation systems have evolved for these traits in countries such as Sweden, Finland, Denmark, Norway, Canada, Germany and the UK, although scales of recording differ. For instance, Holstein UK, and recording agencies in Germany and Canada operate a 5-point scoring system for cow temperament and ease of milking; Sweden, Finland and Denmark use a scale of 1 to 9, while Norway uses a scale of 1 to 3. Currently, INTERBULL computes MACE proofs for about 13 countries for milking speed and temperament. Table 8.16 shows estimates of heritabilities for these traits from several countries. These traits are incorporated into indexes of overall economic merit in several countries (Miglior *et al.*, 2017).

Feed intake, feed efficiency, live weight and body condition

The importance of feed costs in the overall profitability of dairying was highlighted earlier. However, feed intake has been ignored in most improvement programmes until recently. This is partly because of the difficulty of recording feed intake in commercial herds. Some of the modern facilities for automated measurement of individual feed intake such as the Insentec Roughage Intake Control System, GrowSafe and Calan Broadbent Feeding System were described in Chapter 5; these are still mostly used in research farms or nucleus herds. However, the use of these facilities in selected herds that are connected to the whole cow population could enable the application of genomic selection at the population level, as discussed below.

In addition to the difficulty of recording intake, there is also a fairly strong genetic correlation between yield and gross efficiency, which means that selection for yield is expected to lead to improvements in efficiency. So, many testing agencies have relied on this correlated response rather than undertake direct selection. Several studies have demonstrated that food intake is fairly highly heritable (0.16–0.44; van Arendonk *et al.*, 1995; Berry *et al.*, 2007) and that, at least under *ad libitum* feeding of a complete diet, feed intake is not entirely a function of yield (Persaud *et al.*, 1991). Also, total intake over the whole lactation can be predicted fairly well from several weeks of intake recording (Persaud and Simm, 1991). Most of the studies and estimates of heritabilities are based on data from research or experimental farms due to the difficulty of measuring feed intake on commercial farms. However, similar levels of heritability were obtained by Vallimont *et al.* (2010) from monthly recording of feed intake in commercial tie-stall barns in the USA. They reported heritability estimates of 0.18 ± 0.06 for dry-matter intake (DMI), 0.15 ± 0.06 for crude protein intake and 0.18 ± 0.07 for net energy of lactation. The genetic correlations among the three intake traits and fat-corrected milk yield, body weight, and stature were moderate to high (0.52–0.63). The authors concluded that feed intake measured in commercial tie-stalls once per month was sufficiently accurate to enable genetic improvement. Genetic evaluations for DMI were introduced in the Netherlands in 2014, based on DMI data collected from several farms, and DMI predicted for cows with no direct DMI records from milk, fat and protein yields and body weight (de Jong *et al.*, 2016). The heritabilities for DMI were 0.28, 0.25 and 0.20 for first, second and later lactations,

Table 8.16. Some estimates of heritability for temperament and milking speed of dairy cattle.

Trait	Temperament	Milking speed	Source
Canada	0.128 (±0.014)	0.139 ± 0.012	Sewalem *et al.* (2011)
Germany	0.07	0.28	Rensing and Ruten (2005)
Australia	0.16	0.25	Beard (1993)
United Kingdom	0.10	0.11	INTERBULL (2019)
Denmark, Sweden, Finland	0.11	0.22	INTERBULL (2019)
Norway	0.08	0.20	INTERBULL (2019)
Netherlands	0.12	0.23	INTERBULL (2019)

respectively. In an attempt to increase the amount of data on DMI, there has been co-operation among several countries (Australia, UK and the Netherlands) to improve the accuracies of genetic parameters and evaluations (de Haas *et al.*, 2012). The estimates of heritabilities and genetic correlations among the countries using pedigree and genomic information is shown in Table 8.17. Note that there was no pedigree information to link the data from the three countries, hence only the genomic information was used to estimate the genetic correlations. The accuracy of genomic prediction using data from the three countries increased by up to 5.5% compared with univariate models within country (i.e. from on average 0.33 within country to 0.35 using a three-country reference population).

The main purpose of measuring feed intake is to increase the efficiency of feed utilization. Traditional measures used for feed efficiency include feed conversion ratio – the ratio of output (e.g. milk yield) to feed consumed, or the inverse which is feed conversion efficiency (FCE), used more widely in dairy cattle. Estimates of the heritability of FCE in dairy cattle vary from 0.14–0.37 (Pryce *et al.*, 2014). Given the difficulties of directly measuring feed intake, some countries such as Australia, New Zealand, Netherlands and the USA have incorporated gross feed efficiency into their selection indexes indirectly by including milk production and live weight (or predictions of live weight) to predict energy requirements for maintenance and productivity. Pryce *et al.* (2014) explained that accounting for feed costs in a selection index slows down the rate of genetic gain in cow size by increasing maintenance requirements at a slower rate than milk production requirements, leading to improved feed efficiency. Harris *et al.* (2007) reported that using the index Breeding Worth – which includes a measure of feed efficiency – in New Zealand, over 10 years, increased genetic gain for milk and fat plus protein yield by 27% and reduced live weight by 3.1 kg, compared to the rate of genetic gain in the 10 years before the index was introduced.

There is an indication that the above indexes, based on energy requirements predicted from milk production traits and live weight, do not capture all the variation in actual energy requirements (calculated directly from DMI) among animals. Thus, there has been interest more recently in residual feed intake (RFI), also referred to as net feed intake. RFI is the difference between actual and predicted DMI and is calculated as the residual after regressing DMI on energy requirements for milk production traits and maintenance. Thus, RFI is assumed to be a measure of metabolic efficiency of animals because it is thought to capture differences among animals in various activities, including protein turnover, digestibility and heat increment of fermentation. In a review, Pryce *et al.* (2014) reported heritabilities of RFI in growing dairy heifers ranging from 0.22–0.38 and in lactating dairy cows ranging from 0.01–0.32. However, measuring actual DMI is expensive and thus the main focus has been to implement genomic selection for RFI so that the genetic evaluations can be extended to the whole population. This requires DMI to be recorded in a group of cows, with RFI calculated from these measurements, followed by genomic prediction to obtain accurate SNP solutions. These SNP solutions can then be used to estimate genomic breeding values for young genotyped animals without measuring RFI on them. Estimates of accuracies of genomic prediction for RFI in dairy cows vary from 0.30–0.40 (see Price *et al.* (2014) for a review). RFI

Table 8.17. Genetic parameters (heritabilities and genetic correlations) for standardized DMI in Australia (AU), Europe (EU), United Kingdom (UK) and the Netherlands (NL), estimated with a pedigree or genomic relationship matrix (SE in parentheses).

	Heritability		Genetic correlations	
Relationship matrix	Pedigree	Genomic	Genomic AU	Genomic UK
Overall	0.37 (0.069)	0.34 (0.048)		
AU	0.19 (0.102)	0.41 (0.091)		
EU	0.51 (0.089)	0.43 (0.072)	0.47 (0.206)	
UK	0.39 (0.123)	0.38 (0.119)	0.74 (0.341)	
NL	0.71 (0.117)	0.59 (0.098)	0.36 (0.221)	0.50 (0.281)

is a relatively new trait in dairy cattle and studies are currently underway to investigate relationships with other traits, with the ultimate aim of incorporating it into breeding objectives.

It is common for most mammals to lose weight (mainly fat) during lactation. In general, dairy cows experience negative energy balance (EB) for 2 to 4 months after calving, when nutrient requirements for milk production, maintenance and activity exceed the ability of the cow to consume enough feed. The cow consequently mobilizes body tissue reserves to meet her energy requirement. Over the past two decades or so, there has been concern that at least when very high-yielding North American Holsteins are kept in some lower-input systems, the increasing milk yields of high genetic merit cows are being 'fuelled' by progressively greater losses of body condition, rather than by higher feed intake. Thus the duration and magnitude of negative EB has increased in these high-yielding cows. Direct measures of EB are based on individual animal feed intake and milk production. However, given the limitations of recording feed intake in commercial farms, indirect indicators of EB such as body condition score (BCS) are used. BCS is a subjective measure by field officers or type classifiers and it represents a measure of body energy stores. Different countries use different scales for recording BCS, but low values generally reflect emaciation and high values reflect obesity. For example, the UK uses a scale of 1 to 9 to record BCSs with 1 regarded as poor, 5 as intermediate and 9 as grossly fat. BCS is regarded as a useful trait to customize feeding strategies and manage dairy cow fertility and health. In a review, Bastin and Gengler (2013) reported heritability estimates of BCS from 0.05–0.79 and average genetic correlations of –0.37, –0.27 and –0.31 with milk, fat and protein yields, respectively. Estimates of genetic correlations with interval fertility traits (that is, number of days between events such as calving or insemination) are mostly negative varying from –0.38 to –0.84. In the UK, BCS is used as an indirect predictor of fertility in genetic evaluations (Banos and Coffey, 2010).

Climate change mitigation and adaptation traits

Successive reports from the Intergovernmental Panel on Climate Change and national bodies such as the UK Committee on Climate Change have presented the evidence for anthropogenic (human-induced) climate change, called for urgent action to reduce emissions from agriculture, and for adaptation to unavoidable climate change. We discuss the wider context for animal production in Chapter 14. Here we review a few of the potential mitigation and adaptation traits in dairy cattle breeding.

METHANE EMISSIONS Mitigation of enteric methane emissions in dairy cattle has become an important area of research, because methane is a potent greenhouse gas. In Chapter 5 some of the tools for measuring methane were outlined. Negussie *et al.* (2017) presented a review of some indirect or proxy measures for methane emissions; these include feed intake and feeding behaviour, milk production and composition, rumen morphology and rumen metabolites, or microbiome profiling. Proxies related to body weight or milk yield and composition are relatively simple, inexpensive and easier to implement in practice, while those related to rumen function are more challenging. However, the latter may prove more useful in the long run if they succeed in addressing methane production independently of dry-matter intake and production. The estimates of heritability for methane emissions are low to moderate, ranging from 0.12–0.45 (de Haas *et al.*, 2011; Lassen and Løvendahl, 2016; Breider *et al.*, 2019). While routine measurements of methane production are not currently commonplace, research is ongoing, with the aim of including such measurements in national selection indexes. Consequently, advances in methods for measuring methane directly or indirectly are expected.

MILK UREA NITROGEN One of the environmental challenges from dairy farming is the leakage of nitrogen from the urine of cattle grazing in pasture-based systems into groundwater and the resultant pollution. One of the possible mitigation steps is to breed cattle for lower urinary nitrogen (UN) excretion but this is difficult to measure. As mentioned in Chapter 5, milk urea nitrogen (MUN) concentration is a potential proxy trait which is easy to measure. Several studies have shown that when cows are fed diets differing in nitrogen content indoors, MUN is positively associated with UN (Beatson *et al.*, 2019). Under pasture grazing conditions, measurement of UN is more difficult. A study in New Zealand (Hendriks, 2016) indicated that UN increases linearly with MUN. Heritability estimates for MUN with stall-fed cows summarized by Beatson *et al.* (2019) varied from 0.13–0.59, indicating that it is possible to breed cattle for lower MUN. Some studies (e.g. Stoop *et al.*, 2007) have reported MUN to be positively correlated with milk protein percentage, raising the concerns that decreasing MUN may lead to reductions in milk protein yield and percentage. Beatson *et al.* (2019) indicated a small positive relationship with body weight, fat and protein yields (0.02–0.14) but negative correlations with traits associated with fertility (–0.09 to –0.12) and body condition (–0.13 to –0.28).

HEAT TOLERANCE Climate change has prompted research on breeding more robust dairy cows; this is likely to increase in importance over time. The availability of public websites (e.g. aWhere, 2019) make it possible to obtain the climatic conditions associated with a milk test yield record of any animal worldwide. The temperature–humidity index (THI) has been used as a tool to examine potential loss in productivity as a result of climate change. THI is calculated as function of dry bulb temperature (°C) but accounts for relative humidity (see Nguyen *et al.*, 2016), and so is likely to be of more physiological relevance to animals. Hayes *et al.* (2003) have shown that THI on the test day and 1, 2, 3, and 4 days before the test day had significant effects on herd test-day milk production yields. The change in productivity as a result of a unit change in the average THI on the test day and 1, 2, 3, and 4 days before the test day is regarded as a measure of the heat tolerance of the animal. The heritability of heat tolerance for milk, fat and protein yields reported by Nguyen *et al.* (2016) were 0.19, 0.17 and 0.17 in Holsteins and 0.24, 0.18 and 0.18 in Jerseys, respectively. Using data from up to three parities, these values were 0.22, 0.20 and 0.23 in Holsteins and 0.33, 0.26 and 0.27 in Jerseys, respectively. Hence, there appears to be considerable scope for selection to improve heat tolerance in temperate dairy breeds.

Methods and results of genetic evaluation

Milk production traits

Early methods used to evaluate bulls were based on the comparison of the performance of a bull's daughters with that of their dams. In the 1950s and 1960s, the emphasis changed to comparing a bull's daughters with their contemporaries, milked in the same herd, year and season. This has continued to be the basis of genetic evaluation, although there have been major increases in sophistication, in particular the development of the BLUP procedures and more recently the application of genomic methods described in Chapter 7. BLUP procedures have been adopted by most major dairying countries and progressively upgraded over the last few decades. For example, in the UK, sire-maternal grandsire model BLUP evaluations were first introduced in 1979. This improved the accuracy of evaluations compared to earlier methods by recognizing that not all cows were of equal merit, and hence the daughters of bulls being evaluated could be at an advantage or disadvantage, as a result of having a genetically good or bad mother. However, this BLUP model only accounted for differences in the merit of cows via their sire and maternal grandsire. Indexes were produced for cows by combining their sire's and maternal grandsire's PTA with their own production records. Individual animal model BLUP evaluations were introduced in the UK in 1992, providing PTAs directly for bulls and cows. This BLUP animal model for milk production traits was based on milk, fat and protein yields at 305 days, which were computed from the monthly milk records of each cow. Each of these milk traits were regarded as the same trait across various parities for each cow. This was referred to as the individual animal repeatability model. However, in the mid-1990s, a new approach was developed that directly analysed the milk traits measured at monthly intervals by fitting a curve to describe the pattern of production from the beginning until the end of lactation. Also, the records from each lactation were generally treated as separate traits. This method was called the test-day model (TDM; Schaeffer and Dekkers, 1994) as mentioned earlier in this chapter and in Chapter 7. The TDM made it possible to calculate PBVs for any period of the lactation and also calculate the genetic and phenotypic correlations between any two different periods in the lactation for milk traits. While the TDM continues to be used for milk traits and other traits that are repeatedly recorded, the individual animal model is used for most other traits such as type and fertility traits.

The steps involved in producing genetic evaluations, and key features of these, include:

- Collation and checking of milk records by milk-recording agencies and transfer of these, together with the relevant pedigree information, to the agency responsible for genetic evaluation (if this is different). In most countries there is more than one genetic evaluation per annum, so this step is repeated. (For example, in the UK at the time of writing three evaluations are done per annum by EGENES.) There is a trend towards more frequent evaluations, especially genomic evaluations. For example, genomic predictions for newly-genotyped young bulls are carried out monthly in the UK, Germany, USA and Canada. These allow breeding organizations and producers to make their selection decisions earlier and on the basis of better information, although there are obviously extra costs in doing evaluations more frequently.

- In the past, evaluations were often based on heifer lactation records only. However, increasing computer power has led to more lactations being included in evaluations. This was accompanied by the inclusion of test-day milk records from incomplete lactations for heifers that were still in progress, to allow earlier prediction of breeding values for bulls. In the UK, heifers with a progressing lactation with a minimum of three official test-day milk records were included in evaluations from January 1995 until the introduction of the TDM in the mid-2000s. However, with the introduction of the TDM, heifers and cows with at least three test-day yields in any lactation up to the fifth lactation are now used for evaluations in most countries. (For example, up to five lactations for each cow are included in UK evaluations. Completed lactation records collected since 1977 and test-day records since 1990 are included in the evaluation. Pedigree information goes back much further, for example to the 1950s in the case of the Holstein Friesian breed. Table 8.18 shows the total number of records involved in the July 2019 evaluations of dairy breeds in the UK.)

Table 8.18. The number of lactation records and the number of bulls and cows evaluated in the July 2019 genetic evaluation of dairy breeds in the UK by EGENES.

Breed	Number of lactations	Number of cows	Number of bulls
Holstein Friesian	26,884,964	9,302,363	108,543
Ayrshire	821,398	309,592	9,360
Jersey	790,954	268,489	7,730
Guernsey	316,384	113,897	2,637
Dairy Shorthorn	236,456	83,904	2,236
Brown Swiss	67,318	23,526	969
Montbéliarde	74,827	26,846	967

- Multi-trait evaluations are now common, especially for type, fertility and calving traits. Single traits such as milk yields in the various parities are usually treated as separate traits. In the UK, for instance, milk yield or fat yield in the first three parities are treated as separate traits with the fourth and fifth parities regarded as repeat measurements of parity three. However, in other countries (e.g. Canada) the multi-trait model regards milk, fat and protein as different traits within and across parities.
- Evaluations are usually carried out for one breed at a time. However, across-breed evaluations have been introduced in several countries recently, including New Zealand, UK and USA. This is most feasible in countries where herds comprising several breeds and crosses are common.
- In most countries the BLUP animal models are based on completed lactations of test-day yield (TDM) now including all known environmental (e.g. year and season of calving) and management (e.g. the date of milk recording, age at calving, parity number, calving interval) effects in the model. This means that there is no pre-adjustment for environmental or management factors affecting milk traits before BLUP evaluations are carried out.
- Breeding values or transmitting abilities are then predicted. Increasingly, dairy cattle breeding values or transmitting abilities are predicted using individual animal model BLUP using test-day records which includes all relationships between relatives and predicts breeding values for all animals. The statistical model used in the BLUP evaluations accounts for differences in management between and within herds by assigning animals to contemporary groups. An animal's milk record is usually assigned to a different contemporary group depending on the herd, year and day in which the test yield occurred. (For example, in the UK, the test-day milk yield record of animals are assigned to a herd test-day consisting of the herd in which the cow is milked and year, month and day on which the milk yield was measured. However, when the milk-recording agent visits the farm to record the milk yield on a particular date, some cows will be at the beginning of their lactation, others in mid or late lactation. This difference in different stages of lactation for milk records documented on the same day is corrected by fitting a

regression for days in milk. Factors such as age and season of calving are also included in the model and because these factors vary over time, they are nested within herd-calving year classes. The breed composition of crossbred animals is taken into account by fitting heterosis and recombination in the analysis within each lactation. The model also accounts for permanent environmental effects, which were described in Chapter 7.)

- Unknown parents are usually assigned to *genetic groups*. (For example, in the UK unknown parents are assigned to groups according to the year of birth and sex of their offspring, and their own sex and country of origin.)
- In countries with wide use of imported animals or semen, the foreign information is incorporated through INTERBULL MACE (see Chapter 7) which accounts for the genetic correlations among the countries. The INTERBULL code of practice requires that bulls have at least 150 daughters in 50 herds in the importing country for the Holstein breed, and at least 80 daughters in 20 herds for numerically smaller breeds such as the Ayrshire and Jersey, before the local information from the importing country is incorporated in MACE with the foreign information. However, countries may vary these requirements based on their national rules for publishing evaluations for bulls. In the UK, for example, local information is sent to INTERBULL to be incorporated into MACE for foreign Holstein bulls when they have at least 75 daughters in 50 UK herds. When the local information for bulls does not meet the INTERBULL requirements, countries either opt to officially publish the MACE evaluations for such bulls excluding local information, or (as in the UK) they may choose to combine the MACE and local information before publication. Such proofs are designated in the UK as 'combined proofs' with the emphasis on foreign versus local information proportional to the reliabilities of the two proofs. In the case of cows with both foreign and local information, the procedure is slightly different. There are no MACE proofs for cows, so the importing country usually obtains cows' proofs from the exporting country, which are converted to the local scale. The INTERBULL conversion factors are used as described in Chapter 7. Foreign and local proofs are combined by weighting each proof in proportion to its reliability. In the UK combined proofs are produced for cows only when the proof of the cow has a minimum reliability of 30% for milk production traits. The proofs of progeny of cows or bulls with a combined proof are correspondingly adjusted to account for the additional information in their parents.
- PBVs or PTAs (and indexes based on them) of the animals evaluated are expressed relative to some reference population of animals called the base. In most dairy cattle evaluations, results are expressed relative to a fixed base which is updated every few years. For example, at the time of writing the base used in the UK is the average merit of cows born in 2010 and PTAs expressed relative to this are denoted PTA10. This base was introduced in 2015. Bulls or cows which have positive PTA10 for any of the five milk production traits are expected to have genetically higher yields or percentages for the traits concerned compared to the average merit of cows born in 2010. Bulls or cows with negative PTA10 are expected to have genetically lower values than those born in 2010. For example, a bull with PTA of +800 kg milk, +35 kg fat, +30 kg protein, −0.05% fat and 0.00% protein is expected to leave daughters which yield 800 kg more milk, 35 kg more fat and 30 kg more protein with 0.05% lower fat content and the same protein content as the average of cows born in 2010. The alternative to a fixed base is a *rolling base*, such as that used in Canada, as discussed in Chapter 7.
- The results of the evaluations for bulls and cows which have achieved some threshold level of reliability are sent to the owners of the animals concerned, milk-recording agencies, breed societies, breeding companies and other interested parties. (Usually results with low reliability are restricted to the owners and recording agencies.) In the UK, evaluation results are published for bulls and cows which have minimum reliabilities of 50% and 30%, respectively, for milk production traits. In most countries, PTAs are published for kg milk, kg fat, kg protein, % fat, % protein and also for calving traits, health traits and fertility traits.
- In many countries, selection index scores are produced and published as well as PBVs or PTAs. These are of three main types: (i) economic indexes based on PBVs or PTAs for milk production traits only, accounting for expected differences in market values of milk, fat and protein, and possibly for different costs of production; (ii)

broader economic selection indexes including direct measures or predictors of traits such as longevity, fertility, disease resistance or live weight as well as milk production (e.g. the £PLI index used in the UK which, at the time of writing, includes production PTAs for milk, fat and protein yields, plus PTAs for fertility, udder health, leg health, calving ability, survival and efficiency – see Table 8.19); and (iii) indexes which use arbitrary weightings to combine PBVs or PTAs for milk production and type traits. In the second type of index milk production and other traits are combined in an objective way, based on the strength of the genetic associations with traits in the breeding goal and the relative economic values of these. The principles of economic selection indexes were introduced in Chapter 7, but more detailed examples are given later in this chapter.

Other traits

As indicated earlier, a growing number of traits other than milk production traits are being recorded and evaluated in the main temperate dairying countries. Type assessment takes place in virtually all of these countries, and there is increasing interest in recording and evaluating traits associated with reproduction, health, workability and longevity. In some countries there is also interest in traits associated with live weight, feed intake and body condition. Table 8.20 shows the extent to which these other traits are recorded and evaluated in various countries.

In some countries a single agency is responsible for genetic evaluation of all traits, in others a number of organizations are involved. For example, breed societies are responsible for the genetic evaluation of type traits in many countries. Obviously, the more agencies involved in the recording and evaluation of traits, the greater the importance of good communication and co-ordination.

The principles and methods of genetic evaluation of these traits are usually similar to those for milk production traits. In some cases the methods used are less sophisticated than those used for milk traits, since the volume of data is less as such traits may not be collected on all animals, or they are collected less frequently, or the traits are considered to be less important. In other cases, the smaller size of the data sets involved permits the use of more sophisticated methods. For example, genetic evaluations for linear-type traits scored by the Holstein UK in Britain and Ireland are carried out at EGENES using multi-trait animal model BLUP, although the analyses are performed for groups of associated traits, rather than all traits simultaneously, to reduce computing requirements. So, all udder traits are evaluated simultaneously, feet and leg traits are evaluated simultaneously, and so on.

The nature of many non-production traits means that they require some form of transformation before analysis, or special consideration of the method of presentation of PTAs. For example, the units of measurement for linear-type traits are arbitrary (usually scores from 1 to 9) so the results of genetic evaluations for type traits are often presented in standard deviation units rather than in the units of measurement. Hence, breeding values range from about −3 to about +3 standard deviations around the base. Figure 8.16 gives an example of the usual method of presentation. Traits such as

Table 8.19. An example of the way PTAs are presented for bulls. The bulls shown were the top 5 Holstein Friesian bulls from the July 2019 evaluation in the UK, ranked on their £PLI index.

Name of bull	£PLI reliability %	Predicted transmitting abilities (PTA95)					PLI £
		Milk kg	Fat kg	Protein kg	Fat %	Protein %	
VH Balisto Brook	73	437	36.3	24.0	0.23	0.12	794
Bomaz Altatopshot	71	1187	35.4	35.8	−0.13	−0.03	766
Co-op Robust Cabriolet	95	651	42.0	26.4	−0.19	0.06	755
Larcrest Commend	86	316	28.4	25.1	−0.20	0.18	752
Siemers Bloomfield	69	452	39.6	17.2	0.26	0.03	749

Table 8.20. Summary of some traits, other than milk production and type, evaluated for dairy sires in various countries in 2019. Note that this provides only a 'snapshot' of evaluations in countries in INTERBULL. Full details of trait definitions and evaluation procedures and the breeds concerned can be obtained from INTERBULL (2019).

Country	Reproduction				Health			Workability			Longevity
	Calving ease[a]	Calf mortality[a]	Non-return rate[b]	Other cow fertility	Somatic cell count	Mastitis	Other disease	Milking speed	Temperament	Other	
Australia	✓ (d)			✓	✓			✓	✓	✓	✓
Belgium	✓(d)			✓	✓						✓
Canada	✓ (d, m)		✓(c)	✓	✓	✓	✓	✓	✓		✓
Croatia					✓						
Czechia				✓	✓						
DFS[c]	✓ (d, m)	✓ (d, m)		✓	✓	✓	✓	✓	✓	✓	✓
Estonia					✓						
France	✓(d, m)	✓(d, m)		✓	✓	✓		✓	✓		✓
Germany[d]	✓ (d, m)	✓ (d, m)	✓ (b, c)	✓	✓			✓	✓		✓
Hungary	✓(d)				✓						✓
Ireland	✓ (d)	✓ (d)		✓	✓			✓	✓		✓
Israel	✓(d)	✓(d)		✓	✓						✓
Italy	✓ (d)		✓(b, c)	✓	✓			✓			✓
Japan					✓						
Latvia					✓						
Lithuania					✓						
Netherlands[e]	✓ (d, m)	✓(d, m)	✓ (b, c)	✓	✓			✓	✓		✓
New Zealand	✓(d)			✓	✓			✓	✓	✓	✓
Norway	✓ (d, m)	✓ (d, m)	✓ (c)	✓	✓	✓	✓	✓	✓	✓	✓
Poland				✓	✓						✓
Portugal					✓						
Rep. of Korea					✓						
South Africa				✓	✓						✓
Slovenia					✓			✓			✓
Slovak Rep.					✓						
Spain	✓(d, m)			✓	✓						✓
Switzerland	✓(d, m)	✓(d, m)	✓(b, c)	✓	✓	✓		✓	✓		✓
UK	✓(d, m)		✓(c)	✓	✓	✓	✓	✓	✓		✓
Uruguay				✓							
USA	✓ (d, m)	✓(d, m)		✓	✓	✓	✓				✓

[a] d, direct; m, maternal.
[b] b, bull; c, cow.
[c] DFS is a joint evaluaton for Denmark, Finland and Sweden.
[d] Germany, Austria and Luxembourg.
[e] Netherlands (including Belgium Flemish region).

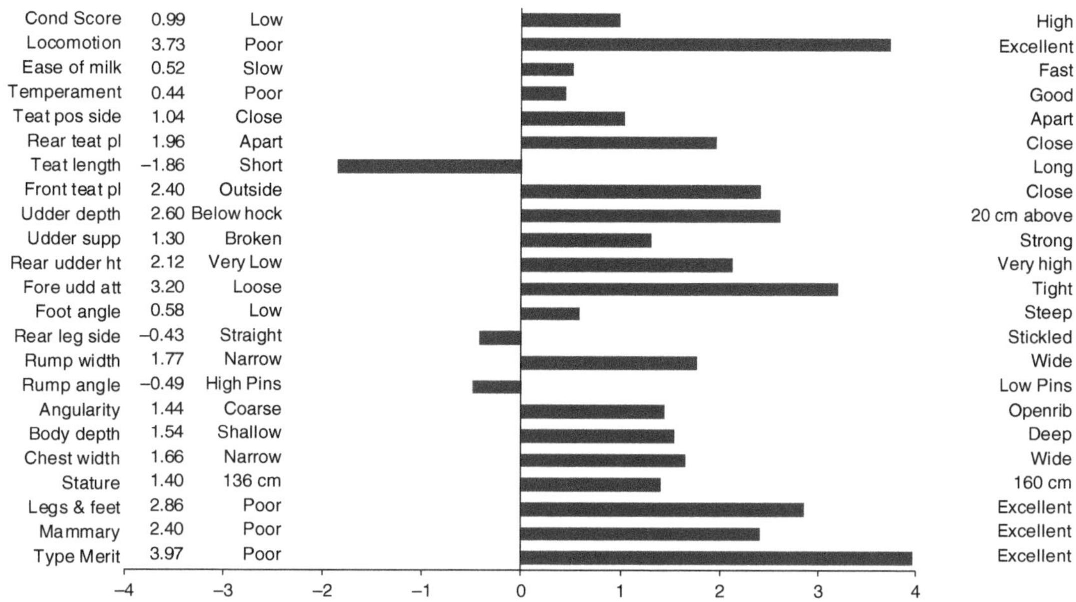

Fig. 8.16. An example of how breeding values for linear-type traits are usually presented (Holstein UK).

ease of calving, disease incidence and some measures of fertility are recorded on a categorical scale. That is, there are only a small number of discrete categories into which the records fall. As a result, the distributions of these traits may differ from the normal distribution on which the conventional methods of predicting breeding values depend. So, records of these traits are often transformed in some way prior to analysis, as mentioned in Chapter 2. Similarly, somatic cell counts usually show an 'extended' distribution, caused by a few animals or herds having very high counts. So, predictions of genetic merit are usually based on transformed data, often logarithms of the actual cell counts. PTAs can either be transformed back to the cell count scale or, perhaps more usefully, expressed in terms of the expected % increase or decrease in cell counts expected in a bull's daughters.

Apart from milk production and most type traits, many of the traits mentioned above have low heritabilities. This means that much larger daughter groups are needed to get reliable progeny test results. For example, to achieve a progeny test with a reliability of 0.8 requires records from around 40 daughters for a trait with a heritability of 0.35 (e.g. first lactation milk production), but over 150 daughters for a trait with a heritability of 0.1 (e.g. some measures of reproduction and resistance to disease). Since the resources available for testing are limited, this means that fewer bulls can be tested if the aim is to produce reliable progeny test results for traits which have a low heritability. However, even if progeny testing is geared towards higher heritability traits, moderately reliable evaluations of these other traits on young bulls are still better than none. One of the major advantages of genomic selection is that high reliabilities can be obtained even for young bulls for traits of low heritability. A requirement, however, is that an initial set of bulls with high reliability evaluations are available as the reference population (see Chapter 7) to compute the SNP solutions for such traits. Then these SNP solutions can be used to compute GEBVs for young bulls with high reliabilities. In the UK, for example, the reliability for GEBV for a young bull for longevity with a heritability of 0.06 is 0.54, which is roughly equivalent to a young bull having about 80 daughters in a conventional progeny test.

The lack of uniformity in recording non-production traits initially hindered the objective use of information across countries. Great strides have been made in 'harmonizing' the way linear-type traits are scored in different countries, and which traits are scored; however, a few differences remain. The problem was largely overcome with the introduction of MACE for international evaluations. This method treats the type traits from the various countries as different traits and includes the genetic correlations among the bulls for these traits in the analysis. For example, in the INTERBULL MACE evaluation in August 2019, the genetic correlations for foot angle between UK and Canada, UK and Italy, USA and Canada, and France and USA were 0.83, 0.73, 0.88 and 0.84, respectively. This approach increases the accuracy of type evaluations for bulls that are used across several countries.

Indexes of overall economic merit

In the past, most dairy cattle breeding schemes worldwide have been geared towards increasing output. There is now growing interest in 'broader' selection goals, stimulated by at least four factors. The first of these is the surplus of dairy products in many temperate countries. Quotas or price constraints in some countries have made higher production *per se* less attractive and reducing costs of production more attractive. Secondly, there is growing public concern for the health and welfare of farm animals, as well as a wider appreciation of the direct economic consequences of disease. There is evidence from several countries that selection for milk production alone tends to lead to a deterioration in udder quality, a higher incidence of mastitis and some other diseases, and poorer reproductive performance. While some of these problems can be offset by improved management, it makes sense to try to breed healthier cows in the first place. Thirdly, the formation of nucleus herds in some countries has facilitated direct recording of some additional traits for selection (e.g. feed intake and health events). Fourthly, the availability of genomic methodology to obtain more accurate predictions for some of the low heritability traits has facilitated the inclusion of some of these in indexes.

Economic indexes which combine production PTAs have become quite widely used in many countries since the 1990s in an attempt to address the first of the issues listed above (e.g. the PIN index in the UK, INET in the Netherlands, INEL in France and PFT in Italy). The PIN index in the UK (phased out in 2014) was fairly typical of this type of production index. PIN was based on PTAs for kg milk, kg fat and kg protein, each weighted by their expected future economic value. These weightings took into account the increasing value of protein compared to fat (a relative value of 1.5:1 was used in PIN as of 1995), the extra transport and cooling costs of high volume-low solids milk, and the cost (at that time) of leasing extra quota to match the higher productivity of daughters of high PTA bulls.

Farmers have long appreciated the need for 'balanced' breeding objectives, and have sought to breed cows which will be functionally sound as well as productive. In many countries there are combined production and type indexes in use in dairy cattle breeding with this aim in mind. However, until recently, most of these have been based on arbitrary weightings on production and type. There is now growing interest in extending production indexes to include measures of reproduction, health, workability and longevity, with components of these overall indexes weighted according to sound economic and scientific principles. In some of these indexes type traits feature as predictors of traits contributing to profit, in others functional type traits (i.e. those relating to the mammary system or feet and legs) are given direct economic value. Table 8.21 gives some examples of this type of index in use in several countries in 2019. This table gives only a 'snapshot' of what is a fast-changing field as countries strive to develop indexes that underpin sustainable, higher welfare dairy production systems.

The development of ITEM, the first broader dairy cattle breeding index in the UK – developed in 1995 by the Scottish Agricultural College (now Scotland's Rural College) and the University of Edinburgh – provides a good example of some of the issues involved in producing broader indexes. ITEM (index of total economic merit) was based on exactly the same principles as PIN and attached the same economic values to PTAs for kg milk, fat and protein as those used in PIN. It is relatively straightforward to calculate the economic values of higher production, but more difficult to assess the benefits of longevity. Detailed studies of costs and returns in dairy herds,

Table 8.21. Examples of several indexes of economic merit in use in 2019. Note that this provides only a 'snapshot' of indexes in some countries with evaluations in INTERBULL. Full details of actual weights on traits can be obtained from INTERBULL. (After INTERBULL, 2019).

Country	Index	Traits included in index						
		Milk, protein, or fat production (one or more yields or %)	Reproduction	Health (including SCC)	Workability	Longevity	Type traits (in own right, or as predictors)	Beef production/ growth
Canada	Total Economic Value	✓		✓	✓	✓	✓	
DFS	Nordic Total Merit Index	✓	✓	✓	✓	✓	✓	✓
Norway	Total Merit Index	✓	✓	✓	✓		✓	✓
UK	£PLI	✓	✓	✓		✓	✓	✓
USA	USDA Net Merit $	✓	✓	✓		✓	✓	

and computer-based simulation, indicated that the net effect of improving longevity by 1% (i.e. 1% fewer cows culled involuntarily in the first 4 lactations) was around £3.37 per cow per annum (Veerkamp *et al.*, 1995). This arises through lower heifer rearing, replacement and culling costs, and having more cows producing at the mature yield level.

The version of ITEM used from 1995 to 1997 included breeding values for four linear-type traits associated with cow longevity. These were udder depth, teat length, angularity and foot angle. The choice of type traits to go into ITEM was based on an analysis of all available linear-type assessment records (Brotherstone and Hill, 1991 and unpublished results). This analysis examined the longevity of cows in relation to linear-type scores; the best possible 'test' of the value of these scores in measuring the functional soundness of cows under practical dairy farming conditions. The four type traits chosen had the closest genetic associations with longevity once the effects of differences in milk production were removed. Genetically shallower udders, shorter teats, greater angularity and steeper foot angles were all associated with longer herd life. Several other traits were linked more weakly to longevity but they added little to the overall picture once these four main traits had been accounted for.

After further research, in 1999, ITEM was modified with the addition of direct measures of the lifespan of bulls' daughters. This modified index was called Profitable Lifetime Index (£PLI). This was based on the same principles as ITEM but the evaluations for lifespan were more accurate. These were based on a direct measure of the longevity in terms of the number of lactations the daughters of the bull have completed and indirect predictions based on type traits (fore-udder attachment, legs and feet composite, mammary composite) and somatic cell count. The £PLI value represents the additional profit a high £PLI bull is expected to return from each of its milking daughters over her lifetime compared to an average bull of £0 PLI.

In the early 2000s, £PLI was expanded further to include more traits associated with profitability and cow welfare. The latest (at the time of writing) version of £PLI, introduced in 2018, includes mastitis, lameness, fertility and efficiency. Mastitis is accounted for indirectly using somatic cell count and the type trait, udder composite; calving interval and non-return rate at 56 days are used as measures of fertility. Locomotion is used as an indirect measure of lameness and body weight is used as a measure of efficiency in utilization of feed resources for maintenance. Table 8.22 shows the different traits in £PLI and their relative weights. £PLI was intended for use for selecting bulls within the various breeds and it was expressed on a different base for each breed. However, due to an increasing trend towards crossbreeding in the UK, to address the fertility problems mentioned and tighten calving patterns, new indexes have been produced that allow comparison across breeds (Holstein Friesian, Ayrshire, Jersey, Guernsey, Brown Swiss, Shorthorn). The Spring Calving Index (£SCI) was introduced in August 2014 and is intended for UK farmers operating a spring block calving system, making extensive use of grass and targeting production of around 6,000 kg/yr. Similarly in August 2018, the Autumn Calving Index (£ACI) was introduced for farmers operating an autumn block calving system, with a higher requirement for winter feeding and targeting production of around 7500 kg/yr. £PLI, £SCI and £ACI are expressed on different genetic bases, so index scores cannot be compared across the different index types. Table 8.22 shows the different traits in £SCI and £ACI and their relative weights.

The international nature of dairy industries, with many AI bulls used worldwide, implies that an increasing array of performance information is becoming available on bulls from different countries. Therefore, broader indexes have become more important, providing a means to combine many more pieces of information with the appropriate emphasis. The development and wider use of the sort of index described here should simplify selection, and help breeding organizations and individual producers to breed cows which are both

Table 8.22. The relative weights on the different components of the three economic indexes used in the UK. (After AHDB, 2019b).

Traits groups	£PLI	£SCI	£ACI
Production	34.4	27.4	30.4
Fertility	15.3	24.8	21.4
Survival	15.1	11.6	18.0
Udder health	13.7	11.6	10.9
Efficiency	11.8	18.4	14.1
Leg health	8.1	4.0	3.3
Calving ability	1.6	2.2	1.9

healthier and more profitable. Figure 8.17 illustrates the relative emphasis on various traits in the national indexes of several European countries. In addition, Figs 8.18 and 8.19 summarize the relative weight and the proportionate estimates of response worldwide for the major traits in the national economic indexes for dairy cows from 1917 to 2017 (Miglior *et al.,* 2017). The figures illustrate that the main emphasis was on selecting for production, and to a lesser extent conformation, in the early years. In more recent years, the relative emphasis on health and fertility has increased at the expense of that on production and conformation.

Evidence of genetic improvement and its value

In several countries selection experiments in dairy cattle have shown that substantial rates of improvement can be achieved by selection on PTAs or their equivalent. In several cases rates of genetic change of about 2% per annum have been achieved (Smith,1984). While these experiments served a useful purpose in the early days of progeny testing and national genetic evaluation schemes, there is now more direct evidence available. The widespread use of AI in most countries has created strong genetic links across herds and years. Hence, the mean PTAs or PBVs from national BLUP evaluations, for animals born in successive years, provide estimates of national genetic trends. These show direct evidence of the rates of genetic improvement that are being achieved in practice.

For example, Fig. 8.20 shows the genetic trends in milk, fat and protein production in milk-recorded Holstein Friesian cows in the UK and the US over a 42-year period. The graph shows cumulative change in cows' predicted breeding values, which equates to the expected genetic change in performance of the cows themselves. Substantial rates of genetic change of over 79 kg milk per annum were sustained in the US over this 42-year period (García-Ruiz *et al.*, 2016; Council on Dairy Cattle Breeding, 2019). The equivalent trend in the UK was about 39 kg per annum over the whole period, but rates of change in PBVs were very low until the mid-1980s. The genetic trends in the USA from 2011 to 2015, since the introduction of genomic selection for milk, fat and protein yields, were 109 kg, 6.0 kg and 4.1 kg, respectively (García-Ruiz *et al.*, 2016). The genetic change in length of productive life was +1.17 months over the same period.

Rates of genetic change in production have accelerated in many countries over the last few decades following the importation of North American genetic material. Figure 8.21 shows the trends in genetic merit of bulls for milk and protein yields in some major dairying countries. The convergence of genetic merit over the last decade is largely due to these importations, but also to improvements in local testing programmes and the implementation of genomic selection in most dairying countries.

Clearly, achieving genetic improvements in yield is only useful if it leads to improved profitability. In the UK, the economic index £PLI has been in use for over 20 years; as explained earlier, it represents the additional profit a high £PLI bull is expected to return from each of its milking daughters over her lifetime compared to an average bull with a value of zero. In the last 9 years, the rate of change in £PLI has been around £62 per year (Marco Winters, AHDB; personal communication). The profit potential of using bulls of high £PLI has been demonstrated from a variety of farm costings. Work undertaken in 2011 by consultancy company Promar (a division of Genus plc), showed that each £PLI point was worth £4.21 in additional margin per cow per year with appropriate management. This translates to £24,000 extra margin per year through better genetics alone, in a top £PLI herd of 100 cows, compared with an average £PLI herd (FarmingUK, 2020).

Probably the longest-running cattle breeding experiment in the world commenced in the mid-1970s at the University of Edinburgh, the East of Scotland College of Agriculture and the Animal Breeding Research Organisation, in the Langhill herd. It continues today at SRUC's Dairy Cattle Research Centre in Dumfries. The herd was initially intended to demonstrate that farmers could have confidence in choosing AI bulls based on their progeny test results – AI use in Scotland was relatively low at the time. However, subsequent research in the herd investigated a wide range of production, feed intake, efficiency, health, welfare, economic and environmental consequences of selection, and contributed to the development of broader breeding goals and indexes in the UK and beyond. From the outset, cows in the Langhill herd were bred to bulls with the highest possible PTAs for kg fat plus protein. From the mid-1970s a control herd was maintained using frozen semen from bulls of around

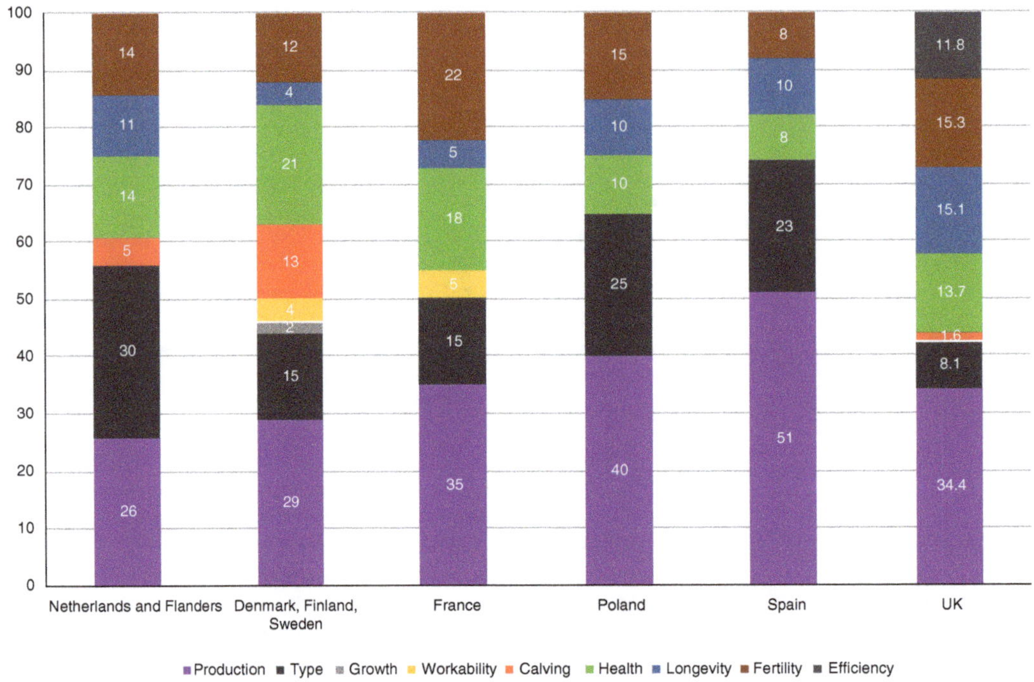

Fig. 8.17. The relative emphasis given to several trait groups in various European dairy indexes. (After Eurogenomics, 2019; AHDB, 2019b.)

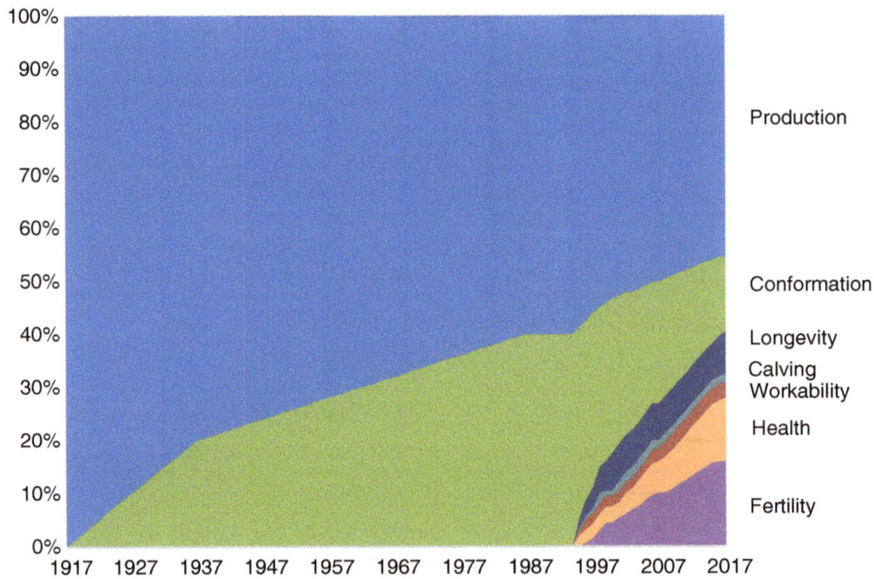

Fig. 8.18. A worldwide summary of the relative weights for the various major traits in national economic indexes for dairy cows from 1917 to 2017. (After Miglior *et al.*, 2017.)

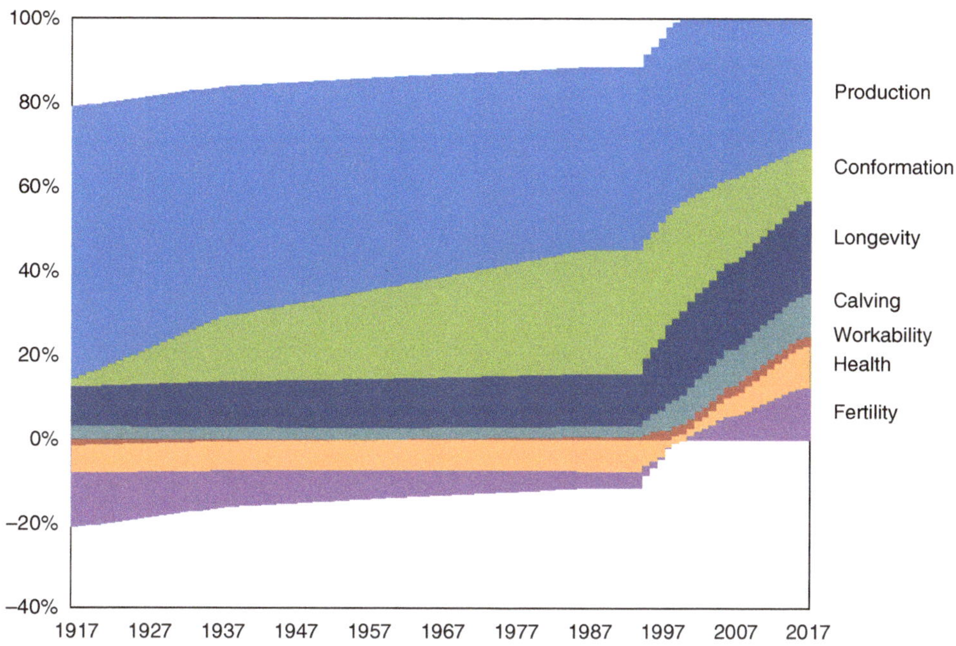

Fig. 8.19. The proportionate estimates of response worldwide for the various major traits in the national economic indexes for dairy cows from 1917 to 2017. (After Miglior *et al.*, 2017.)

national average merit for kg fat plus protein at the time. However, the control bulls were mainly British Friesian bulls, and the national herd was increasingly made up of North American Holstein bulls. So, from the late 1980s control bulls of around national average merit for fat and protein production were used, chosen to have a similar proportion of Holstein genes to selection line bulls. Both selection and control line cows at Langhill have been fed during the winter housing period on complete diets, with feed intake measured on a portion of the herd (Fig. 8.22). Since the mid-1990s, the two lines have been evaluated under two contrasting feeding systems. Most recently these have been systems based on either home-grown forage (with an average dry-matter content of about 324 g/kg and average ME of about 12 MJ/kg DM) or by-products (with an average dry-matter content of about 417 g/kg and average ME of about 13 MJ/kg DM). Table 8.23 shows the performance of animals in the two lines on the two systems between 2016 and 2018. These results demonstrate that, in both high- and lower-input systems, cows of high genetic merit generally have higher economic performance than their contemporaries of only average genetic merit.

Genotype-by-environment interactions

The long-running debate on the importance of genotype-by-environment interactions (whether you need to breed 'horses for courses') has been refuelled by the massive importation of North American Holstein semen into many other countries since the 1980s. In the past, most experimental studies have indicated that, in temperate dairying systems, breed or strain-by-feeding system interactions are of little or no importance, at least for production per cow. In other words, the breeds or strains rank similarly in different feeding systems (Jasiorowski *et al.*, 1983; Holmes, 1995), although the ranking of individual sires may still change.

The bigger the difference in performance between breeds or strains, and the bigger the difference between the environments in which they are compared, the greater the likelihood of finding important interactions. The differences between typical milk production systems in Canada and New Zealand are

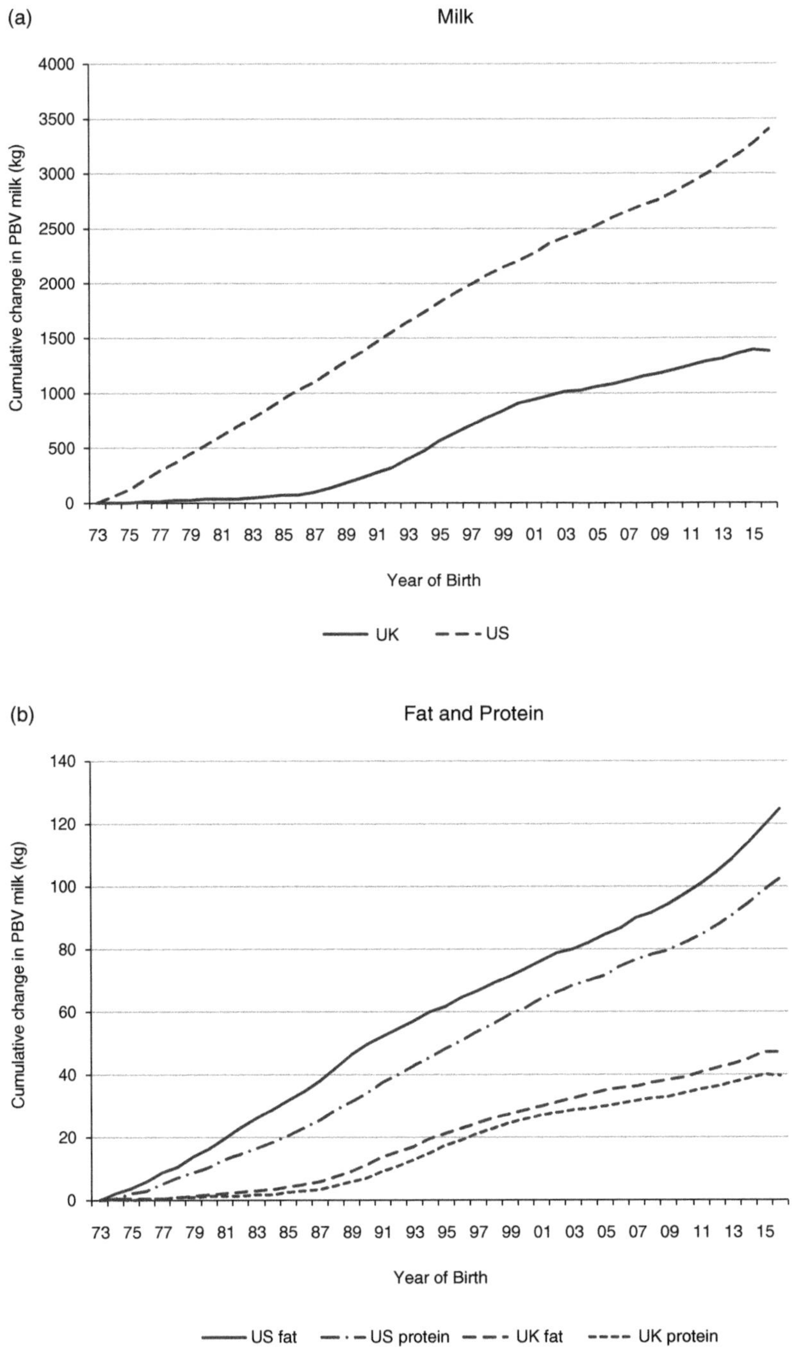

Fig. 8.20. Genetic trends in milk, fat and protein production in milk-recorded Holstein Friesian cows in the UK and the US from 1973 to 2016. (After García-Ruiz *et al.*, 2016; Council on Dairy Cattle Breeding, 2019; EGENES, 2019.)

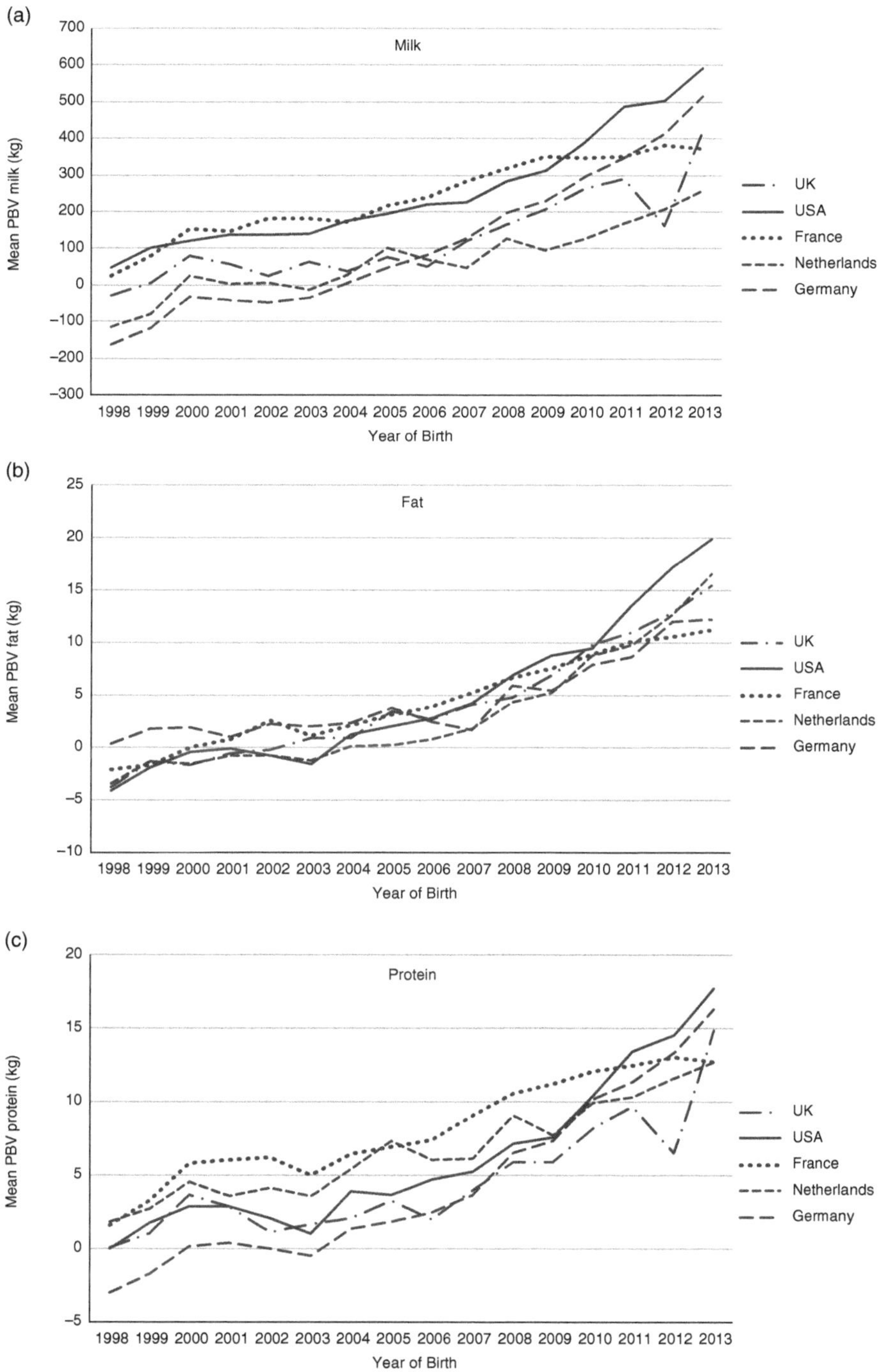

Fig. 8.21. Trends in the genetic merit of bulls for (a) milk, (b) fat and (c) protein yields in UK scale for some major dairying countries 1998 to 2013. (After EGENES, 2019; INTERBULL, 2019.)

Table 8.23. Performance of selection and control line animals from the Langhill trial over a 3-year period (2016–2018).

	Home-grown feeding system		By-product feeding system	
	Selection	Control	Selection	Control
Milk yield (kg)	8726	8292	11312	9781
Fat %	4.26	3.86	3.80	3.49
Protein %	3.32	3.12	3.28	3.11
Fat plus protein yield (kg)	662	579	809	646
Average daily dry-matter intake (kg)	17.65	16.19	22.03	20.07
Live weight (kg)	613	619	638	624
Condition score (5-point scale)	2.17	2.31	2.21	2.34
Productive Life Index (£PLI)	356	–3	366	7

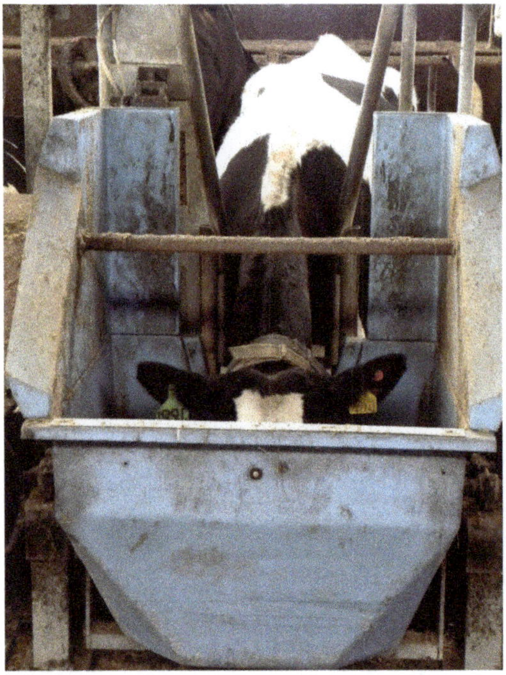

Fig. 8.22. A cow at the Langhill Dairy Cattle Research Centre in Scotland feeding through a HOKO gate which permits monitoring of individual cow intakes. (Courtesy of Scotland's Rural College.)

among the widest in temperate areas. Most dairy herds in Canada are fed relatively high levels of concentrates, while most in New Zealand, until recently, were fed none at all. For this reason, there was particular interest in the results of a trial to compare the performance of the progeny of Canadian and New Zealand Holstein Friesian sires in each of these two countries. Some of the results of this trial, which began in 1984/1985, are shown in Table 8.24. There were major differences in milk production and live weight between heifers reared in the two countries, but these were largely due to differences in management and environment. Compared to the daughters of NZ sires, the daughters of Canadian sires produced slightly more milk of lower fat and protein content, and were slightly heavier and taller at 18 months of age (though not at some other ages) in both Canada and New Zealand. So, there was no evidence of a strain × environment interaction for production apart from first lactation protein yield and percentage protein (Charagu, 1997). Similarly, there were no interactions for other traits such as calving interval, length of productive life or numbers of lactations completed, and economic efficiency in terms of profitability up to the end of lactation or over the productive life of cows. However, despite the similar rankings of strains in the two environments, there were poor correlations between individual sire proofs estimated within each country. In other words, individual sires re-ranked, depending on the country in which they were evaluated.

Mwansa (1997) studied two measures of longevity or survival in the same population to examine the possible genotype-by-environment interaction. The study found some evidence of a genotype-by-environment interaction for survival traits and recommended that the traits should be considered as separate traits in the different environments.

Results from the Langhill trial in Table 8.23 show some evidence of a genotype-by-feeding system interaction, but comparing the average production of the four groups of animals is a fairly crude test. The mean 305-day milk yield, fat plus protein yield and £PLI index are generally higher for the selected lines in the high energy diet

Table 8.24. A comparison of the performance of heifers sired by Canadian or New Zealand Holstein Friesian bulls, and born, reared and milked in Canada or New Zealand. (After Kakwaya and Peterson, 1991; Peterson, 1991; Holmes, 1995; Charagu, 1997; Mwansa, 1997.)

	Nationality of dam and country in which daughters were reared			
	Canada		New Zealand	
	Canadian sires	NZ sires	Canadian sires	NZ sires
Milk yield (kg)	6,699[a]	6,392	3,389[a]	3,155
Fat yield (kg)	241	242	139	138
Protein yield (kg)	215	212	108[a]	105
Fat content (%)	3.64[a]	3.85	4.12[a]	4.38
Protein content (%)	3.22[a]	33.4	3.20[a]	3.33
Live weight at 18 mo. (kg)	447[a]	445	357[a]	347
Height at 18 mo. (cm)	131[a]	129	120[a]	118
No. of completed lactations	2.5[a]	2.2	3.8[a]	4.5
Calving interval (days)	425	377	376	372
Economic efficiency over productive life in $/1,000 M	267	262	121[a]	123
Length of productive life (d)	864[a]	703	1,214[a]	1,456

[a]Means within a row/country significantly different at $P < 0.05$.

compared to the low energy diet. Table 8.25 shows the rate of genetic change for several production traits calculated as regressions of PTAs on year of birth (1996 to 2016) of the Langhill selection line animals managed in the two different feeding systems. None of the differences between the two lines were significant, but the rates of change in the home-grown feeding system tended to be lower than those in the high-input system. (Similar results for milk yield have been reported in a study in Australia (Fulkerson *et al.*, 1996).) This may indicate some degree of genotype-by-feeding system interaction. It appears that cows selected for production in high-input feeding systems may be unable to eat enough low energy feed to keep pace with their potential extra milk yield. Despite mobilizing more body tissue, they are still unable to match the increase in yield seen in their contemporaries on a higher concentrate diet. The question is whether these interactions are large enough to warrant the development of new breeding strategies which increase emphasis on feed intake, rather than tissue loss, to 'fuel' future increases in yield. While research at Langhill, and elsewhere, will continue to monitor the levels of these interactions, the implementation of broader selection indexes in several countries with reduced emphasis on milk yield and more emphasis on fitness traits may reduce the potential impact of genotype-by-environment interactions in practice.

The wider use of international MACE evaluations, described earlier, will also be helpful where

Table 8.25. Change in PTAs per year for production traits in Langhill cows born from 1996 to 2016 managed under two feeding systems. (Source: EGENES, 2019.)

	Change in PTAs for production traits (regression coefficients with standard errors in brackets)	
	Home-grown diet	By-product diet
Milk yield (kg/year)	26.47 (2.5)	31.98 (2.4)
Fat %	−0.0002 (0.0001)	−0.002 (0.001)
Protein %	−0.00005 (0.0004)	−0.002 (0.001)
Fat yield (kg/year)	1.05 (0.01)	1.12 (0.01)
Protein yield (kg/year)	0.86 (0.08)	0.90 (0.07)

genotype-by-environment interactions are important. These evaluations allow for different genetic correlations between performance in different countries. This should ensure that the ranking of imported sires, based on MACE proofs, is more closely tailored to the average production system in the country concerned. Also, in countries that import a high proportion of dairy sires for breeding from other countries, the impact of interactions may be reduced through the use of broader indexes including affected traits (e.g. reproduction, feed intake).

One of the approaches that has been attempted for improving dairy productivity in developing countries involves importing improved breeds such as the

Holstein into small-holder systems, either for cross breeding or to be raised as pure breeds. Given the huge differences in management between large-scale temperate and small-holder systems, high levels of genotype-by-environmental interaction are expected. Studies examining the degree of genotype-by-environment interactions between developed countries and small-holder systems are rare due to the lack of adequate data. Ojango and Pollott (2002) estimated a genetic correlation between first lactation milk yield in UK and Kenya of 0.49 ± 0.06, implying a genotype-by-environment interaction in milk yield. The range of genetic correlations published by INTERBULL between dairy systems in South Africa and other countries for milk yield varies from 0.69 to 0.84, further indicating genotype-by-environment interactions. Also, pure breeds from temperate countries often have very low survivability in tropical environments, therefore it is becoming more common to cross indigenous breeds (that are typically well adapted to the local environment conditions but have low productivity) to improved exotic breeds (that are typically poorly adapted to the local environmental conditions but highly productive), to create animals that are intermediate in terms of both adaptation and productivity (Marshall *et al.*, 2016; African Dairy Genetics Gains Project, 2019).

Practical Guidelines on Selection

Pedigree breeders often have strong views on the sort of animal they wish to breed. They also have the interest and knowledge to wade through the vast quantities of information available, in an increasingly international market, to find animals suited to their breeding programme. It is generally healthy to have individualists and risk-takers in this sector of a livestock breeding industry, as long as there are universal yardsticks available for their customers to compare their products (e.g. the PTAs and indexes described above).

In contrast, many commercial dairy farmers are interested in a simpler set of rules to help them make sense of the advertising material, to become better informed in discussions with persuasive semen sales staff, and ultimately to breed more profitable cows. Although the tools available for selection are being updated continually, some general guidelines for selection to improve profitability are given below. These are aimed primarily at commercial herds, but most are equally relevant to pedigree breeders whose priority is to improve overall merit in commercially-important traits:

- Check that the breed, breed type or cross that you are using is the most appropriate for your production circumstances, by examining the results of objective breed comparisons and recording schemes such as those outlined in this chapter.
- Always use progeny-tested AI bulls with reliable proofs, or genomically evaluated young AI bulls with reliable proofs, to breed replacement heifers.
- Make a shortlist of bulls ranked in descending order on an appropriate index of overall economic merit (e.g. £PLI, £SCI or £ACI in the UK).
- If you firmly believe that your future markets will differ from 'the mainstream', for example because of a special milk payment scheme, or a strong trade for surplus heifer calves, then eliminate bulls from this list which have unfavourable production PTAs or type characteristics, or 'promote' those with favourable characteristics. Similarly, if you have a particularly high incidence of mastitis you may wish to pay particular attention to bulls with favourable PTAs for SCC. However, this second-stage screening should be fairly light, or the benefits of ranking bulls on an economic index will be severely diluted.
- Eliminate bulls from the list if their semen is very highly priced relative to their genetic merit.
- From the remaining animals select a few (e.g. 2 to 4) reliably proven progeny-tested bulls (reliabilities over 75%), or young genomically evaluated bulls, or use bulls of both types. In theory, a single reliably tested bull is sufficient, but selecting more bulls gives scope to avoid matings between close relatives and reduces the risks of all of the semen coming from a chance low-quality batch.
- Avoid matings between close relatives (see Chapter 4 for more details). (Breed societies, recording agencies or breeding companies may provide a service for members, to produce mating lists to help avoid matings between cows currently in the herd and a nominated panel of bulls.)
- Manage the herd to achieve high fertility and, where appropriate, a compact calving pattern. This will maximize the opportunity to breed replacements from the top heifers and cows in the herd, as identified by PTAs or indexes from recording/

evaluation agencies. Use of sexed semen will further increase female selection intensities. It also allows a higher proportion of the herd to be mated to a beef bull, where appropriate.

- If there are extra heifer calves available as potential replacements, use the most appropriate PTAs/indexes available for youngstock and select those with the most favourable scores.

Summary

- Returns from milk production are the most important returns in both high- and low-input dairying systems. Feed costs are the most important variable costs in both high and low-input systems, although the relative importance of concentrate versus forage costs differs substantially between systems.
- Generally, the highest-yielding breeds, and the highest-yielding individuals within breeds, have the highest gross efficiency of conversion of feed energy to milk energy, and produce the highest margins over feed (and other) costs. While production per cow is a major component of profitability in higher-input dairying systems, production per hectare is usually more important in lower-input pastoral systems. The ranking of breeds on production per hectare is less clear than that on production per cow.
- In most temperate dairying countries, the Holstein breed is predominant. However, the Jersey breed is also numerically important in some countries with mainly pastoral production, like New Zealand and Australia. Over the last few decades, the local strains of black-and-white cattle in many temperate countries have been largely substituted by higher-yielding North American Holstein strains. In most temperate countries, there has been only a modest level of use of crossbreeding between dairy breeds, other than to enable breed substitution. New Zealand and Australia are exceptions, with higher use of crossing. However, this appears to be increasing in other temperate countries, especially to increase cow robustness. Crossing between exotic and indigenous breeds is common in tropical countries.
- In the past most within-breed selection programmes have concentrated on increasing yield, with some attention being paid also to the type or conformation of cows. However, there is now increasing interest in broader breeding goals and indexes because of: (i) the increased emphasis in payment schemes in many countries on the yield (or content) of components, particularly protein; (ii) the introduction of milk quotas in some countries; and (iii) the actual or perceived deleterious effect of selection for yield on the health, fertility and welfare of cows.
- Progeny testing schemes have been central to genetic improvement of dairy cattle in most dairying countries since the mid-1900s. The basis of progeny testing schemes is the comparison of the milk production of the daughters of young bulls being tested with the daughters of other bulls recorded in the same herd, year and season. Results are then combined across herds, years and seasons and used to predict the genetic merit of the bulls being tested, and of other animals in the recorded population.
- The main advantage of progeny testing is that it produces accurate predictions of a bull's genetic merit, based on the performance of daughters in commercial herds. The disadvantages are that progeny testing schemes are costly to run, and the results take many years to materialize. Progeny testing schemes also depend on access to a large population of milk-recorded cows, and so they are difficult to sustain in numerically small breeds.
- In the late 1970s and early 1980s, nucleus breeding schemes using multiple ovulation and embryo transfer (MOET) and sib testing were proposed as an alternative to progeny testing. Production records from a bull's sisters are available much sooner than that on his offspring. These schemes reduced generation intervals substantially compared to those possible in progeny testing, but they also reduced the accuracy of selection on males. However, on balance, the gains from shorter generation intervals outweighed the losses from lower accuracy, and the proposed schemes were predicted to give higher rates of genetic gain.
- MOET nucleus schemes were established in several countries in the 1980s and later. However, most schemes evolved into 'fast track' testing schemes which became integrated into progeny testing schemes, rather than replacing them as originally proposed.
- Ongoing MOET nucleus schemes have evolved further to incorporate genomic selection. Well-designed open nucleus schemes provide a good mechanism to record difficult-to-measure traits in a smaller population, enabling genomic selection to be implemented for these traits across cow populations in the countries concerned (and beyond).

- Progeny testing schemes for dairy bulls in most countries have been based on national or regional milk-recording schemes. Traditionally, milk records of cows have only been used for genetic evaluation once lactations are complete. Currently most countries used the test-day milk yield obtained at various intervals in the computation of the genetic merit of bulls using the test-day model. This model better corrects for the environmental effects in play when the milk yield record was obtained. It allows for the relationship among different stages of the lactation to be accounted for. This can reduce substantially the time lag between making test inseminations from a young bull and getting an initial proof as daughters with at least three test-day milk yield can be included in the evaluation.
- Yields of milk, fat and protein are all moderately highly heritable, while fat and protein content are both highly heritable. There are high genetic correlations among milk, fat and protein yields, indicating that selection for any one of these three traits is expected to lead to increases in the other two. However, there are negative genetic correlations between all three yield traits and protein percentage, and between yields of milk and both protein and fat percentage, indicating that selection for yield is likely to lead to a reduction in protein or fat content, or both.
- Assessments of type or conformation are widely used in dairy cattle breeding. Most schemes now use linear assessment, in which the characteristics of the cow are scored in relation to biological extremes. The results of linear assessment are more repeatable, and more amenable to scientific analysis than those from earlier schemes. Most linear-type traits have moderately high heritabilities, and many are useful predictors of traits of economic importance.
- A growing number of countries are recording and evaluating various measures of reproduction, health, workability and longevity, or traits associated with them. Most of these traits have relatively low heritabilities. However, there are unfavourable associations between some of them and production, so genetic evaluations are valuable. PTAs for these traits are incorporated into indexes of overall economic merit in several countries. In a few countries, measurements of feed intake, live weight and body condition, or predictors of these traits, are also being used in indexes, or are being investigated with this in mind.
- There is growing interest in recording claw diseases traits in many countries due to welfare concerns and economic impact. Recording systems are well established in Nordic countries and are expanding to the rest of Europe. These traits are of low heritability and are usually combined into a claw health index for use in breeding programmes.
- BLUP methods of predicting breeding values or transmitting abilities for milk production have been adopted by most major dairying countries over the last couple of decades. Individual animal model BLUP is used with a test-day model in most cases This includes all relationships between relatives and predicts breeding values for all animals. Evaluations are usually based on multiple lactations.
- Genomic selection is increasingly used in many temperate dairy countries for the selection of young bulls into AI studs, and for selection of bull dams. This involves initially calculating the relationship between SNPs and various performance traits in a reference population. The equations derived are then used to calculate the genomic breeding values of young bulls (with no recorded daughters) for selection for widespread use in AI, or of heifers (with no records) for selection as bull dams. The opportunity to select animals at a very young age has reduced the generation interval and increased the rate of genetic progress in many dairy populations. Hence, genomic selection is superseding progeny testing in many countries.
- The principles and methods of genetic evaluation of type, reproduction, health, workability and longevity traits are usually similar to those for milk production traits. The nature of many non-production traits means that they require some form of transformation before analysis, or special consideration on the method of presentation of PTAs.
- In countries with widespread use of imported animals or semen, foreign information plays an important rôle in dairy cattle breeding. International evaluations or converted foreign production proofs for production are often used before local information becomes available, or they are combined with local information. Procedures for using foreign information are already well developed for milk production traits, are under development for type traits, and are the least developed for traits other than production and type.
- In many countries, PTAs on individual traits are combined using selection indexes. As the array of information available on AI bulls worldwide

increases, it is becoming more important to have these different pieces of information combined into indexes which gives them appropriate emphasis. The development and wider use of indexes of overall economic merit should simplify selection and help to breed cows which are both healthier and more profitable.

- Selection experiments in dairy cattle have shown that substantial rates of genetic improvement in production (about 2% per annum) can be achieved by selection on PTAs or their equivalent. Lower, but still substantial, rates of change have been made for several decades in some industry populations, e.g. in North America and New Zealand. Estimates of industry genetic trends were much lower in many other countries (e.g. the UK) until the 1990s. In many countries trends increased as a result of importation of genetic material (mostly directly or indirectly from North America), improvements in local breeding programmes, or both. More recently, the uptake of genomic selection is dramatically increasing rates of genetic change. Most studies show that these changes in production are associated with higher margins over feed and other costs.
- Most experimental studies indicated that, in temperate dairying systems, breed or strain × feeding system interactions are of little or no importance for production. However, several studies show that the ranking of sires, or the scale (but not the direction) of the response to selection, differs between feeding systems or environments. There are also some indications of interactions for traits other than milk production, including reproduction, health and feed intake. In the absence of progeny tests in the relevant environment, the impact of such interactions may be reduced through the use of broader indexes including affected traits (e.g. reproduction, feed intake) or predictors of these, and the use of MACE international evaluations. Studies show that interactions are much more important when breeds or sires from temperate countries are used in tropical systems. Hence, it is important in tropical systems that choice of breed, cross or sire is made on the basis of evaluations in the relevant environment.

References

Abdelsayed, M., Haile-Mariam, M. and Pryce, J.E (2017) Genetic parameters for health traits using data collected from genomic information nucleus herds. *Journal of Dairy Science* 100, 9643–9655. DOI: 10.3168/jds.2017-12960.

Abernethy, D.A., Upton, P., Higgins, I.M., McGrath, G., Goodchild, A.V. *et al.* (2013) Bovine tuberculosis trends in the UK and the Republic of Ireland, 1995–2010. *Veterinary Record* 172, 312. DOI: 10.1136/vr.100969.

African Dairy Genetic Gains Project (2019) Available at: https://africadgg.wordpress.com/category/adgg/ (accessed 21 October 2019).

AHDB (2015) *Dairy Statistics: An Insider's Guide.* Agriculture and Horticulture Development Board, Kenilworth, UK. Available at: https://www.academia.edu/34984904/Dairy_statistics_An_insiders_guide_2015 (accessed 21 October, 2019).

AHDB (2019a) Available at: https://ahdb.org.uk/ (accessed 21 October 2019).

AHDB (2019b) Breeding and Genetics. Available at: https://dairy.ahdb.org.uk/technical-information/breeding-genetics/#.XWsbQigzZPZ (accessed 21 October 2019).

aWhere (2019) Available at: https://www.awhere.com/ (accessed 21 October 2019).

Banos, G. and Coffey, M.P. (2010) Genetic association between body energy measured throughout lactation and fertility in dairy cattle. *Animal* 4, 189–199. DOI: 10.1017/S1751731109991182.

Banos, G., Winters, M., Mrode, R., Mitchell, A.P., Bischop, S.C. *et al.* (2017) Genetic evaluation for bovine tuberculosis resistance in dairy cattle. *Journal of Dairy Science* 100, 1272–1281. DOI: 10.3168/jds.2016-11897.

Bastin, C. and Gengler, N. (2013) Genetics of body condition score as an indicator of dairy cattle fertility. A review. *Biotechnologie, Agronomie, Société et Environnement* 17, 64–75. Available at: https://popups.uliege.be/1780-4507/index.php?id=9570 (accessed 5 September 2020).

Beard, K. (1993) Genetic evaluation for milking speed, temperament, likability and survival in Australia. *Proceedings of the Open Session of the INTERBULL Annual Meeting,* Arhus, Denmark 19–20 August 1993. No 8. Available at: https://journal.interbull.org/index.php/ib/article/view/165 (accessed 21 June 2020).

Beatson, P.R., Meier, S., Cullen, N.G. and Eding, H. (2019) Genetic variation in milk urea nitrogen concentration of dairy cattle and its implications for reducing urinary nitrogen excretion. *Animal* 13, 2164–2171. DOI: 10.1017/S1751731119000235.

Berry, D.P., Buckley, F., Dillon, P., Evans, R.D. and Veerkamp, R.F. (2004) Genetic relationships among linear type traits, milk yield, body weight, fertility and somatic cell count in primiparous dairy cows. *Irish Journal of Agriculture and Food Research* 43, 161–176.

Berry, D.P., Horan, B., O'Donovan, M., Buckley, F., Kennedy, E. *et al.* (2007) Genetics of grass dry matter intake, energy balance, and digestibility in grazing Irish dairy cows. *Journal of Dairy Science* 90, 4835–4845. DOI: 10.3168/jds.2007-0116.

Berry, D.P., Bermingham, M.L., Good, M. and More, S.J. (2011) Genetics of animal health and disease in cattle. *Irish Veterinary Journal* 64, 5. DOI: 10.1186%2F2046-0481-64-5.

Boelling, D. and Pollott, G.E. (1997) The genetics of feet, legs and locomotion in cattle. *Animal Breeding Abstracts* 65, 1–11.

Boelling, D. and Pollott, G.E. (1998) Locomotion, lameness, hoof and leg traits in cattle II: Genetic relationships and breeding values. *Livestock Production Science* 54, 205–215. DOI: 10.1016/S0301-6226(97)00173-5.

Breider, I.S., Wall, E. and Garnsworthy, P.C. (2019) Heritability of methane production and genetic correlations with milk yield and body weight in Holstein-Friesian dairy cows. *Journal of Dairy Science* 102, 7277–7281. DOI: 10.3168/jds.2018-15909.

Brotherstone, S. (1994) Genetic and phenotypic correlations between linear type traits and production traits in Holstein-Friesian dairy cattle. *Animal Science* 59, 183–187. DOI: 10.1017/S0003356100007662.

Brotherstone, S. and Hill, W.G. (1991) Dairy herd life in relation to linear type traits and production. 2. Genetic analyses for pedigree and non-pedigree cows. *Animal Production* 53, 289–297. DOI: 10.1017/S0003356100020286.

Bryant, A.M. (1993) Friesians and Jerseys. *Dairying Research Corporation, Hamilton, Research Update, June* 1993, pp. 3-4.

Bryant, A.M., Cook, M.A.S. and MacDonald, K.A. (1985) Comparative dairy production of Jerseys and Friesians. *Proceedings of the New Zealand Society of Animal Production* 45, 7–11.

Bundesverband Rind und Schwein (2018) *Rinder- und Schweineproduktion in Deutschland 2018*. BRS, Germany. Available at: https://www.rind-schwein.de/brs-news/brs-statistikbroschuere-rinder-und-schweineprodukt.html (accessed 6 November 2019).

CDN (2019) Genomic Young Bulls: Accelerating Genetic Progress. Available at: https://www.cdn.ca/images/uploaded/file/Genomic%20Young%20Bulls%20Article%20-%20September%202017.pdf. (accessed 29 June 2020).

Charagu, P.K (1997*)*. Economic efficiency of Canadian and New Zealand sires in Canada and New Zealand dairy herds and its relationship with other traits. PhD thesis. University of British Columbia, Canada.

Coffey, E.M., Vinson, W.E. and Pearson, R.E. (1986) Potential of somatic cell concentration in milk as a sire selection criterion to reduce mastitis in dairy cattle. *Journal of Dairy Science* 69, 2163–2172. DOI: https://doi.org/10.3168/jds.S0022-0302(86)80649-X.

Cole, J.B., Wiggans, G.R., VanRaden, P.M. and Miller, R.H. (2007) Stillbirth (co)variance components for a sire-maternal grandsire threshold model and development of a calving ability index for sire selection. *Journal of Dairy Science* 90, 2489–2496. DOI: 10.3168/jds.2006-436.

Copeland, L. (1927). Inheritance of butterfat percentage in Jersey cows. *Journal of Dairy Science* 10, 344–352. DOI: 10.3168/jds.S0022-0302(27)93850-8.

Copeland, L. (1937) Persistency of production in Jersey cows and its practical application. *Journal of Dairy Science* 20, 151–158. DOI: 10.3168/jds.S0022-0302(37)95677-7.

Council on Dairy Cattle Breeding (2019) Genetic and Phenotypic Trend. Available at: https://queries.uscdcb.com/eval/summary/trend.cfm (accessed 29 June 2020).

Cunningham, E.P. (1983) Structure of dairy cattle breeding in Western Europe and comparisons with North America. *Journal of Dairy Science* 66, 1579–1587.

Datagene (2018) *Australian Dairy Herd Improvement Report 2017*. Datagene, Southbank, Victoria, Australia. Available at: https://datagene.com.au/sites/default/files/DirectoryPage/Herd%20Improvement%20Report/2017%20Australian%20Dairy%20Herd%20Improvement%20Report.pdf (accessed 6 November 2019).

de Haas, Y.J., Calus, W.M., Dijkstra, J., De Haan, M., Bannink, A. and Veerkamp, R. (2011) Genetic parameters for predicted methane production and potential for reducing enteric emissions through genomic selection. *Journal of Dairy Science* 94, 6122–6134. DOI: 10.3168/jds.2011-4439.

de Haas, Y., Calus, M.P.L., Veerkamp, R.F, Wall, E., Coffey, M.P. *et al.* (2012) Improved accuracy of genomic prediction for dry matter intake of dairy cattle from combined European and Australian data sets. *Journal of Dairy Science* 95, 6103–6112. DOI: 10.3168/jds.2011-5280.

de Jong, G., van der Linde, R., de Haas, Y., Schopen, G.C.B. and Veerkamp, R.F. (2016) Genetic evaluation for feed intake in the Netherlands and Flanders, impact on efficiency and responses. *INTERBULL Bulletin* 50, 1–4. Available at: https://journal.interbull.org/index.php/ib/article/view/1390 (accessed 5 September 2020).

de Oliviera, H.R., Brito, L.F., Lourenco, D.A.L., Masuda, Y., Misztal, I. *et al.* (2018). Application of ssGBLUp using random regression models in the Ayrshire and Jersey breeds. *Joint INTERBULL/EEAP meeting*, Dubrovnick, Croatia. Available at: https://interbull.org/ib/2018_itb_eaap_presentation (accesses 16 November 2019).

Distl, O., Koorn, D.S., McDaniel, B.T., Peterse, D., Politiek, R.D., and Reurink, A. (1990) Claw traits in cattle breeding programmes: report of the EAAP working group "Claw quality in cattle". *Livestock Production Science* 25, 1–13. DOI: https://doi.org/10.1016/0301-6226(90)90037-7.

Druet, T., Schrooten, C. and de Roos, A.P.W. (2010) Imputation of genotypes from different single nucleotide polymorphism panels in dairy cattle. *Journal of Dairy Science* 93, 5443–5454. DOI: 10.3168/jds.2010-3255.

Eaglen, S.A.E., Coffey, M.P., Woolliams, J.A., and Wall, E. (2012) Evaluating alternate models to estimate genetic parameters of calving traits in United Kingdom Holstein-Friesian dairy cattle. *Genetics Selection Evolution* 44, 23. DOI: 10.1186/1297-9686-44-23.

EGENES (2019) Available at: https://www.sruc.ac.uk/info/120275/egenes (accessed 21 October 2019).

Emanuelson, U. (1988) Recording of production diseases in cattle and possibilities for genetic improvements. A review. *Livestock Production Science* 20, 89–106. DOI: 10.1016/0301-6226(88)90055-3.

Eurogenomics (2019) Available at: http://www.eurogenomics.com/genomic-breeding-values/eurogenomics-rankings.html (accessed 06 November 2019).

FarmingUK (2020) Available at: https://www.farminguk.com/news/good-genetics-are-worth-24-000gbp-in-extra-margin-per-100-cows_21150.html (accessed 1 October 2020).

FAO (2019) FAOSTAT. Available at: http://www.fao.org/faostat/en/#data/QL (accessed 5 May 2019).

Fulkerson, W., Davison, T. and Goddard, M. (1996) The genetic merit by level of feeding study at Wollongbar. *Research to Farm.* NSW Agriculture, Wollongbar, Australia.

García-Ruiz, A., Cole, J.B., VanRaden, P.M., Wiggans, G.R., Ruiz-López, F.J. and Van Tassell, C.P. (2016) Changes in genetic selection differentials and generation intervals in US Holstein dairy cattle as a result of genomic selection. *Proceedings of the National Academy of Science, USA* 113, E3995–4004. DOI: 10.1073/pnas.1519061113.

Genus (1996) *Genus Milkminder Annual Report 1995-96*. Genus Management, Wrexham, UK.

Groen, A.F., Hellinga, I., and Oldenbroek, J.K. (1994) Genetic correlations of clinical mastitis and feet and legs problems with milk yield and type traits in Dutch Black and White dairy cattle. *Netherlands Journal of Agricultural Science* 42, 371–378. Available at: https://library.wur.nl/ojs/index.php/njas/article/view/595 (accessed 5 September).

Guinan, F.L., Norman, D. and Dürr, J. (2019) Changes occurring in the breed composition of U.S. dairy herds. *Proceedings of the 2019 INTERBULL Meeting*, 55, 11–16.

Harris, B.L., Pryce, J.E. and Montgomerie, W.A. (2007) Experiences from breeding for economic efficiency in dairy cattle in New Zealand. *Proceedings of the Association for the Advancement of Animal Breeding and Genetics* 17, 434–444. Available at: http://www.aaabg.org/livestocklibrary/2007/harris434.pdf (accessed 1 October 2020).

Hayes, B.J., Carrick, M., Bowman, P. and Goddard, M.E. (2003) Genotype x environment interaction for milk production of daughters of Australian dairy sires from test-day records. *Journal of Dairy Science* 86, 3736–3744. DOI: 10.3168/jds.S0022-0302(03)73980-0.

Hayes, J.F., Cue, R.I. and Monardes, H.G. (1992) Estimates of repeatability of reproductive measures in Canadian Holsteins. *Journal of Dairy Science* 75, 1701–1706. DOI: 10.3168/jds.S0022-0302(92)77927-2.

Hazel, L.N. (1943) The genetic basis for constructing selection indexes. *Genetics* 28, 476–490.

Hendriks, S. (2016) The effect of dietary nitrogen on nitrogen partitioning and milk production in grazing dairy cows. M Animal Science thesis, Massey University, Palmerston North, New Zealand.

Hinks, C.J.M. (1978) The use of centralised breeding schemes in dairy cattle improvement. *Animal Breeding Abstracts* 46, 291–297.

Hoekstra, J., van der Lugt, A.W., van der Werf, J.H.J. and Ouweltjes, W. (1994) Genetic and phenotypic parameters for milk production and fertility traits in upgraded dairy cattle. *Livestock Production Science* 40, 225–232. DOI: 10.1016/0301-6226(94)90090-6.

Holmes, C.W. (1995) Genotype x environment interactions in dairy cattle: A New Zealand perspective. In: Lawrence, T.L.J., Gordon, F.J. and Carson, A. (eds), *Breeding and Feeding the High Genetic Merit Dairy Cow*. Occasional Publication No. 19, *British Society of Animal Science*, pp. 51–58.

Holstein Friesian Society of Great Britain and Ireland. (1995) Focus on type. *Holstein Friesian Journal* 77, 50–59.

Holstein UK (2019) Available at: http://holstein-uk.org/ (accessed 21 October 2019).

Hutchison, J.L., Cole, J.B. and Bickhart, D.M. (2014) Short communication: use of young bulls in the United States. *Journal of Dairy Science* 97, 3213–3220. DOI: 10.3168/jds.2013-7525.

ICAR (2019a) *Yearly Survey on the Situation of Milk Recording Systems (Years 2016, 2017 and 2018) in ICAR Member Countries for Cow, Sheep and Goats*. International Committee for Animal Recording, Rome.

ICAR (2019b) Available at: https://www.icar.org/index.php/publications-technical-materials/technical-series-and-proceedings/atlas-claw-health-and-translations/ (accessed 21 October 2019).

INTERBULL (2019) Available at: https://interbull.org/ib/geforms (accessed 21 October 2019).

Jamrozik, J., Fatehi, J., Kistemaker, G.J. and Schaeffer, L.R. (2005) Estimates of genetic parameters for Canadian Holstein female reproductive traits. *Journal of Dairy Science* 88, 2199–2208. DOI: 10.3168/jds.S0022-0302(05)72895-2.

Jasiorowski, H., Reklewski, Z. and Stolzman, M. (1983) Polish experiment on the comparison of ten Friesian cattle strains. *International Dairy Federation,* document 165, 7–19.

Jenko, J., Wiggans, G.R., Cooper, T.A., Eaglen, S.A.E., Luff, W.G. de L. *et al.* (2016) Cow genotyping strategies for genomic selection in a small dairy cattle population. *Journal of Dairy Science* 100, 439–452. DOI: 10.3168/jds.2016-11479.

Johansson, K., Eriksson, J., Nielsen, U.S., Pösö, J. and Aamand, G.P. (2011) Genetic Evaluation of Claw Health in Denmark, Finland and Sweden. *INTERBULL Bulletin* 44, 224–228. Available at: https://journal.interbull.org/index.php/ib/article/view/1223 (accessed 5 September 2020).

Johnson, K.R. (1957) Heritability, genetic and phenotypic correlations of certain constituents of cow's milk. *Journal of Dairy Science* 40, 723–731.

Jorjani, H., Jakobsen, J., Nilforooshan, M.A., Hjerpe, E., Zumbach, B. *et al.* (2011). Genomic Evaluation of BSW Populations InterGenomics: Results and Deliverables. *INTERBULL Bulletin* 43, 5–8.

Kakwaya, D. and Peterson, R.G. (1991) Comparison of Canadian and New Zealand Holstein heifers for growth traits in Canadian herds. *Journal of Dairy Science* 74, Supplement 1, 231.

Kasbergen, C. (2013) Comparison of profitability Jerseys vs. Holsteins, including benchmarks comparisons for production, reproduction, health and costs of production. BSc. dissertation the Faculty of the Dairy Science Department California Polytechnic State University, San Luis Obispo, USA. Available at: http://digitalcommons.calpoly.edu/cgi/viewcontent.cgi?article=1080&context=dscisp (accessed 6 November 2019).

Lassen, J. and Løvendahl, P. (2016) Heritability estimates for enteric methane emissions from Holstein cattle measured using noninvasive methods. *Journal of Dairy Science* 99, 1959–1967. DOI: 10.3168/jds.2015-10012.

Ledinek, M., Gruber, L., Steininger, F., Fuerst-Waltl, B., Zottl, K. *et al.* (2019) Analysis of lactating cows on commercial Austrian dairy farms: the influence of genotype and body weight on efficiency parameters. *Archives Animal Breeding* 62, 491–500.

Malchiodi, F., Koeck, A., Mason, S., Christen, A.M., Kelton, D.F. *et al.* (2017) Genetic parameters for hoof health traits estimated with linear and threshold models using alternative cohorts. *Journal of Dairy Science* 100, 2828–2836. DOI: 10.3168/jds.2016-11558.

Marshall, K., Tebug, S., Juga, J., Tapio, M. and Missohou, A. (2016) Better dairy cattle breeds and better management can improve the livelihoods of the rural poor in Senegal. *ILRI Research Brief 65*. ILRI, Nairobi. Available at: https://cgspace.cgiar.org/handle/10568/72865 (accessed 6 November, 2019).

Medic, D., Veselinovic, S., Veselinovic, S., Ivkov, V., Grubac, S. *et al.* (1999) MOET program in improvement of genetic basis in nucleus herd of dairy cattle. *Proceedings of the Meeting: 7th Conference for Ovine and Caprine Production & 5th Symposium on Animal Reproduction,* 8–11 September 1999, Ohrid, Macedonia.

Meijering, A. (1984) Dystocia and stillbirth in cattle - a review of causes, relations and implications. *Livestock Production Science* 11, 143–177. DOI: 10.1016/0301-6226(84)90057-5.

Meyer, K. and Burnside, E.B. (1987) Scope for a subjective assessment of milking speed. *Journal of Dairy Science* 70, 1061–1068. DOI: 10.3168/jds.S0022-0302(87)80112-1.

Miglior, F., Muir, B.L. and Van Doormaal, B.J. (2005) Selection indices in Holstein cattle of various countries. *Journal of Dairy Science* 88, 1255– 1263. DOI: 10.3168/jds.S0022-0302(05)72792-2.

Miglior, F., Allison, F., Malchiodi, F., Brito, L.F., Pauline, M. and Baes, C.F. (2017) A 100-Year Review: Identification and genetic selection of economically important traits in dairy cattle. *Journal of Dairy Science* 100, 10251–10271. DOI: 10.3168/jds.2017-12968.

Mrode, R.A., Swanson, G.J.T. and Winters, M.S. (1995) Genetic parameters for somatic cell counts (SCC) for three dairy breeds in the United Kingdom. *Animal Science* 60, 545. DOI: 10.1017/S0308229600028944.

Mrode, R., Brotherstone, S., White, I., Swanson, G., Coffey, M. *et al.* (2005) Random regression model for the genetic evaluation of production traits of dairy cattle in the UK. *INTERBULL Bulletin* 33, 211–214.

Mwansa, P.B. (1997) Genetic analysis of longevity in the Canadian and New Zealand dairy herds. PhD thesis, University of British Columbia, Canada.

Negussie, E., de Haas, Y., Dehareng, Y.F., Dewhurst, R. J., Dijkstra, J. *et al.* (2017). Invited review: Large-scale indirect measurements for enteric methane emissions in dairy cattle: A review of proxies and their potential for use in management and breeding decisions. *Journal of Dairy Science* 100, 2433–2453. DOI: 10.3168/jds.2016-12030.

New Zealand Dairy Statistics (2018). Available at: https://www.dairynz.co.nz/publications/dairy-industry/new-zealand-dairy-statistics-2017-18/ (accessed 6 November 2019).

Nguyen, T.T., Bowman, P.J., Haile-Mariam, M., Pryce, J.E. and Hayes, B.J. (2016). Genomic selection for tolerance to heat stress in Australian dairy cattle. *Journal of Dairy Science* 99, 2849–2862. DOI: 10.3168/jds.2015-9685.

Nicholas, F.W. (1979) The genetic implications of multiple ovulation and embryo transfer in small dairy herds. Paper presented at the *Annual Conference of the European Association for Animal Production*, Harrogate, UK.

Nicholas, F.W. and Smith, C. (1983) Increased rates of genetic change in dairy cattle by embryo transfer and splitting. *Animal Production* 36, 341–353. DOI: 10.1017/S0003356100010382.

Ødegård, C., Svendsen, M. and Heringstad, B. (2013) Genetic correlations between claw health and feet and leg conformation in Norwegian Red cows. *Journal of Dairy Science* 97, 4522–4529. DOI: 10.3168/jds.2013-7837.

Ojango, J.M.K. and Pollott, G.E. (2002) The relationship between Holstein bull breeding values for milk yield derived in both the UK and Kenya. *Livestock Production Science* 74, 1–12. DOI: 10.1016/S0301-6226(01)00282-2.

Oldenbroek, J.K. (1986) The performance of Jersey heifers and heifers of larger dairy breeds on two complete diets with different roughage contents. *Livestock Production Science* 14, 1–14. DOI: 10.1016/0301-6226(86)90092-8.

Oldenbroek, K. and van der Waaij, L. (2015) *Textbook Animal Breeding and Genetics for BSc Students.* Centre for Genetic Resources, The Netherlands and Animal Breeding and Genomics Centre, Groen Kennisnet, Netherlands.

Pander, B.L., Hill, W.G. and Thompson, R. (1992) Genetic parameters of test day records of British Holstein-Friesian heifers. *Animal Production* 55, 11–21. DOI: 10.1017/S0003356100037211.

Persaud, P. and Simm, G. (1991) Genetic and phenotypic parameters for yield, food intake and efficiency of dairy cows fed *ad libitum*. 2. Estimates for part lactation measures and their relationship with 'total' lactation measures. *Animal Production* 52, 445–450. DOI: 10.1017/S0003356100013015.

Persaud, P., Simm, G. and Hill, W.G. (1991) Genetic and phenotypic parameters for yield, food intake and efficiency of dairy cows fed *ad libitum*. 1. Estimates for 'total' lactation measures and their relationship with live-weight traits. *Animal Production* 52, 435–444. DOI: 10.1017/S0003356100013003.

Peterson, R.G. (1991) Evidence of a GxE with Canadian and New Zealand Holsteins. *Paper presented at the Annual Conference of the European Association for Animal Production*, 16–19 September 1991, Berlin, Germany.

Philipsson, J. (1981) Genetic aspects of female fertility in dairy cattle. *Livestock Production Science* 8, 307–319. DOI: 10.1016/0301-6226(81)90049-X.

Philipsson, J. and Lindhé, B. (2003) Experiences of including reproduction and health traits in Scandinavian dairy cattle breeding programmes. *Livestock Production Science* 83, 99–112. DOI: 10.1016/S0301-6226(03)00047-2.

Philipsson, J. Foulley, J.L., Lederer, J., Liboriussen, T. and Osinga, A. (1979) Sire evaluation standards and breeding strategies for limiting dystocia and stillbirth. Report of an EEC/EAAP working group. *Livestock Production Science* 6, 111–127. DOI: 10.1016/0301-6226(79)90013-7.

Philipsson, J., Ral, G. and Berglund, B. (1995) Somatic cell count as a selection criterion for mastitis resistance in dairy cattle. *Livestock Production Science* 41, 195–200. DOI: 10.1016/0301-6226(94)00067-H.

Pollak, E.J. and Freeman, A.E. (1976) Parameter estimation and sire evaluation for dystocia and calf size in Holsteins. *Journal of Dairy Science* 59, 1817–1824. DOI: 10.3168/jds.S0022-0302(76)84442-6.

Pritchard, T., Coffey, M., Mrode R. and Wall, E. (2013) Genetic parameters for production, health, fertility and longevity traits in dairy cows. *Animal* 7, 34–36. DOI: 10.1017/S1751731112001401.

Pryce, J.E., Royal, M.D., Garnsworthy, P.C. and Mao, I.L. (2004) Fertility in the high-producing dairy cow. *Livestock Production Science* 86, 125–135. DOI: 10.1016/S0301-6226(03)00145-3.

Pryce, J.E, Wales, W.J., de Haas, Y., Veerkamp, R.F. and Hayes, B.J. (2014) Genomic selection for feed efficiency in dairy cattle. *Animal* 8, 1–10. DOI: 10.1017/S1751731113001687.

Pryce, J.E., Parker Gaddis, K.L., Koeck, A., Bastin, C., Abdelsayed, M. *et al.* (2016) Invited review: Opportunities for genetic improvement of metabolic diseases. *Journal of Dairy Science* 99, 6855–6873. DOI: 10.3168/jds.2016-10854.

Pryce, J.E., Douglas, P., Reich, C.M., Chamberlain, A.J., Bowman, P.J. *et al.* (2017) Reliability of Australian dairy genomic breeding values increase through the addition of genotyped females with excellent phenotypes. *Proceedings of the Association for the Advancement of Animal Breeding and Genetics* 22, 133–136.

Rendel, J.M. and Robertson, A. (1950) Estimation of genetic gain in milk yield by selection in a closed herd of dairy cattle. *Journal of Genetics* 50, 1–8. DOI: 10.1007/BF02986789.

Rensing, S. and Ruten, W. (2005) Genetic evaluation for milking speed in German Holstein population using different traits in a multiple trait repeatability model. *INTERBULL Bulletin* 33, 163–166. Available at: https://journal.interbull.org/index.php/ib/article/view/895 (accessed 5 September 2020).

Robertson, A. and Rendel, J.M. (1950) The use of progeny testing with artificial insemination in dairy cattle. *Journal of Genetics* 50, 21–31. DOI: 10.1007/BF02986791.

Schaeffer, L.R. and Dekkers, J.C.M. (1994) Random regression in animal models for test-day production in dairy cattle. *Proceedings 5th World Congress Applied to Livestock Production*. Guelph, Canada XVIII, pp. 443-446. Available at: http://www.wcgalp.org/proceedings/1994 (accessed 16 June 2020).

Sewalem, A., Miglior, F. and Kistemaker, G.J. (2011) Short communication: Genetic parameters of milking temperament and milking speed in Canadian Holsteins. *Journal of Dairy Science* 94, 512–516. DOI: 10.3168/jds.2010-3479.

Shook, G.E. (2006) Major advances in determining appropriate selection goals. *Journal of Dairy Science* 89, 1349–1361. DOI: 10.3168/jds.S0022-0302(06)72202-0.

Silva, M.V.G.B., Paiva, L.C., Cembranelli, M.A.R., Martins, M.F., Freitas, A.F. *et al.* (2012) *Programa de Melhoramneto Genético da Raça Girolando- Sumário de Touros- Resultado do Teste de Progênie* Julho/2012. Juiz de For a: Embrapa Gado de Leite, 52 pp. (Embrapa Gado de Leite, Documentos, 154)

Silva, M.V.G.B., Martins, M.F., Cembranelli, M. de R., Paiva, L. de C., Panetto, J.C. do C. *et al.* (2017) Girolando Breed Genetic Improvement Program - Sire Summary - Progeny Test Results – June 2017. Available at: https://www.embrapa.br/en/busca-de-publicacoes/-/publicacao/1080947/girolando-breed-genetic-improvement-program---sire-summary---progeny-test-results---june-2017 (accessed 14 November 2019).

Simm, G. (1998) *Genetic Improvement of Cattle and Sheep*. CAB International, Wallingford, UK.

Simm, G., Veerkamp, R.F. and Persaud, P. (1994) The economic performance of dairy cows of different predicted genetic merit for milk solids production. *Animal Production* 58, 313–320. DOI: 10.1017/S0003356100007236.

Smith, C. (1984) Rates of genetic change in farm livestock. *Research and Development in Agriculture* 1, 79–85.

SRUC (2018) *SRUC Farm Management Handbook 2018/2019*. Scotland Rural College, Edinburgh, UK.

Stock, K.F, Reinhardt, F. and Swalve, H.H. (2017) The importance of claw health traits and implications for future genetic evaluation in German Holstein dairy cattle. *15th Conference of the European Holstein and Red Holstein Confederation*, 18 September 2017, Budapest. Available at: http://www.euholsteins.com/info/documents/KFStock_et_al_ClawHealth_EHRC2017handout.pdf (accessed 6 November, 2019).

Stoop, W.M., Bovenhuis, H. and van Arendonk, J.A.M. (2007) Genetic parameters for milk urea nitrogen in relation to milk production traits. *Journal of Dairy Science* 90, 1981–1986. DOI: 10.3168/jds.2006-434.

Swalve, H.H., Topf, C. and Langholz, H.-J. (1992) Estimation of genetic parameters for differently recorded fertility data in dairy cattle. *Journal of Animal Breeding and Genetics* 109, 241–251. DOI: 10.1111/j.1439-0388.1992.tb00403.x.

Vallimont, J.E., Dechow, C.D., Daubert, J.M., Dekleva, M.W., Blum, J.W. *et al.* (2010) Genetic parameters of feed intake, production, body weight, body condition score, and selected type traits of Holstein cows in commercial tie-stall barns. *Journal of Dairy Science* 93, 4892–4901. DOI: 10.3168/jds.2010-3189.

van Arendonk, J.A.M., Groen, A.F., van der Werf, J.H.J. and Veerkamp, R.F. (1995) Genetic aspects of feed intake and efficiency in lactating dairy cows. *Proceedings of Symposium on Utilization of Local Feed Resources in Dairy Cattle. Perspectives of Environmentally Balanced Production Systems*. European Association for Animal Production publication, Wageningen Institute of Animal Science, Wageningen, Netherlands.

van der Beek, S. (2007) The Future of Dairy Cattle Nucleus Breeding. Available at: http://www.euholsteins.com/info/conferences/ehc2007/11%20The%20future%20of%20Dairy%20Cattle%20Nucleus%20Breeding.pdf (accessed 21 October 2019).

van der Linde, C., de Jong, G., Koenen, E.P.C. and Eding, H. (2010) Claw health index for Dutch dairy cattle based on claw trimming and conformation data. *Journal of Dairy Science* 93, 4883–4891. DOI: 10.3168/jds.2010-3183.

Veerkamp, R.F., Hill, W.G., Stott, A.W., Brotherstone, S. and Simm, G. (1995) Selection for longevity and yield in dairy cows using transmitting abilities for type and yield. *Animal Science* 61, 189–197. DOI: 10.1017/S1357729800013710.

Visscher, P.M. and Thompson, R. (1992) Univariate and multivariate parameter estimates for milk production traits using an animal model. I. Description and results of REML analyses. *Genetics, Selection, Evolution* 24, 415–430.

Vosman, J., de Jong, G., Eding, H. and Knijn, H. (2015) Genetic evaluation for ketosis in the Netherlands based on FTIR measurements. *INTERBULL Bulletin* 42, 1–5. Available at: https://journal.interbull.org/index.php/ib/article/view/1365 (accessed 5 September 2020).

Wiggans, G.R. (2019) *Genomic selection in the USA*. Seminar slides from University of Liverpool, Institute of Veterinary Science, Diploma Bovine Reproduction. Module 615 (Genetics of Cattle) seminar, September 2019. Available at: https://www.uscdcb.com/wp-content/uploads/2019/10/Wiggans-DBRM_UK_Sept2019.pdf (accessed 15 November 2019).

Wiggans, G.R., Misztal, I. and Van Tassell, C.P. (2003) Calving ease (co)variance components for a sire-maternal grandsire evaluation model. *Journal of Dairy Science* 86, 1845–1848. DOI: 10.3168/jds.S0022-0302(03)73771-0.

Wilmink, J.B.M. (1987) Adjustment of test day milk, fat and protein yield for age, season and stage of lactation. *Livestock Production Science* 16, 335–348. DOI: 10.1016/0301-6226(87)90003-0.

Woolliams, J.A. and Smith, C. (1988) The value of indicator traits in the genetic improvement of dairy cattle. *Animal Production* 46, 333–345. DOI: 10.1017/S0003356100018948.

Recommended Reading

Animal (formerly *Animal Science* and *Animal Production*; Journal of the British Society of Animal Science).

Groen, A.F., Sölkner, J., Strandberg, E. and Gengler, N. (compilers) (1996) *Proceedings International Workshop on Genetic Improvement of Functional Traits in Cattle,*

Gembloux, Belgium January 1996. INTERBULL Bulletin No. 12, International Bull Evaluation Service, Department of Animal Breeding and Genetics, SLU, Uppsala, Sweden.

Groen, A.F., Steine, T., Colleau, J.-J., Pedersen, J., Pribyl, J. and Reinsch, N. (1997) Economic values in dairy cattle breeding, with special reference to functional traits. Report of an EAAP working group. *Livestock Production Science* 49, 1–21. DOI: 10.1016/S0301-6226(97)00041-9.

INTERBULL Bulletins. International Bull Evaluation Service, Department of Animal Breeding and Genetics, SLU, S-750 07 Uppsala, Sweden.

Journal of Animal Science (Journal of the American Society of Animal Science).

Journal of Dairy Science (Journal of the American Dairy Science Association).

Livestock Production Science (Journal of the European Association for Animal Production).

McGuirk, B. (2020) A Bovine Thriller. A History of the Dairy Cattle Breeding Industry in Great Britain. ISBN 978-1-5272-6744-2.

Owen, J.B. and Axford, R.F.E. (eds) (1991) *Breeding for Disease Resistance in Farm Animals*. CAB International, Wallingford, UK.

Philipsson, J., Banos, G. and Arnason, T. (1994) Present and future uses of selection index methodology in dairy cattle. *Journal of Dairy Science* 77, 3252–3261.

Proceedings of the Australian Association of Animal Breeding and Genetics.

Proceedings of the New Zealand Society of Animal Production.

Proceedings of the World Congresses on Genetics Applied to Livestock Production. Available at: wcgalp.org (accessed 16 June 2020).

Visscher, P.M., Bowman, P.J. and Goddard, M.E. (1994) Breeding objectives for pasture based dairy production systems. *Livestock Production Science* 40, 123–137. DOI: 10.1016/0301-6226(94)90042-6.

Wiggans, G.R., Misztal, I. and Van Vleck, L.D. (1988) Implementation of an animal model for genetic evaluation of dairy cattle in the United States. *Journal of Dairy Science*, 71, Supplement 2: 54–69. DOI: 10.1016/S0022-0302(88)79979-8.

9 Beef Cattle Breeding

Introduction

The aim of this chapter is to discuss the breeding goals, the breeds and crosses used, the selection criteria and the methods of testing and genetic evaluation used in beef cattle breeding. Figure 9.1 shows world production of beef by continent. The Americas have the highest production at about 46.8% of the world total, and Asia follows with 23.4% of global production. Figure 9.2 shows more details of the world's 15 highest-producing countries. The USA has by far the highest production, followed by Brazil and China. Several European countries also appear in the list.

Beef cattle breeding in temperate countries is less homogeneous than dairy cattle breeding, so it is worth setting the scene a bit further now. In many European countries over half of beef production is from pure dairy or dual-purpose breeds, either from cull cows, from male calves or from surplus female calves not required as dairy herd replacements (Simm, 1998; TEAGASC, 2019). So, this chapter includes discussion of beef breeding goals and criteria in dairy and dual-purpose breeds, as well as considering these topics in specialized beef breeds. There is also an important contribution to beef production through crossing of dairy cows to beef bulls. This produces beef × dairy calves for slaughter and, in some countries, beef x dairy suckler cows (i.e. cows kept solely for rearing beef calves).

Many European countries have only a small specialized beef cattle breeding industry; in many cases this comprises purebred terminal sire breeds to supply beef bulls for crossing in dairy or dual-purpose herds. In contrast, pure beef breeds account for a high proportion of total production in France and, to a lesser extent, in Italy and Spain. In Britain and Ireland, suckler herds of beef × dairy cows, derived as a by-product of the use of beef bulls in dairy herds, make an important contribution to total output. In other major temperate beef-producing countries, such as the US, Canada, parts of South America, New Zealand and parts of Australia, beef production is based on extensively grazed or ranched cows, mainly of pure British beef breeds, like the Hereford, Aberdeen Angus and Shorthorn, crosses among them, or composites based on these and other breeds (see Figs 9.3 and 9.4). In some of these countries, like the US, Canada and parts of Australia, this extensive pre-weaning regime is usually followed by a more intensive finishing period in feedlots (see Fig. 9.5). Hence, there is a much wider range of production systems, breeding goals and testing programmes than those in temperate dairy cattle breeding. The more extensive nature of most production systems, and the widespread use of crossbred animals in the commercial sector of most beef industries, means that performance recording and genetic improvement are concentrated in a much smaller sector of the population than in dairy cattle breeding.

Beef systems are even more heterogeneous in tropical and sub-tropical regions. For example, in Africa, beef cattle can be kept in smallholder to (less commonly) large-scale mixed crop-livestock or pastoral systems. In some cases, the animals will be settled (in one location), while in others some or all of the herd may be transhumant, moving locations in search of pasture and water. Large-scale tropical or sub-tropical beef production units also exist in Brazil and northern Australia.

Breeding Goals

From the brief introduction above it is apparent that there are two broad categories of beef production in many countries: (i) beef production from dairy and dual-purpose herds; and (ii) beef production from specialized beef herds. Within the specialized beef sector, there is further differentiation into terminal sire and maternal breeds, crosses or lines. Terminal sire breeds are also used in dairy and

Genetic Improvement of Farmed Animals (G. Simm *et al.*)
DOI: 10.1079/9781789241723.0009

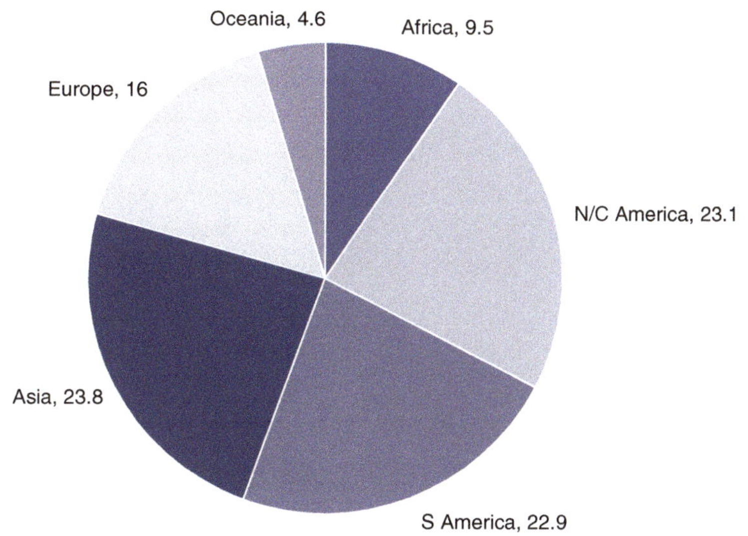

Fig. 9.1. Proportion of world beef and veal production by continent in 2017 (%). (After FAO, 2019.)

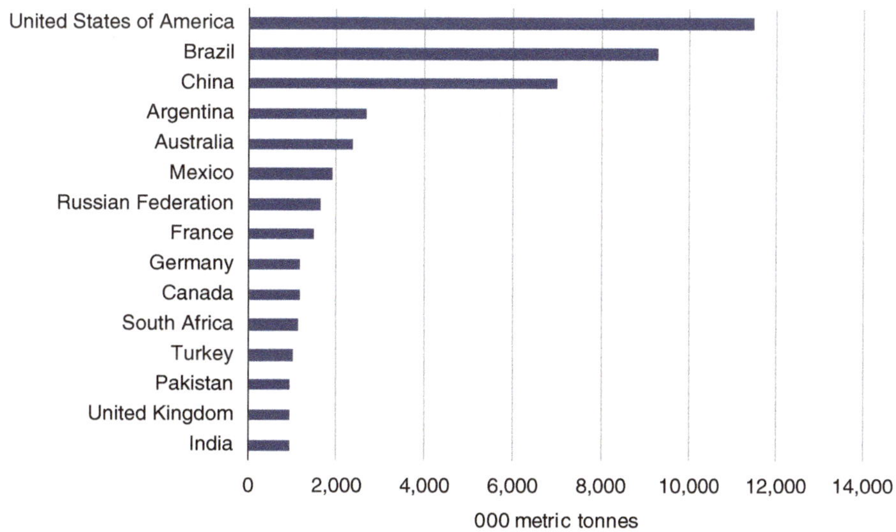

Fig. 9.2. Beef and veal production in 2017 in the world's 15 highest-producing countries. (After FAO, 2019.)

dual-purpose herds. Each of these categories of use requires a distinct set of beef breeding goal traits, or at least different priorities, and these are discussed in more detail below. Individual enterprises may be involved in breeding, rearing and finishing phases, or only a subset of these, which influences the breeding goal traits of most relevance. Carcass value, a function of carcass weight and quality, per breeding cow *per annum* is a major determinant of profitability, influenced by reproductive and maternal performance, as well as growth and carcass traits. Feed costs are the major variable cost in beef production, with health costs being another major contributor (e.g. Fuller, 2018; QMS, 2018).

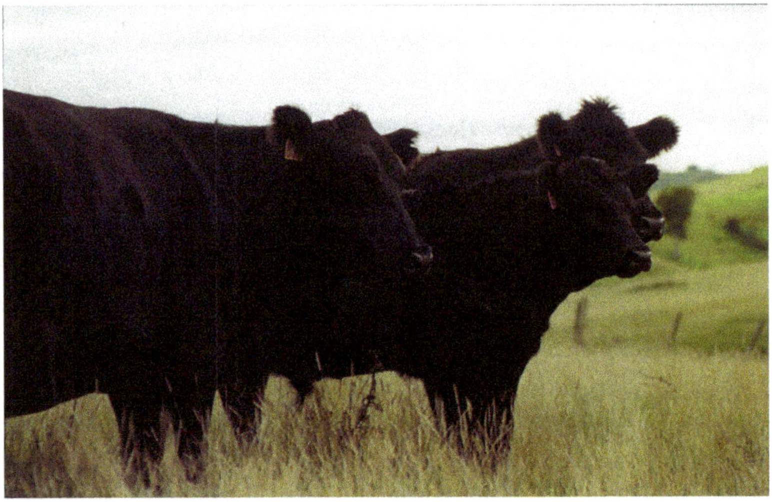

Fig. 9.3. Angus cattle near Wanganui, New Zealand.

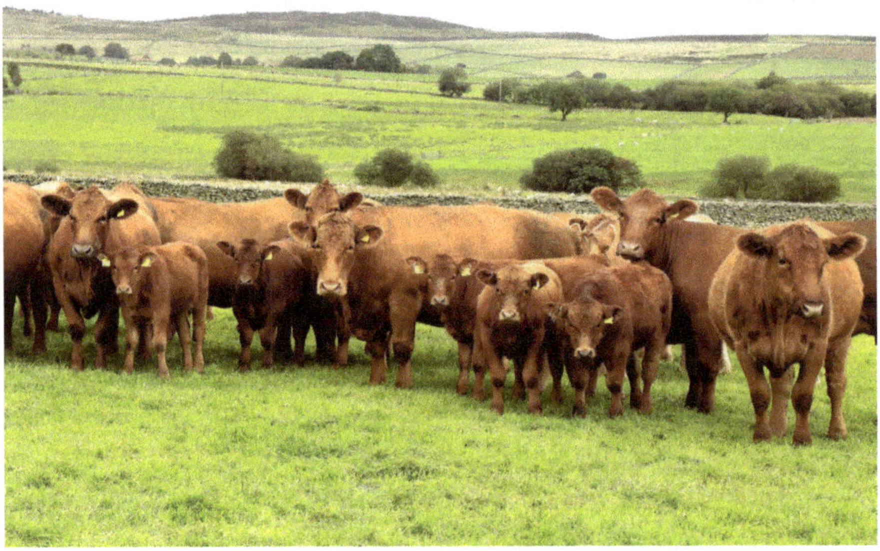

Fig. 9.4. Stabiliser composite cows and calves. (Courtesy of Richard Fuller.)

As discussed in more detail in Chapter 14, there is growing concern globally about the contribution of agriculture to greenhouse gas emissions. Methane emissions from ruminants are especially important, accounting for around 80% of all livestock emissions, with cattle responsible for the majority of these (Gerber *et al.*, 2013). Addressing this challenge is one of the most pressing issues in ruminant livestock production globally. Genetic improvement in individual animal growth and feed conversion efficiency, and in overall beef system efficiency, has reduced emissions per unit product (emissions intensity) over the last few decades. However, there is evidence of differences among beef breeds and sire progeny groups in methane emissions (e.g. Roehe *et al.*, 2016), and a great deal of interest in

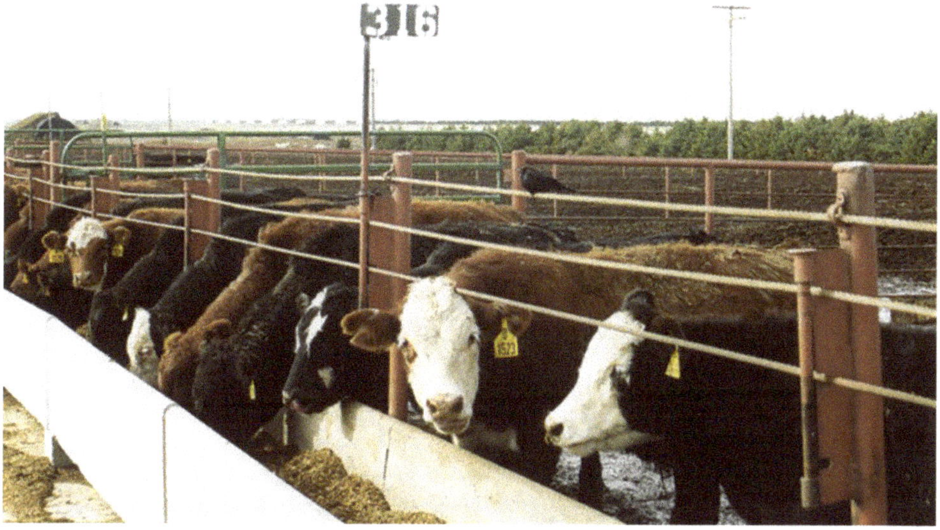

Fig. 9.5. Beef cattle in a feed lot in Nebraska, USA.

more direct approaches to reduce these by selection in terminal and maternal lines.

Beef breeding goals in dairy and dual-purpose breeds

At first sight it seems efficient to breed for both milk and meat production from the same type of animal. This is probably true in small-scale production systems, but it appears to be less true in large, specialized farming systems. Most of the evidence suggests that there is an unfavourable genetic correlation between milk production and growth or carcass characteristics (see Pirchner (1986) for early evidence). In other words, selection for either milk or beef merit tends to cause a deterioration in the other characteristics. It is possible to select for improvement in both characteristics at once, but the rate of progress which can be achieved is much lower than that possible with single-trait selection, or selection for two traits which are favourably correlated (as explained in Chapters 4 and 7).

Some breeds or strains, like the Simmental strains in several continental European countries, have achieved fairly high productivity in both milk and beef traits, as a result of many generations of selection. Even for these strains, it is difficult to compete nationally and internationally with both specialized milk and specialized beef breeds. As a result, there has been a trend towards milk production from more specialized dairy cattle breed types. In some countries, there is an attempt to limit the expected deterioration in beef merit by performance testing dairy bulls for growth and conformation, and preselecting bulls on these traits prior to progeny testing for milk production. In other countries, the deterioration in beef merit of the specialized dairy strains is compensated for, at least partially, by crossing those females not required to breed replacement dairy heifers to specialized beef breeds. Over the last few decades, in temperate dairying countries with large-scale specialized industries, breeding goals in dairy breeds have had little or no emphasis on beef traits; and, in dual-purpose breeds, the emphasis on beef traits has been secondary to that on milk traits. The emphasis given to beef traits in dairy breeds is being reconsidered in some countries, driven by ethical concerns over the practice of culling pure dairy bull calves, because of their perceived low beef value, and the resource inefficiency and environmental cost of this. In some countries with a strong history of using dual-purpose breeds (e.g. Switzerland), additional support has been introduced to maintain their rôle in traditional farming systems.

Terminal sires for use in dairy herds and specialized beef herds

Terminal sire beef breeds (i.e. those specially selected to sire the slaughter generation of animals) are used in dairy herds, for two main purposes. The first is to mate to dairy heifers to reduce the risk of calving difficulties, compared to that following matings to a dairy sire. The second is to mate to mature dairy cows which are not required to breed replacement dairy heifers.

The main priority of dairy farmers selecting a beef bull for use on heifers is calving ease. Difficult calvings are costly, both directly and because they delay rebreeding, depress milk production and compromise both cow and calf welfare and survival. Hence, dairy heifers have often been mated to bulls from one of the easier-calving beef breeds, such as the Hereford, Aberdeen Angus and Limousin. However, mating dairy heifers to a beef bull is becoming less common as more dairy producers realize that their heifers are typically the highest genetic merit animals in the herd, and hence valuable as dams of replacements. Also, the wider availability of calving ease evaluations in dairy breeds means that it is easier to select a dairy sire suitable for mating to heifers.

Although calving ease is still important when beef sires are mated to mature dairy cows, the incidence of calving difficulties is lower in mature cows than heifers. Hence, there is more scope to select beef bulls for other attributes to maximize returns from calf sales. Many beef-cross calves born on dairy farms are sold at a young age. So, increasing calf weight and conformation (muscularity or shape) are important breeding goals for dairy farmers choosing a beef breed, or individual beef sire, though increasing weight and conformation tends to conflict with the aim of reducing calving difficulties.

The performance of beef-cross calves in later life is of little direct concern to most dairy farmers, although, in theory, sire breeds or individual sires with high genetic merit for later performance ought to result in higher rewards in the market place. These market signals work reasonably well at the level of sire breed, especially if these produce easily recognized, colour-marked calves. There is less widespread discrimination among sires within a breed, although in some artificial insemination (AI) companies, beef breed societies or recording agencies there are schemes to identify and promote beef sires for use in dairy herds which combine acceptable calving ease with good growth and carcass characteristics. More widespread, unique identification of cattle, together with the adoption of improved technologies for storing and transferring performance records and breeding values, are helping to improve communication and market signals between different sectors of the industry. Ireland has one of the most modern and comprehensive systems for capturing data from commercial herds for use in beef breeding programmes (Wickham *et al.*, 2012; ICBF, 2020).

In many of the specialized beef production systems in temperate countries, there is widespread use of crossbreeding. Often this is to achieve complementary use of breeds, as explained in Chapter 3. Usually small- or medium-sized breeds or crosses are used as dam lines, and larger breeds are used as terminal sires. Larger breeds are valuable as terminal sires as they usually have faster growth rate and produce leaner carcasses at a given weight than smaller breeds. (Generally, as animals grow towards maturity, they get fatter. When different breeds are compared at similar degrees of maturity in live weight, say when each breed reaches 60% of its expected mature weight, they tend to have similar proportions of fat. However, breeds differ in fatness quite markedly when they are compared at the same weight. At a given slaughter weight, progeny of larger breeds, or larger sires within a breed, tend to be leaner. Alternatively, at a given level of fatness, progeny of larger breeds, or larger sires within a breed, generally produce heavier carcasses.) Although ease of calving is still important when terminal sire breeds are used in specialized beef breeding herds, their main rôle is to improve the growth and carcass characteristics of their crossbred offspring. Hence, there is interest in growth, carcass merit and calving ease whether terminal sire breeds are being used in dairy or beef herds, but the emphasis on these traits varies between these uses.

The definition of carcass merit depends to some extent on whether commercial animals are sold at live auctions, or directly to abattoirs, but it usually encompasses some measure of weight, fatness and conformation. In theory, good communication between sectors of the industry should mean that breeding goals are similar whether animals are marketed dead or alive. However, in practice they often differ. For example, in the UK a premium per kg liveweight is paid in live markets for animals of continental breeds and crosses, and especially those with good conformation. Except in extreme cases, fatness is a secondary concern, although buyers use breed, weight or age and sex as indirect indicators of fatness. For animals sold directly to abattoirs, overall returns will depend largely on carcass weight and visual (human- or machine-derived) scores for fatness and conformation, although breed and sex may modify the carcass price per kg. Increasingly, video image analysis is being used, in place of human visual appraisal, to automatically classify carcasses (Craigie *et al.*, 2012). In Ireland, over 90% of beef carcasses are classified in this way (Department of Agriculture, Food and the Marine, 2019). Video image analysis can improve the repeatability of assessment and the precision of prediction of saleable meat yield/carcass value. Table 9.1 shows a generalized version of the grid used to classify fat and conformation of beef carcasses in the EU, and the regions of the grid that typically attract the highest prices. Average price differentials paid for carcasses in different fat and conformation classes are often used to derive economic values for selection indices for beef cattle.

In general, the relative economic value for conformation derived from market information is lower than the value perceived by breeders and, to some extent, lower than the value attached to conformation in live markets. This may be explained partly by the value of conformation scores in the live animal in predicting killing-out percentage but it probably also reflects the widely held belief in many meat industries that high conformation is of direct value, apart from its value as a predictor of additional meat yield. In many North American and Australasian markets, a premium is paid for high marbling, i.e. high levels of visible intramuscular fat in the eye muscle. Particularly in North America, this premium for marbling is based on its value as an indicator of good eating quality. Recently, interest in marbling in several exporting countries has been fuelled by its importance in the lucrative Japanese beef market.

Meat-eating quality is becoming an increasingly important issue with consumers and the meat industry, in wealthier countries especially. The post-slaughter treatment of carcasses, especially chilling rate, ageing and method of hanging, are known to have important effects on eating quality (Dikeman, 1990; Cuthbertson, 1994; Lambe and Simm, 2004). However, there is less information on pre-slaughter effects on beef eating quality, such as breed, breeding value within breed, or production system. The information that is available suggests that there are breed differences in indirect measures of meat quality, especially marbling, colour and fibre type. There are differences in tenderness between breed types: double-muscled breeds generally have the most tender meat, followed by other *Bos taurus* breeds, with *Bos indicus* breeds ranking lowest. There are less consistent differences in tenderness between the non-double-muscled *Bos taurus* breeds, or between any of the breed types, in juiciness and flavour. Despite this, there are consistent reports of substantial within-breed genetic variation in both indirect and direct measures of eating quality, indicating that there is scope for improvement through within-breed selection (Kemp, 1994).

Table 9.1. A generalized version of the grid used to classify fat and conformation of beef carcasses in the EU. Classes that typically attract the highest prices are in the darkest shade. In some countries the most common classes are further subdivided.

		Fat class → Fatter				
Conformation class		1	2	3	4	5
	E					
	U					
↓	R					
	O					
Poorer conformation	P					

Breeding replacement females for specialized beef herds

The main breeding goals for cows in specialized beef herds, in addition to adequate growth and carcass merit, are good fertility, ease of calving, good maternal ability (which includes adequate milk production and good mothering ability) and low or intermediate mature size, to reduce cow maintenance requirements. These individual goals are sometimes aggregated into measures like *weight of calf weaned per cow per annum*, or *weight of calf weaned per kg cow mature weight per annum*.

The ability of animals to withstand extreme climates, and to tolerate low-quality feed and periods of feed shortage, is also important in some areas and there is often concern about possible genotype × environment interactions for these 'adaptation' traits. These traits are often difficult to define, and the most practical route for within-breed improvement is often simply to record and select on performance in the harsh environment concerned (Simm *et al.*, 1996; Fig. 9.6) The emphasis on each of these traits will vary depending on the production system and breed or crossbred type of cow used. In some cases, the traits of importance will be best improved by selection, in others they will be best improved by crossbreeding. For instance, the fertility of crossbred

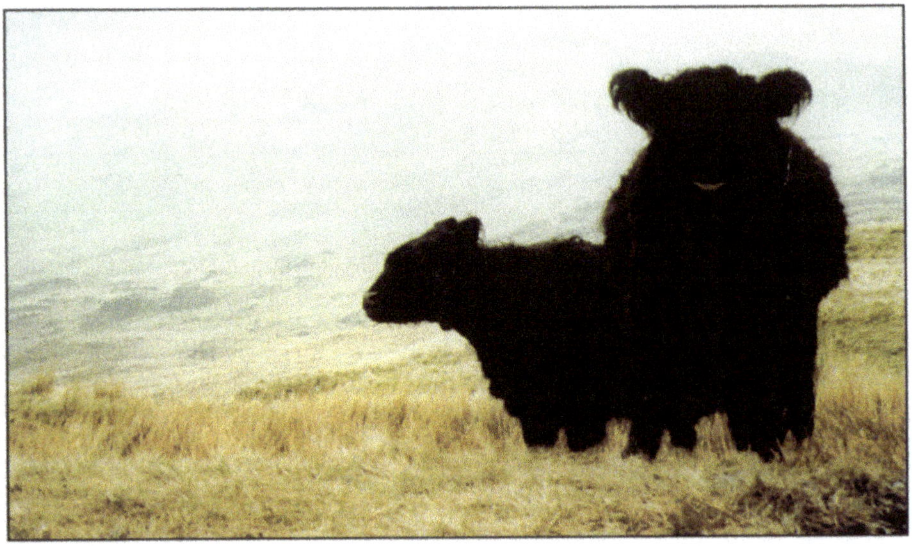

Fig. 9.6. Hardy beef breeds such as the Galloway have undergone many years of natural and artificial selection for adaptation to harsh environments. (Courtesy of Professor Peter Amer.)

cows is usually high as a result of heterosis, and so it is of less concern in selection within the component breeds. Also, in beef × dairy suckler cows, milk production is usually adequate and so other traits assume greater importance in the overall breeding goal. The mature size of specialized beef cows is usually kept in check by choosing a small- or medium-sized breed for use either in the purebred form, or as a component breed of the final cross.

Beef × dairy heifers have made an important contribution to suckler herds in Britain, Ireland and some other countries, in the past. However, these heifers have been produced largely as a by-product of crossing dairy cows to beef bulls to reduce calving difficulties, or to produce calves with improved growth and carcass merit for finishing, rather than to produce breeding beef females per se. The widespread use of Holstein sires in dairy herds in many temperate dairying countries has led to an increase in the size and a reduction in the beef conformation of dairy cows. Also, the number of dairy cows in many European countries is declining as a result of increasing production per cow (AHDB, 2019b). At the same time, there is wider use of large continental beef breeds as crossing breeds in dairy herds, rather than traditional British beef breeds. Together these factors threaten the traditional supply of medium-sized, well-conformed replacement beef × dairy females. This has created opportunities for some breeds or individual breeders to concentrate on breeding goals relevant for beef sires to cross to the more specialized dairy cow in use today. Also, more beef herds in these countries are breeding their own replacements through the use of one of the rotational crossing systems described in Chapter 4, or switching to a specialized composite breed (Fuller, 2018).

Despite these apparently different rôles for beef cattle, in practice many beef breeds and individual breeders have attempted to fulfil all of them. Greater clarity about breeding goals, use of objective information on the merits of different breed types and wider use of tools to select individual animals within breeds will help producers to match breeds and sires to particular rôles more effectively, and to improve the efficiency of beef production. Some developments in these areas are discussed later in this chapter.

Smallholder and pastoral systems in lower income countries

Traditionally, cattle in smallholder and pastoral systems within lower income countries fulfil multiple functions (see Chapter 1). Typically, these have been of indigenous breeds that are well adapted to the local environmental conditions, and have been selected on an informal, visual basis. However, in some cases improved breeds are used, such as the improved Boran cattle of East Africa. Also, for some systems, where there is an increasing emphasis on milk production, crossbreeding with exotic dairy breeds is becoming more common. Productivity in these systems is typically lower than that of larger-scale systems found elsewhere, due to a variety of factors, including the multiple objectives for keeping cattle (that do not necessarily incentivize high productivity), poor levels of animal management and harsh environmental conditions.

Breeds and Crosses Used in Beef Production

The breeds and crosses used in beef production, and how they match the breeding goals mentioned above, are discussed in this section. The strategies used for within-breed selection for these goals, the heritabilities of traits in beef breeding goals and the genetic correlations among them are examined in a later section.

It is difficult to differentiate between many beef, dairy and dual-purpose breeds at the international level. The FAO (2015) survey of domesticated animal breeds identified 1019 local and 205 transboundary cattle breeds. Of these, 184 were extinct and only 285 were *not* considered to be at risk of extinction. Clearly there is a large number of breeds that contribute to beef production worldwide.

The predominance of black-and-white strains in the dairy industry in many countries (as discussed in Chapter 8) means that they too are major contributors to beef output. This happens both directly through surplus calves and cull cows and, in some countries, indirectly through their contribution to the genetic makeup of suckler cows. However, the increasing specialization for milk production in black-and-white strains means that their predominance is often seen as a disadvantage in beef production. Because of the economic incentive towards specialization for milk production in most temperate countries, one of the biggest opportunities to improve beef output from dairy breeds is through crossing those females not required to breed replacement dairy heifers to specialized beef breeds. The proportion of dairy cows available for such crossing is increased by the growing use of sexed dairy semen. In the future, some of the emerging technologies discussed in Chapter 5 may also have a wider rôle in improving the efficiency of beef production from dairy herds.

In Europe, it is more difficult to assess the relative contribution of different breeds and crosses to beef production than it is for dairying. This is partly because of the contribution which dairy and dual-purpose breeds make to beef output, the widespread use of crossbreeding and the generally poorer systems for recording and collating national data on breed use. The French specialized beef breeds, particularly the Charolais and Limousin, and to a lesser extent the British breeds, particularly the Angus and Hereford, predominate in the major European beef-producing countries (see Fig. 9.7 and Simm, 1998). The popularity of the French breeds is probably due to their high growth rates and high lean meat yield, while the popularity of the British breeds is probably due to their relatively low incidence of calving difficulties. Also, the traditional British breeds, especially the Aberdeen Angus, have had a renaissance recently, because of perceived benefits in eating quality. The results of one comparison of the growth and carcass attributes of these breeds were shown in Table 3.4. For other examples, see Thiessen *et al.* (1984), Gregory *et al.* (1991) and Amer *et al.* (1992).

As mentioned earlier, a relatively high proportion of beef produced in France and Italy is from purebred specialized beef herds. In France, the Charolais, Limousin, Blonde d'Aquitaine and Salers breeds are most numerous, while the Piemontese, Marchigiana and Chianina breeds are most numerous in Italy. The breed composition of cows in specialized beef herds in the UK is rather poorly documented.

The increased use of the specialized French breeds as terminal sires in Europe, often at the expense of the traditional British breeds, is mirrored in many other temperate beef-producing countries. However, the British breeds remain important in breeding herds, either as purebreds or as components of crossbred maternal lines, in many of these countries (e.g. the US, Canada, Australia, New Zealand). In some of these countries the traditional supremacy of the British breeds in this maternal rôle is being challenged by new composite breeds, often based on some of these pure breeds.

Often less numerous breeds have a disproportionate influence through the use of AI, especially in dairy herds. For example, in the UK there are relatively small numbers of purebred Belgian Blue cattle, but the breed is widely used through AI due to its ability to leave high-conformation crossbred calves, with acceptable levels of calving ease, when mated to dairy cows.

As mentioned above, the Brazilian beef industry is one of the largest globally. The industry was established several hundred years ago, based on European taurine breeds, but over the last century, and especially in the last 50 years, it has been dominated by the tropically adapted *Bos indicus* Nelore breed, originally imported from India (Fig. 9.8; Mudadu *et al.*, 2016).

Tropically adapted composites based on *Bos indicus* breeds such as the Brahman and Boran, tropically adapted *Bos taurus* breeds (e.g. Afrikaner, Tuli, Belmont Red, Bonsmara, Senepol) and British

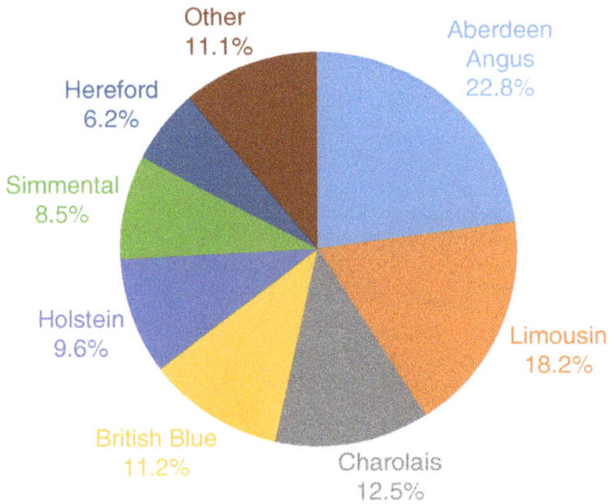

Fig. 9.7. Sire breed of cattle slaughtered in the UK in 2017. (Personal communication: Abbygail Wells and Professor Mike Coffey, SRUC, based on British Cattle Movement Service data.)

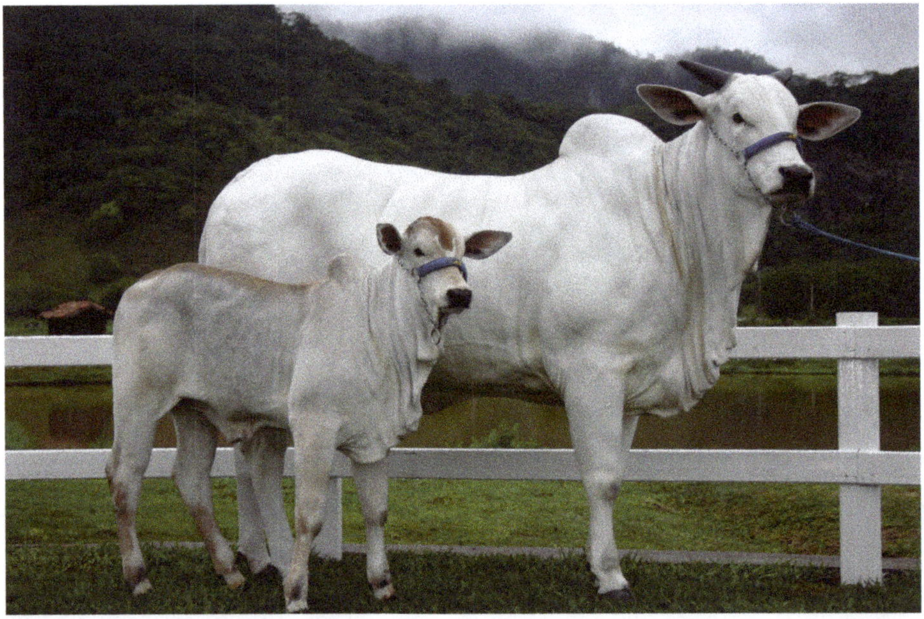

Fig. 9.8. Nelore cow and calf. (Under licence https://pixabay.com/service/license/.)

Bos taurus breeds are used by pastoral companies in northern Australia to optimize productivity in this harsh environment (Beef CRC, 2019a).

As mentioned above, indigenous breeds of cattle are important in multi-functional smallholder and pastoral systems in lower income countries. In some cases, improved breeds, such as the Boran, are being more widely used (see Fig. 9.9).

Selection within breeds

Systems of testing

Historically, most beef cattle genetic improvement programmes have been based on performance testing or progeny testing. The distinction between these is becoming less obvious now, with the use of genomic selection and the wider collection of records from progeny and other relatives from commercial systems. However, it will help to understand the opportunities for further enhancement to look at features of performance testing and progeny testing as originally practised. Both of these depend on performance recording. Essentially, this involves recording the identity, pedigree, birth date, sex and performance (e.g. live weights) of individual animals, plus any major management groupings or treatments likely to influence performance. In performance testing schemes, these records are then used to predict the genetic merit of the recorded animals themselves, as explained in Chapter 7. In progeny testing schemes, the records are usually used to predict the genetic merit of sires. The key features of these two main types of testing are described below.

Performance testing

Since many of the traits of interest in beef cattle can be recorded in both sexes, prior to sexual maturity, there is a long history of performance recording and performance testing in beef breeding. This dates from the 1940s and 1950s in the US, and to slightly later in many other countries. Recording associations were often established specifically to operate early performance recording schemes. Today it is usually the responsibility of breed associations (e.g. in the US), government departments or agencies receiving some government support (e.g. in many European countries), industry bodies or private agencies, either alone or in partnership with each other. In some countries (especially where herds are large and geographically dispersed), performance is usually measured by the breeders themselves and then sent to the recording agency. In others, such as some European countries, some or all of the measurements are made by field staff from the recording agency. The approach used also depends on the value breeders and their customers attach to independent authentication of records.

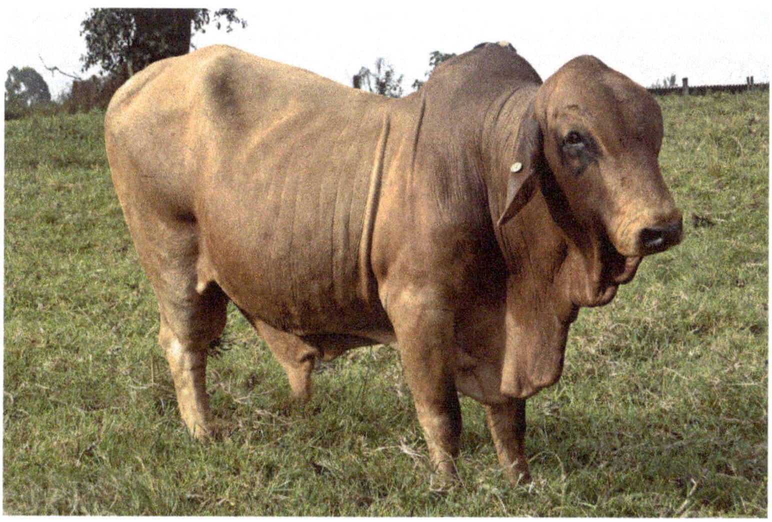

Fig. 9.9. A Boran bull. (Courtesy of ILRI/Susan MacMillan.)

Compared to the situation in dairy cattle breeding, a relatively low proportion of beef cattle are performance recorded (e.g. <2% in the US, Australia and the UK; Simm, 1998). This is partly because of the greater distinction between commercial and breeding herds than in the dairy industry, especially in countries where crossbreeding is widespread. However, even within the purebred sector, there is usually a much lower proportion of recording than in the dairy sector. This is partly due to the greater additional effort involved in recording beef cattle. It is also due to the less direct route for the rewards to accrue; milk recording helps to improve the profitability of milk production directly on the recording farm. In contrast, most of the economic benefits of performance recording beef cattle come through improved sales of breeding stock. In the past, the less widespread conviction of the benefits of recording among beef cattle breeders and their customers has affected the size and consistency of these rewards. However, there is a growing awareness of the value of performance recording in many countries, not least because of the wider use of the modern methods of predicting breeding values discussed in Chapter 7.

Most performance testing schemes involve recording the pre-weaning performance of all animals on-farm. In some countries, postweaning performance continues to be measured on-farm. In others, central performance testing is used. Central testing of beef cattle has been quite widely used worldwide since the 1950s, especially in the US, Canada and Europe. It involves submitting some animals, especially higher-performing bulls, from the breeders' own farms to a central station where they are compared with bulls from other herds in a uniform environment. Disentangling true genetic merit from the effects of good feeding and management was particularly difficult before the availability of best linear unbiased prediction (BLUP) methods and central testing was designed to reduce this problem. Also, it can create larger groups of contemporary animals for comparison; small pedigree herd sizes in many countries limit selection intensities. Central testing also allows more comprehensive measurements of performance, e.g. of feed intake.

Despite the potential benefits of central testing, the correlations between the performance of bulls in central stations and the subsequent performance of their progeny is often lower than expected. In other words, central test results can be a poor indicator of a bull's breeding value. This is often attributed to large pre-test environmental effects. These may be reduced by starting tests at younger ages and putting greater emphasis on traits measured later in the testing period (Andersen *et al.*, 1981; Simm *et al.*, 1985). Partly because of these complications, the central testing of beef bulls has ceased in some countries. Later results from France show reasonable correlations between the weight of bulls tested in central stations and the live weight of their progeny. There were higher correlations still between sire and progeny performance for skeletal and muscular development (see Table 9.2). This may reflect more uniform rearing conditions on French farms in the regions concerned than in other studies. It is also likely that muscular development is less affected by the rearing environment than is live weight.

Progeny testing

Even when the emphasis is on selection on individual animals' performance records there is an automatic, but often slow, accumulation of progeny records from the sires used in performance-recorded herds. However, in many countries there is a more deliberate strategy of first performance testing, then progeny testing bulls, with selection at each stage. As with performance testing, progeny testing schemes either operate on-farm or at central testing stations.

Sequential testing is particularly well organized in the specialized beef breeds in France (see Fig. 9.10 and France Génétique Elevage, 2019). Large numbers

Table 9.2. Genetic correlations between the performance of Charolais bulls in French central testing stations, and the subsequent performance of their progeny in test stations. (After Journaux and Renand, 1992; Bonnett *et al.*, 1994.)

1. Trait measured on bulls in central performance test station	2. Trait measured on 30 male progeny	Genetic correlation between 1 and 2
Weight at approx. 480 days	Weight at 500 days	+0.40
Muscular development (live)	Muscular development (live)	+1.00
Muscular development (live)	Muscular development (carcass)	+0.97
Skeletal development	Skeletal development	+0.75

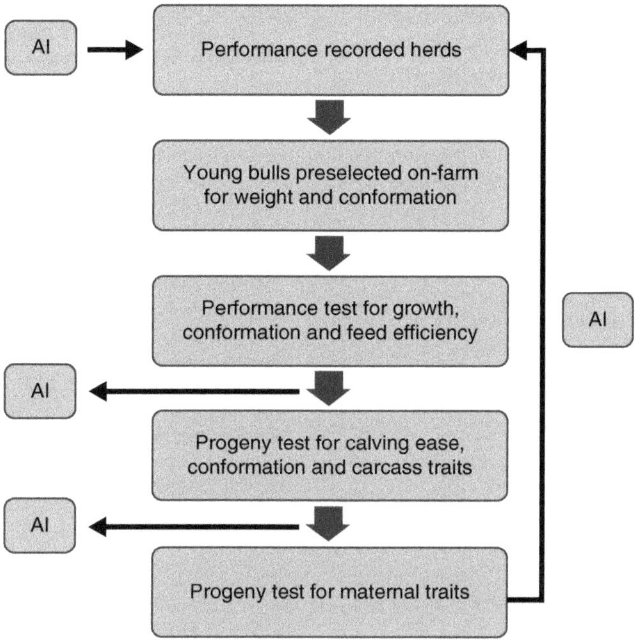

Fig. 9.10. The sequential testing of beef bulls as practised in specialized beef breeds in France. (After Ménissier, 1988.)

of purebred animals are performance-recorded on-farm for weights at birth, 120 and 210 days, and for muscular and skeletal development at weaning. The best males from on-farm recording are brought to central testing stations after weaning and tested further from 8 to 14 months of age. Most of these are selected on the basis of their performance in central test stations. The best of these bulls go on to be progeny tested to assess their daughters' maternal ability, in central progeny test stations.

There has been a recent resurgence of interest in central progeny testing schemes in some countries, including New Zealand and Australia (Beef and Lamb NZ, 2019; MLA, 2019b). Where multiple breeds of sires are involved, these tests can allow fair comparison of progeny and also create data of great value in across-breed genetic evaluations.

A significant development recently has been the use of records from crossbred progeny from commercial meat processing plants to allow prediction of accurate sire breeding values for carcass merit (which might be considered an opportunistic rather than formally designed progeny test). For instance, ICBF (2020) have introduced a comprehensive national scheme in Ireland operating across several sire breeds. The British Limousin Cattle Society (2019) also produces carcass trait estimated breeding values (EBVs) in this way.

In countries where beef bulls are widely used in dairy herds, breed societies or AI organizations often support progeny tests of beef bulls in dairy herds, evaluating calving ease, growth and carcass traits (see e.g. Genus ABS, 2020).

Other breeding schemes

Although most breeding schemes revolve around performance testing or progeny testing, as outlined above, there are some variations which deserve special mention here. The first of these are co-operative breeding schemes, such as group breeding schemes and sire referencing schemes (Simm, 1998). The benefits of these schemes were outlined in Chapter 3. Perhaps because of the relatively high legal and financial commitment required, and the growth in uptake of national across-herd genetic evaluation procedures, there appears to have been a decline in interest in cattle co-operative breeding schemes in temperate countries over the last couple of decades. However, these are of potential value in community-based breeding programmes, which are of growing importance in small ruminants in lower income countries (Mueller *et al.*, 2015).

The potential value of multiple ovulation and embryo transfer (MOET) in accelerating response to selection was first reported for beef cattle by Land and Hill (1975). They estimated that responses to selection for growth rate could be doubled by the use of MOET, albeit with higher rates of inbreeding. As in dairy cattle, these original estimates of the benefits of MOET are now believed to be on the high side. Later estimates suggest that 30% extra progress is possible, compared to a conventional scheme of similar size and with the same rate of inbreeding (Villanueva *et al.*, 1995). While MOET has been used widely in beef cattle as a means of importing and exporting genetic material, and to multiply newly imported breeds or valuable individuals more rapidly than possible with natural reproduction, it has not been used widely in structured breed improvement programmes to date. The theoretical benefits of central nucleus herds using MOET and a few early examples of use were described by Simm (1998).

Traits recorded

Generally, on-farm performance recording schemes around the world have concentrated on measuring live weights at regular intervals (or growth rates between these), together with visual scores of muscularity and measurements or scores of height or skeletal development. The development of mobile, reasonably accurate ultrasonic scanners in the 1970s and 1980s allowed measurements of fat and muscle depths or areas to be included in some on-farm recording schemes. Typically, these ultrasonic measurements are taken on or over the eye muscle at one of the last ribs, or in the loin region of animals, at about a year or 400 days of age. At least in theory, one of the benefits of central testing is that it permits more frequent and more comprehensive measurements to be made. For example, it is rarely practical to measure feed intake of individual animals on farms (see AHDB (2019a) for recent work on this in the UK) but it is fairly common in central performance test stations. Similarly, progeny testing allows direct carcass measurements to be obtained.

Table 9.3 gives examples of the traits typically recorded in beef improvement programmes. For more details of individual programmes, see, for example, American Angus Association (2019), Breedplan (2019), British Limousin Cattle Society (2019) and Signet (2019a). In several countries, EBVs for various components of meat-eating quality are available, based on live animal predictors of eating quality (e.g. ultrasound measures of intramuscular fat), direct or indirect carcass measurements (e.g. laboratory or taste-panel measures) from planned progeny tests or progeny available through commercial meat processing plants, molecular genetic information (individual genes/markers or many single nucleotide polymorphisms via genomic predictions), or combinations of these (see Breedplan, 2019; British Limousin Cattle Society, 2019; MLA, 2019a; Signet, 2019; ICBF, 2020). These tools for assessing genetic merit in meat-eating quality are of growing interest in countries like Brazil and Australia, with a major exporting beef industry based on *Bos indicus* breeds (e.g. Mudadu *et al.*, 2016).

Table 9.3. Traits commonly (or in brackets, less commonly) recorded in beef cattle breeding schemes

Traits recorded
Calving difficulty
(Birth weight)
Weaning weight or 200-day weight
Yearling weight or 400-day weight
(Later weights, e.g. 600-day and adult cow)
Ultrasonic measures of fat and muscle depth or area (and marbling)
(Direct (e.g. taste panel) or indirect (e.g. ultrasonic) measures of meat-eating quality)
Visual scores of muscularity/conformation
(Food intake)
(Scrotal circumference)
(Calving interval)
(Temperament)
(Methane emissions or proxies of these)

Generally, terminal sire characteristics have dominated beef breeding schemes in Europe. With the exception of some breeding schemes in France, few of the maternal characteristics mentioned earlier, like fertility, have been recorded widely. As a result, what little objective selection there has been for maternal characteristics has been on traits like calving ease, birth weight and 200-day weight, which are of importance in both terminal sire and maternal lines. However, until fairly recently, methods of separating direct and maternal genetic influences on these traits have not been in widespread use. Maternal traits have received more attention in North America, Australia, New

Zealand and Brazil, where specialized beef herds account for a far higher proportion of beef output. Genetic evaluations for scrotal size (which is an indicator of both male and female fertility, and age at puberty) and female fertility (measured as days from the start of the mating period to calving) are available for some breeds in Australia and New Zealand. Evaluations for scrotal size and mature cow weight have been introduced for some breeds in the USA.

The following series of tables shows means, standard deviations and estimates of the heritabilities of many of the traits mentioned as breeding goals or criteria, together with estimates of phenotypic and genetic correlations among some of them. These are from a comprehensive review of the international scientific literature (Koots *et al.*, 1994a,b). An important finding of this review was that there are significant effects of breed and country on estimates of heritabilities and correlations. If very reliable local estimates are available, these should be used to design breeding schemes and criteria and perform genetic evaluations. In other cases, it would be better to use published values, or to combine local estimates with the overall means of published estimates.

Table 9.4 shows heritability estimates for reproductive traits. These are often shown separately for heifers and older cows. This is because the traits concerned are believed to be affected by different genes in heifers and cows, or have different incidences, or both, and so heritabilities may differ. Also, in this and some of the following tables, both direct and maternal estimates of heritabilities are shown. As mentioned in Chapter 6, direct heritabilities refer to the trait as measured on the animals recorded. For instance, the direct heritability of calving ease is a measure of the genetic variation in calving ease due to the size and shape of calves themselves, the direct influence calves have on gestation length, plus any other calf factors affecting calving ease. In contrast, the maternal heritability of calving ease is a measure of genetic variation among cows in traits affecting calving ease, such as cow pelvic size and shape, body condition, and maternal influence on gestation length. It is important to make a distinction between direct and maternal genetic influences in evaluating and selecting animals because they can be antagonistic. For example, selecting a smaller bull may improve calving ease when this bull's offspring are born. However, when the bull's daughters

Table 9.4. Means, phenotypic standard deviations and weighted mean estimates of heritabilities for a range of reproductive traits in beef cattle. These come from an extensive review of published values but estimates of means, s.d.s and heritabilities are not necessarily from the same source. The standard errors (s.e.) of heritability estimates provide a measure of their reliability and a means to test whether or not estimates are significantly different from zero, or from each other. See the original review for sources and full details of the methods used to weight estimates and obtain standard errors. (Koots *et al.*, 1994a,b.)

Trait	Unit of measurement	Mean	Phenotypic s.d.	Mean heritability (s.e.)
Age at first calving – direct	days	682	39	0.06 (0.020)
Age at first calving – maternal				0.19 (0.035)
Conception rate – cows, direct	% calving	76	47	0.17 (0.015)
Conception rate – heifers, direct				0.05 (0.010)
Conception rate – cows, maternal				0.02 (0.019)
Conception rate – heifers, maternal				0.02 (0.009)
Calving ease – cows, direct	% unassisted	90.6	15.7	0.13 (0.002)
Calving ease – heifers, direct		91.2	26.7	0.10 (0.002)
Calving ease – cows, maternal		98.2	15.3	0.12 (0.002)
Calving ease – heifers, maternal		90.6	31.7	0.09 (0.002)
Pelvic area, constant age	cm^2	221	58	0.58 (0.058)
Perinatal mortality – cows, direct	% mortality	3.1	20.9	0.10 (0.001)
Perinatal mortality – heifers, direct		9.8	31.7	0.15 (0.003)
Perinatal mortality – cows, maternal		4.2	20.3	0.11 (0.001)
Perinatal mortality – heifers, maternal		6.9	41.3	0.11 (0.001)
Calving rate	% calves weaned	–	–	0.17 (0.010)
Scrotal circumference, constant age	cm	33.9	2.7	0.48 (0.019)

calve themselves, calving ease may deteriorate in the herd, because they are smaller adults as well as smaller calves. Table 9.4 shows that many of the traits concerned with reproduction have fairly low heritabilities. However, many are economically important, and there is substantial variation in them, so there is both the incentive and scope for genetic improvement.

Table 9.5 shows mean estimates of the heritabilities of growth traits. Direct heritabilities tend to be moderately high, while maternal heritabilities tend to be slightly lower. Also, the direct heritability of live weights tends to be fairly high at birth, lower at weaning and higher again at yearling or later ages. Table 9.6 shows the heritabilities of a range of carcass measurements. These tend to be even higher than those for growth traits. However, they have to be assessed either indirectly on live candidates for selection (e.g. by ultrasonic measurements), or directly on progeny or other relatives of the candidates for selection, so they are not as easy to improve as it seems at first sight.

Table 9.7 shows mean estimates of phenotypic and genetic correlations between some reproduction, growth and carcass traits. There are unfavourable associations between several reproduction and growth traits, which complicates selection for dual-purpose characteristics. Generally, there are strong phenotypic and genetic associations between weights at different ages: the closer the age, the stronger the association.

Table 9.5. Means, phenotypic standard deviations and weighted mean estimates of heritabilities for a range of growth traits in beef cattle. These come from an extensive review of published values, but estimates of means, s.d.s and heritabilities are not necessarily from the same source. See the original review for sources and full details of the methods used to weight estimates and obtain standard errors. (After Koots *et al.*, 1994a,b.)

Trait	Unit of measurement	Mean	Phenotypic s.d.	Mean heritability (s.e.)
Birth weight - direct	kg	35.1	4.3	0.31 (0.003)
Birth weight - maternal		34.9	4.4	0.14 (0.002)
Weaning weight - direct	kg	203	25	0.24 (0.002)
Weaning weight - maternal		217	29	0.13 (0.002)
Yearling weight - direct	kg	345	38	0.33 (0.004)
Postweaning gain	kg/day	0.978	0.134	0.31 (0.004)
Yearling gain - direct	kg/day	0.852	0.082	0.34 (0.017)
Feed intake	kg DM/day	6.48	0.62	0.34 (0.025)
Feed conversion ratio (feed (or energy)/ gain)	kg (or unit energy)/kg	6.00	0.66	0.32 (0.024)
Mature cow weight	kg	446	54	0.50 (0.021)

Table 9.6. Means, phenotypic standard deviations and weighted mean estimates of heritabilities for a range of carcass traits in beef cattle. These come from an extensive review of published values, but estimates of means, s.d.s and heritabilities are not necessarily from the same source. See the original review for sources and full details of the methods used to weight estimates and obtain standard errors. (After Koots *et al.*, 1994a,b.)

Trait	Unit of measurement	Mean	Phenotypic s.d.	Mean heritability (s.e.)
Backfat depth, constant age[a]	mm	10.6	2.6	0.44 (0.019)
Carcass weight, constant age	kg	313	19	0.23 (0.011)
Carcass weight, constant finish	kg			0.36 (0.111)
Dressing %, constant age	%	60.1	1.9	0.39 (0.021)
Cutability (meat yield), constant age	%	54.8	20.1	0.47 (0.024)
Lean:bone ratio	–	4.07:1	0.29	0.63 (0.041)
Lean %	%	62.3	2.8	0.55 (0.028)
Marbling, constant age	score	7.36	2.51	0.38 (0.034)
Eye muscle area, constant age	cm^2	68.9	7.0	0.42 (0.023)
Tenderness	Warner-Bratzler shear force	5.48	1.00	0.29 (0.038)

[a]For most traits, heritability estimates at a constant weight or finish are similar.

Table 9.7. Mean estimates of phenotypic and genetic correlations between pairs of traits in beef cattle from an extensive review of published values. Correlations with age at calving are unweighted, all others are weighted. See the original review for sources and full details of the methods used to weight estimates. (After Koots *et al.*, 1994a,b.)

		Mean correlation between traints	
Trait 1	Trait 2	Phenotypic	Genetic
Age at first calving, direct	Birth weight, direct	0.05	−0.14
	Postweaning gain	0.10	0.48
	Mature cow weight	−0.36	−0.10
Calving ease, direct	Calving ease, maternal	–	−0.30
	Birth weight, direct	−0.28	−0.74
	Weaning weight, direct	0.04	−0.21
	Postweaning gain	−0.09	−0.54
	Yearling weight, direct	0.01	−0.29
	Mature cow weight	−0.03	−0.23
Birth weight, direct	Birth weight, maternal	–	−0.35
	Weaning wt, maternal	0.34	−0.14
	Weaning wt, direct	0.46	0.50
	Postweaning gain	0.19	0.32
	Yearling wt, direct	0.38	0.55
	Mature cow weight	0.34	0.67
Weaning weight, direct	Birth weight, maternal	0.34	−0.05
	Weaning wt, maternal	–	−0.16
	Postweaning gain	0.09	0.44
	Yearling wt, direct	0.71	0.81
	Food intake	0.47	–
	Food conversion ratio	0.00	−0.50
	Mature cow weight	0.45	0.57
Yearling weight, direct	Postweaning gain	0.74	0.81
	Food intake	0.64	0.16
	Food conversion ratio	−0.46	−0.60
	Mature cow weight	0.54	0.72
Market weight, constant age	Dressing %, const. age	0.06	−0.23
	Backfat, constant age	0.19	0.00
	Eye muscle, const. age	0.33	0.43
	Marbling, const. age	0.15	0.34
	Cutability, const age	−0.22	−0.19

This means that selection for growth characteristics alone usually leads to unfavourable responses in birth weight (i.e. increased birth weight which generally leads to more difficult calving) and heavier mature cow weight. Unfavourable responses in birth weight can be reduced by selecting individual animals with EBVs which depart from this general trend (e.g. low birth weight EBVs, but high EBVs for later weights) or by including birth weight and later weights in an index with negative and positive economic values, respectively. Similar approaches can be used to reduce unfavourable responses in cow mature weight although using separate terminal sire and maternal breeds or crosses is probably more efficient.

Methods and results of genetic evaluation

Overview

Methods of genetic evaluation were described in general in Chapter 7. The purpose of this section is to outline the status of their use in beef cattle. Until the early 1970s, the genetic evaluation methods employed in beef cattle in most countries were fairly simple. These usually produced adjusted records of performance, contemporary comparisons or predicted breeding values which could only be compared within herd (or within a central test team). However, from the 1970s onwards BLUP methods of evaluation began to be adopted. BLUP provides more accurate prediction of breeding values than other methods. Also, BLUP predicted breeding values (PBVs) can be compared across herds and years, providing that there are genetic links between herds and years. This is particularly important in countries where pedigree beef herd sizes are small, and so selection intensities are usually low.

Sire model BLUP evaluations for beef cattle across herds and years were first used in the early 1970s in the USA (Benyshek and Bertrand, 1990). National animal model BLUP evaluations, producing PBVs for all animals, not just sires, are the norm now in most wealthier countries. Similarly, most of these countries use multi-trait evaluations. A growing number of countries are involved in international evaluations. Likewise, there is growing use of genomic information to enhance the accuracy of EBVs and provide earlier information on genetic merit in traits that are difficult or expensive to measure, occur late in life or in one sex. (See Breedplan (2019), British Limousin Cattle Society (2019), and ICBF (2020) for examples of genomic breeding values (GEBVs) for a range of traits).

The results of beef evaluations are expressed as PBVs or EBVs, predicted (or estimated) transmitting abilities (PTAs or ETAs), expected progeny differences (EPDs) or, increasingly, GEBVs. As explained in Chapter 7, PBVs, EBVs or GEBVs express genetic merit in terms of the recorded animal itself, while PTAs, ETAs or EPDs all express merit in terms of the expected performance of progeny (i.e. a PTA, ETA or EPD for any trait is half the PBV, EBV or GEBV for that same trait).

We identified earlier that beef breeds or breeders often have different breeding goals, with different emphasis on terminal sire (e.g. growth and carcass) versus maternal traits. There are often unfavourable associations between these. Hence, genetic evaluations usually distinguish between direct and maternal components of breeding values for key traits, especially calving ease and weaning or 200-day weight, sometimes referred to as 200-day milk, as the maternal component of breeding values for weaning weight is assumed to be mainly influenced by the dam's genetic merit for milk yield (see, for example, Breedplan, 2019; Signet, 2019b). Because of the longer time needed to record maternal performance traits, the fact that some, such as 200-day milk, are based on indirect information, and their lower heritabilities, accuracies for these traits are often low in young bulls (see Table 9.8).

While BLUP EBVs are already scaled to take account of their accuracy, accuracies are still a useful guide to the risk that an individual animal's EBV will change in future. They are particularly useful in distinguishing between animals whose EBVs are based mainly on ancestors' records, or indirect measurements, and those with direct information recorded. Table 9.9 illustrates this. Low accuracy figures imply that the eventual very accurate EBV for milk, obtained after collecting lots of records, *could* be quite different from the initial EBV. This leads many breeders to ask 'why bother publishing low accuracy EBVs?' The answer is that they are still the best guide available, and that across a group of animals, they will be right, on average.

Table 9.8. Typical accuracies of EBVs for different traits from multi-trait animal model BLUP evaluations for bulls with different sources of records available. (After Dr R.E. Crump, personal communication.)

Trait	Young bull with own record only, in a group with five contemporaries	Young bull with no records itself, but with five recorded progeny	Widely used bull with no records itself, but 50 recorded progeny
Birthweight	51%	60%	92%
200-day milk	21%	29%	69%
200-day growth	42%	52%	89%
400-day growth	51%	60%	92%
Backfat depth	43%	53%	89%
Muscling score	40%	50%	88%

Table 9.9. Possible range of final very accurate EBVs for an animal with a current EBV for 200-day milk of +10 kg (see Fig. 7.10 also). (After Dr R.E. Crump, personal communication.)

Accuracy of current EBV	95% chance that final EBV is in range
20 %	−8 to +28
40 %	−7 to +27
60 %	−4 to +24
80 %	−1 to +21
90 %	+2 to +18
100 %	10

Results of evaluations are available to individual breeders after each new evaluation. Usually these include summaries of the predicted merit of the current calf crop, and the sires and dams they represent. Also, national or international sire summaries are usually produced for each breed, after each evaluation. These national sire summaries list EBVs/GEBVs (or EPDs) and accuracies for sires which are currently in use, and whose EBVs/GEBVs (or EPDs) have accuracies above an agreed threshold level. Lists of 'trait leaders' (sires ranked on EBVs/GEBVs) are usually presented for most traits. Additionally, these national summaries sometimes give details of promising young bulls and top cows. Table 9.10 shows the typical layout of information in sire summaries. See also websites of major breed societies or evaluation agencies for current examples.

Evaluations across herds, breeds and countries

To be able to compare BLUP PBVs fairly across contemporary groups and years, genetic links are needed between groups and years, as explained in Chapter 7. In dairy herds, strong links occur automatically because of the very widespread use of AI. In some countries there is little use of AI in specialized beef breeds, and this has limited the effectiveness of national across-herd genetic evaluations. AI use is higher in other countries, especially those with smaller herds where bull ownership is less cost effective than AI, and where a high turnover of bulls is needed to control inbreeding. For example, between 20% and 50% of births in pedigree herds of the major beef breeds in Britain are the result of AI (Simm, 1998). Also, the recent introduction of foreign breeds to a country, or the popularity of imported strains within a breed, tend to increase the use of AI.

Table 9.10. An example of the typical layout of information in beef sire summaries.

Bull name Sire Dam	Breeder / owner / herd prefix	Identity no. / Date of birth		Birth weight (kg) (+ = heavier)	200-day weight - maternal (kg) (+ = heavier)	200-day weight - direct (kg) (+ = heavier)	400-day weight - (kg) (+ = heavier)	Ultrasonic fat depth (mm) (+ = fatter)	Ultrasonic muscle depth (mm) (+ = deeper)
Glendale Bill									
Glendale Fred	A. Smith	ABC1567	**EBV or**						
Glendale Mary	Glendale	20/03/12	**GEBV**	+2.0	−1.5	+20.5	+35.5	−0.1	+0.3
			Accuracy	45%	20%	40%	50%	39%	40%
Glendale Bob									
Glendale Fred	A. Smith	ABC1569	**EBV or**						
Glendale Daisy	Glendale	27/03/12	**GEBV**	−1.0	+1.0	−0.5	−5.5	−0.2	−0.3
			Accuracy	40%	18%	38%	45%	38%	39%
High Farm Felix									
Glendale Fred	B. Brown	DEF1234	**EBV or**						
High Farm Sue	High Farm	15/02/12	**GEBV**	+4.0	−3.5	+25.0	+40.0	+0.3	+0.5
			Accuracy	47%	21%	41%	52%	40%	42%
Newfield Superman									
Newfield Ted	G. White	GHJ3456	**EBV or**						
Newfield Blossom	Newfield	11/03/10	**GEBV**	+2.5	−1.0	+22.5	+37.5	0.0	+0.4
			Accuracy	92%	69%	89%	92%	89%	85%

In such cases there will often be strong enough genetic links between herds and years to make reliable comparisons of EBVs across herds and years. Similarly, a major technical limitation to performing evaluations across breeds is that animals of different breeds are rarely kept as contemporaries under similar management and feeding systems. However, across-breed evaluations are becoming feasible using information from crossbred animals from designed breed comparisons, together with estimates of genetic trends in each of the purebred populations since the breed comparison was made (Benyshek and Bertrand, 1990; Amer *et al.*, 1992), or from central performance or progeny tests with different breeds represented. Dealing properly with heterosis when records from crossbred animals are used is another requirement of across-breed genetic evaluations.

Compared to the situation in dairy cattle, there has been less work on developing international conversions of EBVs or EPDs for beef cattle, or performing international genetic evaluations. However, there is growing interest in this area. For example, international conversions have been produced for some beef breeds in use in Canada and the US. Also, INTERBEEF (2019), a working group of the International Committee on Animal Recording, has been producing across-country evaluations for several breeds in Europe, Australia and South Africa since 2015 (ICAR, 2019).

As national beef cattle data sets are typically much smaller than those for dairy cattle, and as computing power has increased dramatically, across-country genetic evaluation of beef cattle is usually based on actual phenotypic records for both bulls and cows. Individual countries send phenotypic records and pedigree records to INTERBEEF and the across-country genetic evaluations are done, accounting for the genetic correlations among the countries, as explained in Chapter 7. INTERBEEF first produced international evaluations for adjusted weaning weight in the Limousin breed; these are now also available in the Charolais and Simmental breeds. Also, international evaluations are available for additional traits such as birth weight and calving ease. INTERBEEF carries out two official evaluation runs per year and this now involves about ten countries. There is on-going research to develop evaluations for fertility and carcass traits. International evaluations help to address the issue of low accuracy EBVs, at least in relatives of bulls used across countries, by pooling data and so increasing accuracy of resulting EBVs or GEBVs.

Indexes of overall economic merit

The theoretical benefits of using selection indexes were described in Chapters 4 and 7. Briefly, these apportion selection emphasis in the most appropriate way, based on the relative economic importance of traits in the breeding goal, and on the strength of genetic associations between measured traits and breeding goal traits (if these differ).

Much of the emphasis in early beef improvement programmes was on producing indexes for terminal sire growth and carcass characteristics. These have become more sophisticated with a wider range of traits being recording.

Until recently, fewer indexes were available for maternal breeds or lines (i.e. including EBVs for fertility, maternal component of calving ease, direct and maternal components of weaning weight, mature size). The simplest index of this type is to combine direct and maternal EBVs for weaning weight. The weight of calf weaned by daughters of bulls in a maternal breed or line will be maximized by selecting bulls on their maternal EBV for weaning weight (or 'milk' EBV) plus *half* their direct EBV for weaning weight (this is because calves benefit from *all* of their mother's genes for milk but they only benefit from *half* her genes for growth). However, other important maternal traits need to be considered separately if this approach is used.

In countries with a specialized suckler beef sector, more comprehensive indexes for maternal performance have become more common now. In the UK, for example, Signet offers five indexes for different purposes, as shown in Fig. 9.11 (see also Breedplan, 2019).

Some providers offer software to allow breeders to specify their own breeding objectives and tailor or customize economic values to their own requirements (e.g. BreedObject®, 2019). In theory, unless systems differ dramatically, the use of customized indexes has only a small effect on expected response. However, in practice, the use of customized indexes appears to improve both the understanding and the uptake of indexes.

Evidence of genetic improvement and its value

ESTIMATES OF GENETIC CHANGE In theory, changes of at least 1–2% of the mean *per annum* are possible following selection for weight or growth traits in beef cattle. However, in practice, rates of change are often lower than this. For example, a review of

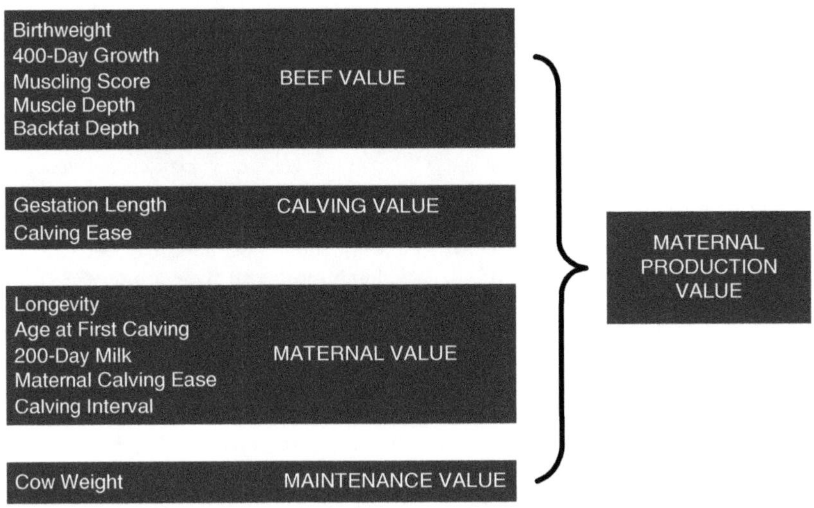

Fig. 9.11. The structure of the indexes produced for Signet recorded pedigree beef herds in Britain. Beef Value ranks animals on genetic merit for growth and carcass traits; Calving Value ranks animals on their predicted genetic merit for direct calving ease. The two indexes can be added together to rank animals on their predicted overall genetic merit for both production and calving ease. Maternal Value and Maintenance Value comprise estimated breeding values for maternal traits of importance in breeding replacement suckler cows. The Maternal Production Value combines terminal sire and maternal traits, using their relative economic values – this includes a weighting for the frequency with which each trait is expressed in the lifetime of a suckler cow and her descendants. (After Signet, 2019b; see also Roughsedge *et al.*, 2005.)

several beef cattle selection experiments showed that average changes of 0.6% and 0.8% per annum were achieved with selection for weaning and yearling weight respectively (Mrode, 1988).

The increased uptake of across-herd BLUP genetic evaluations over the last few decades has permitted more widespread estimation of genetic trends in industry breeding schemes. When evaluations are made within breeds, EBVs and trends cannot be used to compare the *absolute* performance of different breeds. However, they do indicate the genetic *changes* which have occurred within breeds, over a given period of time. Figure 9.12 shows estimated genetic trends in growth traits, Beef Index and Retail Value in the Limousin breed in the UK since 2004. Genetic trends are simply average (G)EBVs plotted by year of birth. They give a useful retrospective view of the changes which have occurred within a breed, providing that the genetic parameters used are appropriate. Hence, these graphs show the breed-wide changes which have occurred as a result of selection on within-herd performance records, as well as other subjective methods of selection.

In the past, industry trends in many breeds have been well below those theoretically possible, and below those actually achieved in selection experiments. When trends are being examined in a single trait, this may be partly due to the fact that selection is increasingly for multiple traits. It may also reflect the relatively low use of objective methods of selection in some breeds or countries. However, as Fig. 9.12 shows, this situation is changing, particularly with the availability of GEBVs.

Genetic increases in birth weight have occurred in many studies of industry trends. This is largely a consequence of selection for higher weights at later ages, rather than a desire to increase birth weights per se. This is a result of the positive genetic correlations between weights at different ages. Most breeders would like to limit increases in birth weight, because of its association with calving difficulties. Multi-trait animal model BLUP EBVs can help to identify individual animals which depart from the general trend, e.g. by having low birth weight EBVs, but high EBVs for later weights.

VALUE OF GENETIC IMPROVEMENT Compared to the situation in dairy cattle, there have been relatively few studies of the value of genetic improvement in beef cattle, though these do show favourable estimates of cost:benefit. A study of the costs and benefits of the implementation of across-herd BLUP and index selection in the terminal sire sector of the British beef industry estimated benefits from 10 years of genetic progress, considering a 20-year time frame, of £4.9 million (Amer *et al.*, 2007). Benefits from genetic progress for growth and carcass characters in dual-purpose beef breeds were £18.2 million after subtraction of costs associated with a deterioration in calving traits. The same study reported an internal rate of return on the combined investment in sheep and beef cattle breeding of 32%. Byrne *et al.* (2018) estimated

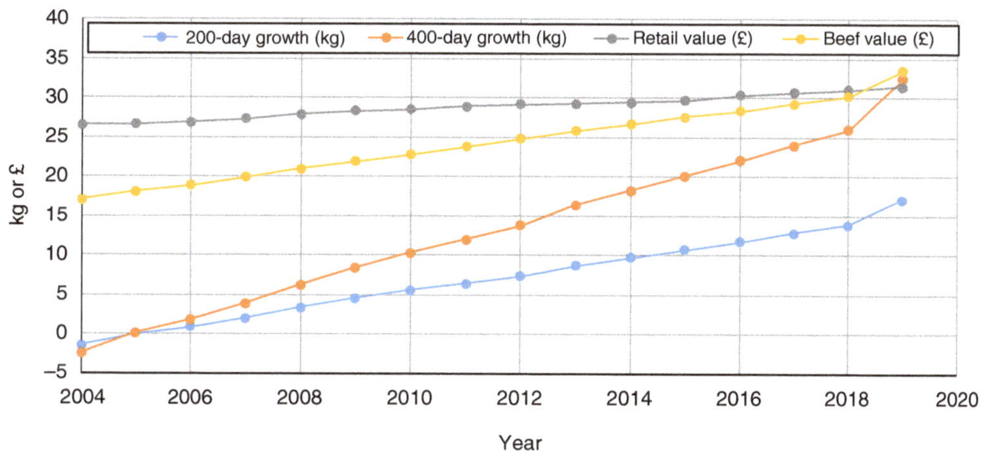

Fig. 9.12. Trends in GEBVs for 200- and 400-day weight and Beef Index and Retail Value in the Limousin breed in the UK since 2004. (After British Limousin Cattle Society Ltd.)

net benefits of €180 million from recent genetic improvement of beef cattle in Ireland – as in the UK, with a benefit from changes in terminal sire traits and a loss from deterioration in maternal traits. It is estimated that research to develop new EBVs for the Australian Beefplan system has generated a return of AU$336 million over the period 1993–2009 (Beef CRC, 2019b).

Despite the slower rates of improvement in beef cattle, compared to that possible in other species, and differences among countries in the scale of the industries, the costs of improvement schemes, and the value of the products, it is likely that there are usually major *national* benefits from beef improvement. However, it is often difficult for *individual* commercial producers to measure the increased margins from genetically superior stock and, in turn, to pay an appropriate premium to breeders of replacement stock. In Britain, an early Meat and Livestock Commission study relating the economic performance of crossbred cattle to the index scores of sires helped to convince producers of the value of within-breed selection. The study involved pairs of high- and low-index bulls of several breeds, selected on within-herd indexes prior to the introduction of BLUP evaluations. A high index natural service bull, producing about 120 offspring over his working life, was expected to leave progeny worth a total of about £2500 more than a low-index sire (Lewis, 1992). The availability of across-herd BLUP evaluations means that high merit animals should now be identified more accurately, and much higher selection intensities can be achieved. Hence, the financial benefits of within-breed selection should be even higher than this study identified. The expected benefits in a commercial herd from selecting bulls ranked in the top 40% on overall merit in the Signet beef indexes mentioned earlier, are shown in Table 9.11. See Beef and Lamb NZ (2019) for a more recent investigation of the benefits of high EBV sires.

Table 9.11. Expected responses following selection of bulls ranked in the top 40% on combined merit in two beef indexes being used in Britain. The relative contributions of Calving Value and Beef Value to overall merit in this example were 16:84. (After Professor Peter Amer, personal communication.)

Profit trait	Economic response (£)
Carcass weight (kg)	2.38
Carcass conformation (pts)	0.51
Carcass fatness (pts)	–0.05
Gestation length (days)	0.15
Calving ease (units)	0.41
Total economic response per calf (£)	3.39

Genotype × Environment Interactions

There have been a number of experiments and analyses of field data to investigate genotype × environment interactions in beef cattle (e.g. Bishop, 1983; Bertrand *et al.*, 1985; Morris *et al.*, 1993). Several studies indicate that small- or medium-sized breeds have higher overall productivity or profitability in extensive grazing systems than larger breeds. But larger breeds tend to do best in more intensive systems with high levels of concentrate feeding. These differences may be most pronounced in composite traits such as weight of calf weaned per cow mated, or per unit of cow weight.

In general, if there is a big enough difference between genotypes, or environments, or both, then it is likely that interactions will be found. The overall message as far as interactions are concerned is: (i) to be aware that they can exist; (ii) to take action if there is sound evidence that they exist in the traits of interest in the breed or system that concerns you (e.g. by restricting the choice of sires to those measured in similar conditions, or those evaluated in a wide range of conditions); and (iii) not to let the possibility of interactions in some cases detract from the value of genetic improvement in most cases.

Practical Guidelines on Selection

Some practical guidelines on selection to improve performance in objectively measured traits are given below. Most of these are equally relevant in purebred and commercial herds, and whether the selection is for carcass or maternal traits. However, pedigree breeders often wish to pay more attention to individual trait EBVs than commercial producers. Also, they may be willing to take greater risks by selecting animals with low accuracy EBVs, or by selecting occasional unrecorded animals if levels of recording are low in the breed concerned. The guidelines on selection between breeds or crosses are aimed primarily at commercial producers, since most pedigree breeders will already be firmly committed to their current breed.

Selection between breeds or crosses

- Clearly define the rôle of the animals you are selecting and identify the animal characteristics which are economically important. Choose an appropriate breed or cross, based on the sort of objective comparisons of performance discussed earlier.

Selection of bulls (or semen) for use in a purebred herd

- Set your breeding objective; the priority should be on traits expected to be of most economic (or other) importance in a few (cattle) generations time. Identify the selection index or set of EBVs/GEBVs which is most relevant for your breeding objective.
- Produce a shortlist of bulls which can be fairly compared, nationally or internationally, ranked on this index or on EBVs/GEBVs for the most important individual traits.
- If there are no national across-herd evaluations in the breed of your choice, select bulls from co-operative schemes or individual herds which have a history of using objective selection for the index or set of EBVs most relevant to your breeding goal.
- If there are economically-important traits in your breeding goal which are not included in the index available, or for which no EBVs are available, then eliminate any animals which do not meet your minimum standards. Culling for these secondary traits should be in proportion to the economic (or other) importance of the trait, and the scope for genetic change in them. Selection for traits of minor economic importance, or traits which have a small genetic component will dilute overall progress.
- Eliminate any animals which are not functionally sound. Culling should be confined to important characteristics which have a genetic component.
- If accuracies are available for the index or EBVs of your choice, and you are concerned about the risk of using low accuracy bulls, eliminate those with very low values, or spread the risk by using more bulls.
- Choose the highest index bull left on the list that you can afford and is likely to deliver economic benefit.
- Avoid matings between close relatives. Where available via the recording agency or breed society, use computer programs to optimize mate selection.
- Genetic gain will be maximized by replacing bulls whenever a bull of higher merit is available within this herd, or elsewhere. (Though this may conflict with shorter-term profitability.)

Selection of replacement females in a purebred herd

- When breeding replacement females to maximize genetic gain in a pedigree herd, rank them in a similar way to that outlined for bulls, for the relevant breeding goal (e.g. terminal sire traits or maternal traits, depending on the rôle of the breed concerned).
- Rank the potential female replacements on the chosen index, or on the individual BLUP EBVs/GEBVs of most relevance. Genetic gain will be maximized by replacing cows of any age which have low EBVs by replacements which have higher EBVs.
- If BLUP EBVs are not available, then it is difficult to compare the genetic merit of cows of different ages. The simplest policy is to calculate the optimum female generation interval to maximize genetic progress in your breeding goal (as explained in Chapter 4), and then cull cows on age to achieve this.
- Similar rules on culling for functional fitness, or traits of secondary economic importance, to those described above for bulls should be applied.

Selection of replacement bulls and cows for a commercial herd

- Genetic progress in commercial herds will be maximized by following similar guidelines on bull selection to those above.
- Usually, crossbred suckler cows do not have EBVs available. In choosing cows to breed replacement females, rank animals on half their sires' EBVs/GEBVs for important traits, if these are available. Alternatively rank them on their actual performance, adjusting where possible for age, etc. Whenever there is scope to do so, try to breed replacements from the highest-ranking cows on this list, subject to functional soundness.

- In selecting cows to breed replacements there may be a conflict between maximizing genetic progress and maximizing short-term economic performance in commercial (and pedigree) herds. For example, it may be more profitable in the short term to select replacements which are likely to calve at the optimum time, rather than to select strictly on estimated genetic merit. Hence, most scope for genetic improvement will be through selection of bulls, and initial selection of the breed or cross of cows to be used.

Summary

- Beef cattle breeding in temperate countries is less homogeneous than dairy cattle breeding. In most European countries a high proportion of beef production is from pure dairy or dual-purpose breeds. In other major temperate beef-producing countries, beef production is based on extensively grazed or ranched cows, mainly of pure British beef breeds like the Hereford, Aberdeen Angus and Shorthorn, crosses among them, or composites including them. In tropical systems, indigenous tropically adapted breed types are widely used.
- There are two broad categories of beef production in many countries: (i) beef production from dairy and dual-purpose herds; and (ii) beef production from specialized beef herds. Within the specialized beef sector, there is further differentiation into terminal sire and maternal breeds, crosses or lines. Terminal sire breeds also get used in dairy and dual-purpose herds. Each of these categories has distinct beef-breeding goals, or at least different priorities.
- While it may be efficient to breed for both milk and meat production from the same type of animal in small-scale production systems, it appears to be less efficient in large, specialized farming systems. As a result, there is a general trend towards milk production from more specialized dairy cattle breeds and strains.
- Terminal sire beef breeds are used in dairy herds, for two main purposes. The first is to mate to dairy heifers to reduce the risk of calving difficulties, compared to that following matings to a dairy sire. The second is to mate to mature dairy cows which are not required to breed replacement dairy heifers.
- In many of the specialized beef production systems there is widespread use of crossbreeding – often to achieve complementary use of breeds. Although ease of calving is still important when terminal sire breeds are used in specialized beef-breeding herds, their main rôle is to improve the growth and carcass characteristics of their crossbred offspring.
- The main breeding goals for cows in specialized beef herds, in addition to adequate growth and carcass merit, are good fertility, ease of calving, good maternal ability and low or intermediate mature size, to reduce cow maintenance requirements. The ability of animals to withstand extreme climates, and to tolerate low-quality feed and periods of feed shortage is also important in some areas. Some traits of importance are best improved by selection, others by crossbreeding.
- The predominance of black-and-white strains in the dairy industry means that they are major contributors to beef output both directly through surplus calves and cull cows and, in some countries, indirectly through their contribution to the genetic makeup of suckler cows. In many temperate countries the predominant specialized beef breeds are the French breeds, particularly the Charolais and Limousin, and to a lesser extent the British breeds, particularly the Hereford and Angus. However, several less numerous breeds have a disproportionate influence through the use of AI, especially in dairy herds.
- Historically, most beef cattle genetic improvement programmes have been based on performance testing or progeny testing. The distinction between these is becoming less obvious now, with the use of genomic selection, and the wider collection of records from progeny and other relatives from commercial systems. Most performance-testing schemes involve recording the preweaning performance of all animals on-farm. In some countries postweaning performance continues to be measured on-farm. In others, central performance testing is used. Even when the emphasis is on selection on individual animals' performance records, there is an automatic accumulation of progeny records from the sires used in performance-recorded herds. However, in some countries there is a more deliberate strategy of first performance testing,

then progeny testing bulls, with selection at each stage. As with performance testing, formal progeny testing schemes either operate on-farm or at central testing stations.

- Generally, on-farm performance recording schemes around the world have concentrated on measuring live weights at regular intervals (or growth rates between these), together with visual scores of muscularity and measurements or scores of height or skeletal development. Ultrasonic measurements of fat and muscle depths or areas are also widely used. More frequent and more comprehensive measurements are often made in central tests. There is much research interest in breeding approaches to reduce methane emissions.
- Reproductive traits have fairly low heritabilities. However, many are economically important, and there is substantial variation in them, so there is both the incentive and scope for genetic improvement. Direct heritabilities of growth traits tend to be moderately high, while maternal heritabilities tend to be slightly lower. The heritabilities of carcass measurements tend to be even higher than those for growth traits. However, they have to be assessed either indirectly on live candidates for selection (e.g. by ultrasonic measurements), or directly on progeny or other relatives of the candidates for selection, so they are not as easy to improve as it seems at first sight.
- There are unfavourable associations between several reproduction and growth traits, which complicates selection for dual-purpose characteristics. Generally, there are strong phenotypic and genetic associations between weights at different ages – the closer the age, the stronger the association. This means that selection for growth characteristics alone usually leads to unfavourable responses in birth weight (i.e. increased birth weight which generally leads to more difficult calving), and heavier mature cow weight.
- Multi-trait animal model BLUP evaluations are common in temperate and some tropical regions. There is growing use of genomic information to enhance the accuracy of EBVs and provide earlier information on genetic merit in traits that are difficult or expensive to measure, occur late in life or in one sex.
- The results of evaluations are usually expressed as EBVs, GEBVs or EPDs.
- To be able to compare BLUP PBVs fairly across contemporary groups and years, genetic links are needed between groups and years. In some countries there is little use of AI in specialized beef breeds, and this has limited the introduction of national across-herd genetic evaluations. There is growing effort on international genetic evaluations for key traits in beef cattle.
- In theory, changes of 1–2% of the mean per annum are possible following selection for weight or growth traits in beef cattle. However, in practice, rates of change in selection experiments and in industry are often lower than this. The wider use of more effective genetic evaluation techniques and genomic selection will allow more rapid improvement in a wider range of traits in future.
- It is likely that there are major *national* benefits from genetic improvement of beef cattle in many countries. However, it is difficult for *individual* commercial producers to measure the increased margins from genetically superior stock and, in turn, to pay an appropriate premium to breeders of replacement stock. Experimental evidence of these benefits is helping to increase awareness of the value of genetic improvement among producers.

References

AHDB (2019a) Beef Feed Efficiency Programme. Available at: https://ahdb.org.uk/beef-feed-efficiency-programme (accessed 1 October 2020).

AHDB (2019b) Beef Production from the Dairy Herd. Available at: https://ahdb.org.uk/knowledge-library/beef-production-from-the-dairy-herd (accessed 1 October 2020).

Amer, P.R., Kemp, R.A. and Smith, C. (1992) Genetic differences among the predominant beef cattle breeds in Canada: An analysis of published results. *Canadian Journal of Animal Science* 72, 759–771. DOI: 10.4141/cjas92-088.

Amer, P.R., Nieuwhof, G.J., Pollott, G.E., Roughsedge, T., Conington, J.E. and Simm, G. (2007) Industry benefits from recent genetic progress in sheep and beef populations. *Animal* 1, 1414–1426. DOI: org/10.1017/S175173110700078X.

American Angus Association (2019) Available at: http://www.angus.org/ (accessed 7 February 2019).

Andersen, B.B., de Baerdemaeker, A., Bittante, G., Bonaiti, B., Colleau, J.J. *et al.* (1981) Performance testing of bulls in AI: report of a working group of the Commission on Cattle Production. *Livestock*

Production Science 8, 101–119. DOI: 10.1016/0301-6226(81)90015-4.

Beef and Lamb NZ (2019) Beef Progeny Test. Available at: https://beeflambnz.com/news-views/topics/Beef-Progeny-Test (accessed 7 February 2019).

Beef CRC (2019a) Appendix 6 - Economic Value of Crossbreeding and Grain-finishing tropically Adapted Cattle. Available at: http://www.beefcrc.com/documents/products/exit-report/Beef-CRC-Exit-Report-Appendix-6-Northern-crossbreeding.pdf (accessed 23 January 2019).

Beef CRC (2019b) Appendix 5 – New Traits in BREEDPLAN (Developed in CRCI and II). Available at: http://www.beefcrc.com/documents/products/exit-report/Beef-CRC-Exit-Report-Appendix-5-New-traits-in-BREEDPLAN.pdf (accessed 23 January 2019).

Benyshek, L.L. and Bertrand, J.K. (1990) National genetic improvement programmes in the United States beef industry. *South African Journal of Animal Science* 20, 103–109. Available at: https://www.ajol.info/index.php/sajas/article/view/138855.

Bertrand, J.K., Berger, P.J. and Willham, R.L. (1985) Sire x environment interactions in beef cattle weaning weight field data. *Journal of Animal Science* 60, 1396–1402. DOI: 10.2527/jas1985.6061396x.

Bishop, S.C. (1993) Grassland performance of Hereford cattle selected for rate and efficiency of lean gain on a concentrate diet. *Animal Production* 56, 311–319. DOI: 10.1017/S0003356100006346.

Bonnett, J.N., Journaux, L., Mocquot, J.C. and Rehben, E. (1994) Breeding cattle for the next millennium. *British Cattle Breeders Club Digest* 49, 10–18.

BreedObject® (2019) Available at: http://breedobject.com/ (accessed 7 February 2019).

Breedplan (2019) Available at: https://breedplan.une.edu.au/ (accessed 4 October 2020).

British Limousin Cattle Society (2019) Performance Programmes. Available at: https://limousin.co.uk/performance-programmes/ (accessed 10 August 2019).

Byrne, T., Amer, P., Kirk, T., Hely, GF. and Cromie, A. (2018) 20 years of genetic improvement. *ICBF and Sheep Ireland Genetics Conference: 'Sustainable Farming – Progress Through Genetics'*, 5 December 2018. Available at: https://www.icbf.com/wp/wp-content/uploads/2018/12/Amer_20-years-of-ICBF.pdf (accessed 24 February 2019).

Craigie, C.R., Navajas, E.A., Purchas, R.W., Maltin, C.A., Bünger, L. *et al.* (2012) A review of the development and use of video image analysis (VIA) for beef carcass evaluation as an alternative to the current EUROP system and other subjective systems. *Meat Science* 92, 307–318. DOI: 10.1016/j.meatsci.2012.05.028.

Cuthbertson, A. (1994) Enhancing beef eating quality. *British Cattle Breeders Club Digest* 49, 33–37.

Department of Agriculture, Food and the Marine (2019) EU Beef Carcase Classification Scheme. Available at: https://www.agriculture.gov.ie/farmingsectors/beef/eubeefcarcaseclassificationscheme (accessed 23 January 2019).

Dikeman, M.E. (1990) Genetic effects on the quality of meat from cattle. *Proceedings of the 4th World Congress on Genetics Applied to Livestock Production* XV, 521–530. Available at: http://www.wcgalp.org/proceedings/1990 (accessed 16 June 2020).

FAO (2015) *The Second Report on the State of the World's Animal Genetic Resources for Food and Agriculture*, Scherf, B.D. and Pilling D. (eds) FAO Commission on Genetic Resources for Food and Agriculture Assessments, Rome. Available at: http://www.fao.org/3/a-i4787e.pdf (accessed 4 October 2019).

FAO (2019) FAOSTAT. Available at: http://www.fao.org/faostat/en/#data/QL/visualize (accessed 10 August 2019).

France Génétique Elevage (2019) France, the Country of Beef Breeds. Available at: http://en.france-genetique-elevage.org/IMG/pdf/fge_beef_breeds_selection.pdf (accessed 15 January 2019).

Fuller, R. (2018) *Suckler Beef - A Practical Guide to Profitability*. Context, Packington, UK.

Genus ABS (2020) *2020-21 Beef in Focus Sire Directory*. Available at: https://www.absglobal.com/uk/wp-content/uploads/sites/31/2020/07/1973-Beef-InFocus-Directory-2020-2021-FINAL.pdf (accessed 4 October 2020).

Gerber, P.J., Steinfeld, H., Henderson, B., Mottet, A., Opio, C. *et al.* (2013) Tackling Climate Change Through Livestock – A Global Assessment of Emissions and Mitigation Opportunities. Food and Agriculture Organization of the United Nations (FAO), Rome. Available at: http://www.fao.org/3/a-i3437e.pdf (accessed 30 June 2019).

Gregory, K.E., Cundiff, L.V. and Koch, R.M. (1991) Breed effects and heterosis in advanced generations of composite populations for preweaning traits of beef cattle. *Journal of Animal Science* 69, 947–960. (Also, see other papers by the same authors in Volumes 69 and 70.)

ICAR (2019) INTERBEEF Working Group. Available at: https://www.icar.org/index.php/technical-bodies/working-groups/interbeef-working-group/ (accessed 7 February 2019).

ICBF (2020) About ICBF. Available at: https://www.icbf.com/wp/ (accessed 18 June 2020).

INTERBEEF (2019) Available at: https://www.icar.org/index.php/technical-bodies/working-groups/interbeef-working-group/ (accesses 21/10/19).

Journaux, L. and Renand, G. (1992) Genetic relationship between station performance testing and station progeny testing of Charolais bulls. *Book of Abstracts from the 43rd Annual Meeting of the European Association for Animal Production*, Madrid, Spain, Paper G.Va.37, p. 210.

Kemp, R.A. (1994) Genetics of meat quality in cattle. *Proceedings of the 5th World Congress on Genetics Applied to Livestock Production* 19, 439–445. Available at: http://www.wcgalp.org/proceedings/1994 (accessed 16 June 2020).

Koots, K.R., Gibson, J.P., Smith, C. and Wilton, J.W. (1994a) Analyses of published genetic parameter estimates for beef production traits. 1. Heritability. *Animal Breeding Abstracts* 62, 309–338.

Koots, K.R., Gibson, J.P. and Wilton, J.W. (1994b) Analyses of published genetic parameter estimates for beef production traits. 2. Phenotypic and genetic correlations. *Animal Breeding Abstracts* 62, 825–853.

Lambe, N. and Simm, G. (2004) Animal breeding and genetics/Traditional animal breeding. In: Jensen, W.K., Devine, C. and Dikeman, M. (eds), *Encyclopedia of Meat Sciences*. Elsevier, Oxford, Volume 1, pp. 11–19.

Land, R.B. and Hill, W.G. (1975) The possible use of superovulation and embryo transfer in cattle to increase response to selection. *Animal Production* 21, 1–12. DOI: 10.1017/S000335610003035X.

Lewis, W.H.E. (1992) Beef index validation - national results from suckler herds. *British Cattle Breeders Club Digest* 47, 24–27.

Ménissier, F. (1988) La sélection des races bovines à viande spécialisées en France. *Proceedings of the 3rd World Congress on Sheep and Beef Cattle Breeding*, 2, pp. 215–236. Dunmore Press, New Zealand.

MLA (2019a) Meat Standards Australia. Available at: https://www.mla.com.au/marketing-beef-and-lamb/meat-standards-australia/ (accessed 10 August 2019).

MLA (2019b) Progeny Testing of Elite Sires for Profitability Traits. Available at: https://www.mla.com.au/research-and-development/search-rd-reports/final-report-details/Productivity-On-Farm/Progeny-testing-of-elite-sires-for-profitability-traits/677 (accessed 10 August 2019).

Morris, C.A., Baker, R.L., Hickey, S.M., Johnson, D.L., Cullen, N.G. and Wilson, J.A. (1993) Evidence of genotype by environment interaction for reproductive and maternal traits in beef cattle. *Animal Production* 56, 69–83. DOI: 10.1017/S0003356100006176.

Mrode, R.A. (1988) Selection experiments in beef cattle. Part 2. A review of responses and correlated responses. *Animal Breeding Abstracts* 56, 155–167.

Mudadu, M.A., Porto-Neto, L.R., Mokry, F.B., Tizioto, P.C., Oliveira, P.S.N. *et al.* (2016) Genomic structure and marker-derived gene networks for growth and meat quality traits of Brazilian Nelore beef cattle. *BMC Genomics* 17, 235. DOI: 10.1186/s12864-016-2535-3.

Mueller, J., Rischkowsky, B., Haile, A., Philipsson, J., Mwai, O. *et al.* (2015) Community-based livestock breeding programmes: essentials and examples. *Journal of Animal Breeding and Genetics* 132, 155–168.

Pirchner, F. (1986) Evaluation of industry breeding programs for dairy cattle milk and meat production. *Proceedings of the 3rd World Congress on Genetics Applied to Livestock Production* Vol IX, 153–164. Available at: http://www.wcgalp.org/proceedings/1986 (accessed 16 June 2020).

QMS (2018) Cattle and Sheep Enterprise Profitability in Scotland. Available at: https://www.qmscotland.co.uk/sites/default/files/qms_cattle_sheep_enterprise_2018_0.pdf (accessed 1 October 2020).

Roehe, R., Dewhurst, R.J., Duthie, C.A., Rooke, J.A., Mckain, N. *et al.* (2016) Bovine host genetic variation influences rumen microbial methane production with best selection criterion for low methane emitting and efficiently feed converting hosts based on metagenomic gene abundance. *PloS Genetics* 12, 20. DOI: 10.1371/journal.pgen.1005846.

Roughsedge, T., Amer, P.R., Thompson, R. and Simm, G. (2005) Development of a maternal breeding goal and tools to select for this goal in UK beef production. *Animal Science* 81, 221–232. DOI: 10.1079/ASC50230221.

Signet (2019a) Signet Breeding Services. Available at: http://www.signetfbc.co.uk/ (accessed 10 August 2019).

Signet (2019b) Breeding Indexes. Available at: https://www.signetdata.com/technical/beef-genetic-notes/breeding-indexes/ (accessed 4 October 2020).

Simm, G. (1998). *Genetic Improvement of Cattle and Sheep*. Farming Press, Ipswich, UK.

Simm, G., Smith, C. and Prescott, J.H.D. (1985) Environmental effects on bull performance test results. *Animal Production* 41, 177–185. DOI: 10.1017/S0003356100027835.

Simm, G., Conington, J., Bishop, S.C., Dwyer, C.M. and Pattinson, S. (1996) Genetic selection for extensive conditions. *Applied Animal Behaviour Science* 49, 47–59. DOI: 10.1016/0168-1591(95)00667-2.

TEAGASC (2019) Dairy Calf to Beef. Available at: https://www.teagasc.ie/animals/beef/dairy-calf-to-beef/ (accessed 7 February 2019).

Thiessen, R.B., Hnizdo, E., Maxwell, D.A.G., Gibson, D. and Taylor, C.S. (1984) Multibreed comparisons of British cattle. Variation in body weight, growth rate and food intake. *Animal Production* 38, 323–340. DOI: 10.1017/S0003356100041520 (Also, see other papers by the same authors in later volumes of *Animal Production*.)

Villanueva, B., Simm, G. and Woolliams, J.A. (1995) Genetic progress and inbreeding for alternative nucleus breeding schemes for beef cattle. *Animal Science* 61, 231–239. DOI: 10.1017/S1357729800013758.

Wickham, B.W., Amer, P.R., Berry, D.P., Burke, M., Coughlan, S. *et al.* (2012) Industrial perspective: capturing the benefits of genomics to Irish cattle breeding. *Animal Production Science* 52, 172–179.

Recommended Reading

Animal (formerly *Animal Production* and *Animal Science*; Journal of the British Society of Animal Science).

Canadian Journal of Animal Science (Journal of the Agricultural Institute of Canada/Canadian Society of Animal Science).

Journal of Animal Science (Journal of the American Society of Animal Science).

Livestock Production Science (Journal of the European Association for Animal Production).

Proceedings of the Australian Association of Animal Breeding and Genetics.

Proceedings of the New Zealand Society of Animal Production.

Proceedings of the World Congresses on Genetics Applied to Livestock Production Available at: http://www.wcgalp.org/ (accessed 16 June 2020).

10 Sheep and Goat Breeding

Introduction

Sheep are probably the most versatile of the domestic animal species. In temperate countries today, they are kept mainly for the production of meat, wool and milk. However, particularly in some of the world's poorest countries, they have additional, important rôles, including the provision of pelts, fertilizer and fuel, providing a four-legged form of financial investment, and using resources unsuitable for other forms of agriculture.

Figures 10.1 to 10.3 show the world's major producers of sheep meat, milk and wool by continent. Asia has the highest production of meat, milk and wool, with Africa being the second highest producer of meat, Europe of milk and Oceania of wool. Figures 10.4 to 10.6 show the 15 highest-producing countries for each commodity. China, Australia and New Zealand head the list of individual countries producing the most meat and wool. China, Turkey and Greece head the list of countries producing the most sheep milk.

In Northern Europe, despite their historical importance as wool producers – a rôle in which they had a major impact on the social and industrial shape of Britain in particular – sheep are kept primarily for meat production today. For example, wool accounts for only about 2.7 to 4.8% of average gross output from sheep enterprises in Britain (SAC, 2017) and there is a small but growing tendency to keep wool-shedding breeds, since some producers consider the costs of producing wool to be higher that its returns. In several Southern European countries and in parts of Asia and Africa, sheep are kept primarily for milk production and meat is produced as a by-product, albeit a valuable one. Although most wool is used in the Northern hemisphere, a large proportion of production is in the Southern hemisphere – but China is now the single largest wool-producing country. Australia has the world's largest specialized wool production industry, but meat is an important by-product – especially indirectly, with dual-purpose F_1 ewes resulting from crosses of Merino ewes being mated to meat-producing rams. In New Zealand, the substantial sheep industry is based largely on dual-purpose breeds and many home-produced composites for the production of both meat and wool.

The aim of this chapter is to discuss the breeding goals, the breeds and crosses, the selection criteria, and the methods of testing and evaluation used in sheep breeding in both temperate and tropical areas. The emphasis is on sheep meat and wool production, but both milk and multi-purpose production are discussed briefly too.

Goat production and breeding are commonly dealt with together with sheep, since they are both small ruminants, have similar structural and biological characteristics, and are often found in similar locations. The major products from goats are meat, milk and, to some extent, fibre. World 2017 production of goat meat was 5.8 Mt compared to the 9.3 Mt for sheep. However, the distribution between continents favours Asia (72%) and Africa (23%) with little being produced elsewhere (FAO, 2018). World goat milk production was 18.7 Mt in 2017 compared to 10.4 Mt for sheep, but the distribution across continents was similar to sheep's milk with 57% in Asia, 24% in Africa and 15% in Europe. China, India, Pakistan, Nigeria and Bangladesh were the top five goat meat-producing countries, and India, Bangladesh, Sudan, Pakistan and France were the top five milk-producing countries. No FAO statistics are available for fibre.

In this chapter, we will concentrate mainly on sheep breeding but give some goat-breeding examples where the differences are notable. Comprehensive goat-breeding schemes are much rarer than for those involving sheep, and so fewer examples are available to describe here. One exception is in France, where goat milk production is a major activity.

Genetic Improvement of Farmed Animals (G. Simm *et al.*)
DOI: 10.1079/9781789241723.0010

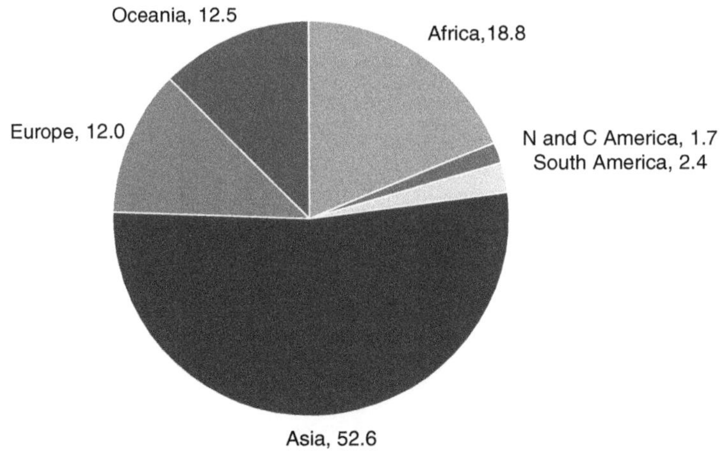

Fig. 10.1. Proportion of world production of mutton and lamb by continent in 2016 (%). (After FAO, 2018.)

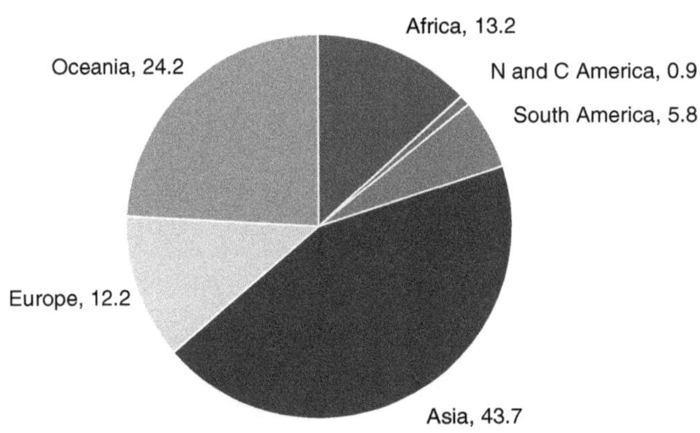

Fig. 10.2. Proportion of world production of greasy wool by continent in 2013 (%). (After FAO, 2018.)

Breeding goals

Meat production

Figure 10.7 summarizes the contribution of different measures of performance to the superiority in net margin of the top 25% of commercial flocks recorded by AHDB Beef and Lamb in Britain. This chart helps to identify the animal characteristics which affect profitability in UK meat sheep production systems.

Although the relative importance of these varies between systems, and between countries, the key animal characteristics are:

- **The number of lambs reared to slaughter per ewe per annum.** Lamb sales per ewe are obviously strongly influenced by litter size and lamb survival. There is variation both between and within breeds in litter size, and to a lesser extent survival. Also, these two characteristics are related at the phenotypic level, as higher litter sizes generally result in smaller individual lamb birth weights and higher rates of lamb mortality. Hence, there is usually an intermediate optimum number of lambs born for a given production system. For example, in UK lowland meat production systems, the optimum number of lambs reared per litter may be two or higher, but in very harsh hill or range conditions it may be closer to one lamb reared. In most sheep production systems ewes lamb once per annum. However,

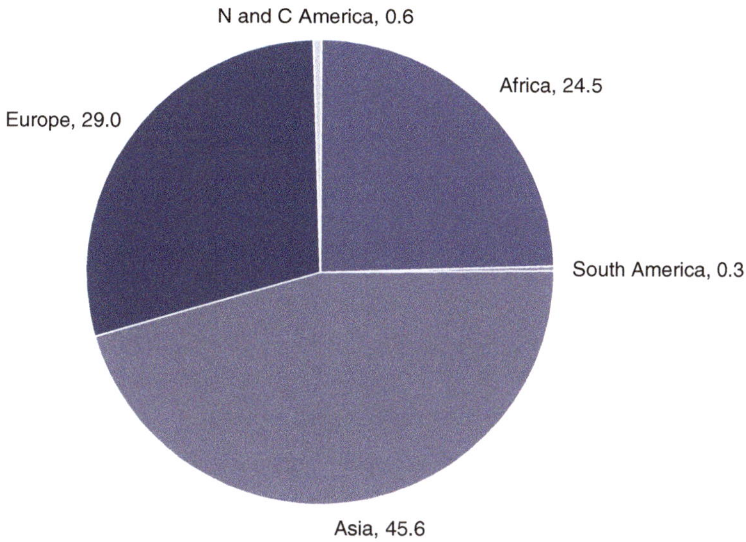

Fig. 10.3. Proportion of world production of sheep milk by continent in 2016 (%). (After FAO, 2018.)

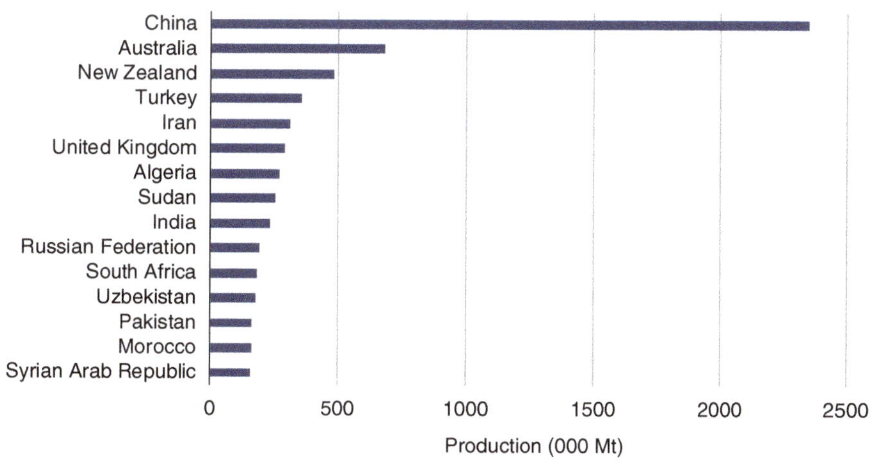

Fig. 10.4. Production of sheep meat by the 15 highest-producing countries in the world in 2016. (After FAO, 2018.)

because of a relatively short gestation length, there is an opportunity to increase output by lambing more than once per annum, and frequent-lambing systems have been adopted in a few areas (the targets are usually three lambings in 2 years, or five lambings in 3 years). Sheep are seasonal breeders in countries with varying day length but there is variation both between and within breeds in the onset and the duration of the breeding season. These animal characteristics influence the ability to lamb more frequently and also affect output in conventional systems.

- **The average value of the lambs produced.** In some countries and production systems, some or all of the lambs are sold after weaning for finishing on other farms (or in feedlots). The proportion of lambs which are sold directly for slaughter, rather than sold for finishing elsewhere, is an important factor affecting profitability. For example, in Britain, the

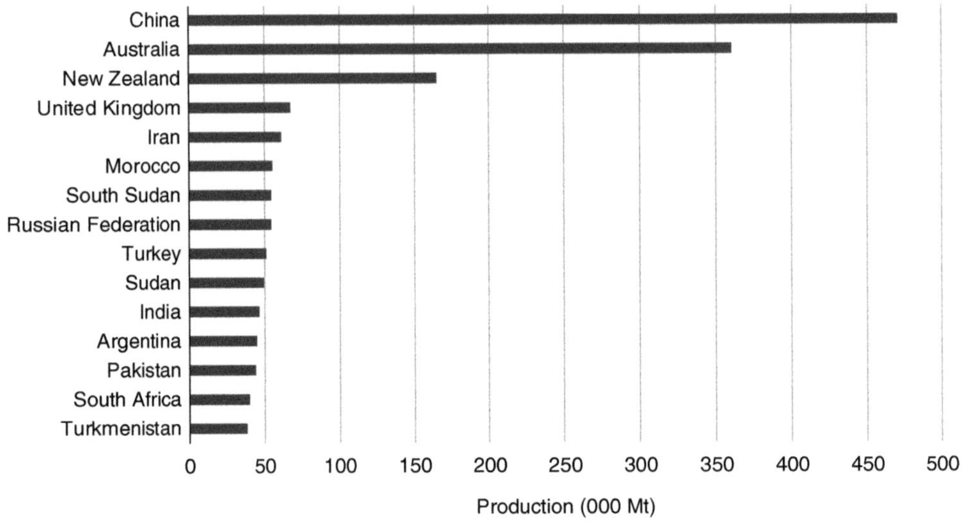

Fig. 10.5. Production of greasy wool by the 15 highest-producing countries in the world in 2013. (After FAO, 2018.)

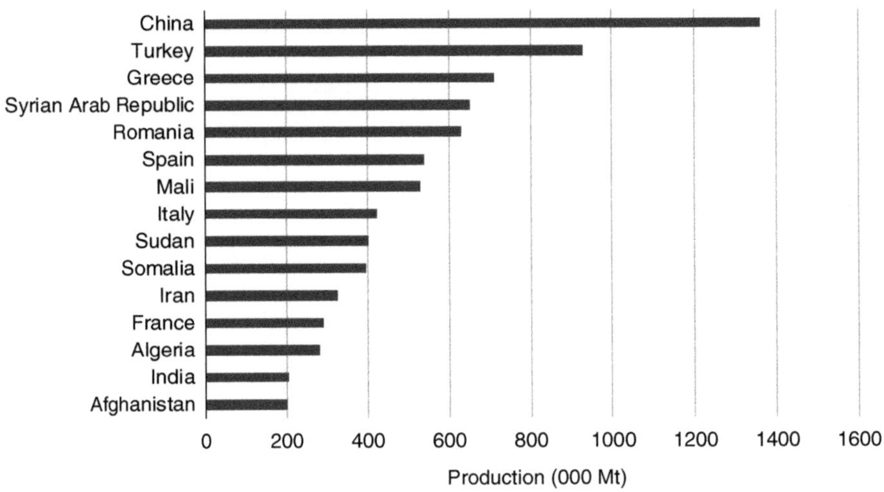

Fig. 10.6. Production of sheep milk by the 15 highest-producing countries in the world in 2016. (After FAO, 2018.)

results from commercial flocks consistently show that flocks achieving a higher proportion of lambs sold directly for slaughter produce higher returns per lamb. Obviously, there are many management and environmental influences on the proportion of lambs sold for slaughter, but lamb growth and carcass composition are important animal factors which also influence it.

In systems producing lambs directly for slaughter, carcass value has an important impact on *gross margins*. Carcass value is usually a function of carcass weight, fatness and conformation, although breed, age and sex can also influence carcass prices in their own right. The relative importance of these measures of carcass value varies between regions and countries. Often there are strong local preferences for carcasses of a certain

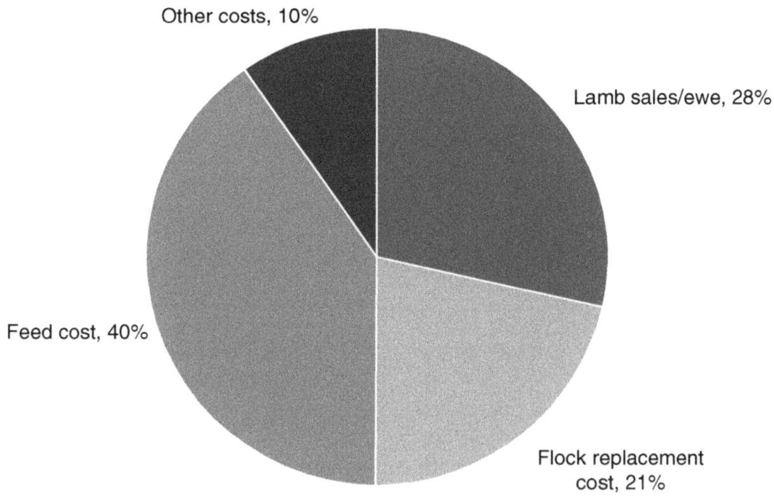

Fig. 10.7. Contribution to top 25% superiority in net margin per ewe for AHDB Stocktake recorded flocks in 2016/17. (After AHDB, 2016.)

weight, fat or conformation range, and those falling outside this range will be penalized. For example, in Britain most lamb carcasses fall in the weight range of 16–22 kg. In Mediterranean countries the preference is for much lighter, leaner carcasses. This market for lighter carcasses has, historically, led to a large increase in exports of carcasses from the smaller hill breeds in Britain.

In many Western countries, consumers have shown a strong preference for leaner meat over the last few decades. Hence, for these countries, efficient production of *lean* meat is a primary breeding goal. It may not be biologically or economically efficient to attempt to match consumer preferences precisely in the live animal, but they are often too far apart. Historically, for example, the average lamb carcass in Britain contained 20 percentage units of fat in excess of that desired by consumers (Kempster *et al.*, 1986). More recently there has been some improvement in the composition of carcasses produced. Some payment schemes discriminate strongly between carcasses of different fatness classes, but in other cases there is still a mismatch between consumer demand and market supply.

In many countries, carcasses are scored visually for fat cover and conformation. For example, Table 10.1 shows the fat and conformation grid used to classify lamb carcasses by MLC Services Ltd (MLCSL) in Britain, together with the proportions of carcasses falling into each cell, in 2017. This method of classification is based on a standard one employed across the EU, but fat classes 3 and 4 are subdivided into low and high bands in the British version. The target specification for most major buyers in Britain is for carcasses in the leaner fat classes 1, 2 and 3L and in conformation classes E, U or R. While there has been a steady improvement in the proportion of carcasses falling in the target sector, this was still only 54.7% in the sample classified by MLCSL in 2017 (AHDB, 2018a). To some extent, price differentials reflect consumer preference for leaner meat. But the 'true' market signals for leaner meat are blunted by overcapacity in the British abattoir sector, which means that achieving high throughput of animals often overrides payment on quality.

The fat content of carcasses is not the only concern that consumers have towards sheep meat. There is increasing interest in the consumption of animal products which have been produced and marketed in a sustainable way. This trend affects consumer thinking, especially in wealthier countries. This can be at odds with the pressure to increase the quantity and efficiency of meat production to meet the likely rise in demand for food. These issues are discussed by Montossi *et al.* (2013).

Choosing a breeding goal to select between or within terminal sire breeds is complicated by the association between mature size and carcass

Table 10.1. The EU sheep carcass classification grid used in Britain, showing the distribution (%) of lamb carcasses classified in 2017. Fat classes range from 1, the leanest, to 5 the fattest. Conformation is scored on a 5-point scale, from E, the highest conformation class to P, the poorest. (After AHDB, 2018a.)

		Fat class			→	Fatter		
		1	**2**	**3L**	**3H**	**4L**	**4H**	**5**
Conformation	**E**	–	0.9	3.1	1.5	0.4	0.1	0.0
class	**U**	–	2.6	12.2	6.6	1.5	0.3	0.1
↓	**R**	0.3	8.6	29.3	14.4	3.0	0.5	0.1
Poorer	**O**	0.5	3.8	7.2	2.4	0.3	0.1	0.0
conformation	**P**	0.2						

composition. Generally, as all animals grow towards maturity, they get fatter. Breeds differ in fatness quite markedly when they are compared at the same weight. However, when they are compared at similar degrees of fatness, most of the differences in saleable meat yield disappear (Massender *et al.*, 2019). Differences in mature size may also explain much of the within-breed variation in carcass composition at a given weight. So, the simplest way to breed leaner lambs is probably to select larger terminal sire breeds, and larger sires within these breeds. (This assumes that all progeny are slaughtered – if some female progeny are kept for breeding then there will be a penalty because of their larger mature size and hence higher maintenance costs.)

Although mature size is a useful concept when considering breeding goals, it is difficult to apply in practice in within-breed selection because of the time and expense involved in keeping animals until they are mature before making selection decisions. In practice, early growth rates are usually used as indicators of eventual mature size. Also, although mature size is important, it does not explain *all* of the differences in fatness so it is worth paying attention to levels of fatness in immature animals too (Simm, 1992). Hence, the breeding goal is often to increase the rate of gain of lean tissue to an immature weight, or to increase the proportion of lean in the carcass at an immature weight. While these broad definitions of breeding goals have been applied to breeds used in a range of production systems so far, they could be refined to match particular systems more closely in future. For example, some breeds or sectors of a breed may choose to go for rapid early lean growth to produce maximum returns from early grass-based finishing systems. The danger with this approach is that lambs may be produced with too little fat. In this case, growth rate or mature size may be more important than fatness in the overall breeding goal. Others may opt for maximizing returns from longer finishing systems, in which case controlling fatness may be more important than growth rate or mature size.

Carcass conformation may be a useful indicator of differences in saleable meat yield among breeds. However, most studies *within* breeds, except 'double-muscled' breeds or strains, show that conformation is closely associated with fatness, and is of little or no value in predicting saleable meat yield, or proportion of higher-priced cuts (Simm, 1994). Despite this, payment schemes in many countries include premiums and penalties for high- and low-conformation carcasses respectively, so it can be argued that conformation has a direct economic value.

- **Feed consumption.** As with other livestock, feed costs are the most important variable costs in sheep meat production. In some countries or regions, or in some seasons, sheep meat production is based on concentrate feeding of lambs, and so lamb growth and feed conversion efficiency can have a big influence on profitability, e.g. early lamb production in the UK. However, in most countries sheep meat production is based on extensive grazing of grass or forage crops. Feed costs and feed efficiency are still important here, but they are most commonly measured indirectly via output of lamb per hectare, and the stocking rate of ewes achieved. Stocking rate has an important effect on gross margin per hectare. Although the stocking rate achieved is probably mainly a function of land type and grassland management, animal characteristics such as ewe mature weight and litter size also have an important effect on it (i.e. because feed requirements are proportional to weight, it is easier to achieve high stocking rates with ewes of low mature weight, than those of higher mature weight).

- **Health and longevity.** Figure 10.7 shows that flock replacement costs have an important bearing on net margins achieved by better producers. Ewe longevity is affected by a wide range of both management and animal factors, including voluntary or involuntary culling due to disease (e.g. tooth loss, mastitis). Sheep are noted for the large number of diseases to which they can succumb, and so veterinary and medicine costs also have a direct effect on profitability. There is genetic variation between and within breeds in susceptibility to many common diseases.

Hence, the profitability of sheep meat production is affected by a mixture of maternal characteristics such as ewe fertility, litter size, rearing ability, mature size and milk production, and terminal sire characteristics such as growth and carcass quality. In some countries, such as France, these breeding goals are often pursued together in the same pure breeds. In other countries, especially Britain, there is widespread use of crossbreeding to achieve the complementary use of breeds with different growth and reproductive characteristics, and to allow the pursuit of different breeding goals in specialized maternal and terminal sire breeds.

Examples of goat meat breeding objectives are rare, but the Australian Kidplan scheme has some interesting parallels with equivalent sheep schemes (Sheep Genetics, 2019).

Community breeding programmes have recently become the most successful method for genetic improvement of sheep and goats in sub-Saharan Africa, especially in Ethiopia (Haile *et al.*, 2019). This involves treating sheep flocks or goat herds across several communities as a single population. A selection committee, usually composed of three to five members elected by the community, are involved in the selection of the breeding rams or bucks. Two stages of ram/buck selection are usually involved: initial screening when sales of young lambs/kids occur traditionally (at 4–6 months of age) and final selection for breeding. Breeding goals include growth performance (assessed via birth weight, 3-month weight, 6-month weight, yearling weight), twinning rate and (for sheep) fleece weight. Males are selected on estimated breeding values (EBVs) or indexes. The rams and bucks for breeding are then screened from the selected set based on factors such as conformation, coat colour, presence or absence of horns, horn type and tail type.

Wool production

The main uses of wool are in the production of garments, furnishing or other fabrics, fillings and carpets. The fibre diameter and staple length (the length of the shorn fibres) are the main wool characteristics determining the end-use, and hence the price of wool. Table 10.2 illustrates the typical fibre diameter of wool from different categories, as well as giving examples of the major breeds which produce each type, and the end-uses of the wool. The

Table 10.2. Typical fibre diameter of wool of different categories, examples of the major breeds which produce each type, and end-uses of the wool. (Source: Ponzoni *et al.*, 1990.)

Wool category	Fibre diameter (microns)	Major breeds	End-use of wool
Fine	Up to 25	Merino, Polwarth	Garment manufacture: light-weight, high-quality clothing fabric; high-quality knitwear
Medium	25 to 30	Corriedale, other dual-purpose breeds (usually 50% Merino)	Garment manufacture – medium-weight clothing fabric Machine and hand knitting yarns
Coarse	30 and over	Romney, Coopworth, Perendale, Border Leicester	Garment manufacture: heavy-weight clothing fabric e.g. Tweeds Blankets Thick machine and hand knitting yarns Furnishing fabric Carpets
Speciality carpet	Medullated, mean 40	Drysdale, Tukidale, Carpetmaster, Elliotdale, Scottish Blackface	Carpets Upholstery fillers

table illustrates the clear demarcation between breed types in terms of fibre diameter, but there are also big differences in fleece weight. For example, Merinos typically produce fleeces weighing about 7 kg (fleece weight as shorn, prior to scouring), compared to fleece weights of about 3–4 kg for dual-purpose breeds like the Coopworth, and 2–2.5 kg for the larger of the British hill breeds.

Only the finest wool is suitable for use in garment manufacture, and it is this type of wool which is most valuable. The vast majority of wool produced for garment manufacture comes from Merino sheep, or derivatives of this breed. Within this fine-wool sector there are further strong links between fibre diameter and price. Coarser wool from dual-purpose breeds or meat breeds is less valuable and gets used for the other purposes mentioned. The coarsest wool of all gets used in the manufacture of carpets because of its hard-wearing properties. An additional important property of speciality carpet wool from some breeds, such as the Drysdale or Scottish Blackface, is the high proportion of medullated fibres – fibres with a hollow core of large fragile cells, within a sheath of the normal dense cortical cells (Ponzoni *et al.*, 1990). Medullation affects the appearance of dyed wool, and the wool-handling characteristics – medullated fibres feel 'crisp' rather than soft. Although fibre diameter is important in determining the category of use, there is little or no premium for finer fibre *within* these non-garment sectors.

The main factors affecting income in specialized garment wool production systems are mean fleece weight and mean fibre diameter. Fleece weight is either expressed as greasy or clean. Greasy fleece weight is the weight as clipped. Clean fleece weight is the weight after scouring to remove natural oils and vegetable matter, dust, etc. The two measures are highly correlated genetically. Clean fleece weight expressed as a percentage of greasy fleece weight is termed yield – typically this is about 68%, but it can vary markedly depending on the environment in which the sheep are kept. There is also substantial genetic variation in yield within a given environment. The mean fibre diameter is important because it determines both the weight of the fabric (finer fibres produce lighter weight cloth) and its comfort (finer fibres result in a 'softer' finish, which is especially important for fabrics worn next to the skin). Figure 10.8 shows the relationship between fibre diameter and price in Australia during 2018. Other wool characteristics such as the range in fibre diameter, staple length, staple strength, 'style' (visual characteristics of the fleece associated with processing quality), fibre curvature, comfort factor, spinning fineness, wool colour and level of contamination can also be important, although several of these are related to fibre diameter. Other animal factors, such

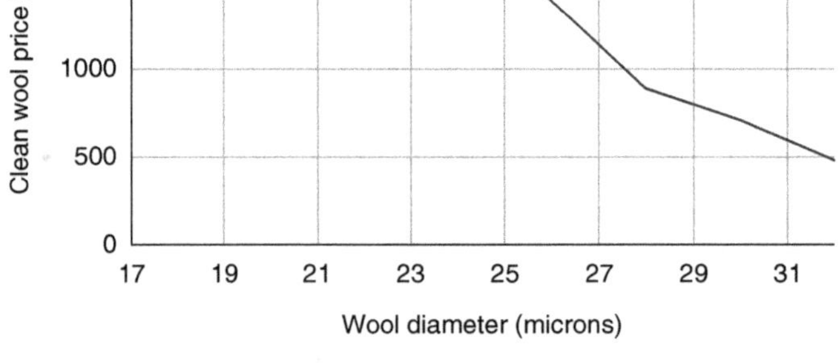

Fig. 10.8. The average relationship between wool fibre diameter and price in Australia between July and November 2018. (After Australian Wool Exchange, 2018.)

as the incidence of fleece rot, fly strike and internal parasitism, are important in certain areas – either because they reduce productivity and welfare, or in extreme cases, cause higher mortality.

Historically, most Merino breeding programmes have focused on increasing fleece weights, while maintaining fibre diameter. However, the trend towards lighter weight fabrics in garment manufacture means that fibre diameter has become more important. One of the fundamental problems in setting and achieving breeding goals for fine-wool production is that there is a moderately antagonistic relationship between fleece weight and fibre diameter, both across strains and within strains. In other words, higher-producing strains or individuals tend to produce wool of higher fibre diameter. This is illustrated in Fig. 10.9 which shows both the average fleece weight and the average fibre diameter of groups of wethers (castrated males) from different Merino studs in New South Wales, Australia.

Goat fibre production is a much less developed industry than wool production in sheep. Angora goats are a good example of a specialized goat breed for fibre production, originating in Turkey but being imported into a number of other countries. Visser and Van Marle-Köster (2014) outline key breeding goals for Angora goats in South Africa which has focused on traits related to fitness, body weight and fibre production.

Fibre from cashmere goats is also a source of income in some countries where the fine fibres produced are equivalent to the fine-wool from Merino sheep. Breeding objectives are to increase fibre production and reduce fibre diameter to produce more of the finer type of cashmere. Breeding goals for cashmere goats in Australia are outlined by Ponzoni and Gifford (1990) and include fibre diameter and fibre yield.

Milk production

Sheep milk production in Mediterranean countries usually involves out-of-season lambing from October to January, rather than the more typical season in Northern Europe of March to April. Lambs are usually reared on their mothers for a month or so, and then weaned. Most lambs are slaughtered at weaning, but in some countries they are reared for slaughter at heavier weights. In most systems, milking of ewes commences after weaning, but in others, ewes are also milked during the suckling period. Ewes are milked for up to 7 months after weaning. Most sheep milk produced in the EU is used for further processing, especially the manufacture

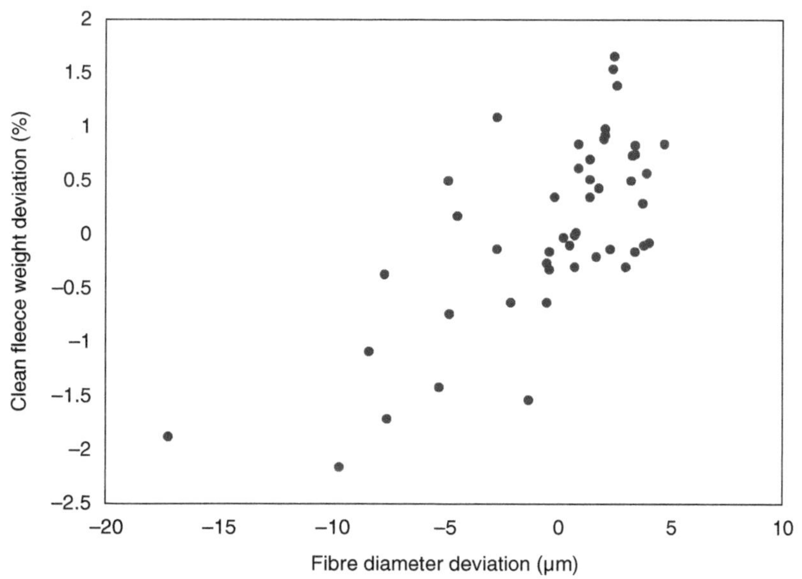

Fig. 10.9. The average fleece weight and the average fibre diameter of groups of wethers from different Merino studs in New South Wales. (After Atkins *et al.*, 2005.)

of cheese, and so compositional quality of the milk is important. In the main milk-producing countries in the EU, the contribution of milk sales to total income ranges from about one-third in those countries, systems or breeds with lower milk yields, up to two-thirds of total income when milk yields are high (see, for example, Milán *et al.*, 2014).

Hence, the animal factors influencing profitability in milk production systems include the ability to lamb out of season, the yield and quality of milk produced, the number of lambs weaned and, to a lesser extent, the growth rate of these lambs.

Goat milk production has similar goals to that of sheep milk. However, goats have the ability to prolong lactation to a much greater extent than sheep. For dairy goats in the UK, Desire *et al.* (2018) reported lactation lengths of up 520 days. Analysing records from over 200,000 French dairy goats, Arnal *et al.* (2018) describe five basic types of lactation curves of goats and analyse the factors determining the various types. In the UK, the Edinburgh Genetic Evaluation Services (EGENES) undertakes genetic evaluation for two of the major goat farms producing genomic breeding values (GEBVs) for production traits, milk, fat and protein, conformation traits such as udder furrow, udder depth, udder attachment, teat form, teat incline, teat placement and back leg form, and also feed intake. These traits are included in a selection index for the selection of parents for breeding.

Additional breeding goals

The key production traits associated with profitability in sheep production have been discussed above. In several sophisticated sheep systems further traits have been considered either to reduce costs, improve health or reduce greenhouse gas emissions. These are discussed here.

Several health traits have been considered for inclusion in breeding goals in different sheep industries. The use of anthelmintic drenches against gastrointestinal (GIT) parasites has been a key feature of many sheep systems. However, the development of resistance to these medicines by many parasite species has led to the investigation of breeding for increased parasite resistance in sheep. Researchers in Australia demonstrated the efficacy of this approach by breeding for high and low parasite resistance in two research lines using faecal egg count (FEC) as the indicator trait; low FEC being a proxy for increased GIT parasite resistance. Such measurements subsequently spread to commercial flocks and it has been demonstrated that the genetic control of this trait in resource flocks is similar to that in commercial animals (e.g. Pollott and Greeff, 2004a). Subsequently, GIT parasite resistance has been included as a breeding objective in several industries worldwide. Other health traits that have been considered in breeding programmes include resistance to facial eczema, foot rot and mastitis.

The health traits discussed above could also be considered to be methods to reduce production costs. In some industries, notably in the UK and Australia, attention in the coarse-wool breeds has turned towards eliminating wool shearing since in many cases the direct and opportunity costs of wool production outweigh the returns to the breeder. This has led to the use of breeds of sheep which shed their wool naturally in some systems. A number of tropical, temperate and primitive breeds shed their wool naturally; this is a trait of the original wild sheep domesticated to produce modern breeds. Primitive breeds such as the Soay have retained their ability to shed wool while more modern breeds, such as the Wiltshire Horn, have been bred to shed their wool using genes inherited from breeds used by the Romans (Fig. 10.10; Ryder, 1983). Further composite breeds like the Easycare have been developed in the UK to incorporate wool shedding into a type of sheep which lambs on its own and has been selected to reduce production costs. Recent studies on wool-shedding breeds have demonstrated that a major gene with a dominant mode of inheritance is involved in some of these

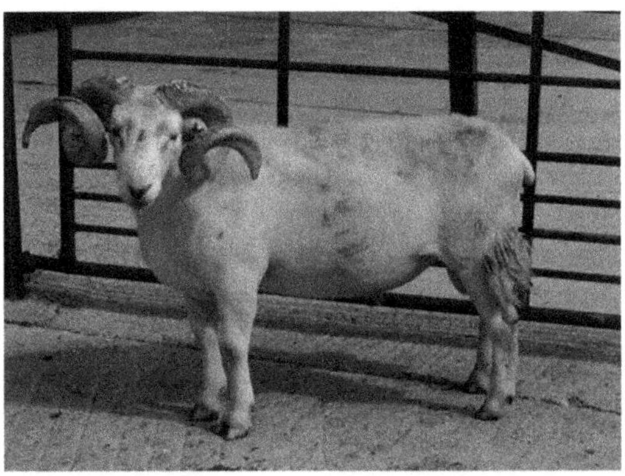

Fig. 10.10. A Wiltshire Horn ram shedding its wool naturally. (Courtesy of Mr Tim White.)

breeds (Pollott, 2011). This gene may be introgressed into other breeds and have an immediate effect on the carriers.

Multi-purpose breeding goals

The profitability of animal production usually depends on an array of animal characteristics, rather than any one alone. The options for selection for more than one trait were discussed in Chapters 3, 4, 6 and 7. For within-breed selection, the most efficient option is usually to select on a multi-trait index, where the breeding goal comprises the sum of breeding values for all important traits, each weighted by its relative economic value. So, for sheep enterprises where any combination of meat, milk and wool production is important, it is sensible to consider index selection for this combination. In multi-purpose or maternal breeds, crosses or lines, it is important to consider lifetime profitability, to account for differences in the timescale over which traits are expressed, and the number of expressions of each trait. For instance, in dual-purpose breeds producing meat and wool, meat output is a function of the number and value of lambs reared at each lambing over the ewe's lifetime, together with her cull value. In a breed which averages 1.5 lambs reared, and typically has 5 lamb crops, ewes would rear an average of 7.5 lambs in their lifetime. So, the economic value of a trait which genetically improves value per lamb needs to be multiplied by 7.5 to account for multiple expressions, but then divided by 2 to account for the fact that the ewe contributes only half the genes of her lambs.

Wool traits have multiple expressions too, probably five or six shearings per ewe lifetime in this example, so the economic value of improvement per fleece needs to be multiplied by 5 or 6 to account for this. Since genetic improvements in wool traits are expressed by the ewe herself, the relative economic values remain on this scale, rather than dividing by 2 as for offspring traits. Similarly, for selection between breeds or crosses, it is sensible to compare these for lifetime physical performance in each of the important characteristics, weighted by the economic values – in other words, ranking breeds or crosses on their expected total lifetime profit.

In addition to these traits directly influencing returns from meat, milk or wool, there are other important animal characteristics worth considering, both in specialized and multi-purpose breeding goals. Reproduction traits obviously have an important bearing on both meat and milk production. The number of lambs born and, especially, the number of lambs reared has an important influence on profit in meat and milk production. In both meat and milk production, regularity of breeding is an important goal also and where there is parasite resistance to drugs, selection for sheep which are resistant to parasites is likely to be an important part of the breeding goal.

Reducing greenhouse gas emissions has become a key topic in ruminant production. Breeding objectives to increase productivity have commonly been linked to reduced greenhouse gas (GHG) emissions per unit of output produced (Jonker *et al.*, 2018). This double-win situation may be relevant for many highly managed sheep systems; however, for more extensive systems this may not be feasible. Alternative approaches looking at host (i.e. sheep) genetic influences on rumen microbiology are relatively novel and may prove to be useful in addressing GHG production concerns. How and when such measures can be introduced to breeding goals remains to be seen.

Sheep are often kept in harsh environments, whether these are the cold and wet conditions typical of the hills and mountains of Britain, or the hot and dry conditions typical of many sheep-producing areas of Australia. It is likely that through a combination of natural and artificial selection, some breeds have become better adapted to these harsh conditions than others. A better understanding of the traits involved in adaptation to harsh environments is needed, both to prevent possible deleterious effects of selection for production alone, and possibly to allow more objective genetic improvement in future. For example, it is likely that a range of physical (e.g. lamb birth coat and adult fleece types), behavioural (e.g. lamb vigour and sucking behaviour, maternal behaviour and grazing behaviour) and disease resistance traits is important in conferring good adaptation to harsh environments. A better knowledge of the heritabilities of the traits involved, and the genetic associations among them, and with other production traits, helps in developing more sustainable breeding goals.

Some of the approaches matching breeds and crosses to particular breeding goals are discussed in the next section. Within-breed selection for the goals identified in the last few sections is discussed in the section after that.

Breeds and Crosses Used in Sheep Production

The FAO (2015) lists 2544 pure breeds of sheep involved worldwide in the production of meat, milk and wool. In addition to the large number of breeds involved, the frequent use of crossbreeding between them makes a comprehensive discussion here impossible. Instead, the aim is to outline briefly some of the breeds, crosses and industry structures involved in a few major sheep-producing countries.

Meat production

The UK has one of the largest specialized sheep meat production industries in the world, with a breeding flock of around 16.6 million ewes in 2017. Comprehensive surveys of the British sheep industry have been undertaken in 1971, 1987, 1996, 2003 and 2012. The latter survey showed that, while there are many regional variations, the much-publicized stratification of the industry remains important (EBLEX, 2014). This stratified system involves largely purebred flocks of the hill breeds in harsher areas, which are usually bred pure for the first four lamb crops. Older ewes of these breeds are then drafted to better ground for crossing, particularly with longwool sires such as the Bluefaced Leicester, but also with some terminal sire breeds such as the Texel. The resulting crossbred ewes form the basis of the sheep industry in much of the uplands and lowlands and are usually mated to rams of the terminal sire breeds.

This system has evolved for a variety of reasons over the decades. But, as discussed in Chapter 3, it does make very efficient use of the complementarity of breeds, and of both maternal and individual heterosis. The hardiness and relatively small mature size of hill breeds is complemented by the larger size and greater prolificacy of the longwool crossing breeds, to create an F_1 female of intermediate size with good maternal characteristics, which shows heterosis for survival and reproduction. These ewes, in turn, are mated to rams from larger terminal sire breeds with improved growth and carcass attributes, to produce a three-way crossbred lamb which itself shows heterosis for survival.

Table 10.3 shows the number of ewes of the six most numerous British hill breeds, which alone account for around 37% of the national flock. Table 10.4 shows that the majority of hill ewes are bred pure. A small proportion are crossed to other hill breeds, but more commonly crosses are to longwool sires, or to terminal sires, to produce lambs for further breeding or slaughter, respectively. Statistics for the most numerous crossbred ewe types are shown in Table 10.5. North Country Mule ewes, derived from Swaledale ewes (Fig. 10.11) crossed to Bluefaced Leicester rams, are the most numerous crossbred type. Their popularity is probably due to the higher number of lambs weaned than by competitors, as outlined in Chapter 4. Other crossbred ewes resulting from matings with Bluefaced Leicester rams are also numerous in Britain. The survey also showed the importance of terminal sire breeds in the British sheep industry. Despite accounting for only about 3.7% of the breeding ewe flock, rams from the terminal sire breeds sired 68% of all lambs slaughtered in Britain. The most numerous terminal sire breeds were Texel, Suffolk and Charollais.

Table 10.3. Estimated total number of ewes mated in the most numerous hill sheep breeds in Britain in 2003 and 2012. (After EBLEX, 2014.)

	Total number of ewes mated ('000)		
Breed	2003	2012	No. ewes mated as a % of national flock (2012)
Scottish Blackface	1686	1125	11
Welsh Mountain	1563	966	10
All Cheviots	502	439	4
Swaledale	1047	721	7
Hardy Speckled Face	276	134	2
Beulah	498	144	3
Total	5572	3529	37

Table 10.4. Mating structure of purebred hill ewes in Britain in 2012. (After EBLEX, 2014.)

Ewe type	Ram type	% of hill ewes mated to this ram type
Hill ewes	Same hill breed	62.5
	Other hill breed	2.9
	Longwool/crossing breed	20.9
	Terminal sire breed	10.4
	Other	3.2

In contrast to the UK situation, most specialized meat production in other European countries is from purebred sheep. In many of these countries there are strong regional allegiances to local meat breeds, such as the Ile de France, Berrichon du Cher, Charollais, and the hardy Prealpes du Sud in France.

Table 10.5. Estimated number of crossbred ewes of the most numerous types mated in Britain in 2003 and 2012. (After EBLEX, 2014.)

Crossbred type	Total number of ewes mated ('000)		
	2003	2012	No. ewes mated as a % of national flock (2012)
Longwool × hill			
North Country Mule (BfL × Sw)	1915	1636	13
Welsh Mule (BfL × WM)	738	576	4
Scotch Mule (BfL × SB)	610	469	4
Greyface (BL × SB)	212	91	1
Welsh Halfbred (BL × WM)	130	41	< 1
Scottish Halfbred (BL × Ch)	100	44	< 1
F_1 hill breeds			
Hill × hill	239	116	1
Suffolk × hill	81	27	< 1
Texel × hill	92	61	1
Total	4117	3061	26

BfL, Bluefaced Leicester; Sw, Swaledale; WM, Welsh Mountain; SB, Scottish Blackface; BL, Border Leicester; Ch, Cheviot.

Wool production

In most specialist wool-producing countries, the vast majority of wool production is from Merino ewes and wethers (Fig. 10.12). Specialized wool breeds are believed to have originated in the Middle East, and to have been spread around the Mediterranean by Phoenicean, Greek and Roman traders (McMaster, 1995). After the fall of the Roman Empire, they survived in the Iberian Peninsula. There, under the influence of the Moors and later the Spanish aristocracy, these Merinos became the major source of high-quality woollen cloths for the expanding economies and populations of Europe. Exports of Merinos were strictly controlled, but elite flocks were established elsewhere in the late Eighteenth Century by way of royal favour. At about this time famous flocks were established at Rambouillet, France and in Saxony. The Peninsular War in the early 19th century broke the Spanish monopoly on fine wool and led to a decline in the local woollen industry. As a result of this, and the growing demand for fine wool by textile mills in Britain and elsewhere, large numbers of Spanish Merinos were driven across the Pyrenees to France. Even greater numbers were

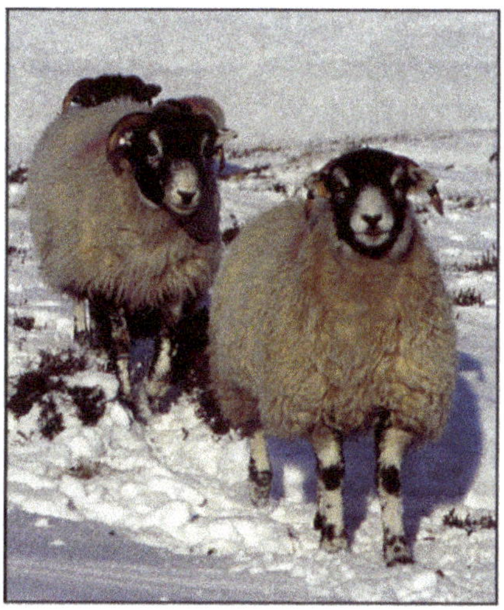

Fig. 10.11. Hill sheep breeds such as the Swaledale have undergone many years of natural and artificial selection for adaptation to harsh environments.

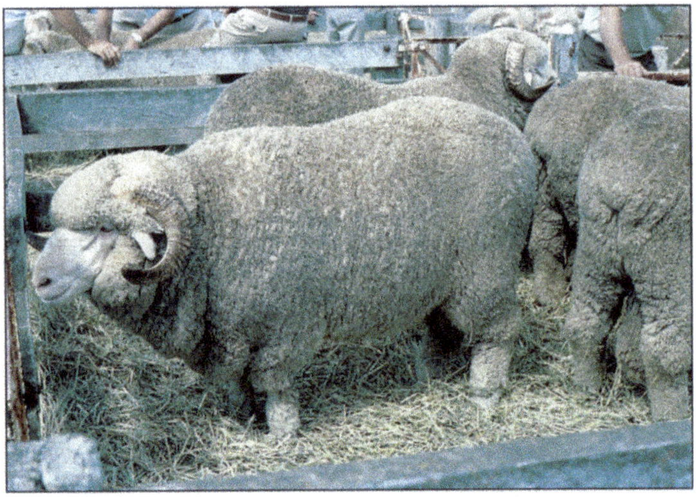

Fig. 10.12. South Australian strain Merino stud ram, housed and fed in preparation for showing and sale; Mt. Bryan, mid-north South Australia. (Courtesy of Dr Sandra Eady.)

shipped to North and South America, South Africa and Australia, where their influence remains today, either directly or indirectly.

There were, and still are, many strains of Merinos with different production capabilities. There are meat-producing and dual-purpose strains (e.g. the German Mutton Merino and the South African Dohne Merino, respectively), but it is the specialized wool-producing strains which are the most numerous worldwide today. The largest population of specialized wool-producing Merinos occurs in Australia (about 26.7 million ewes and 13 million wethers in 2017). There, and elsewhere, the main groups of strains are classified as fine-, medium- or broad-woolled, with typical fibre diameters of about 20, 22 and 24 microns (μ), respectively. However, there are many more subdivisions of these groups, down to the level of *bloodlines*, which are effectively animals from the same stud. Traditionally, commercial wool producers in Australia have shown great loyalty to particular studs, and so they have been 'tied' to producing a particular type of wool. There has been a great deal of extension effort in Australia to encourage commercial producers to become more mobile in their choice of stud, to exploit the large differences in fibre diameter and fleece weight between bloodlines. Similarly, there are efforts to encourage stud breeders to use both between- and within-bloodline selection to accelerate improvements in wool quality while maintaining fleece weight and profitability (Atkins *et al.*, 2005).

Dual-purpose meat and wool production

Both New Zealand and Australia have large populations of sheep used in dual-purpose production of meat and wool. Merinos were introduced to New Zealand from New South Wales in 1842 (Ryder, 1983). However, these were not very well suited to the wetter climate and improved pastures of much of New Zealand. So, only around 5% of the current sheep population comprises purebred Merinos (Corner-Thomas *et al.*, 2013) but they contributed to the formation of several synthetic breeds, such as the Corriedale. This was developed in the mid to late 1800s by crossing the Merino primarily with the Lincoln breed. The majority of the approximately 31 million breeding ewes in New Zealand are purebred dual-purpose sheep that produce relatively high fleece weights of intermediate quality (e.g. for the production of heavier garments and furnishings), as well as producing lambs for meat production. The majority of these dual-purpose sheep are Romney, Coopworth, Perendale and Merino ewes, with the Corriedale falling out of favour. Recent developments have seen a dramatic increase in the number of composites found in New Zealand. More than 40% of flocks comprise composites, mainly based on the Romney breed but

Coopworth and Perendales were also used as the basis for the new types (e.g. Highlander, Ezicare). These flocks also contain a proportion of Texel, Finnish Landrace and East Friesian genetics, the latter reflecting a move towards improved maternal breeds. Typically, New Zealand flocks are bred pure, or part of the flock is crossed to terminal sires. Historically, the Southdown was the most important of these crossing sire breeds, but the demand for larger, leaner carcasses has led to substitution by other breeds such as the Texel and to a lesser extent Suffolk. (In Australia, New Zealand and other major wool-producing nations, white breeds are generally preferred for crossing in situations where some females may be retained for breeding, because of the penalties for coloured fibres in fleeces.)

In Australia, about 33% of Merino ewes are mated to sires of other breeds (MLA, 2017), especially Border Leicester sires, in a system which is analogous to the crossing of draft hill ewes in Britain. The resulting F_1 females form the backbone of the commercial lamb production industry in Australia, which is concentrated in the wetter parts of the country. Typically, these F_1 ewes are mated to terminal sire breeds such as the Poll Dorset, Suffolk and Texel. As in Britain, this system allows complementary use of breeds – for wool traits in the case of the Merino, and reproduction traits in the case of the Leicester – as well as maximizing the benefits of maternal and individual heterosis. A smaller proportion of the Australian national flock comprises dual-purpose breeds like the Corriedale and Polwarth. (The Polwarth is also a synthetic breed, developed in Australia by backcrossing the Corriedale to the Merino.) These dual-purpose breeds are either bred pure or, as with Merino crossbred ewes, a proportion are crossed to terminal sires. As in New Zealand, there is an increase in the use of composite ewes. A small (~4%), but growing proportion of ewes belong to the 'cleanskin' breeds. These are wool-shedding breeds where, clearly, meat is the primary focus of production.

Milk production

In Southern Europe, most sheep milk production, and associated meat production, is from pure breeds with strong regional ties. The main output from European sheep dairy flocks is local cheese with a strong Protected Designation of Origin status. For example, the Lacaune breed from the Massif Central area of France (Figs 10.13 and 10.14) is famous for the production of Roquefort cheese. In Greece, Italy, Spain and Portugal, the most numerous breeds include the Sarda (Italy), Churra (Spain), Manchega (Spain), Latxa (Spain), Serra da Estralla (Portugal), Karagouniki and Chios (both Greece; De Rancourt and Carrère, 2011). Importations of the highly productive Awassi, and its composite derivative the Assaf, from Israel has occurred in a number of European countries. Their impact has been such that Milán

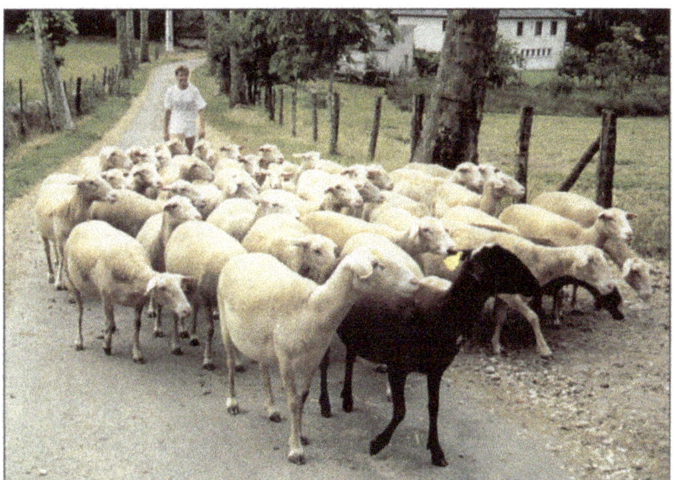

Fig. 10.13. Lacaune dairy ewes in south-central France. (Courtesy of Professor David Thomas.)

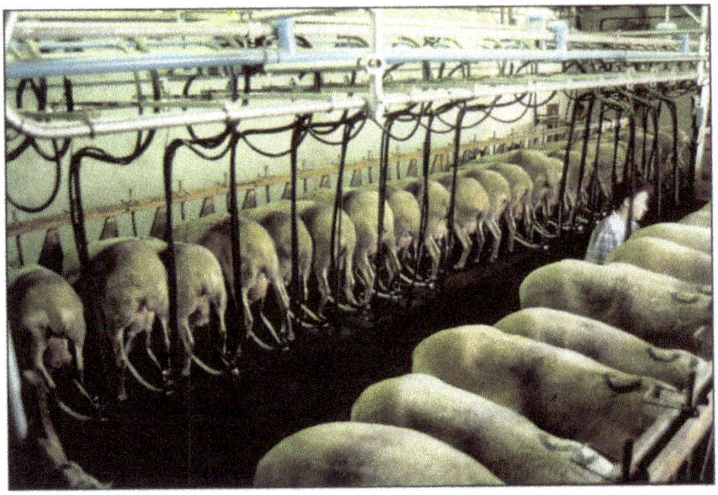

Fig. 10.14. Lacaune dairy ewes in the milking parlour on a farm in south-central France. (Courtesy of Professor David Thomas.)

et al. (2014) suggest that the Assaf is now the most important dairy sheep in Spain. There are smaller numbers of dairy sheep enterprises in Northern Europe. These are usually based on Friesian ewes, or derivatives of this breed such as the British Milksheep – a synthetic breed formed from crosses with the Bluefaced Leicester, Lleyn, Polled Dorset and other breeds.

Goat Breeds

The FAO summary of world animal genetic resources (FAO, 2015) lists 576 local goat breeds (Fig. 10.15). Many of these are outside of breeding schemes based on objective scientific improvement. However, certain breeds form the basis of improvement programmes in several countries. The majority of improved breeds are kept for milk, including the Saanen, Toggenburg (Fig. 10.16) and Anglo Nubian. The Boer goat from South Africa is a specialized meat breed, with breeds such as the Angora and Cashmere being kept for fibre.

Selection Within Breeds

Meat production

Systems of testing

In many respects, the development of breeding programmes and testing systems for specialized meat breeds, or for meat traits in dual-purpose breeds, has shadowed the development of the equivalent systems in beef cattle, which were discussed in the last chapter. Historically, central performance tests of potential sires were found in many countries. These have largely been abandoned due to both cost and the low coverage of animals and flocks involved. The majority of improvement programmes are now based on on-farm recording of performance.

The development of on-farm recording in Britain is probably fairly typical of that in most meat or dual-purpose sheep industries. National recording of sheep began in the early 1970s, shortly after the formation of the Meat and Livestock Commission (MLC), and most individual animal performance recording of sheep breeds in Britain remained under the auspices of the MLC until 1995. Since then Signet, now part of the Agriculture and Horticulture Development Board (AHDB Beef and Lamb), has taken over operation of these services. Currently the AHDB Signet Sheepbreeder scheme is based on on-farm recording of pedigree information, litter size, live weights at a range of ages from weaning to breeding ages – these are used as measures of both direct and maternal performance – and ultrasonic measurements of carcass merit. Breeders are responsible for recording pedigree and birth details and records of weights, while ultrasonic measurements are made by Signet staff. Additional traits are recorded in some cases, including

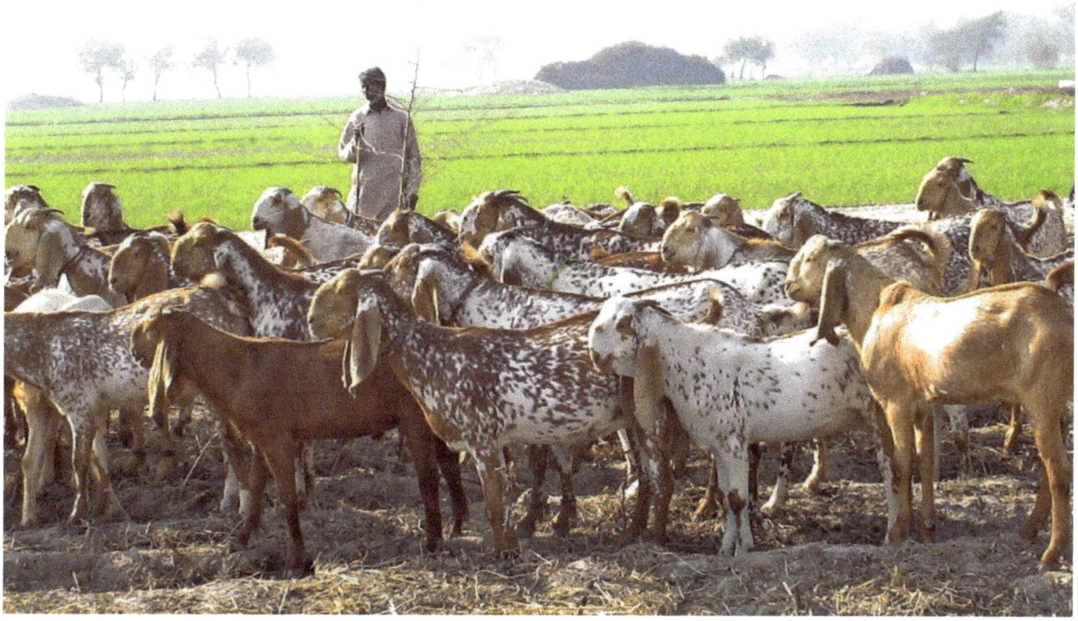

Fig. 10.15. A herd of Makhi Cheeni goats near Hasilpur, Bahawalpur, Pakistan. (After ILRI/M Sajjad Khan.)

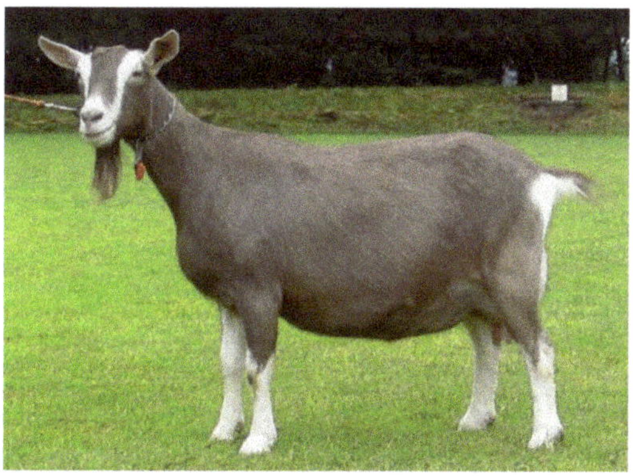

Fig. 10.16. An example of a European dairy goat breed, a Toggenburg. (After Teunie at Dutch Wikipedia.)

computed tomography (CT) scanning information, faecal egg counts, and so on.

About 40 breeds participate in the Signet scheme in Britain. The majority of recorded flocks are from the terminal sire breeds. The average size of recorded flocks in these breeds is about two to three times larger than the average non-recorded flock. There are smaller numbers of performance-recorded hill flocks, but these have larger average flock sizes. Few flocks from the traditional long-wool crossing breeds are performance recorded. In total, less than 1% of purebred ewes are performance recorded in Britain, although around 8–15% of pedigree registered sheep in the main terminal sire breeds are recorded. A relatively low proportion of sheep are performance recorded in most other major lamb-producing countries too.

There are several reasons for this low level of performance recording. There is probably less conviction of the benefits of genetic improvement of objective measures of performance among pedigree sheep breeders and their customers, than among pig, poultry and dairy farmers. This often results in stock of high predicted genetic merit being undervalued. Also, the additional effort and indirect costs involved in recording individual ewe and lamb performance are probably greater than those in dairy or beef cattle. Extra input is needed at lambing time, and other key measurement times, to ensure that accurate records of pedigree and performance are obtained. Often recording has to be undertaken outdoors, which requires additional commitment, especially in extreme climates. In both sheep and beef cattle recording schemes, the fact that terminal sire breeds are the most commonly recorded breed type is partly a function of the more or less single-purpose rôle, and hence relatively simple selection goal, in these breeds. Also, recording is often easier due to more favourable locations and smaller flock or herd sizes.

Co-operative breeding schemes, such as group breeding schemes and sire-referencing schemes, have been important in several countries. Group breeding schemes were initiated in the 1960s by commercial sheep and beef producers in New Zealand and Australia, who were dissatisfied with the quality of breeding stock produced by 'elite' studs. In their heyday, several million sheep and cattle were involved in these schemes in New Zealand and Australia – including one Australian Merino group alone with over a million ewes. These schemes usually involve the creation of a nucleus flock of elite animals, drawn from co-operating members' flocks (or elsewhere). The nucleus may then be closed to the importation of males or females from other flocks (e.g. to help maintain high health status), or it may remain open to further importations of animals of sufficiently high merit (James, 1977; Roden, 1994). Animals in the nucleus flock are comprehensively performance recorded and intensely selected, to maximize rates of genetic gain. Usually, the purpose of the nucleus flock is to breed high genetic merit replacement breeding stock, especially rams, for use in members' own flocks. The screening of elite animals into the nucleus, the more comprehensive recording, and the larger size of the nucleus, usually mean that rates of gain are higher than that which could be achieved by individual members, especially when their flocks are small.

The success of these original schemes in the 1960s and 70s led to the establishment of similar schemes elsewhere. For example, group breeding schemes were established in several sheep breeds in Britain. The longest established group was the CAMDA Welsh Mountain group breeding scheme in North Wales (Fig. 10.17). The scheme started in 1976 when ten Welsh Mountain breeders formed a nucleus flock of 400 ewes after recording their individual flocks with MLC for 2 years. An open nucleus was maintained until 1983 when the flock was closed for health reasons. Two 50-ewe control flocks were also established, one 'commercial' control using industry rams, and one conventional genetic control to allow genetic improvement to be measured over time. The group finally closed in

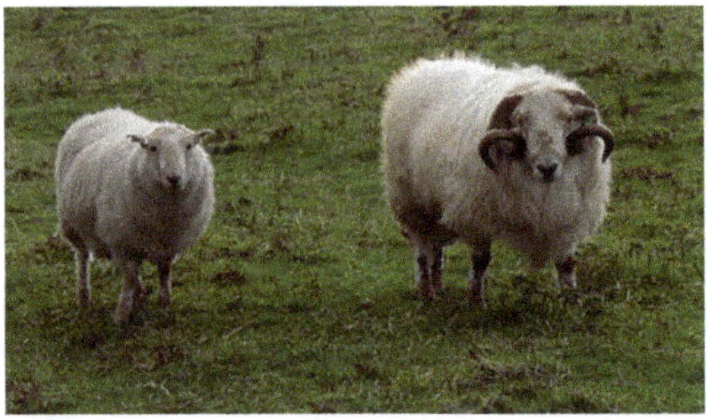

Fig. 10.17. Welsh Mountain ewe and ram typical of those from the CAMDA group breeding scheme nucleus flock in North Wales. (Copyright John Haynes.)

2011 with the sale of the nucleus flock. Several smaller group breeding schemes were established in Britain during the 1970s and 80s but most of them ceased to operate by the early 2000s.

While group breeding schemes can undoubtedly help to accelerate genetic improvement, there has been a relatively low involvement in this type of scheme in many countries, compared to that seen originally in New Zealand and Australia. Even in these countries, the popularity of these schemes declined (Parker, 1993). This may be due in part to the high level of co-operation and the financial and legal commitment required to make the schemes work. However, some of these obstacles may be overcome by sire-referencing schemes. In several cases sire-referencing schemes have evolved from what were previously group breeding schemes.

Sire-referencing schemes have similar aims to group breeding schemes, but they do not require the formation of central nucleus flocks, which can be expensive to maintain. Instead, genetic links are created across members' flocks by the use of a panel of artificial insemination (AI) rams on a portion of the ewes in each flock (see Fig. 10.18), or by sharing rams across flocks. Because of these links between flocks, across-flock best linear unbiased prediction (BLUP) methods can then be used to produce EBVs which can be compared fairly across co-operating flocks (see Chapter 7). Sire-referencing schemes operated in sheep or beef cattle in Australia, New Zealand, USA, South Africa, France and the UK for many years. The development of these schemes has been assisted in several countries by improvements in AI techniques for sheep, the wider accessibility of BLUP evaluation procedures, and the availability of cheaper, powerful computers.

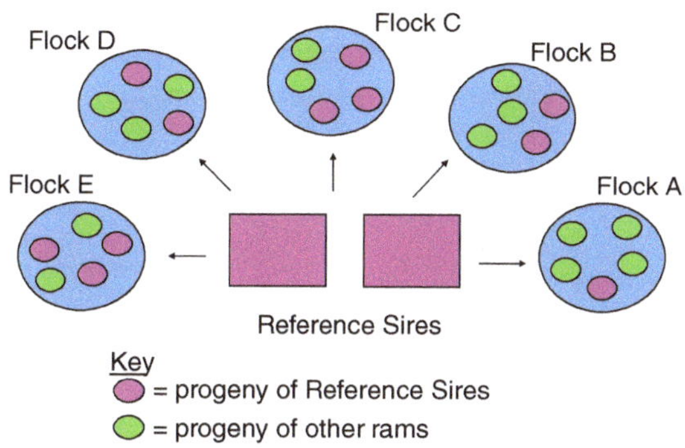

Fig. 10.18. Schematic diagram illustrating the principle of sire-referencing schemes These rely on the creation of genetic links across flocks, usually through the use of a panel of AI rams in common across flocks.

For example, sire-referencing schemes were established in eight sheep breeds in Britain in the 1990s – mainly terminal sire breeds (Macfarlane and Simm, 2008) and increased to about 20 breeds at their peak. These schemes, too, appear to have declined in popularity recently – perhaps partly because of the additional cost and commitment involved; perhaps partly because of the use of new genetic evaluation methods, as discussed below.

The operation of sire-referencing schemes usually involves:

- **Selection of a panel of reference rams for use across members' flocks.** To qualify as potential reference sires, animals must have high EBVs or index scores, and be functionally sound. Qualifying animals may be brought to a central location where all members may gather to view them and vote for their choice, based on their own preferred combination of index score, pedigree, conformation and breed type. A panel of about six reference sires could be in use at any one time, with two or three of these replaced annually, depending on their latest EBVs and popularity with members.
- **Use of several reference sires, by AI or natural mating, on a proportion of the ewes in each member's flock.** In schemes with a wide geographic spread of members, insemination with fresh semen is impractical, and so laparoscopic AI with frozen semen can be used. A total of 30 ewes per flock is usually recommended for mating to reference sires. This number provides a reasonable compromise between maximizing rates of genetic gain and minimizing AI use, or the use of nominated sires (Lewis *et al.*, 1996).
- **Recording performance in appropriate traits via a suitable recording scheme.**
- **Evaluation of performance records using across-flock, multi-trait animal model BLUP.** This produces EBVs which can be compared fairly across flocks and across years. This allows animals of different age groups to be compared, and genetic trends to be estimated (examples of these are given in the next section).
- **Use of these results to select the next generation of potential reference sires and to select sires and replacement females for the individual members' flocks.**

A combination of the cost and complexity of running sire-referencing schemes and the advent of better genetic technologies has led to the demise of sire-referencing schemes in Britain. Initially, greater computing power and the build-up of many years of records allowed the introduction of whole-breed genetic evaluations. These typically involved all recorded flocks in a breed, often supplemented with non-recorded but pedigreed flocks to aid genetic linkage, which were analysed by single-trait or multi-trait BLUP to produce EBVs for the whole breed. These EBVs were used in a range of selection indexes to produce data which breeders could use to sell their breeding stock based on objective measurements and comparable figures. Effectively all EBVs within a breed were directly comparable, for any given trait, allowing buyers to assess the value of a particular replacement ewe or ram in terms of the key traits for the breed.

Many commercial buyers, particularly of terminal sire rams for use in their own flock, are more interested in the quality of the lambs produced rather than being tied to a particular breed. This leads to questions about how EBVs in one breed compare to those in another breed, for the same traits. This led to a further development in sheep testing where animals of known pedigree from different breeds are kept on the same farms and evaluated together. Once this step has been made then it is feasible to operate multi-breed genetic evaluations which use both the whole-breed data plus the links between breeds provided by the animals compared on the same farms from different breeds. Initially, this has been tried with the terminal sire breeds in the UK (Signet, 2019). The same concept has been applied in Australia across eight sites involving the major breeds and crosses used for all commercial traits of interest (Fogarty *et al.*, 2006). This was an extensive programme, called the 'Information Nucleus', which provides a major source of data on EBVs, new traits and genomic methods.

In lower income countries, community-based breeding programmes (CBBPs) for sheep and goats have become the main focus for testing and disseminating improved genetics. These schemes have the ability to dovetail into local farming structures and to support technical changes that may be necessary. One such scheme is illustrated in Fig. 10.19 with groups of herds of goats at the base of what looks like a traditional breeding pyramid. All the recording and selection decisions are carried out in the nucleus and bucks with elite genetics passed down from the nucleus, through a multiplier level to the CBBPs. Selection decisions taken in the nucleus are informed by the owners in the CBBPs resulting in multi-purpose goats suitable for local farmers.

Traits recorded

The animal characteristics important in meat production were identified earlier, and include measures of growth, carcass composition and reproduction. Some of these can be measured directly on candidates for selection. In these cases, the traits in the breeding goal and those actually recorded (the selection criteria) are often the same. For example, records of litter size, number of lambs reared and weights of lambs at various ages can all be obtained relatively easily. However, carcass characteristics have to be measured indirectly, or on relatives of the candidates for selection. Ultrasonic measurements are widely used in several countries to predict the carcass composition of candidates for selection. Computed tomography scanning is also becoming more widely used on a small proportion of the breeding population comprising elite rams.

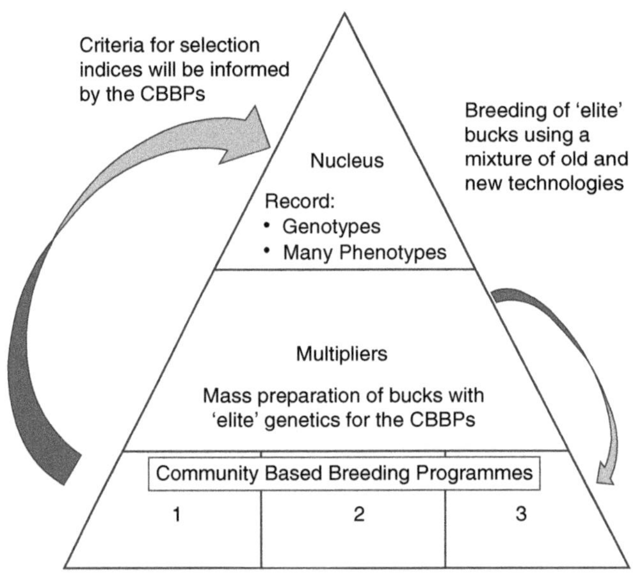

Fig. 10.19. Traditional breeding pyramid adapted to local goat production conditions.

(The assumption in this chapter is that the recording and evaluation schemes are geared towards improving characteristics under the control of many genes, as well as non-genetic effects. However, there has been some interest in single genes with a major effect on carcass composition, such as the *callipyge* gene mentioned in Chapter 2, and quantitative trait loci uncovered by modern molecular genetic techniques such as the myostatin gene.)

The heritabilities of some of the important traits in meat or dual-purpose breeds, and the correlations among them, are shown in Tables 10.6 to 10.9. Generally, growth and carcass traits are moderately variable and moderately to highly heritable. In contrast, most reproductive traits are more variable but have low heritabilities. The repeatabilities of most reproductive traits, except ovulation rate, are fairly low. So, there is scope for increasing the accuracy of selection by using repeated measures of performance when these are available (as explained in Chapter 7). This is reflected in the fact that heritabilities based on the average of several repeated measures of performance are slightly higher than those based on single measures of performance. The correlations among live weights measured at different ages are generally high, especially later in life when the strong maternal influence on birth weights and other early weights has declined. Generally, the shorter the interval between measurements, the higher the correlations are. Correlations between weight and carcass dimensions are usually positive. There are usually small and positive phenotypic correlations between weight and various measures of reproductive performance. The genetic associations between weight and fertility (conception rate and related traits) tend to be negative, but those between yearling or hogget live weight and numbers of lambs born or reared are usually positive.

In Chapter 6 we outlined a number of additional variance components that could be calculated given the right circumstances and data structure. Sheep provide a good example of where maternal influences on productivity can be studied, and both the genetic and permanent environmental effects of the mother can be estimated. In their study of the Suffolk Sire-Referencing scheme in Britain, Maniatis and Pollott (2002) estimated the maternal additive genetic effects and maternal permanent environmental effects on lamb data recorded for 8-week weight, 20-week (scanning) weight, ultrasonic fat depth and muscle depth. This involved a large dataset with over 55,000 records for 8-week weight and

Table 10.6. Estimates of coefficients of variation and weighted mean heritabilities for growth and carcass traits in sheep, from an extensive survey of published results. The number of estimates contributing to the weighted mean heritability, and the standard deviation of estimates, are shown in brackets. The coefficient of variation is a measure of the variation in the trait concerned (see Chapter 2). It is calculated as the standard deviation of the trait, divided by its mean. In this case it has been multiplied by 100 so that it is expressed as a percentage. (After Safari *et al*., 2005)

Trait	Coefficient of variation (%)	Heritability (no., s.d.)	Comments
Birth weight	19	0.15 (6, 0.02)	Meat breeds
	23	0.19 (26, 0.02)	Dual purpose
Weaning weight	18	0.18 (7, 0.04)	Meat breeds
	16	0.18 (40, 0.02)	Dual purpose
Post-weaning weight	11	0.29 (23, 0.03)	Meat breeds
	12	0.26 (26, 0.12)	Dual purpose
Daily gain	20	0.17 (21, 0.01)	Meat breeds
Adult weight	6	0.30 (4, 0.03)	Meat breeds
	11	0.31 (19, 0.03)	Dual purpose
Fat depth, live animal	20	0.26 (27, 0.02)	Unadjusted for weight or age at slaughter
Fat depth, carcass	46	0.30 (6, 0.03)	Unadjusted for weight or age at slaughter
Eye muscle dimensions,[a] live animal	10	0.24 (11, 0.03)	Unadjusted for weight or age at slaughter
Eye muscle dimensions, carcass	11	0.30 (4, 0.03)	Unadjusted for weight or age at slaughter
Lean meat yield	9	0.35 (2, 0.02)	Unadjusted for weight or age at slaughter
Meat pH	6	0.35 (2, 0.02)	Unadjusted forweight or age at slaughter
Meat colour	10	0.16 (2, 0.03)	Unadjusted forweight or age at slaughter

[a]Eye muscle depth, width or area.

Table 10.7. Estimates of coefficients of variation, weighted mean heritabilities and repeatabilities for reproduction traits in sheep, from an extensive survey of published results. Repeatabilities measure the extent to which the performance of an animal is similar at successive recordings, as a result of both genetic effects and permanent environmental effects - see Chapter 4 for more details. The number of estimates contributing to the weighted means, and the standard deviation of estimates, are shown in brackets. (After Safari *et al.*, 2005.)

	Single record of performance		Average of several records of performance		
Trait	CV (%)	Heritability (no., s.d.)	CV (%)	Heritability (no., s.d.)	Repeatability
Ewe fertility	52	0.08 (18, 0.01)	40	0.07 (5, 0.03)	0.09 (27, 0.05)
Ovulation rate	26	0.15 (5, 0.02)	–	–	0.37 (10, 0.15)[a] 0.31 (9, 0.11)[b]
No. lambs born/ewe joined	53	0.10 (19, 0.01)	36	0.15 (18, 0.08)	0.11 (35, 0.04)
No. lambs born/ewe lambing (or litter size)	34	0.13 (49, 0.01)	24	0.21 (9, 0.16)	0.14 (50,0.07)
No. lambs weaned/ewe joined	64	0.07 (11, 0.01)	43	0.15 (14, 0.09)	0.08 (20, 0.04)
No. lambs weaned/ewe lambing	45	0.05 (8, 0.01)	–	–	0.08 (17, 0.03)
Lamb survival (maternal)	47	0.03 (16, 0.01)	36	0.11 (4, 0.10)	0.09 (18, 0.05)
Weight of lamb weaned/ewe joined	48	0.13 (7, 0.03)	43	0.18 (7, 0.11)	0.10 (4, 0.05)
Weight of lamb weaned/ewe lambing	36	0.11 (11, 0.02)	–	–	0.15 (6, 0.04)
Testis diameter (or scrotal circumference)	9	0.21 (6, 0.06)	–	–	–
Worm resistance	31	0.27 (16, 0.02)	–	–	–
Feed intake	20	0.13 (3, 0.03)	–	–	–

[a]Repeatability within a year.
[b]Repeatability across years.

over 28,000 scanning records. They found the heritability of 8-week weight to be 0.30 when analysed with a simple animal model, but when maternal effects were added to the model this reduced to 0.14. The maternal genetic component was 0.10 of the phenotypic variance, almost as high as the heritability and the permanent maternal environmental effect accounted for 0.08 of the phenotypic variance. Not surprisingly, there was a correlation between the additive and the maternal additive genetic effects (–0.36). Weight at scanning (20 weeks) had a heritability of 0.32 with a simple animal model and 0.20 when all effects were included in the model; maternal genetic and permanent environment effects were 0.07 and 0.06, respectively, as a proportion of the phenotypic variance. Clearly, the maternal additive effect plays a lesser rôle as the lambs became older. Despite these additional effects being shown to have a significant effect on the pre-weaning traits measured there is no record at the time of writing of sheep improvement schemes actually using these models in practice.

Selection also takes place for disease resistance, especially resistance to intestinal worms, in meat and dual-purpose breeds in the UK, New Zealand and Australia. This is of growing importance because of the increasing resistance of worms to anthelmintic treatments (Fig. 10.20). Faecal egg counts are often used as an indicator of resistance to intestinal parasites. These have been shown to be a good indicator of worm burdens, and to be heritable (average heritability of 0.27; Safari *et al.*, 2005). Similarly, selection for tolerance to facial eczema, a fungal infection of the skin, is part of the breeding goal in some meat and dual-purpose breeds in affected areas of New Zealand. In animals which have been exposed to the disease agent, either naturally or by an artificial challenge, tolerance can be measured from the concentration of a liver enzyme in the blood. In parts of Australia there is also interest in selection for resistance to fly strike using 'dag scores' (a measure of faecal contamination), body wrinkle score and wool cover. The potential for genetics to counteract health problems is widely recognized but not always simple to implement. In a comprehensive review, Bishop (2015) concluded that:

> the considerable genetic variation that invariably exists for resistance to infections (and infectious disease) suggests that selection for increased resistance can be an attractive option to complement, but not

Table 10.8. Mean estimates of phenotypic and genetic correlations between live weights and carcass characteristics measured at different ages in sheep from an extensive review of published values. Number of studies summarized shown in parentheses. (Source: Safari *et al.*, 2005)

Trait 1	Trait 2	Mean correlation between traits: Phenotypic	Genetic
Birth weight	Weaning weight	0.37 (10)	0.47 (14)
	Post-weaning weight	0.32 (7)	0.29 (8)
	Adult weight	0.26 (5)	0.22 (7)
	Growth rate (g/d)	0.13 (1)	0.27 (6)
Weaning weight	Post-weaning weight	0.70 (9)	0.85 (11)
	Adult weight	0.56 (12)	0.75 (16)
	Growth rate (g/d)	0.16 (1)	0.79 (4)
Post-weaning weight	Adult weight	0.74 (9)	0.93 (11)
	Growth rate (g/d)	–	0.19 (1)
	Fat depth, live	0.36 (9)	0.36 (9)
	Fat depth, carcass	−0.06 (1)	0.34 (6)
	Eye muscle,[a] live	0.33 (6)	−0.12 (1)
	Eye muscle, carcass	0.32 (8)	0.28 (8)
Adult weight	Growth rate (g/d)	0.34 (1)	0.78 (1)
Fat depth, live	Fat depth, carcass	0.51 (1)	0.77 (1)
	Eye muscle, live	0.30 (10)	0.33 (10)
	Eye muscle, carcass	–	–
Carcass weight	Fat depth, carcass	0.54 (2)	0.39 (2)
	Eye muscle, carcass	0.54 (2)	0.54 (2)
Fat depth, carcass	Eye muscle, carcass	−0.05 (2)	−0.33 (2)

[a]Eye muscle depth, width or area

Table 10.9. Mean estimates of phenotypic and genetic correlations between live weights measured at different ages, and reproduction traits in sheep from an extensive review of published values. NB some estimates are based on a small number of studies – see original review for details. Correlations in brackets are with average performance over a number of records. (Source: Safari *et al.*, 2005)

Trait 1	Trait 2	Mean correlation between traits: Phenotypic	Genetic
Weaning weight	Fertility	0.09 (2)	−0.28 (2)
	No. lambs born/ewe joined	0.04 (1)	0.15 (2)
	No. lambs born/ewe lambing	0.06 (5)	0.29 (11)
	No. lambs weaned/ ewe joined	0.03 (1)	0.18 (2)
	No. lambs weaned/ ewe lambing	–	−0.05 (4)
	Weight weaned/ewe joined	0.13 (1)	0.75 (1)
	Worm resistance	−0.03 (5)	−0.03 (5)
Post-weaning weight	Fertility	–	–
	No. lambs born/ewe joined	0.12 (1)	0.23 (1)
	No. lambs born/ewe lambing	0.01 (6)	0.17 (7)
	No. lambs weaned/ ewe joined	0.01 (1)	0.29 (1)
	Weight weaned/ewe joined	0.24 (1)	0.77 (1)
	Worm resistance	−0.08 (4)	−0.24 (4)
Adult weight	Fertility	0.11 (2)	0.40 (2)
	No. lambs born/ewe joined	0.03 (10)	0.15 (10)
	No. lambs born/ewe lambing	−0.02 (1)	0.27 (3)
	No. lambs weaned/ ewe joined	0.09 (4)	0.33 (4)
	No. lambs weaned/ ewe lambing	–	–
	Weight weaned/ewe joined	0.21 (6)	0.70 (6)
	Worm resistance	0.07 (3)	−0.24 (4)

replace, existing control measures. Furthermore, such selection may have additional epidemiological benefits in terms of reducing transmission of infection and possibly extending the sustainability of other control strategies, because using multiple control strategies can reduce pathogen evolution risks. However, the challenge is to define cost effective selection protocols that are attractive to sheep farmers.

Perhaps the most widespread disease-related breeding scheme in sheep is that for scrapie resistance in the UK. Scrapie has been recognized in British sheep flocks for centuries but came into wider public recognition during the BSE ('mad-cow disease') crisis of the 1990s. Both diseases are examples of transmissible spongiform encephalopathies which create modified versions of the prion proteins normally found in the central nervous system. These modified prion proteins appear to cause a neurodegenerative disease in susceptible animals. There is no known cure for scrapie, but it has long been recognized that some sheep are resistant to scrapie. This stimulated a search for genes associated with

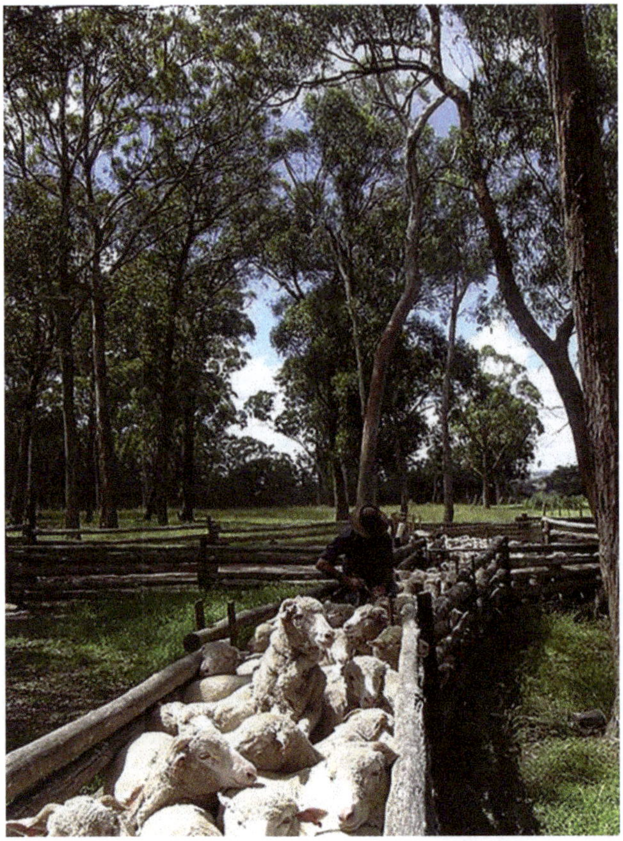

Fig. 10.20. Drenching Merinos in Australia. The resistance of internal parasites to anthelmintics is of major concern in parts of Australia and New Zealand, and increasingly in other sheep-producing countries too. However, selection of sheep for resistance to the parasites appears to be effective. (Courtesy of C. Goodwin; GNU Free documentation license.)

resistance to scrapie in sheep, and the recognition that resistance was conferred on sheep by certain polymorphisms of three alleles in the genes coding for prion proteins (the so-called PrP gene). Animals with one or two copies of the so-called ARR genotype, after the three amino acids produced by the three polymorphisms, were more resistant to scrapie but those with most other genotypes were more susceptible. The UK government set up a National Scrapie Plan (NSP) in 2001 in an attempt to eliminate non-resistant genotypes from the national sheep population (NSP, 2006). Evaluating the outcome of the NSP in 2015, Ortiz-Pelaez *et al.* (2014) estimated that frequencies of the resistant alleles and genotypes had increased between 2002/3 and 2012/3. Correspondingly, susceptible alleles and genotypes had declined over this period. However, this was a relatively small change with ARR allele frequency rising from 43.3% to 52.3% and that of the most susceptible genotypes declining from 6.5% to 3%. Nevertheless, the fully susceptible genotypes accounted for only 28% of sampled animals by 2012/3.

Methods and results of genetic evaluation

Historically, the results of most meat sheep recording schemes were evaluated by contemporary comparisons, or indexes based on these. For example, in Britain, performance records from the MLC/Signet Sheepbreeder recording scheme were allocated to contemporary groups based on lamb sex, litter size and dam age. Records were then standardized within contemporary groups, and the individual animal's performance in each trait was presented as a deviation from its contemporary group mean (in s.d. units; see Chapter 7). Multi-trait indexes were derived from these standardized deviations.

Since the early 1990s, genetic evaluation in many major sheep industries has been based on BLUP methodology. The advantages of BLUP methods were described fully in Chapter 7. In particular, they offer more accurate estimates of breeding value than other methods and a more flexible method of combining information on different traits from different classes of relatives. Also, where sufficiently strong genetic links occur, they allow EBVs to be compared fairly across flocks and years. This has several important benefits. Firstly, the number of candidate animals for selection which can be directly compared is greatly increased. This has direct benefits on the rate of response which can be achieved. Secondly, if relevant estimates of heritabilities and correlations are used, the genetic trend in performance can be charted year-by-year, by comparing the average EBVs of animals born in the breed or flock in successive years. This provides a valuable check on genetic progress, both for breeders themselves and for their customers. However, compared to the situation in dairy and beef cattle, there is relatively little use of AI in sheep in most countries, and so genetic links between flocks are usually weaker. This has limited the impact of across-flock evaluations, except where these links have been created deliberately, such as in sire-referencing schemes or centralized ram comparison schemes.

The steps involved in genetic evaluation of meat breeds, or evaluation of meat traits in dual-purpose sheep and goat breeds are generally very similar to those outlined for beef cattle in the last chapter. Briefly, these include:

- Collation and checking of performance records by the recording agency, and transfer of these to the agency responsible for genetic evaluation, if this is different. (In most countries evaluations are performed by the recording agency itself, a government agency or university.) This step is repeated each time evaluations are performed. Usually this is one or two times per annum for across-flock or national evaluations, and more frequently for within-flock evaluations, but this varies depending on the seasonality of the breed concerned and the timespan over which traits of interest are recorded. If genomic estimated breeding values (GEBVs) are to be estimated, then appropriate young animals are genotyped.
- With BLUP evaluation methods, environmental effects are estimated and breeding values are predicted simultaneously. The statistical model used determines which environmental effects are accounted for. Some of these can be identified explicitly, others are accounted for by assigning animals to contemporary groups.
- BLUP or GBLUP evaluations are then carried out with the single-trait or multi-trait individual animal model as appropriate, where all relationships between animals in the pedigree file are recognized and accounted for, and all animals in the pedigree file get (G)EBVs. Increasingly, BLUP evaluations distinguish between direct and maternal genetic influences on early growth. GEBV evaluations based on the single-trait or multi-trait individual single-step models are currently used for the computation of the genetic merit of goats in two of the largest goat farms in the UK. The single-step approach combines both the pedigree information and genotypes for a subset of animals that are genotyped plus the records to compute GEBVs. This enables genotypic information to contribute for all animals in the analysis.
- EBVs (or GEBVs) are expressed relative to some reference population of animals called the base. In most countries a fixed base is used, i.e. EBVs are expressed relative to those of a group of animals born in a particular year, though this base is updated from time to time, i.e. making a more recent annual cohort the reference population with average EBV of 0.
- In some countries, (G)EBVs for individual traits are combined into indexes of overall economic merit. These are discussed in more detail in the following section.
- Accuracies or reliabilities may be produced for each of the EBVs.
- Results of evaluations are sent to individual breeders after each new evaluation. Usually these include summaries of the predicted merit of the current lamb crop, and the sires and dams they represent. National sire summaries are not yet used as widely as in beef breeds, but this is likely to occur when national evaluations become more widespread.

It is difficult to estimate how many countries are using BLUP methods for the genetic evaluation of sheep. FAO (2015) suggest that 19% of countries use genetic evaluations for sheep but do not specify which method is used. BLUP methods are used in either national or particular meat sheep breeding programmes in Canada, the US, Australia, New Zealand, South Africa, Norway, Finland, Denmark, Sweden, France, Slovakia, Spain, Iceland, Czech Republic, Poland, Ireland and the UK. In those countries which adopted BLUP evaluations relatively early, single-trait sire model evaluations were often used, mainly for within-flock evaluations. However, multi-trait animal model evaluations are widely used now, and these are gradually being extended to across-flock evaluations of groups of flocks or national populations. For example, in the UK, multi-trait animal model BLUP evaluations are performed annually (or more often) for most recorded breeds. Within-flock multi-trait animal model BLUP evaluations are carried out for other recorded flocks. At the time of writing, only two countries are using genomic selection methods although another four will introduce them soon (J. Conington, personal communication).

Use of indexes of overall economic merit

Selection indexes are widely used in meat and dual-purpose breeds. For example, in Britain they have been used since the mid-1980s. Currently, participants in the Signet Sheepbreeder recording scheme have had a choice of five indexes: Terminal Sire, Maternal, Longwool, Welsh/Carcass and Hill (Table 10.10). Since the introduction of multi-trait animal model BLUP evaluations, index scores are derived solely from the animals' own EBVs for the relevant traits (i.e. all available performance information from relatives has already contributed to these EBVs).

Indexes used in Australian meat breeds mirror those described for the UK above. In addition, Australian terminal sire indexes incorporate meat eating quality and shear-force measurements. In New Zealand there are currently two indexes available based around terminal sire breeds and maternal breeds. The main difference to the UK is that wool is included in the maternal index. EBVs for facial eczema and FEC are also available in New Zealand.

Since the mid-1980s ultrasonic measurements of fat and muscle have been obtained in testing programmes in a number of countries. For example, in Britain, MLC launched an ultrasonic scanning service for performance-recorded sheep in 1988. This was based on research at SAC to test scanning techniques and derive and test a selection index for terminal sire breeds, to combine measurements of weight, and fat and muscle depths. The development and testing of this index are described below, as they illustrate some useful general principles.

Table 10.10. Selection objectives, breeds and selection criteria for the five major indexes used in British sheep breeding. (After AHDB, 2018b.)

Index and objective	Main breeds	Selection criteria
Terminal sire – increase carcass lean meat yield but limit the rise in fatness	Charollais, Hampshire Down, Ile de France, Meatlinc, Poll Dorset, Suffolk, Texel, Vendeen	Scanning weight, ultrasonic fat and muscle depths. Used to compute EBV for carcass muscle and carcass fat which are given weightings of +3 and −1 in the index
Maternal – enhance lamb survival and pre-weaning growth rate by improving maternal ability	Lleyn, Poll Dorset	Litter size, 8-week liveweight, mature size and maternal ability. Index weightings vary by breed
Longwool – enhance carcass quality whilst maintaining prolificacy and mature size	Bluefaced Leicester	Scan weight, fat and muscle depths and litter size
Hill – improve overall productivity indicated by number of lambs successfully reared to a heavier carcass weight	Scottish Blackface, North Country Cheviot	Mature weight, longevity, maternal ability and number of lambs reared to weaning
Welsh/carcass index – improve maternal ability, lamb growth and carcass quality	Welsh hill breeds, such a Beulah and Welsh Hardy Speckledface, Lleyn	Lamb liveweight, ewe mature weight, ultrasound measurements

The breeding goal of the terminal sire index comprised carcass lean weight and carcass fat weight at a constant age (Simm and Dingwall, 1989). The selection criteria were live weight, ultrasonic fat depth and ultrasonic muscle depth measured at a constant age. This index was very similar to the one described in Chapter 7 except that, in this case, the relative economic values were chosen to achieve 'desired gains' in the traits in the breeding goal, rather than being based on actual market returns. This approach was chosen because of the weak relationship between carcass price and fatness in Britain at the time the index was derived.

Figure 10.21 shows the expected responses in goal traits from selection on indexes combining the same measurements of live weight, ultrasonic fat and muscle depths on the animal itself, but with a range of different relative economic values for weight of lean and fat in the carcass. All the responses shown are at a constant age. The graph illustrates that with a high penalty on fat compared to the value of lean (the left-hand side of the graph), selection on the index derived will lead to large reductions in weight of fat, but little improvement in weight of lean at a constant age. Conversely, if the penalty for producing fat is low, relative to the value of carcass lean weight (the right hand side of the graph), selection on the index derived will lead to large increases in both carcass lean weight and carcass fat weight. (Although fat *weight* is increasing, fat *proportion* will decrease if there is a large enough increase in lean weight).

These results might be confusing at first sight, but they are a direct consequence of the positive correlations between live weight, carcass fat weight and carcass lean weight. Within a breed, at a constant age, bigger animals generally have more lean *and* more fat. If selection is solely for weight at a constant age, we expect to get more lean and more fat. A selection index can help to restrict the increase in fat weight. But, if fat is heavily penalized, a lot of the potential improvement in lean weight has to be sacrificed, in order to avoid increases in fat weight. If fat is not heavily penalized, increases in fat weight can be tolerated, in order to get greater increases in lean weight.

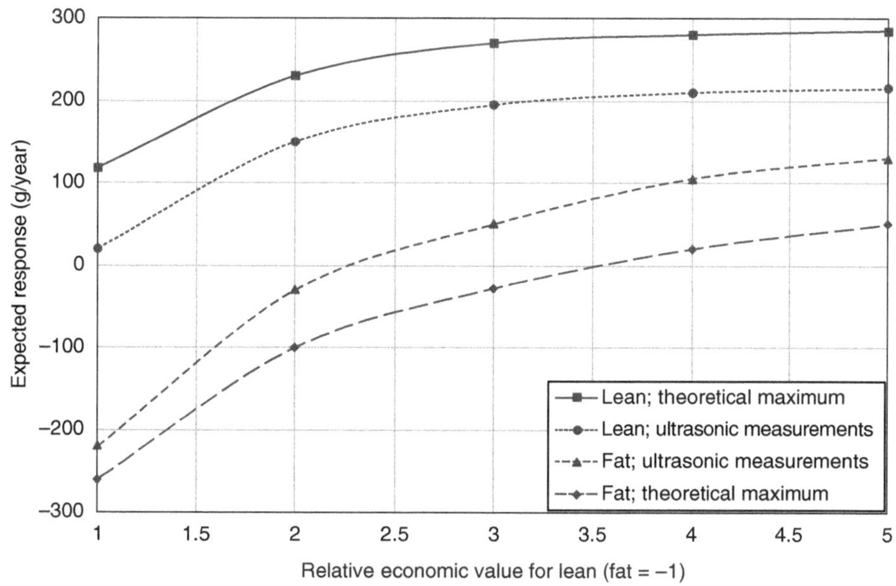

Fig. 10.21. Expected responses in carcass lean weight and carcass fat weight following index selection, when the relative economic values of carcass lean and fat weights range from +1:−1 to +5:−1. Selection is either on indexes combining measurements of live weight, ultrasonic fat depth and ultrasonic muscle depth on the animal itself, or on indexes based on live weight and 100% accurate measurements of fat and lean content of the live animal. This provides an estimate of the theoretical maximum rate of change which could be achieved, e.g. by the use of more advanced scanning methods. (Source: Simm and Dingwall, 1989.)

Intermediate relative economic values of +3 for lean and −1 for fat were chosen for use in a SAC selection experiment in Suffolk sheep, and for use in the Signet Sheepbreeder scheme, as they were expected to give almost maximum responses in lean weight, while heavily restricting changes in fat weight. This is illustrated further in Fig. 10.22, which shows expected responses in lean and fat weights following selection on weight alone, an index combining weight and fat only, the full index described above, or selection on an index with 100% accurate measurements on the live animal. Table 10.11 shows the index weights derived for use on ultrasonic and live weight measurements from candidates for selection alone (i.e. excluding records from relatives), assuming relative economic values of +3 and −1.

Advanced imaging techniques, such as CT (Fig. 10.23), can enhance the level of accuracy of carcass lean and fat EBVs. In the UK, CT measurements have been available since 1997. Two-stage selection programmes are used for sheep, with CT measurements being made on rams with the best EBVs, or index score, for ultrasonic measurements and live weight in on-farm recording programmes. Seven breeds and 250 breeders have been involved with this additional recording programme and have generated about 10,000 scans since 1997. As well as providing more accurate 'carcass' data, CT scanning also allows new traits to be measured such as gigot muscularity, vertebra number, spine length, intramuscular fat percentage and eye muscle area.

The UK Terminal Sire Index changed in 2018 to be based on scanning traits adjusted on a liveweight basis. The rationale for this was that breeders did not want to see leaner animals rewarded at the expense of well-muscled, slightly fatter individuals. Recorded terminal sires, with superior growth and muscling, were already helping to produce leaner commercial lambs and this was taken into account when setting index weightings. Also, when carcass traits are expressed on a weight-adjusted basis, animals with a high yield of muscle in the carcass tend to have less fat, so the index does not need to apply an additional reward for leanness. In fact, a small, positive weighting was applied to both of the weight-adjusted breeding values for fat to avoid the inadvertent selection of ultra-lean genetics in the quest for greater levels of muscling. In the new Terminal Sire Index, about 70% of the emphasis is put on liveweight at scanning, with equal amounts on muscle depth and lean weight, with gigot weight receiving slightly less weight than the two lean measures. Fat depth, fat weight and 8-week

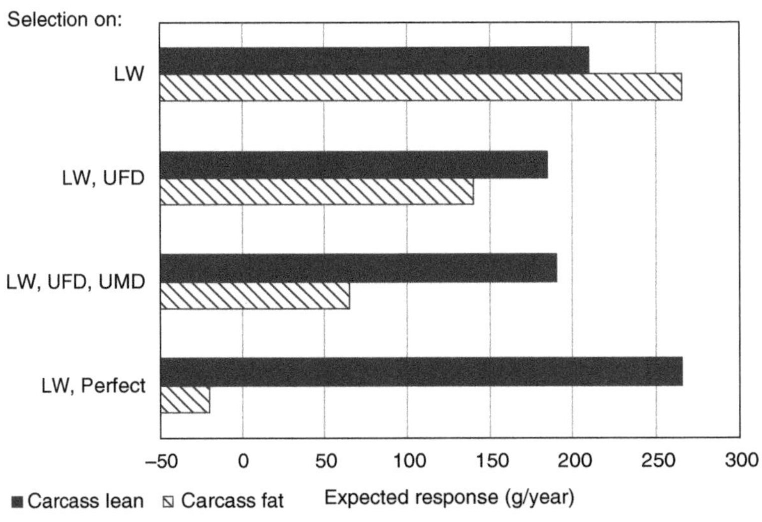

Fig. 10.22. Expected responses in carcass lean weight and carcass fat weight following selection on various combinations of index measurements. Index measurements include live weight (LW), ultrasonic fat depth (UFD), ultrasonic muscle depth (UMD), or hypothetical measurements which produce 100% accurate prediction of fat and lean content of the live animal (Perfect). This provides an estimate of the theoretical maximum rate of change which could be achieved, e.g. by the use of more advanced scanning methods. (Source: Simm, 1992, based on Simm and Dingwall, 1989.)

liveweight also receive some weight, the former to allow some control of fatness.

In order to produce more comprehensive indexes for multi-purpose breeds, e.g. to account for new measurements of carcass merit, estimates of genetic parameters are required for the new traits. Estimates of economic values of new traits will also be required if conventional (rather than 'desired gains') selection indexes are being used. Tables 10.6 to 10.9 indicate recent estimates of genetic parameters for a number of key meat traits and Table 10.12 shows heritabilities for some traits that may become important in the future. These include mastitis traits in meat breeds, greenhouse gas emission traits, skin traits, longevity, postnatal traits and meat quality traits.

Table 10.11. Details of the lean growth selection index used in the SAC Suffolk selection experiment and in the Signet Sheepbreeder recording scheme in Britain (NB the index weights shown are only relevant when selection is based on measurements from candidates only, and not on records from relatives). (Source: Simm and Dingwall, 1989).

Selection goal[a]	Relative economic value
Carcass lean weight	+3
Carcass fat weight	−1
Index measurements[a]	**Index weightings**
Live weight	+0.10/kg = +0.55/s.d.
Ultrasonic fat depth	−0.41/mm = −0.51/s.d.
Ultrasonic muscle depth	+0.26/mm = +0.53/s.d.

[a]All at 150 days of age.

Evidence of genetic improvement and its value

In theory, if there is genetic variation in any animal characteristic, then there is scope for changing it through selection. So, estimates of variances and heritabilities provide evidence of the *potential* for genetic improvement. In practice, however, having evidence that genetic change *has actually been made* is far more convincing for breeders and their customers (and reassuring for scientists and advisers!). In the past, most evidence of this sort has come from self-contained selection experiments, or from related trials sampling animals from industry which have different EBVs or different selection histories. However, with the wider use of BLUP methods in sheep breeding, more evidence of this sort has come from industry breeding schemes themselves, via estimates of genetic trends. Impressive genetic trends from industry schemes are particularly valuable in encouraging wider uptake of objective selection methods, because genetic improvement in these cases has been achieved by breeders on commercial farms rather than in experimental flocks. Some examples of each of these types of evidence are given below.

Selection in the CAMDA Welsh Mountain group breeding scheme, mentioned earlier, was on a selection index designed to increase lamb weight, increase ewe mature size and maintain prolificacy at the initial level (since this was considered to be optimal for the hill environment). Since 1980, a clear divergence in performance of the nucleus and control flocks was achieved as shown in Fig. 10.24.

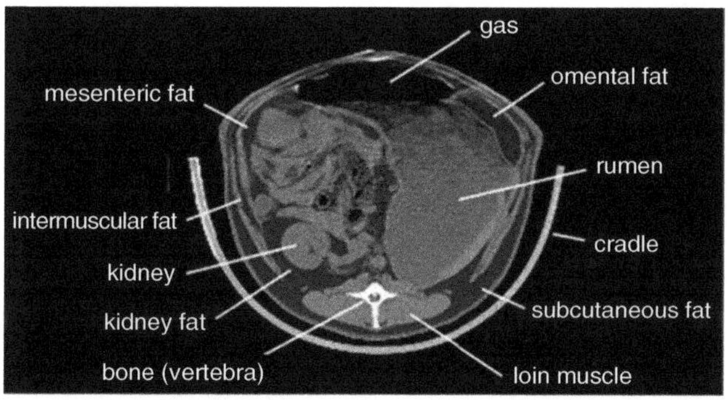

Fig. 10.23. An image obtained by computer tomography (CT), showing a 'cross section' through a sheep lying on its back in a scanning cradle. Air appears black in this image, fat dark grey, muscle light grey and bone white. Key organs and tissues are labelled. Advanced imaging techniques such as CT are very useful tools in research and have the potential to accelerate selection for altered carcass composition.

Table 10.12. The heritabilities of important traits in sheep.

Trait	Heritability	Reference
Average somatic cell score (mid lactation)	0.11 (0.04)	McLaren *et al.* (2018)
Average somatic cell score (late lactation)	0.08 (0.05)	
Sum California mastitis test (mid lactation)	0.09 (0.04)	
Sum California mastitis test (late lactation)	0.12 (0.07)	
Methane production/day	0.29 (0.05)	Pinares-Patino *et al.* (2013)
Methane production/kg dry matter intake (DMI)	0.13 (0.03)	
Dagginess at 3 months	0.44 (0.03)	Pickering *et al.* (2013)
Dagginess at 8 months	0.33 (0.02)	
Breech bareness	0.32 (0.02)	
Stayability	0.087 (0.002)	Lee *et al.* (2015)
Length of productive life	0.10 (0.002)	
Loin pH	0.14 (0.02)	Brito *et al.* (2017)
Marbling score	0.31 (0.03)	
Tenderness score	0.27 (0.03)	
Colour	0.19 (0.02)	
Methane/day	0.23 (0.04)	Jonker *et al.* (2018)
Carbon dioxide per day	0.32 (0.05)	
Methane/kg DMI	0.13 (0.02)	
DMI	0.33 (0.09)	Safari *et al.* (2007)
Dagginess	0.15 (0.03)	O'Brien *et al.* (2017)
Lameness	0.06 (0.02)	
Mastitis	0.04 (0.03)	
Birth difficulty	0.21 (0.05)	Macfarlane *et al.* (2010)
Vigour of lambs	0.34 (0.14)	
Suckling behaviour	0.03 (0.05)	
Hot carcass weight	0.25 (0.04)	Mortimer *et al.* (2014)
Intramuscular fat %	0.48 (0.05)	
Shear force after 5 days of ageing	0.27 (0.04)	
pH	0.08 (0.02)	
Isocitrate dehydrogenase activity	0.20 (0.04)	
Myoglobin concentration	0.25 (0.03)	
Fresh meat redness	0.08 (0.03)	
Fresh meat yellowness	0.10 (0.03)	
Fresh meat lightness	0.18 (0.03)	
Retail display meat redness	0.25 (0.04)	
Retail display meat yellowness	0.10 (0.03)	
Retail display meat lightness	0.41 (0.05)	
Retail display meat oxy/met value	0.27 (0.04)	
Retail display meat hue	0.36 (0.05)	
Retail display meat chroma	0.16 (0.04)	
Iron content of wet muscle tissue	0.21 (0.04)	
Zinc content of wet muscle tissue	0.27 (0.04)	
Eicosapentaeonic acid content of wet muscle (EPA)	0.17 (0.03)	
Docosapentaeonic acid content of wet muscle (DPA)	0.05 (0.02)	
Docosahexaeonic acid content of wet muscle (DHA)	0.22 (0.03)	
EPA + DHA	0.16 (0.03)	
EPA + DPA + DHA	0.08 (0.02)	
Linoleic acid content of wet muscle tissue (LA)	0.22 (0.04)	
Arachidonic acid content of wet muscle tissue (ARA)	0.15 (0.04)	
LA + ARA (mg/100 g tissue)	0.20 (0.04)	

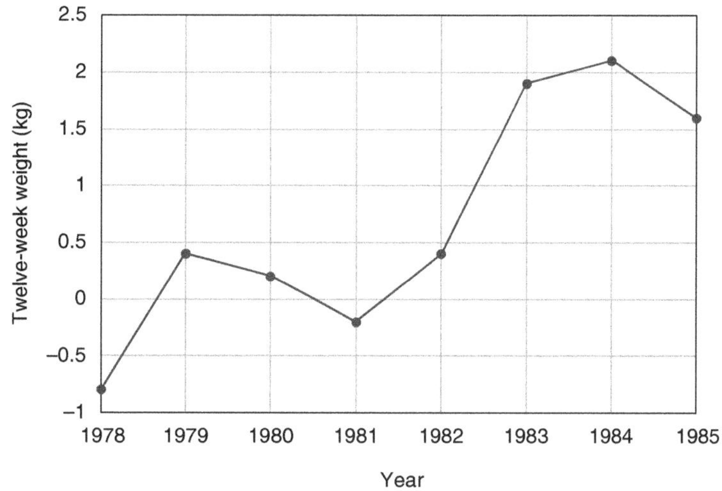

Fig. 10.24. Trends in 12-week weights in the CAMDA Welsh Mountain nucleus flock over the first 8 years of operation. Values shown are the differences between average weights in the nucleus and control flocks. (Source: Meat and Livestock Commission, 1986.)

An average increase of about 0.4 kg per year was achieved in 12-week lamb weights, as a result of selection over the first eight years of operation (Guy *et al.*, 1986) and improvement continued at a similar rate thereafter.

Selection experiments have been established for various carcass traits at a number of locations around the globe, but particularly in New Zealand and the UK. Most of the New Zealand selection lines have been selected for ultrasonic backfat depth, adjusted for live weight. However, index selection has been practised in a number of the more recent experiments in the UK and New Zealand. In most of these experiments, rates of genetic change in excess of 2% per annum have been achieved in fat depth or index score. These responses are close to the maximum expected values for the traits and flock sizes concerned (Simm, 1992, 1994).

One example of this type of experiment was the SAC selection experiment in Suffolk sheep mentioned previously. Selection in the SAC flock was based on the index that combines measurements of live weight, ultrasonic fat depth and ultrasonic muscle depth, all measured at 150 days of age. Compared to unselected control line ram lambs, selection line ram lambs performance tested in 1994, after 9 years of selection, had about 6 kg higher live weight (+10%), 1.0 mm lower ultrasonic fat depth (−13%), 3 mm higher ultrasonic muscle depth (+13%) and 18% higher index score (see Table 10.13 and Fig. 10.25). Similar proportional responses were obtained in ewe lambs.

The estimated genetic trends in three British breeds from 1990 to 2018 are shown in Figs 10.26 and 10.27. Figure 10.26 shows trends in the index for all recorded lambs in Suffolks, Charollais and Dorsets, whereas Fig. 10.27 shows the genetic trends in fat and muscle depth EBVs for all Suffolk lambs. Annual responses in lean growth index appear to be similar to those achieved in the SAC experiment. Because of the much larger size of the industry schemes, they can achieve these similar responses in the index of objectively measured traits, while taking account of visually assessed breed characteristics and conformation. (Also, some breeders used the individual trait EBVs to put particular selection emphasis on a component of the index.)

Often pedigree animals are reared under more favourable conditions than their commercial counterparts. The SAC experiment involved *ad libitum* feeding of a high-energy, high-protein diet, partly to replicate levels of performance achieved in many industry pedigree flocks in Britain, and partly to increase variation in carcass composition, to make it easier to detect differences between animals using ultrasonic scanning.

Table 10.13. Performance test results for ram lambs tested in 1994, after 9 years of selection in the SAC Suffolk selection experiment.

	Selection line	Control line	Difference (Sel-Con) %
Number of rams tested	113	48	
Live weight (kg)	67.0	61.0	+10%
Fat depth (mm)	5.9	6.9	−13%
Muscle depth (mm)	28.7	25.4	+13%
Index score	180	100	+18%[a]

[a]Difference in index score measured before scaling – indexes were scaled so that the average score in the control line each year equalled 100 points, and so that the index had a s.d. of 40 points.

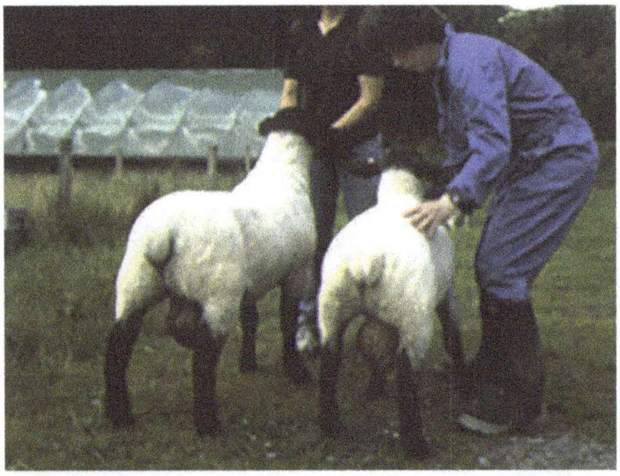

Fig. 10.25. Ram lambs from the SAC Suffolk selection experiment. The larger lamb is from the selection line, the smaller one from the control line.

However, the majority of lambs slaughtered for meat production in Britain are reared at grass. Two experiments were conducted at SAC (now part of Scotland's Rural College, SRUC) that provide evidence of the commercial value of objective genetic improvement programmes in pedigree flocks.

The first of these trials involved high- or low-index Suffolk rams mated to Scottish Mule ewes. Their lambs were reared at grass to produce carcasses of about 16.5, 20.0 or 23.5 kg. Sample-joint dissections on these carcasses showed that the progeny of high index sires had about 1.0% more lean and about 3.5% less fat than the progeny of low index sires (sires differed by 100 index points, or 2.5 standard deviations in index score; Lewis *et al.*, 1996). Another experiment showed significantly higher saleable meat yield from the carcasses of selection line progeny than from control line progeny, both at a constant carcass weight (+0.10 kg) and a constant level of fatness (+0.25 kg). On average, carcasses from selection line sires achieved prices about £1.50 higher than those for controls and were slaughtered 11 days sooner; this earlier slaughter date would save about £0.60 in grazing costs (Simm and Murphy, 1996). This financial advantage is worth up to £600 over the working life of a ram. In both of these experiments the progeny of high index sires had apparently poorer conformation, but this difference appears to be largely due to differences in fatness. More recent work comparing high- and low-index rams on commercial farms was reported by Marquez *et al.* (2013). Differences between the high- and low-index rams was found for a number of traits measured on the live animal.

Estimates of recent genetic trends in recorded traits, industry statistics and published estimates of the economic values of trait changes were used to investigate the value of genetic improvement in the UK sheep industry by Amer *et al.* (2007). Despite rates of genetic change in the relevant performance-recorded breeding populations being substantially less than theoretical predictions, the financial benefits of genetic change were substantial. Over 20 years, the benefits from 10 years of genetic progress at recently achieved rates in recorded hill sheep, sheep crossing sire and sheep terminal sire breeding programmes was estimated to be £5.3, £1.0 and £11.5 million, respectively. If dissemination of genetic material is such that these rates of change are also realized across the entire ram breeding industry, the combined benefits would be £110.8 million. Additional benefits from identification and use of the best animals available from the breeding sector for commercial matings through performance recording and genetic evaluation could not be quantified. When benefits of genetic improvement were expressed on an annual present value basis and compared with lagged annual investment costs to achieve it, the internal rate of return (IRR) on the investment in sheep was 32%.

A similar study looking at the return on the Meat and Livestock Australia investment in Australian sheep genetics (Fennessy *et al.*, 2014) concluded that the IRR was about 27%. This was a substantial increase in value of Australian sheep products resulting from investment in sheep genetics.

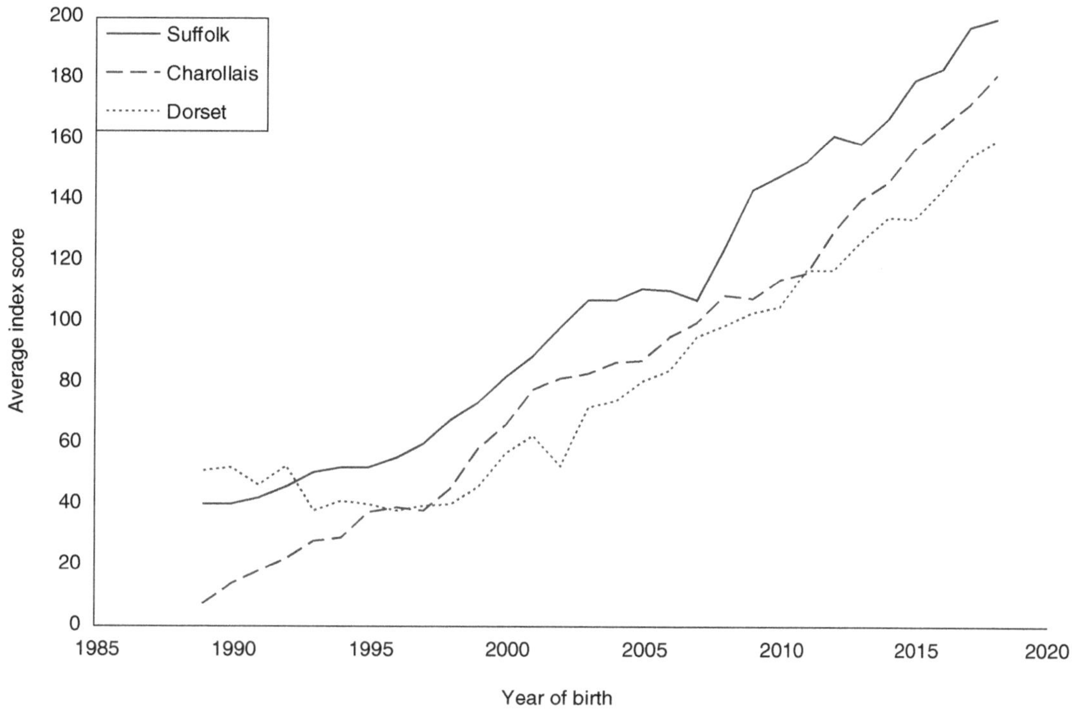

Fig. 10.26. Genetic trends in Terminal Sire index in the Suffolk, Charollais and Dorset breeds in Britain 1990 to 2018. (Source: AHDB/Signet Breeding Services, 2018.)

Wool production

Systems of testing

The improvement of wool traits in specialized wool breeds and dual-purpose breeds is also based on on-farm recording in most countries. The most important objectively measured traits are fleece weight and fibre diameter. Fibre diameter is measured at approved laboratories with sophisticated laser equipment to measure both the mean and coefficient of variation of fibre diameter. Other fleece characteristics such as staple strength, colour, resistance to compression and style (a visual appraisal of manufacturing properties) have usually been assessed subjectively in the past, but objective techniques are now available for most of them (Figs 10.28 and 10.29). These characteristics are all moderately or highly heritable but are of secondary economic importance to fleece weight and fibre diameter (Holman and Malau-Aduli, 2012).

The suitability of most of the important wool traits for objective measurement and selection means that these techniques have become used in most Merino industries. For example, performance recording schemes for wool traits were developed for Merino sheep in Australia in the 1950s with the introduction of fleece measurement services in NSW in the mid-1970s. Other fleece measurement services followed, and a national performance recording scheme was launched in 1987 to provide a framework for the use of objective fleece measurements and a means for calculating EBVs for important wool traits in a standard way. Similar developments have occurred in most of the major finewool-producing countries.

Co-operative breeding schemes are the main method for the genetic improvement of Merino sheep in Australia and elsewhere. Although group breeding schemes have been employed in Australia in the past, sire-referencing schemes were used more recently. Since the inception of the Sheep Cooperative Research Centre programme in Australia in 2001 there has been a

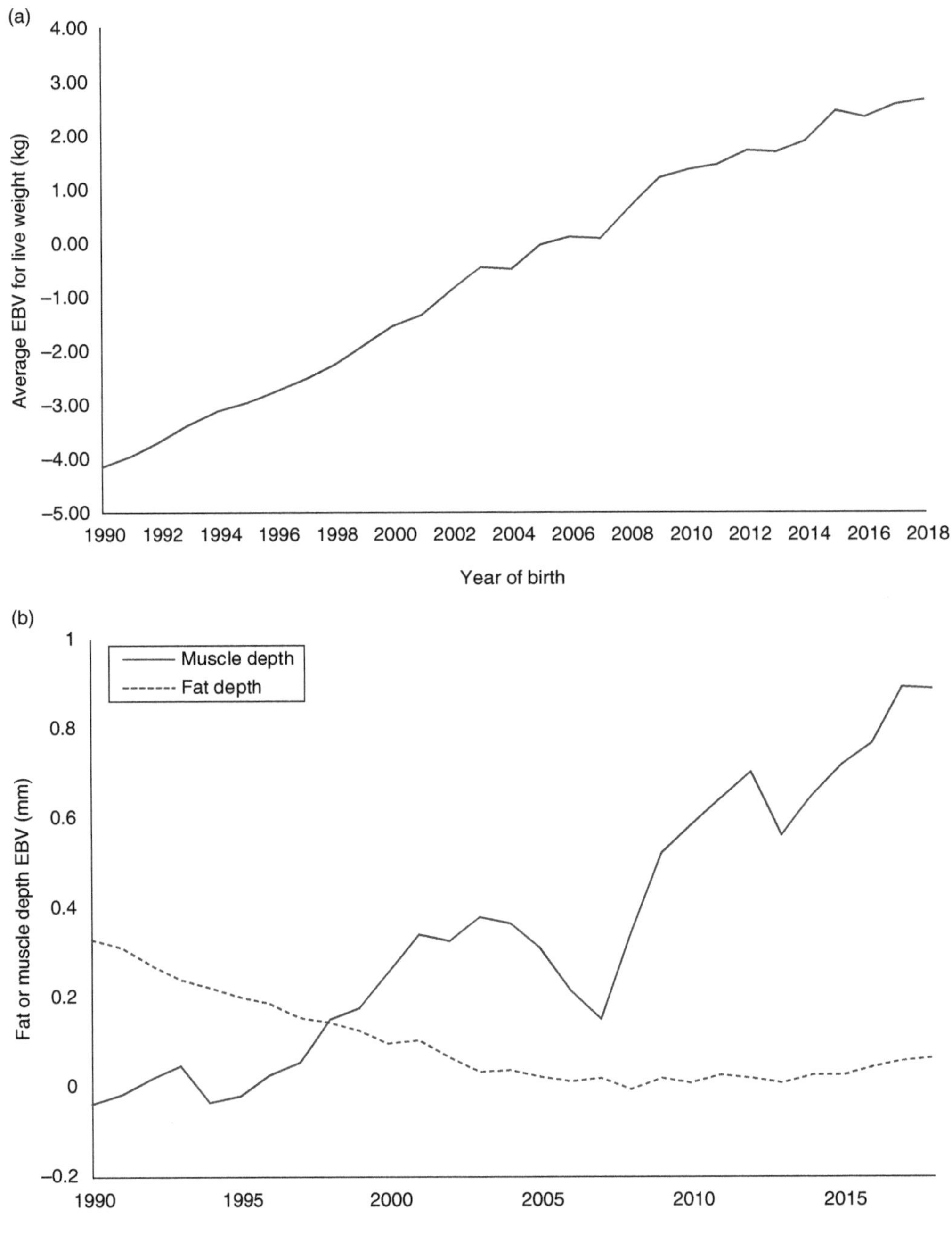

Fig. 10.27. Genetic trends in components of the lean growth index in the Suffolk breed in Britain 1990–2018. (a) Live weight at scanning (about 20 weeks of age), and (b) ultrasonically measured muscle and fat depths. (Source: AHDB/ Signet Breeding Services, 2018.)

move to rationalize wool recording and genetic evaluation schemes in Australian sheep from several more local schemes. This resulted in large across-flock BLUP evaluations for wool traits (Collison *et al.*, 2018).

Traits recorded

Tables 10.14 and 10.15 show the heritabilities of, and correlations among, some of the important characteristics in specialized wool breeds or dual-purpose

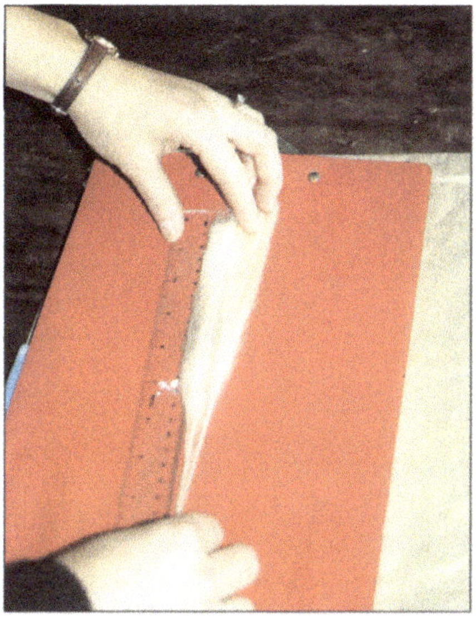

Fig. 10.28. Objective recording of staple length from sheep in the SAC/Roslin Institute Hill Sheep Breeding Project.

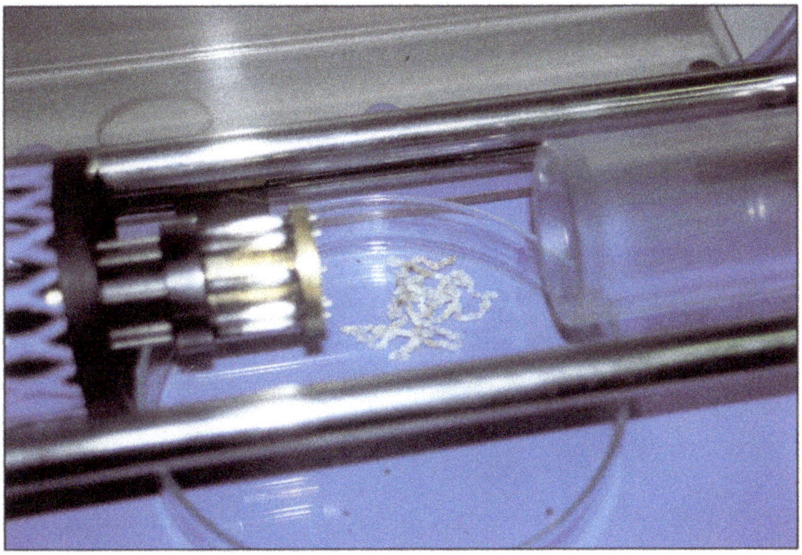

Fig. 10.29. 'Coring' of a fleece sample from a Merino, prior to automatic measurement of fibre diameter.

Table 10.14. Estimates of coefficients of variation and weighted mean heritabilities of wool traits in specialized wool breeds of sheep, from an extensive survey of published results. The number of estimates contributing to the weighted mean heritability, and the standard error of estimates, are shown in brackets. (Source: Safari *et al.*, 2005.)

Trait	Coefficient of variation (%)	Heritability (no., s.e.)
Greasy fleece weight	16.5	0.37 (20, 0.02)
Clean fleece weight	16.2	0.36 (30, 0.03)
Fibre diameter (FD)	7.4	0.59 (27, 0.02)
Coefficient of variation of FD	12.2	0.52 (14, 0.04)
Staple length	11.9	0.46 (15, 0.04)
Staple strength	29.2	0.34 (11, 0.03)
Crimp frequency	16.1	0.03 (11, 0.03)
Incidence of fleece rot	149	0.17 (1, 0.02)
Fleece rot severity	185	0.23 (1, 0.02)
Efficiency of wool growth	29.7	0.25 (3, 0.03)

breeds where wool is an important component. The heritabilities of both greasy and clean fleece weights are moderately high; that of fibre diameter is higher still. There is a positive (i.e. unfavourable) correlation between fleece weight and fibre diameter. Also, there are moderate positive genetic correlations between live weight and fleece weight and lower but mainly positive (i.e. unfavourable) genetic correlations between live weights and fibre diameter. There are generally fairly weak associations between reproductive performance and fleece weight, at both the phenotypic and genetic levels.

In addition to the traits listed in these tables, FEC is being used increasingly by Merino breeders as an indicator of resistance to intestinal parasites. It has been shown to be a good indicator of worm burdens, and to be heritable (heritability of about 0.25–0.3). Recently, much effort has gone into estimating associations with production traits, and exploring ways of including FEC in the overall breeding goal (Pollott and Greeff, 2004a; Fogarty *et al.*, 2006).

Methods of genetic evaluation

The Australian wool industry uses across-flock genetic evaluations to provide EBVs for Merino sheep and their crosses. Since 2005 EBVs for the main wool traits plus others such as breech wrinkle, dag scores, post-weaning age wool traits and reproductive traits have become routine. Flocks are linked by historic central testing sires and those from resource flocks, such as the Information Nucleus programme, resulting in >80% flocks being linked for the wool traits (Collison *et al.*, 2018).

Use of indexes of overall economic merit

Over the last few years, the use of multi-trait indexes in Merino breeding programmes has increased. These indexes are particularly useful in selecting for unfavourably correlated traits, like fleece weight and fibre diameter. Two major indexes are available to wool breeders in Australia: Fibre Production and Dual-purpose. The Fibre Production index concentrates on a balance between increasing wool production and decreasing fibre diameter. The Dual Purpose index includes meat production as well as the wool traits to give a balanced improvement in all traits (Collison *et al.*, 2018).

An additional aid in this area has been the development of computer software which allows the formulation of personalized breeding objectives (Collison *et al.*, 2018). This software allows breeders and their advisers to decide which traits to include in the overall objective. It also calculates relative economic values based on the size and composition of the flock concerned, the quantity and specifications of wool sold, the reproductive performance of the flock, and the age, weight and value of surplus sheep sold. Although there is flexibility in the way breeding objectives are formulated, the modifications have to fall within realistic ranges. Expected responses from selection on these flock-specific economic values can be compared with those expected from selection on a standard index.

Tailoring breeding objectives to an individual breeder's (or group's) requirements is rarely expected to give very different responses from those following selection on a single national index. However, having the software and advisory support to explore the options is usually very informative itself. If it results in greater understanding of the scope and limits of objective selection by breeders, and a greater uptake of these techniques, then usually this will compensate for the cost and complication of having different indexes in use.

Evidence of genetic improvement and its value

Although the estimates of genetic variation and heritabilities indicate the considerable scope for genetic improvement of wool traits, there are only a few examples so far of responses being measured in experimental or industry breeding schemes.

Table 10.15. Mean estimates of phenotypic and genetic correlations between live weights measured at different ages, wool and reproduction traits in sheep from an extensive review of published values. Note: some estimates are based on a small number of studies – see the original review for details. Number of estimates shown in brackets. (Source: Safari *et al*., 2005.)

		Mean correlation between traits	
Trait 1	Trait 2	Phenotypic	Genetic
Birth weight	Greasy fleece weight	0.24 (3)	0.21 (4)
	Clean fleece weight	0.24 (3)	0.11 (3)
	Fibre diameter	−0.05 (2)	0.18 (2)
	Staple length	–	0.05 (1)
Weaning weight	Greasy fleece weight	0.25 (10)	0.24 (12)
	Clean fleece weight	0.31 (7)	0.21 (7)
	Fibre diameter	0.05 (8)	0.05 (9)
	CV of FD[a]	0.05 (1)	0.02 (1)
	Staple length	0.01 (7)	0.17 (7)
	Staple strength	0.06 (2)	0.21 (2)
Post-weaning weight	Greasy fleece weight	0.44 (8)	0.35 (8)
	Clean fleece weight	0.39 (10)	0.24 (10)
	Fibre diameter	0.16 (11)	0.2 (11)
	CV of FD	−0.17 (4)	−0.17 (4)
	Staple length	0.20 (3)	0.16 (3)
	Staple strength	0.22 (1)	0.30 (1)
Adult weight	Greasy fleece weight	0.37 (11)	0.22 (12)
	Clean fleece weight	0.21 (11)	0.35 (11)
	Fibre diameter	0.13 (12)	0.15 (13)
	CV of FD	−0.06 (6)	−0.08 (6)
	Staple length	0.10 (4)	0.01 (4)
	Staple strength	0.04 (2)	−0.11 (2)
No. lambs weaned/ewe joined	Fleece weight	0.00 (4)	−0.12 (5)
	Fibre diameter	0.01 (2)	0.00 (2)
	Staple length	–	−0.20 (1)
No. lambs born/ewe joined	Fleece weight	−0.03 (3)	−0.13 (4)
	Fibre diameter	−0.03 (1)	−0.17 (1)
	Staple length	–	−0.05 (1)
Wt. lambs weaned/ewe joined	Fleece weight	0.01 (8)	0.16 (8)
	Fibre diameter	0.06 (5)	0.15 (5)
	Staple length	–	–
No. lambs weaned/ewe lambing	Fleece weight	–	−0.10 (5)
	Staple length	–	−0.45 (4)
Greasy fleece weight	Fibre diameter	0.31 (15)	0.36 (18)
	CV of FD	0.36 (5)	0.09 (6)
	Staple length	0.32 (5)	0.44 (11)
	Staple strength	0.19 (3)	0.16 (3)
Fibre diameter	CV of FD	−0.09 (10)	−0.10 (11)
	Staple length	0.19 (9)	0.19 (10)
	Staple strength	0.23 (6)	0.37 (6)
CV of FD	Staple length	−0.12 (7)	−0.06 (7)
	Staple strength	−0.38 (5)	−0.52 (5)
Staple length	Staple strength	0.07 (5)	0.05 (5)

[a]CV, Coefficient of variation; FD, fibre diameter.

Fogarty *et al.* (2006) quoted results from the Trangie QPLUS$ selection lines. The relative changes in fleece weight and fibre diameter depended on which of the indexes were used in the different lines. This trial demonstrated that different sets of relative weights could be applied to different sheep lines and each produced the desired response. This ranged from maintaining either fleece weight or fibre diameter and maximizing the change in the other trait or putting equal weight on both traits. Table 10.16 shows the changes in each trait for the different selection indexes. For example, by applying equal weight to both traits it was possible to achieve an increase in fleece weight of 19.6% and a decrease in fibre diameter of −1.62 microns, both desirable outcomes. Table 10.16 also shows that by trying to maintain either trait and change the other, greater gains were possible in the trait being changed but the implication was that the overall economic merit of the outcome was worse than when equal weight was put on both traits.

The value of genetic improvement in the Merino industry in Australia has been estimated to be AU$3500 million over 30 years, in present value (roughly £1750 million; Atkins, 1993). Improvements in the structure of the industry, and realistic levels of uptake of objective selection methods and new breeding technologies could add a further AU$1900 million, at present value, over the next 30 years.

Milk production

The major sheep milk-producing countries of the world lie within the Mediterranean basin, with France, Spain, Italy, Greece and Israel being the main and most innovative ones. Although the main focus of dairy breeding has been on the use of local breeds, there has been a clear division of approach between within-breed improvement programmes and the use of crossbreds or composites. Major European dairy breeds such as the Lacaune in France have used on-farm recording, AI and, more recently, genomic selection, to improve milk yields. On the other hand, countries such as Israel and Spain have favoured the use of crossbreds or composites. The Improved Awassi was developed in Israel from local sheep flocks, and averages over 500 l/lactation, making it the most productive dairy sheep breed in the world. The Assaf – a cross between the Awassi and the East Friesian – was developed in Israel in the 1950s and 1960s.

In purebred selection, rams are selected for further use, or culled, on the basis of their daughters' milk production, milk quality, and associated traits. Milk recording of dairy cattle usually takes place at monthly intervals, and both morning and afternoon milkings are usually recorded on test days. However, the costs of this level of recording are prohibitive for most dairy sheep enterprises and only a relatively small proportion of sheep in the specialized dairy breeds in Europe are recorded. Simplified recording systems for sheep have been approved by ICAR (the International Committee on Animal Recording). These involve recording only a single milking on each test day. The first method involves recording morning and afternoon milkings in alternate months. The second method involves recording at the same time each month, but adjusting records for the difference between morning and afternoon milkings, based on total bulk tank readings. In addition, many dairy sheep systems commence milking after a suckling

Table 10.16. Selection differentials achieved for clean fleece weight and mean fibre diameter by selecting the top 5% of ewes on each trait and three indexes of both traits in the Trangie QPLUS$ lines. (After Taylor, 2006.)

			Realized selection differentials	
Selection criteria	Mean of 600 ewes	Mean of top 5%	Clean fleece weight (%)	Mean fibre diameter (μm)
Clean fleece weight (FW; kg)	4.4	5.6	+27.3	+0.22
Mean fibre diameter (FD; μm)	20.5	17.6	−4.6	−2.89
	Selection objective			
3% index	Maintain FD; increase FW		+25.8	−0.38
8% index	Equal emphasis		+19.6	−1.62
15% index	Maintain FW; decrease FD		+3.3	−2.71

period of variable length. This means that most dairy sheep lactations are recorded during the declining phase of the lactation only, the main exception being in Israel where lambs are weaned at birth and the complete lactation is recorded.

The problem of low levels of recording has been tackled, in France in particular, by attempting to segment the population clearly into nucleus and commercial tiers. Milk recording is then concentrated in the nucleus tier, which comprises 10–20% of the total population (Barillet *et al.*, 2016). Genetic improvement is disseminated to the commercial tier via the sale of rams from nucleus flocks, or via AI from nucleus rams. Most recording systems have focused on milk yield, but fat and protein concentrations are also widely recorded, and other traits such as functional type traits and resistance to mastitis are recorded in France and Spain. Estimates of the heritabilities of the milk production traits and the genetic correlations among them are shown in Table 10.17. These agree very closely with the equivalent estimates for dairy cattle shown in Chapter 8.

As for milk recording, methods of evaluation of dairy sheep have generally followed those used in dairy cattle. Animal model repeatability BLUP evaluations are used for dairy sheep in the major dairying countries. Genomic breeding values have been introduced in France. Genetic trends in milk yield of 2.0% and 2.4% of the mean per annum have been reported for the Manech and Lacaune breeds, respectively, with somewhat lower levels in the Churra breed in Spain (Carta *et al.*, 2009).

Use of genomics in sheep and goat breeding

Genomic studies in sheep and goats became possible with the development of the Ovine 50K single nucleotide polymorphism (SNP) Chip in 2009 and the Illumina Goat 50K SNP Chip in 2014. This was followed by the Ovine 600K SNP Chip more recently, and a low-density panel with 16,301 SNPs for sheep has been developed by the International Sheep Genomics Consortium in 2017. Genomic predictions and selection (see Chapters 6 and 7) have been successfully implemented for production traits such as sheep wool traits, growth traits, muscle and fat depth in New Zealand (Auvray *et al.*, 2014) and Australia (Daetwyler *et al.*, 2010), and for several traits in dairy sheep and goats in France (Carillier *et al.*, 2014) and dairy goats in the UK (Mucha *et al.*, 2015).

The Australian Information Nucleus and Sheep Genetics Resource Flock programmes incorporated data on SNP markers into their programme. This information is combined with ram genotyping in some ram breeding flocks to produce GEBVs for carcass, adult wool and reproduction traits (Brown *et al.*, 2018). In dairy cattle breeding one of the main objectives of genomic selection methods is to predict an animal's genetic merit at, or soon after, birth, to reduce the long generation intervals involved in traditional progeny testing, this is less relevant in meat and wool breeds of sheep. Often lambs have a good estimate in early life of their genetic merit for growth and wool traits. Hence, the main aim of using genomic selection in sheep is to increase the accuracy of GEBVs and to produce GEBVs for 'hard-to-measure' traits (e.g. carcass traits or traits measured in adult animals). Studies on the Australian data suggest that increases in accuracy of between 0–18% are possible, depending on the initial accuracy of EBVs produced from pedigree information only. Interestingly, in a study of possible designs for the French sheep meat industry, Raoul *et al.* (2018) found annual genetic gains of ~18% for several genomic selection designs.

One key limiting factor in the application of genomic selection methods is the size of the reference population used to predict the genotypes of the non-reference animals. This needs to be large enough to increase accuracies significantly. Also, experience in Australia has shown that using single-step GBLUP (see Chapter 7) with multiple traits across breeds

Table 10.17. Estimates of the heritabilities of milk production traits in sheep (on the diagonal, in bold) and the genetic correlations among them. Average of results from 9 reports from Europe. (Source: Carta *et al.*, 2009.)

Traits	Milk yield	Fat yield	Protein yield	Fat %	Protein %
Milk yield	**0.20 to 0.32**				
Fat yield	0.77 to 0.89	**0.16 to 0.26**			
Protein yield	0.88 to 0.94	0.82 to 0.93	**0.18 to 0.27**		
Fat %	−0.43 to −0.56	0.02 to 0.25	−0.18 to −0.28	**0.10 to 0.61**	
Protein %	−0.46 to 0.64	−0.36 to −0.12	−0.01 to −0.15	0.41 to 0.85	**0.31 to 0.69**

requires computing strategies which can optimize the large volume of information available. This becomes even more critical when composites are included in the analysis since SNPs may not be associated with the same levels of performance in animals with differing genetic backgrounds. The characteristics of the current genomic prediction systems for sheep and goats include small reference population sizes ranging from 1900 to 8000, consisting of mostly crossbreeds or multi-breed populations (Rupp *et al.*, 2016). The increase in accuracy provided by molecular information (from 5% to 27%) is somewhat lower than in other species as a result of the smaller reference populations (Mrode *et al.*, 2018).

Two studies report the application of genomic selection to dairy sheep populations. Baloche *et al.* (2014) found that genomic selection in the Lacaune breed using single-step GBLUP could increase accuracies by 20% but considered that the cost of genotyping was more critical in sheep compared to dairy cattle schemes. This was mainly due to the relative value of a single animal from the two species. Usai *et al.* (2018) working on Sarda sheep in Italy also found increases in accuracy from using genomic selection methods. In this case the improvement in accuracy over pedigree-based breeding values was 31%. Currently, it appears that improved accuracies are the main outcome of applying genomic selection in sheep, with cost-effectiveness varying, depending on the value of the additional realized gains and the additional costs incurred.

Genotype × Environment Interactions

There has been as much heated debate, if not more, about genotype × environment interactions in sheep breeding as there has in other species. The golden rule mentioned earlier still applies – if there is a big enough difference between genotypes, or environments, or both, then it is likely that interactions will be found. A good example of this is the fact that most specialized meat breeds selected under intensive management simply would not survive in British mountains or the Australian rangelands. However, within breeds the answers are less clear. The issue of testing meat breeds in Britain under intensive feeding, when their progeny are expected to perform in an extensive environment, was mentioned earlier. Several studies have investigated the extent of within-breed G × E effects and generally they have been found to be real but of a low size. At the time of writing, no country appears to have implemented adjustment of EBVs for different environments.

Interactions may be more important within hill breeds, especially where live weight and fat levels are being measured. A study in Scottish Blackface sheep has shown a low genetic correlation between live weights measured in intensive and extensive feeding systems, and only a moderate genetic correlation between fat depths measured in these two environments (Bishop *et al.*, 1996). Also, the heritability of ultrasonic fat depth measured on improved pastures was about double that measured on unimproved hill land (Conington *et al.*, 1995). These results mean that the optimum environment for selection of hill sheep may vary, depending on the importance of altering weight and reducing or controlling fat in the breeding goal.

In specialized wool breeds, there are few reports of interactions affecting individual production traits, although they are sometimes reported for overall economic merit and secondary traits such as fleece rot and some measures of wool quality (Woolaston, 1987; Atkins and Casey, 1994). In a study of Merino wool traits, Pollott and Greeff (2004b) found evidence of a G × E effect in fleece weight and FEC of about 3% but they concluded that it was of no practical value. Clearly, some rams did show greater changes in these traits across environments. Comparing Merino performance from common sires in Australia and New Zealand, McMillan *et al.* (2018) found that only yearling clean fleece weight showed a real difference in ranking between countries and concluded that testing could take place in either country without a major effect on EBVs.

The overall message as far as interactions are concerned is: (i) to be aware that they can exist; (ii) to take action if there is sound evidence that they exist in the traits of interest in the breed or system that concerns you (e.g. by restricting the choice of sires to those measured in similar conditions, or those evaluated in a wide range of conditions); and (iii) not to let the possibility of interactions in some cases detract from the value of genetic improvement in most cases.

Practical Guidelines on Selection

Some practical guidelines on selection to improve performance in objectively measured traits in sheep and goats are given below. Most of these are equally relevant in purebred and commercial flocks or herds, and whether the selection is for meat, milk or wool/fibre traits. However, pedigree breeders using these methods often wish to pay more attention to individual trait EBVs than commercial producers. Also, they may be willing to take greater risks by selecting animals with low accuracy EBVs, or by selecting occasional unrecorded animals if levels of recording are low in the breed concerned. The guidelines on selection between breeds or crosses are aimed primarily at commercial producers, since most pedigree breeders will already be firmly committed to their current breed.

Selection between breeds or crosses

- Clearly define the rôle of the animals you are selecting and identify the animal characteristics that are economically important. Choose an appropriate breed, breed type or cross, based on the sort of objective comparisons of performance discussed earlier.

Selection of rams, bucks or semen for use in a purebred flock or herd

- Set your breeding objective – the priority should be on traits expected to be of most economic importance in a few (sheep or goat) generations time.
- Identify the selection index or set of (G)EBVs which is most relevant for your breeding objective.
- Produce a shortlist of animals which can be fairly compared, ranked on this index or on EBVs for the most important individual traits.
- Where national across-flock/herd BLUP evaluations are available, this shortlist might be compiled from a national sire summary, or from EBVs presented at ram or buck sales or in semen catalogues. Include homebred rams or bucks on the shortlist if their index scores or EBVs warrant it and they are directly comparable.
- If across-flock/herd evaluations are only available for co-operative breeding schemes, then rank the animals available from the scheme making the best genetic progress in traits relevant to your breeding goal. (Often access to high merit animals, and hence rate of genetic gain in purebred flocks/herds, will be improved by joining an effective co-operative scheme.)
- If there are no across-flock/herd evaluations in the breed of your choice, select rams/bucks from one or more flocks/herds which have a history of using objective selection for the index or set of EBVs most relevant to your breeding goal. (Try to compare the performance of purchased and homebred rams/bucks, or new and existing purchased rams/bucks, by mating them to groups of ewes/does balanced for genetic merit. If the purchased males are inferior to homebred males, change sources, or stick to homebred males.)
- If there are economically important traits in your breeding goal that are not included in the index available, or for which no EBVs are available, then eliminate any animals which do not meet your minimum standards. Culling for these secondary traits should be in proportion to the economic importance of the trait, and the scope for genetic change in them. Selection for traits of minor economic importance, or traits which have a small genetic component will dilute overall progress.
- Eliminate any animals that are not functionally sound, for example, those which have unacceptable locomotion, testicle size or jaw structure. Culling should be confined to important characteristics which have a genetic component.
- If accuracies are available for the index or EBVs of your choice, and you are concerned about the risk of using low accuracy males, eliminate those with very low values, or spread the risk by using more of them. (As explained in Chapter 7, BLUP EBVs already account for accuracy, and so *on average* progress in a flock, herd or breed is maximized by selecting on EBVs regardless of accuracy. However, breeders are often concerned because large sums of money are at stake on *individual* animals. In these situations, the accuracy provides a useful measure of the risk that an EBV will change in future. Choosing high EBV males with high accuracies is a less risky strategy than choosing high EBV males with low accuracy, but if there are few high EBV, high accuracy males available, choosing several animals is less risky than gambling on only one.)
- Within reason, choose the highest index males left on the list that you can afford.
- Avoid making matings between close relatives in purebred flocks or herds. (Computer programs may be available via the recording agency or breed society, to assist with this task.)
- Genetic gain will be maximized by replacing rams or bucks whenever males of higher merit are available within this flock/herd, or elsewhere. If there are no national evaluations to allow you to compare the merit of your own males with others, calculate the male generation intervals which will maximize progress in your breeding goal (as explained in Chapter 4) and aim to replace rams/bucks accordingly.

Selection of replacement females in a purebred flock or herd

- Progress will be maximized by selecting replacement females on the most relevant index or set of EBVs. Choose this index or set of EBVs as described above for rams/bucks.
- Unless the flock/herd is of low genetic merit, it will usually be most cost effective to select among homebred females only, rather than buying in replacement females.
- If BLUP EBVs are available, then the genetic merit of females of all ages within the flock/herd can be compared directly. Rank the potential female replacements on the chosen index, or on the individual BLUP EBVs of most relevance. Genetic gain will be maximized by replacing ewes of any age which have low EBVs by replacements which have higher EBVs. (In a closed flock/herd which has been selecting for a few years, selection of replacement females and culling on BLUP EBVs is unlikely to dramatically alter the age structure of the flock/herd. However, when selection on BLUP EBVs first starts, some attention may need to be paid to the short-term economic effects of dramatic changes in age structure. For example, if it turns out that most older females have very low EBVs, although it would be genetically preferable, it may not be economically justifiable to cull all of these in one year because of the effect this may have on flock/herd output.)
- If BLUP EBVs are not available, then it is difficult to compare the genetic merit of females of different ages. The simplest policy is to calculate the optimum female generation interval to maximize genetic progress in your breeding goal (as explained in Chapter 4), and then cull ewes/does on age to achieve this.
- Apply similar rules on culling for functional fitness, or traits of secondary economic importance, to those described above for rams/bucks.

Selection of replacement males and females for commercial flocks or herds

- Selection of rams for a commercial flock, and bucks for a commercial herd, should follow the same guidelines as those for purebred flocks or herds, except that the choice of index or EBVs should focus on expected market returns over the working life of the ram or buck (pedigree flocks or herds should have longer timescales than this).
- Rams or bucks purchased to breed replacement females in self-replacing flocks or herds should be selected on an index or set of EBVs for traits of importance in their daughters, e.g. litter size, lamb weaning weight, mature size, milk production.
- Crossbred replacement females are unlikely to have EBVs. However, whenever possible, buy replacement females from breeders who use objective information, relevant to your breeding goal, in their own breeding programme.

Summary

- Sheep are kept primarily for the production of meat, wool and milk in temperate countries, and milk and meat in tropical areas. In some countries or systems only one of these products is important, but in others there are multi-purpose production systems, and hence multi-purpose breeding goals.
- Goats are important producers of meat and milk in Asia, Africa and parts of Europe, and important fibre producers in a few countries. Breeding schemes for goats in most countries are less well developed than for sheep, but where they exist, they generally mirror sheep schemes. Both sheep and goat dairy breeding schemes tend to be simplified versions of schemes developed for dairy cattle.
- Reproductive performance, growth and carcass composition are the most important components of the breeding goal for meat production. Fleece weight and fibre diameter are the most important components of the breeding goal for specialized wool production. Reproductive performance, milk yield and milk composition are the most important breeding goal traits for sheep and goat milk production. However, other traits influencing inputs, like feed consumption, disease resistance and longevity, are also important in most cases.
- Specialized sheep meat breeds, such as the Suffolk, Texel, Charollais and Dorset Down are widely used as terminal sires in crossing systems (e.g. in the UK, New Zealand, Australia where they are usually mated to longwool × hill ewes, purebred dual-purpose ewes or composites and longwool ×

Merino ewes, respectively). In other countries (e.g. France and several other European countries) meat production is based on pure breeds.

- Specialized wool production worldwide is dominated by the Merino breed, or breeds or crosses derived from it.
- Sheep milk production is usually based on specialized regional breeds, such as the Lacaune (France), Sarda (Italy), Churra (Spain), and Karagouniki (Greece). Crossbreds or composites are important in some countries (Spain, Israel). In Northern Europe the Friesian breed, or derivatives of it, are often used.
- The majority of improvement programmes in meat-producing sheep breeds are based on on-farm recording of performance. Co-operative breeding schemes are important in several countries and have been replaced by whole-breed evaluations in other countries. Community breeding programmes have recently become the most successful method for genetic improvement of sheep and goats in sub-Saharan Africa.
- The traits recorded in meat sheep breeding programmes usually include litter size, number of lambs reared and weights of lambs at various ages. Also, ultrasonic measurements of fat and muscle depth or area are becoming quite widely recorded.
- Generally, growth and carcass traits are moderately variable and moderately highly heritable. In contrast, most reproductive traits are more variable but have low heritabilities.
- BLUP methods are the method of choice for genetic evaluations. The relatively low use of AI in sheep in most countries means that genetic links between flocks are weaker than those in dairy and beef herds. The use of sire-referencing schemes and of AI has increased the use of across-flock evaluations in some countries. Genomic breeding values are being introduced in some industries where an increase in breeding value accuracy is expected or where there are some 'difficult-to-measure' traits.
- Selection indexes have become widely used in meat and dual-purpose sheep breeds over the last few decades. These usually combine growth and ultrasonic measurements in terminal sire breeds, and often include reproduction or wool traits, or both, in dual-purpose breeds.
- There is evidence of substantial rates of genetic change in growth and carcass traits, in both experimental sheep flocks and industry schemes, in several countries. The national value of genetic improvement schemes has been estimated in several countries, and this is usually high in relation to their cost.
- The improvement of wool traits in specialized wool breeds and dual-purpose breeds is also based on on-farm recording in most countries. Co-operative breeding schemes are also important in some countries.
- The most important objectively measured traits are fleece weight and fibre diameter, but others include staple strength, colour, resistance to compression and style.
- The main fleece characteristics are all moderately or highly heritable, but there is a positive (i.e. unfavourable) correlation between fleece weight and fibre diameter.
- BLUP evaluations are widely used in Merino breeding programmes, but their uptake in some cases is limited by the lack of pedigree information in stud flocks. The increasing use of AI has improved the use of across-flock BLUP evaluations.
- Multi-trait indexes are used in Merino breeding programmes. Uptake is being stimulated in some cases by the availability of advice and software to help farmers formulate personalized breeding objectives.
- The value of genetic improvement in the fine-wool industry in Australia has been estimated to be very high indeed.
- Improvement programmes for dairy sheep usually involve the evaluation of rams in milk-recorded flocks through the use of AI and whole-scheme genetic evaluations.
- Recording systems are similar to those used in dairy cattle. These concentrated on the yield in the past, but in several countries these now include milk quality, somatic cell count and functional type traits.
- The heritabilities of milk production traits are moderately high. Genetic correlations among yield traits are also high, but there are negative correlations between some yield traits and concentration of fat and protein, as in dairy cattle.
- Animal model BLUP evaluations are used for dairy sheep in several countries, and. substantial genetic trends in milk yield have been reported. Genomic breeding values have been introduced in a few countries for sheep and goats.
- Genotype × environment interactions appear to be important in some sectors, but there are well-established guidelines to minimize their impact.

References

AHDB (2016) *Stocktake report 2016*. AHDB, Stoneleigh, UK.

AHDB (2018a) *Sheep yearbook 2018*. AHDB, Stoneleigh, UK.

AHDB (2018b) Breeding Indexes. Available at: https://www.signetdata.com/technical/sheep-genetic-notes/breeding-indexes/ (accessed 28 September 2020).

AHDB/Signet Breeding Services (2018) Terminal sheep Breeds Make Strong Genetic Gains. Available at: hhttps://signetdata.com/news/posts/2016/december/terminal-sheep-breeds-make-strong-genetic-gains/ (accessed 28 September 2020).

Amer, P.R., Nieuwhof, G.J., Pollott, G.E., Roughsedge, T., Conington, J. and Simm, G. (2007) Industry benefits from recent genetic progress in sheep and beef populations. *Animal* 1, 1414–1426. DOI: 10.1017/S175173110700078X.

Arnal, M., Robert-Granié, C. and Larroque, H. (2018) Diversity of dairy goat lactation curves in France. *Journal of Dairy Science* 101, 11040–11051. DOI: 10.3168/jds.2018-14980.

Atkins, K.D. (1993) Benefits of genetic improvement to the Merino wool industry. *Wool Technology and Sheep Breeding* 41, 257–268.

Atkins, K.D. and Casey, A.E. (1994) Recent developments in wool sheep breeding. *Proceedings of the 5th World Congress on Genetics Applied to Livestock Production* 18, pp. 23–30. Available at: http://www.wcgalp.org/proceedings/1994 (accessed 16 June 2020).

Atkins, K.D., Martin, S.J., Casey, A.E., Graham, R.P., Semple, S.J. *et al.* (2005) *Merino Bloodlines: The Comparisons 1994–2004*. NSW DPI PRIMEFACT 75, NSW, Australia.

Australian Wool Exchange (2018) AWEX Wool Market Indicators. Available at: http://www.awex.com.au/market-information/awex-wool-market-indicators/ (accessed 18 November 2018).

Auvray, B., McEwan, J., Newman, S.A., Lee, M. and Dodds, K. (2014) Genomic prediction of breeding values in the New Zealand sheep industry using a 50K SNP chip. *Journal of Animal Science* 92, 4375–4389. DOI: 10.2527/jas.2014-7801.

Baloche, G., Legarra, A., Sallé, G., Larroque, H., Astruc, J-M. *et al.* (2014) Assessment of accuracy of genomic prediction for French Lacaune dairy sheep. *Journal of Dairy Science* 97, 1107–1116. DOI: 10.3168/jds.2013-7135.

Barillet, F., Lagriffoul, G., Marnet, P.-G., Larroque, H., Rupp, R. *et al.* (2016) Breeding objectives and reasoned strategy of implementation at the population level for French dairy sheep breeds. *INRA Productions Animales* 29, 19–40.

Bishop, S.C. (2015) Genetic resistance to infections in sheep. *Veterinary Microbiology* 181, 2–7. DOI: 10.1016/j.vetmic.2015.07.013.

Bishop, S.C., Conington, J., Waterhouse, A. and Simm, G. (1996) Genotype × environment interactions for early growth and ultrasonic measurements in hill sheep. *Animal Science* 62, 271–277. DOI: 10.1017/S1357729800014570.

Brito, L.F., Clarke, S.M., McEwan, J.C., Miller, S.P., Pickering, N.K. *et al.* (2017) Prediction of genomic breeding values for growth, carcass and meat quality traits in a multi-breed sheep population using a HD SNP chip. *BMC Genetics* 18, 7. DOI: 10.1186/s12863-017-0476-8.

Brown, D., Swan, A., Boerner, V., Li, L., Gurman, P. *et al.* (2018) Single step genetic evaluations in the Australian sheep industry. *Proceedings of the World Congress on Genetics Applied to Livestock Production* 11, 460. Available at: http://www.wcgalp.org/proceedings/2018 (accessed 16 June 2020).

Carillier, C., Larroque, H. and Robert-Granié, C. (2014) Comparison of joint versus purebred genomic evaluation in the French multi-breed dairy goat population. *Genetics Selection Evolution* 46, 67. DOI: 10.1186/s12711-014-0067-3.

Carta, A., Casu, S., and Salaris, S. (2009) Invited review: Current state of genetic improvement in dairy sheep. *Journal of Dairy Science* 92, 5814–5833. DOI: 10.3168/jds.2009-2479.

Collison, C., Brown, D., Gill, S., Chandler, H., Apps, R. *et al.* (2018) A decade of sheep genetics: what have we achieved? *Proceedings of the World Congress on Genetics Applied to Livestock Production* 11, 661. Available at: http://www.wcgalp.org/proceedings/2018 (accessed 16 June 2020).

Conington, J., Bishop, S.C., Waterhouse, A.W. and Simm, G. (1995) A genetic analysis of early growth and ultrasonic measurements in hill sheep. *Animal Science* 61, 85–93. DOI: 10.1017/S1357729800013552.

Corner-Thomas, R.A., Kenyon, P.R., Morris, S.T., Greer, A.W., Logan C.M. *et al.* (2013) A survey examining the New Zealand breed composition, management tool use and research needs of commercial sheep farmers and ram breeders. *Proceedings of the Association for the Advancement of Animal Breeding and Genetics* 20, 18–21.

Daetwyler, H.D., Hickey, J.M., Henshall, J.M., Dominik, S., Gredler, B. *et al.* (2010) Accuracy of estimated genomic breeding values for wool and meat traits in a multi-breed sheep population. *Animal Production Science* 50, 1004–1010. DOI: 10.1071/AN10096.

de Rancourt, M. and Carrère, L. (2011) Milk sheep production systems in Europe: Diversity and main trends. In: Bernués A., Boutonnet J.P., Casasús I., Chentouf M., Gabiña D. *et al.* (eds) *Economic, Social and Environmental Sustainability in Sheep and Goat Production Systems*. Zaragoza: CIHEAM/FAO/CITA-

DGA. Options Méditerranéennes: Série A. Séminaires Méditerranéens 100, 107–111.

Desire, S., Mucha, S., Coffey, M., Mrode, R., Broadbent, J. and Conington, J. (2018) Pseudopregnancy and aseasonal breeding in dairy goats – genetic basis of fertility and impact on lifetime productivity. *Animal* 12, 1799–1806. DOI: 10.1017/S1751731117003056.

EBLEX (2014) *The Breeding Structure of the British Sheep Industry 2012*. AHDB, Stoneleigh, UK.

FAO (2015) *The Second Report on the State of the World's Animal Genetic Resources for Food and Agriculture*, Scherf, B.D. and Pilling, D. (eds) FAO Commission on Genetic Resources for Food and Agriculture Assessments, Rome. Available at http://www.fao.org/3/a-i4787e/index.html (accessed 22 June 2020).

FAO (2018) FAOSTAT. Available at: http://www.fao.org/faostat/en/#data/QL/visualize (accessed 5 May 2018).

Fennessy, P., Byrne, T., Amer, P. and Martin, G. (2014) *Evaluating the Impact of Animal Genetics and Genomics RD&E Investment*. MLA, Sydney, Australia.

Fogarty, N.M., Safari, E., Gilmour, A.R., Ingham, V.M., Atkins, K.D. *et al*. (2006) Wool and meat genetics—the joint possibilities. *International Journal of Sheep and Wool Science* 54, No. 1. Available at: http://sheepjournal.net/index.php/ijsws/issue/view/66 (accessed 8 September 2020).

Fogarty, N.M., Banks, R.G., van der Werf, J.H.J., Ball, A.J. and Gibson, J.P. (2007) The information nucleus – a new concept to enhance sheep industry genetic improvement. *Proceedings of the Association for the Advancement of Animal Breeding and Genetics* 17, 29–32.

Guy, D.R., Croston, D. and Jones, D.W. (1986) Response to selection in Welsh Mountain sheep. *Animal Production* 42, 442.

Haile, A., Gizaw, S., Getachew, S., Joaquín, T., Mueller, P. *et al*. (2019) Community-based breeding programmes are a viable solution for Ethiopian small ruminant genetic improvement but require public and private investments. *Journal of Animal Breeding and Genetics* 136, 1–10. DOI: 10.1111/jbg.12401.

Holman, B.W.B. and Malau-Aduli, A.E.O. (2012) A review of sheep wool quality traits. *Annual Review and Research in Biology* 2, 1–14. Available http://sciencedomain.org/abstract/375 (accessed 8 September 2020).

James, J.W. (1977) Open nucleus breeding schemes. *Animal Production* 24, 287–305. DOI: 10.1017/S0003356100011818.

Jonker, A., Hickey, S.M., Rowe, S.J., Janssen, P.H., Shackell, G.H. *et al*. (2018) Genetic parameters of methane emissions determined using portable accumulation chambers in lambs and ewes grazing pasture and genetic correlations with emissions determined in respiration chambers. *Journal of Animal Science* 96, 3031–3042. DOI: 10.1093/jas/sky187.

Kempster, A.J., Cook, G.L. and Grantley-Smith, M. (1986) National estimates of the body composition of British cattle, sheep and pigs with special reference to trends in fatness. A review. *Meat Science* 17, 107–138. DOI: 10.1016/0309-1740(86)90059-8.

Lee, M.A., Cullen, N.G., Newman, S.A.N., Dodds, K.G., McEwan, J.C. and Shackell, G.H. (2015) Genetic analysis and genomic selection of stayability and productive life in New Zealand ewes. *Journal of Animal Science* 93, 3268–3277. DOI: 10.2527/jas.2014-8259.

Lewis, R.M., Simm, G., Dingwall, W.S. and Murphy, S.V. (1996) Selection for lean growth in terminal sire sheep to produce leaner crossbred progeny. *Animal Science* 63, 133–142. DOI: 10.1017/S1357729800028368.

Macfarlane, J.M. and Simm, G. (2008) Genetic improvement programme for meat type sheep: an experience from the United Kingdom. Paper presented at *3rd International Symposium about Goat and Sheep Meat Type*, in João Pessoa, Paraiba, Brazil, November 2007.

Macfarlane, J.M., Matheson, S.M. and Dwyer, C.M. (2010) Genetic parameters for birth difficulty, lamb vigour and lamb suckling ability in Suffolk sheep. *Animal Welfare,* 19(S), 99–105. Available at: https://www.ingentaconnect.com/contentone/ufaw/aw/2010/00000019/a00102s1/art00013 (accessed 28 September 2020).

Maniatis, N. and Pollott, G.E. (2002) Nuclear, cytoplasmic and environmental effects on growth, fat and muscle traits in Suffolk lambs from a sire referencing scheme. *Journal of Animal Science* 80, 57–67. DOI: 10.2527/2002.80157x.

Marquez, G.C., Haresign, W., Davies, M.H., Roehe, R., Bunger, L. *et al*. (2013) Index selection in terminal sires improves lamb performance at finishing. *Journal of Animal Science* 91, 38–43. DOI: 10.2527/jas.2012-5383.

Massender, E., Brito, L.F., Cánovas, A., Baes, C.F., Kennedy, D. and Schenkel, F.S. (2019) A genetic evaluation of growth, ultrasound, and carcass traits at alternative slaughter endpoints in crossbred heavy lambs. *Journal of Animal Science* 97, 521–535. DOI: 10.1093/jas/sky455.

McLaren, A., Kaseja, K., Yates, J., Mucha, S., Lambe, N.R. and Conington, J. (2018) New mastitis phenotypes suitable for genomic selection in meat sheep and their genetic relationships with udder conformation and lamb live weights. *Animal* 12, 2470–2479. DOI: 10.1017/S1751731118000393.

McMaster, J.C. (1995) Breeding for fibres. *Proceedings of the World Sheep and Wool Congress*. Royal

Agricultural Society of England, Kenilworth, UK, Three Counties Agricultural Society, Malvern, UK, National Sheep Association, Malvern, UK.

McMillan, A.J., Ferguson, M.B. and Brown, D.J. (2018) Genotype by environment interaction for Merino sheep in New Zealand and Australia for a range of traits. *Proceedings of the World Congress on Genetics Applied to Livestock Production* 11, 267. Available at: http://www.wcgalp.org/proceedings/2018 (accessed 16 June 2020).

Meat and Livestock Commission (1986) *Sheep Yearbook 1986*. Meat and Livestock Commission, Bletchley, UK.

Milán, M.J., Frendi, F., Gonzalez-Gonzalez, R. and Caja, G. (2014) Cost structure and profitability of Assaf dairy sheep farms in Spain. *Journal of Dairy Science* 97, 5239–5249. DOI: 10.3168/jds.2013-7884.

MLA (2017) *MLA and AWI Wool and Sheepmeat Survey Report – Sheepmeat.* MLA, North Sydney, Australia.

Montossi, F., Font-i-Furnols, M., del Campo, M., San Julián, R., Brito, G. and Sañudo, C. (2013) Sustainable sheep production and consumer preference trends: Compatibilities, contradictions, and unresolved dilemmas. *Meat Science* 95, 772–789. DOI: 10.1016/j.meatsci.2013.04.048.

Mortimer, S.I., van der Werf, J.H.J., Jacob, R.H., Hopkins, D.L., Pannier, L. *et al.* (2014) Genetic parameters for meat quality traits of Australian lamb meat. *Meat Science* 96, 1016–1024. DOI: 10.1016/j.meatsci.2013.09.007.

Mrode, R., Tarekegn, G.M., Mwacharo, J.M. and Djikeng, A. (2018) Invited review: Genomic selection for small ruminants in developed countries: how applicable for the rest of the world? *Animal* 18, 1–9. DOI: 10.1017/S1751731117003688.

Mucha, S., Mrode, R., MacLaren-Lee, I., Coffey, M., and Conington, J. (2015) Estimation of genomic breeding values for milk yield in UK dairy goats. *Journal of Dairy Science* 98, 8201–8208. DOI: 10.3168/jds.2015-9682.

NSP (2006) *National Scrapie Plan for Great Britain*. SVS, Worcester, UK.

O'Brien, A.C., McHugh, N., Wall, E., Pabiou, T., McDermott, K. *et al.* (2017) Genetic parameters for lameness, mastitis and dagginess in a multi-breed sheep population. *Animal* 11, 911–919. DOI: https://doi.org/10.1017/S1751731116002445.

Ortiz-Pelaez, A., Thompson, C.E and Dawson, M. (2014) The impact of the National Scrapie Plan on the PRNP genotype distribution of the British national flock, 2002–2012. *Veterinary Record* 174, 530. DOI: 10.1136/vr.102255.

Parker, A.G. (1993) Application of performance recording in sheep - industry structure. In: Blair, H.T. and McCutcheon, S.N. (eds) *Proceedings of the A.L. Rae Symposium on Animal Breeding and Genetics*. Department of Animal Science, Massey University, Palmerston North, New Zealand, pp. 120–126.

Pickering, N.K., Blair, H.T., Hickson, R.E., Dodds, K.G., Johnson, P.L. and McEwan, J.C. (2013) Genetic relationships between dagginess, breech bareness, and wool traits in New Zealand dual-purpose sheep. *Journal of Animal Science* 91, 4578–4588. DOI: 10.2527/jas.2013-6741.

Pinares-Patino, C.S., Hickey, S.M., Young, E.A., Dodds, K.G., MacLean, S. *et al.* (2013) Heritability estimates of methane emissions from sheep. *Animal* 7, S2, 316–321. DOI: 10.1017/S1751731113000864.

Pollott, G.E. (2011) A suggested mode of inheritance for wool shedding in sheep. *Journal of Animal Science* 89, 2316–2325. DOI: 10.2527/jas.2010-3713.

Pollott, G.E. and Greeff, J.C. (2004a) Genetic relationships between faecal egg count and production traits in commercial Merino sheep flocks. *Animal Science* 79, 21–32. DOI: 10.1017/S1357729800054497.

Pollott, G.E. and Greeff, J.C. (2004b) Genotype by environment interactions and genetic parameters for fecal egg count and production traits of Merino sheep. *Journal of Animal Science* 82, 2840–2851. DOI: 10.2527/2004.82102840x.

Ponzoni, R.W. and Gifford, D.R. (1990) Developing breeding objectives for Australian cashmere goats. *Journal of Animal Breeding and Genetics* 107, 351–370. DOI: 10.1111/j.1439-0388.1990.tb00044.x.

Ponzoni, R.W., Rogan, I.M. and James, P.W. (1990) Genetic improvement of apparel and carpet wool production. *Proceedings of the 4th World Congress on Genetics Applied to Livestock Production* Vol XV, pp. 149–166. Available at http://www.wcgalp.org/proceedings/1990 (accessed 16 June 2020).

Raoul, J., Swan, A.A. and Elsen, J.M. (2018) Assessment of a genomic design for a French meat sheep breeding program. *Proceedings of the World Congress on Genetics Applied to Livestock Production* 11, 79. Available at: http://www.wcgalp.org/proceedings/2018 (accessed 16 June 2020).

Roden, J.A. (1994) Review of the theory of open nucleus breeding systems. *Animal Breeding Abstracts* 62, 151–157.

Rupp, R., Mucha, S., Larroque, H., McEwan, J. and Conington, J. (2016) Genomic application in sheep and goat breeding. *Animal Frontiers* 6, 1, 39–44. DOI: 10.2527/af.2016-0006.

Ryder, M.L. (1983) *Sheep and Man.* Duckworth, London.

SAC (2017) *Farm Management Handbook.* SAC Consulting. Edinburgh, UK.

Safari, E., Gilmour, A.R. and Fogarty, N.M. (2005) A review of genetic parameter estimates for wool, growth, meat and reproduction traits in sheep. *Livestock Production Science* 92, 271–289. DOI: 10.1016/j.livprodsci.2004.09.003.

Safari, E., Fogarty, N.M., Mortimer, S.I., Greeff, J.C., Hatcher, S. *et al.* (2007) Feed intake and its genetic relationship with growth traits in Merino sheep. *Proceedings of the Association for the Advancement of Animal Breeding and Genetics* 17, 199–202.

Sheep Genetics (2019) *Welcome to Kidplan*. Available at: http://www.sheepgenetics.org.au/Breeding-services/KIDPLAN-Home (accessed 3 November 2019).

Signet (2019) *The National Sire Evaluation*. AHDB, Kenilworth, UK.

Simm, G. (1988) *Artificial Insemination and Embryo Transfer: How They Can Help Sheep Breeders*. SAC Technical Note T136. The Scottish Agricultural College, Perth, UK.

Simm, G. (1992) Selection for lean meat production in sheep. In: Speedy, A.W. (ed.) *Recent Advances in Sheep and Goat Research*. CAB International, Wallingford, UK, pp. 193–215.

Simm, G. (1994) Developments in improvement of meat sheep. *Proceedings of the 5th World Congress on Genetics Applied to Livestock Production* 18, 3–10. Available at: http://www.wcgalp.org/proceedings/1994 (accessed 16 June 2020).

Simm, G. and Dingwall, W.S. (1989) Selection indices for lean meat production in sheep. *Livestock Production Science* 21, 223–233. DOI: 10.1016/0301-6226(89)90052-3.

Simm, G. and Murphy, S.V. (1996) The effects of selection for lean growth in Suffolk sires on the saleable meat yield of their crossbred progeny. *Animal Science* 62, 255–263. DOI: 10.1017/S1357729800014557.

Simm, G. and Wray, N.R. (1991) *Sheep Sire Referencing Schemes - New Opportunities for Pedigree Breeders and Lamb Producers*. SAC Technical Note T264. The Scottish Agricultural College, Edinburgh, UK.

Taylor, P.J. (2006) *A Few Selected Lines*. Newsletter of the Trangie QPLU$ Project. Issue 5 April 2006.

Usai, M.G., Salaris, S., Casu, S., Sechi, T., Miari, S. *et al*. (2018) Feasibility of genomic predictions of Sarda breed rams using a female reference population. *Proceedings of the World Congress on Genetics Applied to Livestock Production* 11, 670. Available at: http://www.wcgalp.org/proceedings/2018 (accessed 16 June 2020).

Visser, C. and Van Marle-Köster, E. (2014) Strategies for the genetic improvement of South African Angora goats. *Small Ruminant Research* 121, 89–95.

Woolaston, R.R. (1987) Genotype x environment interactions and their possible impact on breeding programs. In: McGuirk, B.J. (ed.) *Merino Improvement Programs in Australia*. Australian Wool Corporation, pp. 421–425.

Recommended Reading

Animal (formerly *Animal Science* and *Animal Production*; Journal of the British Society of Animal Science).

Livestock Production Science.

Piper, L. and Ruvinsky, A. (eds) (1997) *The Genetics of Sheep*. CAB International, Wallingford, UK.

Proceedings of the Australian Association of Animal Breeding and Genetics.

Proceedings of the New Zealand Society of Animal Production.

Proceedings of the World Congresses on Genetics Applied to Livestock Production. Available at: wcgalp.org (accessed 16 June 2020).

Simões, J. and Gutiérrez, C. (2017) *Sustainable Goat Production in Adverse Environments I: Welfare, Health and Breeding*. Springer International, New York, USA.

Simões, J. and Gutiérrez, C. (2018) *Sustainable Goat Production in Adverse Environments II: Local Goat Breeds*. Springer International, New York, USA.

Thomson, M. and Rowe, J. (eds) (2019) *Concept to Impact: The Story of the Sheep CRC 2001–2019*. Sheep CRC Ltd, Armidale, Australia.

11 Poultry Breeding

Introduction

Poultry species have probably undergone the most dramatic change in production characteristics of all the farmed livestock species. Originally kept as a household food source in both rural and urban areas, poultry are now maintained on an industrial scale in many countries. This change has been dominated by a small, and reducing number of large, multinational breeding companies. Of course, in many countries, small-scale poultry production remains important, but this is overshadowed by the sheer size and scale of the industrial poultry sector. Consequently, poultry production is in the hands of a wide range of producers varying from very large industrialized units in wealthier countries, to very small family-based units, in parts of India and most of Africa and South-East Asia. In this chapter, we explore the way in which poultry breeding companies use genetics to meet consumer demand in the most economical manner. Because the poultry sector is diverse in terms of both the species used, the systems of production and products sold, we concentrate on the major species and products to illustrate how breeding is practised.

The Global Poultry Sector

The global poultry production sector is dominated by chickens, but a number of other species are important in a range of countries, including turkeys, ducks, geese, guinea fowl, pheasants, partridge, quail and pigeons. Data from FAO (2019) show that chicken meat dominates the poultry meat sector with an estimated annual production in 2017 of 109 million tonnes (Mt), followed by turkey meat (6 Mt) then duck meat (4 Mt) and meat from geese and guinea fowl combined (3 Mt).

Figure 11.1 shows the distribution of chicken meat production by world region. Asia dominates this sector with 34.5% of world chicken meat production in 2017. This is followed by North and Central America (23.2%), South America (19.2%) and Europe (16.7%). Within these regions the USA, Brazil and China dominate chicken meat production by country (Fig. 11.2) with over 10 Mt of chicken meat in 2017.

Asia also dominates the chicken egg production sector to an even larger extent than with chicken meat at 62.2% of world production in 2017. The Americas and Europe make up most of the remaining egg production (Fig. 11.3). China produces the most eggs at 500,000 M eggs in 2017, with the USA, India and Mexico as the next largest producers (Fig. 11.4).

With such diverse products and locations, it is not surprising that breeding methods are also diverse. In this chapter we consider the major breeding goals for each of the products and then outline how the breeding and selection methods have been developed appropriately using chicken meat (broiler) and chicken egg sectors as the main examples.

Breeding Goals

Meat production

The 2017 FAO (2019) world figures show that over 66 billion chickens were produced for meat consumption. As in most meat-producing systems, the aim is to produce the optimum amount of meat required by the consumer on a carcass, as efficiently as possible. During the 1950s the chicken industry concentrated on productivity, with growth rate as a key breeding objective, and some emphasis on feed conversion ratio and carcass composition. Since feed is the major cost in poultry systems, it follows that reducing the number of days to slaughter for a given weight of carcass is a key economic driver. Clearly, there is a lower limit to this objective. Following this early emphasis on reducing days to slaughter, experience dictated that health and welfare traits should receive more emphasis in breeding programmes. In addition, the rapid increase

Genetic Improvement of Farmed Animals (G. Simm *et al.*)
DOI: 10.1079/9781789241723.0011

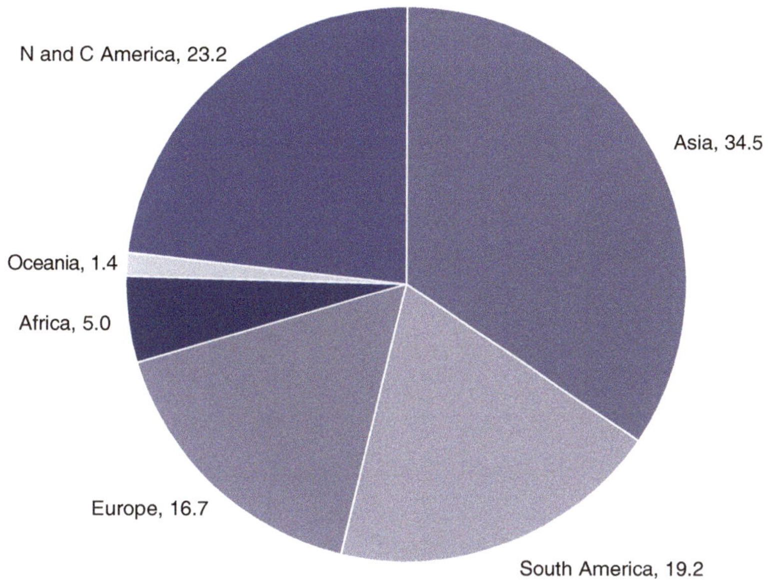

Fig. 11.1. Proportion of world chicken meat production by continent in 2017 (%). (After FAO, 2019.)

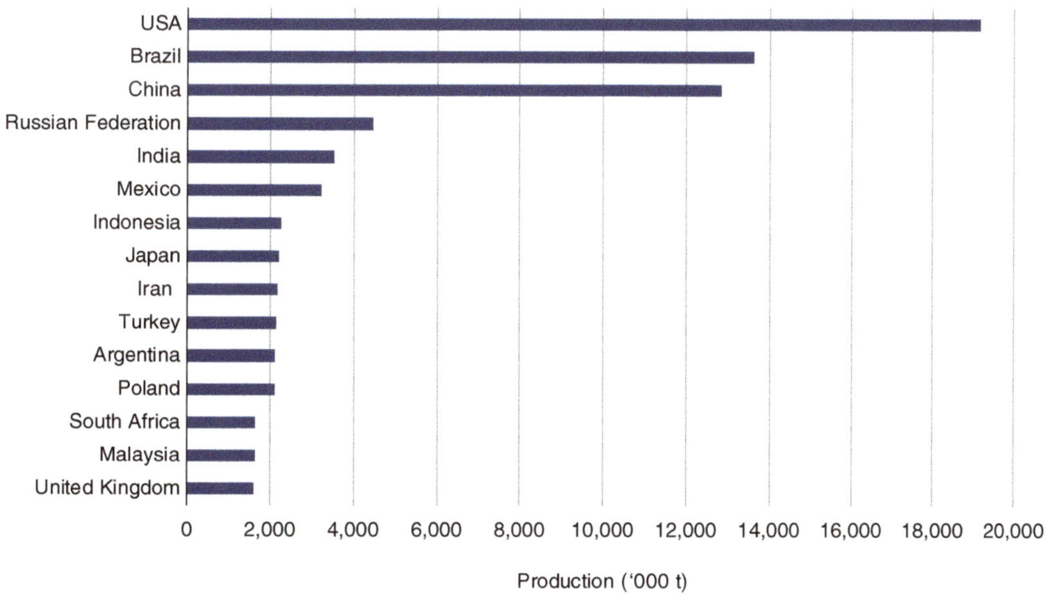

Fig. 11.2. Production of chicken meat by the 15 highest producing countries in the world in 2017. (After FAO, 2019.)

in growth at a young age led to a correlated response in the size of adult breeding birds, which needs to be managed carefully to avoid metabolic problems. Currently, a multi-dimensional breeding goal is common, with an increased emphasis on biological efficiency, reproduction, adaptability, welfare and robustness that focuses on sustainability, product quality and health (Neeteson-van

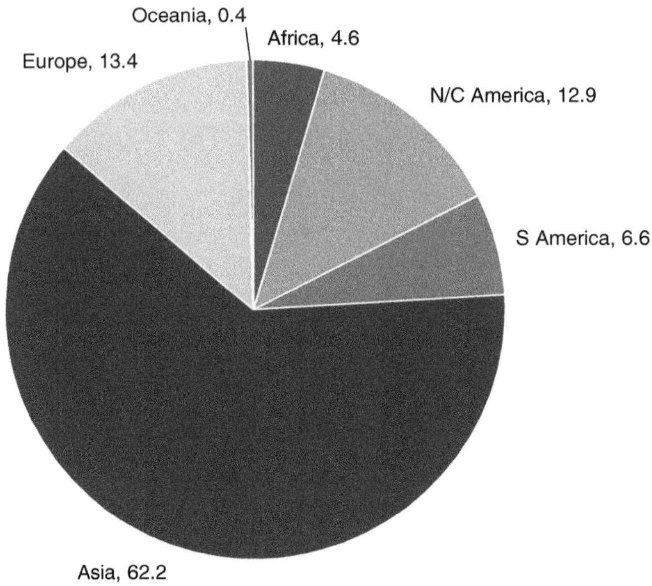

Fig. 11.3. Proportion of world chicken egg production by continent in 2017 (%). (After FAO, 2019.)

Nieuwenhoven *et al.*, 2013). In his review of the breeding goals of this industry, Laughlin (2007) divides the selection objectives for the broiler breeders into ten groups of traits: weight, growth profile, feed conversion, breast meat, meat quality, heart/lung fitness, skeletal integrity, eggs, hatchability and immune response. This more holistic approach includes simultaneously improving antagonistically related traits, such as growth rate and skeletal strength (Kapell *et al.*, 2012a) or yield and meat quality (Bailey *et al.*, 2015).

Not only has the historical change in poultry meat production been dramatic, but forecasts of future demand are equally arresting. The OECD/FAO (2016) forecast that by 2025 global meat production and consumption will increase by 48 Mt, with poultry meat contributing 44% to the total production growth and being equivalent to the additional growth of all other meats. Over 70% of the increase in poultry production is expected to come from low- and middle-income countries while the increase in consumption is expected to occur more evenly across regions and income levels globally.

The bulk of this anticipated increase in demand for chicken meat is likely to be met by an increase in the gene flow originating from birds produced by a small number of global breeding companies. Over recent years there have been number of mergers of broiler breeding companies such that, at the time of writing, there are two main companies: the Aviagen Group comprising the Ross, Rowan Range, Arbor Acres, Indian River, Specialty Males brands and Hubbard, and Cobb-Vantress who market the Cobb and CobbSasso birds.

Selection for early growth, feed conversion and carcass composition

As with all meat-producing livestock species, selection for improved meat production is based on faster early growth of the juvenile. This trait, or weight-for-age, is relatively simple to record and has been shown to be moderately heritable and variable. Thus, as a basis for a selection programme it has much to recommend it. However, several studies have highlighted the tendency to produce fatter animals using this simple selection goal and so additional traits are added to the selection objective to counteract this. In the case of broiler production this has involved the measurement of both feed conversion ratio (FCR; kg of food per kg of weight gain) and breast meat yield. Both traits are also moderately heritable and variable and so lend themselves as breeding objective traits. Compared to other livestock species, these two traits are reasonably easy

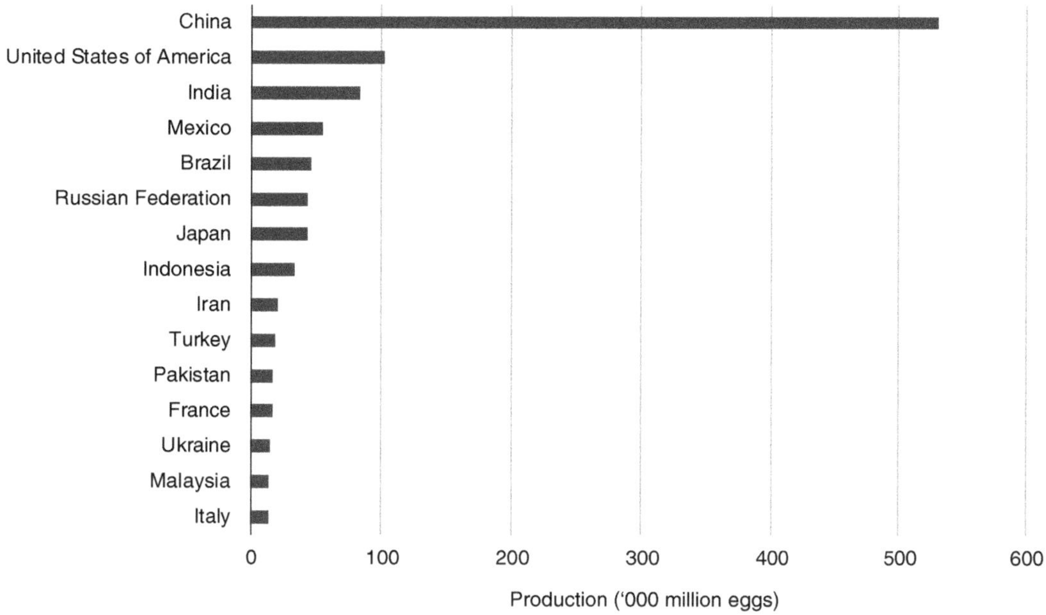

Fig. 11.4. Production of chicken eggs by the 15 highest producing countries in the world in 2017. (After FAO, 2019.)

to measure and include in breeding programmes, due to the small size of the birds, controlled management and high reproductive rate. Large full-sib and half-sib cohorts allow some birds to be used for carcass measurements to add selection accuracy without compromising selection intensity.

A number of alternatives to FCR have been explored in poultry breeding and include residual feed intake (RFI), coefficient of digestibility (CDU) and maintenance efficiency (MEff). Residual feed intake is the difference between the expected feed consumption for a bird of a given size, based on common nutrition equations, and the actual amount of feed that a bird eats in a given time (Koch *et al.*, 1963). More efficient animals have a negative value since they eat less than they are expected to for any given set of production characteristics. However, the risk of selecting for RFI is that birds will attain better FCR through lower feed intake (the genetic correlation between RFI and FI is typically 0.6). Reducing feed intake may compromise the bird's robustness, particularly in sub-optimal environments. The use of CDU attempts to take into account the efficiency of digestion of particular nutrients (protein, starch, lipid, etc.). This is calculated as the difference between the feed composition of the bird and the composition of the excreta, for any given nutrient. Whereas this is a more labour-intensive process, it provides more comprehensive data in terms of the environmental impact of poultry. Alternatively, MEff attempts to measure how efficient an animal is at maintaining body temperature, basal metabolism and basic movement, independently of body weight.

Selection for health and welfare traits

The early dramatic changes made in the growth and feed conversion traits in the broiler industry have come at a cost to the health and welfare of the animals. In particular, there is evidence of unfavourable consequences in broiler chickens for gait/lameness and cardiovascular function if these health traits are ignored in selection. Breeding companies have responded by increasing emphasis on functionality/welfare traits (see Neeteson-van Nieuwenhoven *et al.*, 2013). A number of selection traits have been considered in this area, including leg joint integrity, cardiovascular function, and incidence of ascites and sudden death syndrome. Avendaño and Ralph (2018) outline welfare-related traits in use in breeding programmes, including skeletal support (clinical and sub-clinical leg health and locomotion), contact dermatitis, cardiovascular function and liveability in a broiler breeding programme. Avendaño *et al.* (2017) list a number of additional health and welfare-related traits such as leg bone deformity, gait score, tibial dyschondroplasia, crooked toes and mortality. Katanbaf and Hardiman (2010) indicate that a breeding company like Cobb will record 56 traits per pedigree bird in their broiler breeding programme, over half of them related to health and fitness.

Selection for adult traits

Although the emphasis in broiler breeding is clearly on the performance of birds at a young age (growth rate, FCR, etc.), the adult breeding birds must be considered too. A key trait is the fertility of the adults, as well as liveweight, functional and fitness traits. One consequence of selection for early growth is that older birds are likely to be fatter unless later weight gain is controlled. The major method for achieving this is through restricting the quality and/or quantity of food offered, but this has implications for the welfare of the bird, since they will be consuming less food than their appetite dictates. There may be some scope for selecting broiler breeders on the basis of a change in the shape of the growth curve such that growth is optimal in early life and adult liveweight is genetically restricted.

A crucial adult trait in commercial broilers is the fertility of both males and females and hatchability of the eggs. Clearly broilers are not kept for egg production, but the number of broiler chicks hatched is a key factor in efficiency of the broiler industry. As we will see later, broilers are divided into lines to develop male and female traits, but all lines need to pay some attention to the fertility of both sexes, which is negatively correlated with growth and conformation traits. It is therefore of interest to investigate the way that fertility changes over the laying period in broiler breeders and the relationship between male and female fertility. The fertility of an egg, the basic measured trait in this type of work, is a function of the genotype of the embryo, which in turn is influenced by its parental genotypes. Female contributions to fertility are via egg quality, behavioural and physiological effects, e.g. via the sperm storage tubules. Males will contribute to fertility via sperm quality traits, behaviour and any leg problems. Wolc *et al.* (2009) investigated male and female fertility simultaneously and the relationship between them. They also looked at how this varied over the laying period. Fertility reached a peak at about 35 weeks of age in their study and the heritability of fertility followed a similar pattern in both sexes but that of males was slightly higher than females. The heritability of fertility reached a peak at about 32 weeks of age with male fertility being about 0.02 higher than for females at any given age. Interestingly the genetic correlation between male and female fertility was just less than 1.0.

Egg production

The number of eggs produced annually is shown in Fig. 11.4 and is equivalent to about 75 Mt of eggs by weight. Preisinger (2018) suggests that with a growing world population a further 1 Mt of eggs will be required annually which translates into 50 M extra hens with the potential to provide 20 kg of egg mass per hen, over a laying period from 20 to 76 weeks of age. Egg production varies considerably between countries but the egg sector in different countries varies a great deal in a number of other ways too. These include the legal framework, consumer preferences and a wide variety of housing systems. Not only must layer breeding companies respond to these changing factors but they also have to anticipate future changes since breeding decisions made today may only reach the commercial flocks about five years into the future. Currently there are a small number of layer breeding companies. Hendrix Genetics market the Babcock, Bovans, Dekalb, Hisex, ISA and Shaver brands. Other companies include Hy-Line, Lohmann Tierzucht and H+N International

Legislative framework

The legal context of animal welfare has become a feature of modern intensive production systems and varies around the world. This covers two major features of laying hen production: housing system and controls on animal mutilation. Commercial layer cages have been banned in some countries for a number of years, and public opinion in other countries may make this a more widespread feature of layer production. Regulation of minimum space requirements for animals is common in many countries and behavioural enrichment (e.g. provision of perching in indoor systems or providing outdoor access for free ranging) is provided in some systems. A number of practices have been prohibited in some countries, including beak trimming and the culling of surplus male chicks. Hence, sex determination is carried out on eggs. In addition, the use of genetically modified feed is also banned in some countries. The use of antibiotics as a routine management practice is banned in some countries, and there is a growing call for a general limitation on their use.

Consumer preferences

Traditional consumer preferences have been expressed in terms of the quality and appearance of the product. This is still the case for eggs, with egg colour and size preferences varying throughout the world. So, for example, white eggs are preferred in North and Central America, the Middle East, India, Taiwan and the Philippines, but brown eggs are the colour of choice in China, Europe and Latin America. Interestingly, tinted eggs have a market in China and Japan (Preisinger, 2018).

Recently, consumer preferences have also encompassed animal welfare and environmental impact of different types of production and housing systems. This has been reflected in legislation in some countries, controlling or banning certain housing and production methods.

Housing systems

Housing systems can be divided into cage systems and non-caged systems. Cage systems may be conventional, furnished/enriched or colony cages. Non-caged systems may be single tiered/floor housed, multi-tiered aviaries with or without integrated nest boxes or outdoor free-range systems. The United States and non-EU European countries tend to use conventional systems which comprise up to about ten hens housed together with ~430 cm^2 of space per bird. Muir *et al.* (2014) list a number of advantages of this system, including:

- a stable social hierarchy associated with the small group size;
- low mortality;
- low risk of damaging feather pecking and outbreaks of cannibalism;
- cleaner eggs with low levels of parasitism;
- improved bird health with low levels of infection, bumblefoot, keel bone damage (deformation and fractures), and aerial pollution;
- low risk of predation;
- easy management and care; and
- high economic efficiency.

However, they also list the disadvantages as:

- discomfort and abnormal behaviour resulting from limited space for hens to perform heritable behaviours such as dust bathing, roosting, and pre-laying nesting;
- decreased bone quality (osteoporosis) with high susceptibility to fractures on depopulation; and
- increased body injury from feather pecking and cannibalism, resulting from insufficient space to escape from dominant birds.

These cages can result in increased stress in hens and a reduced quality of life due to a barren environment and overcrowding.

Alternative caged systems have been developed using a range of furnished accommodation for hens. These can range from group houses for 60 or more birds, smaller cages for 15–30 birds and even smaller cages for less than 15 birds. Natural nesting, roosting and scratching behaviour is facilitated by using a variety of perches, dust baths and nesting facilities in the pens. These systems are not without their health and welfare problems, including higher mortality, feather pecking and cannibalism, as well as health problems associated with roosting (Muir *et al.*, 2014).

Non-caged systems have also been developed to try to overcome the problems mentioned above in both caged and furnished systems and to allow birds some freedom to forage, bath in dust, nest and exercise their limbs. The main drawbacks of these systems listed by Muir *et al.* (2014) are:

- unstable hierarchy associated with the large flock group size;
- high levels of mortality resulting from high risks of feather pecking and cannibalism;
- high risk of hens sustaining fractures associated with collision damage with perches, nest boxes and other structures;
- increased risk of smothering;
- increased risk of disease and parasites due to contact with droppings, infective agents and wild birds;
- increased risk from predation; and
- reduced egg production due to high mortality and poor bird welfare, especially in subordinate hens which may have limited access to feed,

water and other provided structures (nest boxes and range) due to aggressive encounters and resource guarding by dominant hens.

The choice of housing systems varies between and within continents, and in some cases is governed by legislation. For example, in Switzerland, Austria, Sweden and Germany, commercial layer cages were banned for a number of years before the EU ban on cages finally came into effect in 2012. Enriched cages, considered by poultry scientists as an acceptable compromise between the demands of the industry, of animal welfare organizations, and of the behavioural needs of laying hens, are used in Europe as an alternative to conventional battery cages. Retailers and animal welfare groups in different countries continue to press for a complete ban on cages. In North America, a change from cage systems to aviary systems is most likely within the next decade.

Clearly, each system has some advantages and some disadvantages that need to be evaluated within the particular legal framework of a given country. Such varied systems provide a challenge for breeders since a range of selection of objectives, or at least different priorities, apply to each situation, and need to be accommodated in breeding programmes.

Layer breeding objectives and criteria

Although the major breeding companies do not publish their breeding objectives and selection criteria for commercial reasons, we can infer what they may be from various sources. For example, Groen (2003) lists a number of key breeding goals for layer production (Table 11.1). These cover the basic production traits but also egg quality, production efficiency, reproductive performance and functional traits associated with welfare, behaviour and disease. Clearly, the exact objectives and goals of any one company will vary but Table 11.1 captures the main priorities of layer breeding programmes.

Table 11.1. Suggested breeding goals for layer production. (After Groen, 2003.)

Type of trait	Recorded trait
Egg production level	Age at first egg Hen-day egg production (eggs/per 100 d) Persistency of production (rate of lay) Pauses (broodiness) Egg size/weight
Egg quality	Outer: Egg deformation Shell thickness, colour, texture, porosity and shape Inner: Albumen quality Blood spots Taste
Efficiency of production	Mature body weight Feed consumption (level and type of feed)
Reproductive performance	Female and male fertility Hatchability of eggs (% hatched)
Functional traits	Disease resistance Leg strength Survival Feeding behaviour Maternal care Cannibalism Temperament (e.g. flightiness)

Selection for egg traits

The production of eggs varies considerably between breeds and individual birds. The key factors in commercial production are the number of eggs per given time period, the length of the laying period and the efficiency of feed conversion to egg weight. Ideally, birds would produce one egg per day, but this varies for a number of reasons, not least the birds' natural tendency towards missing days due to broodiness. The start and finish of the laying period are key parameters and efforts to breed for earlier sexual maturity and longer length of lay are critical to profitable production. Additional egg traits to do with size and quality will vary with the intended market. Egg size/weight, shell, albumen and yolk quality are often included in selection programmes.

Selection for health traits

Modern laying hens tend to have a relatively low body weight, a relatively low food intake and produce many eggs. They deposit a large amount of calcium in eggshells and, consequently, the stores of calcium in the body are often used extensively. This can result in poor bone formation and bone strength, which may result in broken bones. The cost of this to production and welfare has led to some emphasis on measuring and breeding for better bone quality.

All animal systems are subjected to disease outbreaks, which tend to be more acute in intensive systems. One genetic approach is to consider each disease in turn and investigate its heritability and correlations with other key traits. An alternative is to look at the immune systems and select for animals showing certain immunological characteristics. Since disease resistance traits are commonly polygenic it seems more likely that breeding for general disease resistance may be a useful way forward. Bird survival to a specific age or time point in the production cycle is a more general measure of the health of the layer.

Selection for social and behavioural traits

As we have seen, the basic goals in layer breeding are to produce the greatest number of saleable eggs at minimum cost in a specified production period. However, the decision by the EU to ban conventional cages for birds since 2012 has led to cage-free housing systems for layers in Europe and given rise to a number of new challenges when measuring egg production. This change has put more emphasis on the behaviour of laying hens in group-housed facilities as a key focus. Birds have to visit nest boxes to lay and so nesting behaviour is a key trait in such systems. It is still important to produce more eggs per time period, of good quality, but genetic parameters under these conditions may be different from the traditional values derived from caged birds. In order to measure bird activity in cage-free conditions, behaviour can be monitored with transponder-based methods. Icken *et al.* (2012) describe two systems used in cage-free systems and give some genetic parameters of behaviour traits.

The Weihenstephan Funnel Nest Box was developed to record single-hen nesting behaviour in a floor-housing system. The Electronic Pop-Hole was designed to gather information on ranging behaviour of the birds. When combined together, these two systems provide data on laying time, allowing exact oviposition time to be ascribed to each bird. Unlike in cages where the number of eggs laid is the same as the number of saleable eggs, when using floor systems birds may lay their eggs anywhere leading to a number of unsaleable 'floor eggs'. The automatic recording systems allow the number of saleable nest eggs to be recorded per bird as well as nest acceptance characteristics.

Future selection goals

Despite the extensive list of breeding goals shown in Table 11.1, Preisinger (2018) suggests that there are further goals that need to be incorporated into layer breeding programmes. These include extending the length of the production cycle in order to increase the number of saleable eggs per hen, improving egg shell quality, better bone quality to address the leg and other breakages found in free-range, floor and perch environments, and increased hen liveability with consistent feather cover throughout the laying period.

The growing concern over the environmental impact of animal-sourced foods is also stimulating debate on future breeding objectives – though poultry are already among the most efficient livestock. One route whereby layers impact the environment is through the use of land and other resources to grow cereals for feed, and the greenhouse gases emitted in the process. Improvements in feed efficiency have already reduced this impact, but further improvements are possible. Another environmental impact of layers is via the greenhouse gas emissions produced from poultry systems. Improved digestibility of key nutrients by selection could be one approach to reducing this environmental impact.

Breeds, Crosses and Hybrid Lines Used in Poultry Production

In its publication on the state of the world's animal genetic resources, FAO (2015) lists 1729 breeds of chickens worldwide, of which only 212 are considered 'not at risk'. As in most livestock, there has been a proliferation of local breeds, some of which have become common regionally or nationally. Numerous chicken breeds were developed in Europe and North America (e.g., Rhode Island Red, Single-Comb White Leghorn), for use in small backyard flocks, for the production of eggs or meat or both, with others developed as breeds for showing. Many of these went on to have wider global use. Breeding programmes of the major commercial breeding companies were based initially on these breeds, but most selection now takes place within lines originally produced by crossing breeds.

In the 1950s, modern poultry production emerged, with specialized industrial chicken breeds selected intensively for either meat-type (broiler) or egg-type (layer) chickens. All commercial white egg chicken lines are based on the White Leghorn breed

(Fig. 11.5), whereas brown egg chicken lines were initially selected from North American dual-purpose breeds (selected for both meat and egg production), such as Rhode Island Red (Fig. 11.6) and White Plymouth Rock, which originated from crosses between Asian and European breeds. Due to the negative genetic correlation between production (growth) and reproduction (egg number), commercial poultry meat production used crosses among specialized broiler lines. Lines selected primarily for growth traits are referred to as sire or male lines, because only males are used in the final commercial cross. The lines used for the female side of the cross are selected for both reproductive and growth traits and are referred to as dam or female lines. The male lines are derived from Cornish stock, originating from the British Cornish Indian Game breed, having a thick compact body type with a high proportion of breast muscle. The dam lines originate from many of the same dual-purpose breeds used for brown egg production (e.g. Barred Plymouth Rock, White Plymouth Rock, New Hampshire).

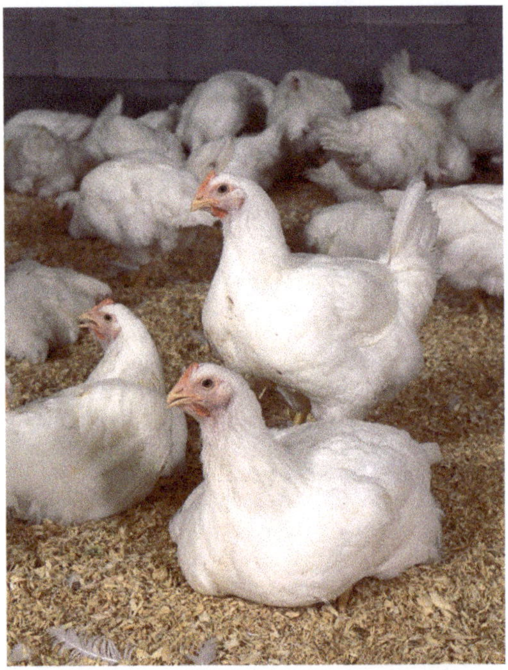

Fig. 11.5. A group of modern broiler chickens. (After K-State Research and Extension; https://www.flickr.com/photos/ksrecomm/ licensed under Creative Commons 2.0.)

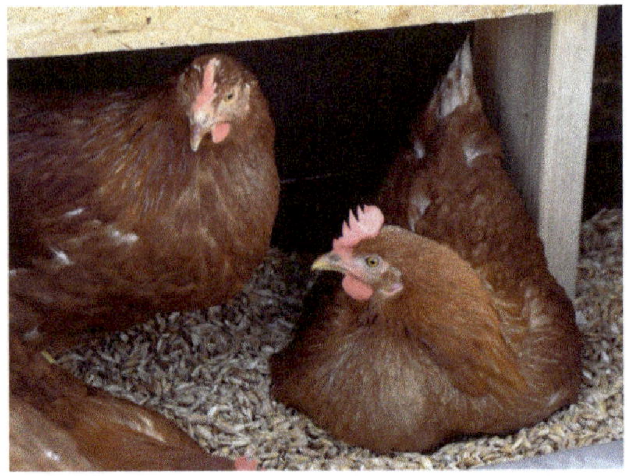

Fig. 11.6. Laying hens in a barn. (Photo by Nadine Trief from Pixabay.)

Genetic Improvement Strategies in Large-Scale Chicken Production Systems

Overview

The change in the poultry industry over recent years from backyard production to industrial methods has been mirrored by changes in the selection methods employed. Early reliance on pedigree recording as the basis for mass selection in the middle of the 20th century was expanded by the later use of artificial insemination (AI). Rapid development of the use of 'lines' or 'strains' and the testing of all possible crosses between them, particularly in the egg-laying types, allowed the identification of offspring with the most desirable combination of characteristics. During the 1970s, FCR testing changed from family-based methods to individually housed approaches. Soon afterwards, companies developed a great-grandparent approach, which involved using several different lines, crossed in a particular combination to develop specific sire and dam lines, based on different selection criteria appropriate to the line. With the introduction of best linear unbiased prediction (BLUP) in the 1990s, breeding values were estimated within lines before production of the final crosses for commercial production. For an extended history of broiler breeding see Tixier-Boichard *et al.* (2012).

Changing consumer expectation and legal changes is some countries has driven the wider use of cage-free systems in egg production. Cage-free systems tend to incur about 20% higher costs, but Preisinger (2018) suggests that this may be offset by new housing systems, smaller flock sizes and increased egg output in these systems. Whatever the system, persistency of lay is an important selection objective implying higher and longer production periods for layers.

Meat production

Meat production traits encompass a range of different aspects of animal performance and carcass characteristics. Live animal traits such as growth/weight are relatively easy to measure, with feed traits requiring more attention. Carcass traits are typically measured on relatives not required for breeding, although in experimental conditions to estimate genetic parameters this is not usually a requirement. Results from a typical study of commercial weight, feed and carcass traits (Morris, 1996) are shown in Tables 11.2 to 11.5.

The basic broiler traits related to early growth tend to contain useful genetic variation which can be used in genetic improvement programmes. Typical genetic parameters are shown in Tables 11.2 and 11.3. Weight for age and food conversion ratio have somewhat higher heritabilities than weight gain on test and feed consumption, but nevertheless they should all respond to selection. Not surprisingly, weight gain and feed consumption have a high genetic correlation but FCR and weight gain have a strong negative genetic correlation; birds that grow more do so with a lower feed requirement per kg of weight gain.

The carcass traits in Table 11.3 tend to show a good level of usable genetic variation. All the carcass traits have a heritability above 0.25. Breast weight, a key trait in broiler production is well correlated with other important carcass components such as thigh weight and wing weight but also bone weight.

The carcass traits are shown as a proportion of the carcass weight in Table 11.4. In this case percentage breast meat is positively genetically correlated with FCR and negatively correlated with % drumstick and wings. This is understandable since, if the breast is a greater proportion of the carcass, then the other components will contribute less.

As we have seen above, there is a strong effect of bodyweight on test with some of the broiler traits. Table 11.5 shows the genetic correlations between feed consumption, adjusted for bodyweight, and broiler traits. In this case higher feed consumption is linked with heavier carcasses, more breast meat, less thigh, drumstick and wing percentage, higher abdominal fat percentage and more bone.

Measurement of feed intake in breeding programmes has allowed the calculation of the heritability of FCR, RFI and CDU traits. All three traits have been shown to be heritable and to contain useful variation for selection programmes. Heritability estimates for FCR ranged from 0.07 to 0.41 in a review of methods by Sell-Kubiak *et al.* (2017) depending on a range of environmental factors. They also quote a range of heritability values for RFI from 0.23 to 0.49 and indicate that the two traits (FCR and RFI) tend to be highly genetically correlated at between 0.74 to 0.93. This indicates that the two traits are largely measuring the same thing and are controlled by similar sets of genes. The CDU trait has been less widely studied, but in the studies reviewed were found to have a similar range of heritability values as the other two traits.

These basic broiler traits underpin most broiler breeding programmes, but the later addition of health and welfare traits have provided a varying focus in broiler breeding programmes.

Health traits in broilers

In order to control the level of common health and welfare conditions in broiler breeding it is important to know if any of the traits are under genetic

Table 11.2. Correlation matrix (standard errors in parentheses[a]) for 34- to 48-day feed traits estimated from a multivariate REML analysis of all animals with complete feed records (Phenotypic correlations above the diagonal; heritability on the diagonal (bold); genetic correlations below the diagonal). (After Morris, 1996.)

Trait	34-day weight	Feed consumption	Weight gain	Feed conversion ratio
34-day weight	**0.51 (0.13)**	0.22	0.10	0.12
Feed consumption	0.11 (0.53)	**0.04 (0.11)**	0.81	−0.06
Weight gain	−0.53 (0.47)	0.68 (0.45)	**0.10 (0.11)**	−0.63
Feed conversion ratio	0.84 (0.17)	−0.21 (0.66)	−0.85 (0.25)	**0.17 (0.08)**

[a]Standard errors for phenotypic correlations ranged between 0.01 and 0.05.

Table 11.3. Correlation matrix for 34- to 48-day feed traits and 52-day carcass traits estimated by multivariate REML analysis of all animals with complete carcass records. Standard errors are in parentheses.[a] (Phenotypic correlations above the diagonal; heritability on the diagonal (bold); genetic correlations below the diagonal.) (After Morris, 1996).

		Trait												
		1	2	3	4	5	6	7	8	9	10	11	12	13
1	34-day weight	**0.83 (0.24)**	0.24	0.12	0.07	0.64	0.63	0.54	0.47	0.33	0.53	0.43	0.16	0.58
2	Feed consumption	−0.02 (0.13)	**0.16 (0.06)**	0.85	−0.24	0.71	0.69	0.60	0.54	0.50	0.50	0.46	0.25	0.59
3	Weight gain	−0.52 (0.14)	0.55 (0.13)	**0.09 (0.02)**	−0.69	0.73	0.72	0.63	0.60	0.53	0.56	0.45	0.20	0.60
4	Feed conversion	0.53 (0.13)	0.58 (0.13)	−0.36 (0.18)	**0.25 (0.06)**	−0.42	−0.42	−0.39	−0.40	−0.33	−0.36	−0.22	−0.02	−0.33
5	Plucked weight	0.71 (0.07)	0.41 (0.19)	0.22 (0.19)	0.29 (0.20)	**0.30 (0.08)**	0.99	0.83	0.80	0.71	0.77	0.64	0.26	0.84
6	Carcass weight	0.71 (0.07)	0.37 (0.21)	0.19 (0.20)	0.28 (0.22)	0.97 (0.01)	**0.28 (0.08)**	0.86	0.81	0.71	0.77	0.65	0.26	0.84
7	Breast weight	0.52 (0.10)	0.32 (0.18)	−0.09 (0.22)	0.47 (0.23)	0.55 (0.11)	0.63 (0.10)	**0.33 (0.07)**	0.71	0.51	0.57	0.43	0.10	0.62
8	Thigh weight	0.53 (0.10)	0.23 (0.26)	0.25 (0.20)	0.08 (0.23)	0.84 (0.09)	0.89 (0.08)	0.50 (0.14)	**0.25 (0.09)**	0.49	0.54	0.41	0.15	0.57
9	Drumstick weight	0.19 (0.11)	0.06 (0.25)	0.48 (0.15)	−0.36 (0.19)	0.60 (0.12)	0.56 (0.13)	−0.11 (0.22)	0.74 (0.11)	**0.25 (0.07)**	0.55	0.41	0.11	0.58
10	Wing weight	0.71 (0.07)	0.14 (0.22)	0.15 (0.18)	0.07 (0.20)	0.94 (0.04)	0.92 (0.05)	0.46 (0.12)	0.80 (0.11)	0.60 (0.13)	**0.45 (0.11)**	0.48	0.17	0.64
11	Skin weight	0.57 (0.12)	0.05 (0.28)	−0.20 (0.26)	0.32 (0.22)	0.47 (0.19)	0.55 (0.18)	0.08 (0.21)	0.39 (0.25)	0.20 (0.23)	0.51 (0.19)	**0.31 (0.12)**	0.52	0.45
12	Abdominal fat weight	0.14 (0.14)	0.22 (0.27)	−0.09 (0.22)	0.40 (0.20)	0.07 (0.25)	0.14 (0.25)	−0.12 (0.20)	0.00 (0.28)	−0.15 (0.25)	0.03 (0.24)	0.70 (0.19)	**0.45 (0.16)**	0.09
13	Bone weight	0.54 (0.08)	0.51 (0.22)	0.42 (0.16)	0.20 (0.23)	0.95 (0.05)	0.89 (0.06)	0.40 (0.16)	0.73 (0.22)	0.66 (0.13)	0.86 (0.13)	0.37 (0.25)	0.03 (0.29)	**0.32 (0.13)**

[a]Standard errors for phenotypic correlations ranged between 0.01 and 0.05

control and how they may be related to production traits. Table 11.6 lists some heritabilities for health traits in broilers. The first two traits relate to the health of the animal in direct response to two common infectious diseases, *Escherichia coli* and *Salmonella enteritidis*. These two traits have a relatively low heritability (< 0.1) but as we saw in Chapter 4, heritability is only one component of the likely response to selection; selection intensity and the variability of the trait are also important. Plasma cardiac troponin T is an indicator of ascites and cardiovascular function, two important traits to monitor in modern broiler breeding programmes, and is moderately heritable. Mortality from *Salmonella* has a low to moderate heritability, while the leg trait tibial dyschondroplasia appears to be moderately highly heritable.

Many of the health traits appear to have arisen in conjunction with the breeding of faster-growing and more efficient broilers. Table 11.7 reflects this to some extent by showing a low to moderate set of genetic correlations with two key broiler traits, bodyweight and breast meat yield. The relationships with bodyweight appear to be stronger than with breast meat yield

Male and female traits in broilers

Although the primary aim of broiler breeding is to produce chicken meat as economically and sustainably as possible some thought must be given to the fertility of the adult birds, a set of traits which are commonly affected by breeding for faster juvenile growth. The genetic parameters of egg production traits in broilers may be different from those in the egg-laying strains and some typical values are shown in Table 11.8. These traits are hen-day rate egg production (EP; the number of eggs laid as a percentage of the number of days in lay from first until last egg), settable eggs (ST; the number of eggs set as a percentage of total eggs laid), fertility (FT; the number of fertile eggs as a percentage of the

Table 11.4. Correlation matrix for 34- to 48-day feed traits, 52-day body weights and 52-day carcass traits adjusted for carcass weight traits estimated by a multivariate REML analysis of all animals with complete carcass records. Standard errors in parentheses.[a] (Phenotypic correlations above the diagonal; heritability on the diagonal (bold); genetic correlations below the diagonal.) (After Morris, 1996.)

		Trait												
		1	2	3	4	5	6	7	8	9	10	11	12	13
1	**Initial test weight**	**0.83**	0.24	0.12	0.07	0.64	0.63	−0.02	−0.06	−0.15	0.08	0.02	−0.01	0.09
		(0.05)												
2	**Feed consumption**	−0.02	**0.15**	0.85	−0.24	0.71	0.69	0.00	−0.04	0.01	−0.04	0.00	0.07	0.01
		(0.13)	**(0.06)**											
3	**Weight gain**	−0.54	0.54	**0.09**	−0.69	0.73	0.72	0.01	0.02	0.04	0.01	−0.04	0.00	−0.02
		(0.18)	(0.18)	**(0.03)**										
4	**Feed conversion**	0.54	0.57	−0.38	**0.26**	−0.42	−0.42	−0.04	−0.09	−0.04	−0.06	0.08	0.09	0.05
		(0.15)	(0.16)	(0.20)	**(0.07)**									
5	**Plucked weight**	0.71	0.41	0.21	0.29	**0.29**	0.99	−0.05	0.00	0.03	0.04	−0.01	0.00	0.02
		(0.07)	(0.22)	(0.25)	(0.26)	**(0.10)**								
6	**Carcass**	0.71	0.35	0.17	0.28	0.97	**0.27**	−0.01	0.00	0.01	0.01	−0.01	0.00	0.01
		(0.08)	(0.23)	(0.27)	(0.28)	(0.01)	**(0.10)**							
7	**Per cent breast**	−0.06	0.07	−0.24	0.27	−0.25	−0.17	**0.82**	0.04	−0.28	−0.27	−0.34	−0.26	−0.39
		(0.08)	(0.20)	(0.18)	(0.20)	(0.17)	(0.18)	**(0.10)**						
8	**Per cent thighs**	−0.15	−0.17	0.20	−0.35	0.02	0.07	−0.17	**0.16**	−0.19	−0.21	−0.26	−0.11	−0.36
		(0.19)	(0.38)	(0.37)	(0.37)	(0.36)	(0.37)	(0.29)	**(0.11)**					
9	**Per cent drumstick**	−0.39	−0.25	0.41	−0.67	−0.13	−0.20	−0.63	0.61	**0.36**	0.00	−0.10	−0.11	−0.03
		(0.13)	(0.17)	(0.19)	(0.16)	(0.18)	(0.19)	(0.11)	(0.26)	**(0.05)**				
10	**Per cent wings**	0.57	−0.15	0.04	−0.17	0.71	0.65	−0.45	−0.05	0.04	**0.28**	−0.05	−0.05	−0.01
		(0.14)	(0.27)	(0.24)	(0.23)	(0.25)	(0.27)	(0.15)	(0.40)	(0.17)	**(0.10)**			
11	**Per cent skin**	0.16	−0.26	−0.49	0.24	−0.21	−0.14	−0.40	−0.26	−0.17	−0.04	**0.37**	0.48	−0.24
		(0.14)	(0.33)	(0.28)	(0.24)	(0.27)	(0.28)	(0.17)	(0.37)	(0.17)	(0.29)	**(0.16)**		
12	**Per cent abdominal fat**	0.00	0.11	−0.20	0.38	−0.16	−0.09	−0.26	−0.27	−0.29	−0.24	0.74	**0.48**	−0.25
		(0.14)	(0.29)	(0.28)	(0.23)	(0.28)	(0.28)	(0.19)	(0.37)	(0.16)	(0.27)	(0.19)	**(0.17)**	
13	**Per cent bone**	0.00	0.51	0.58	−0.03	0.44	0.26	−0.51	−0.26	0.36	0.32	−0.27	−0.19	**0.24**
		(0.18)	(0.31)	(0.31)	(0.31)	(0.28)	(0.31)	(0.22)	(0.45)	(0.21)	(0.38)	(0.34)	(0.33)	**(0.14)**

[a]Standard errors for phenotypic correlations ranged between 0.01 and 0.05.

Table 11.5. Genetic (r_g) and phenotypic (r_p) correlations between feed consumption adjusted for initial and final body weights and growth, feed and carcass traits. Heritability for adjusted feed consumption was 0.38 (0.12). (After Morris, 1996.)

Trait	r_g	s.e.	r_p	s.e.
Initial test weight	0.21	0.14	0.11	0.04
Feed consumption	0.81	0.10	0.44	0.03
Weight gain	−0.04	0.26	−0.08	0.04
Feed conversion	0.91	0.03	0.73	0.02
Plucked weight	0.19	0.26	0.03	0.05
Carcass weight	0.16	0.27	0.01	0.05
Percent breast	0.30	0.21	−0.02	0.05
Percent thigh	−0.35	0.37	−0.10	0.04
Percent drumstick	−0.57	0.15	−0.02	0.04
Percent wings	−0.34	0.24	−0.11	0.04
Percent skin	0.05	0.28	0.07	0.05
Percent abdominal fat	0.31	0.26	0.13	0.05
Percent bone	0.15	0.32	0.04	0.05

number of eggs set) and hatchability (HT; the number of hatching eggs producing viable chicks as a percentage of the number of eggs found to be fertile at the 18 day inspection).

There are strong genetic correlations between egg production and settable eggs and also between fertility and hatchability. The relationships between juvenile body weight at 30 days of age and a range of broiler and egg traits is shown in Table 11.9. Both fertility and hatchability are correlated with body weight but in opposite directions; fertility declines as bodyweight increases, but hatchability increases with increased juvenile bodyweight. This is the reason why body weight, fertility and hatchability are included in the breeding goal as part of a balanced breeding programme.

Fertility of broiler breeders is known to change over a typical laying period from 29 to 57 weeks of age, and both males and females are known to

Table 11.6. Heritability of broiler health traits. (After Szwaczkowski, 2003; Kapell *et al.*, 2012a.)t

Trait	Heritability	Reference
Antibody response to *E. coli*	0.03–0.10	Yonash *et al.* (1996)
Cecal carrier state of *S. enteritidis*	0.06	Berthelot *et al.* (1998)
Plasma cardiac troponin T	0.19	Bautista-Ortega *et al.* (1999)
Salmonella mortality %	0.12	Janss and Bolder (2000)
Tibial dyschondroplasia (4 weeks of age)	0.37	Kuhlers and McDaniel (1996)
Tibial dyschondroplasia (7 weeks of age)	0.42	Kuhlers and McDaniel (1996)
Tibial dyschondroplasia	0.10–0.27	Kapell *et al.* (2012a)
Long bone deformity	0.04–0.07	Kapell *et al.* (2012a)
Crooked toes	0.01–0.10	Kapell *et al.* (2012a)
Hock burn	0.06–0.09	Kapell *et al.* (2012a)

Table 11.7. Typical genetic correlation ranges between bodyweight (BW) and breast meat yield (BMY) with a range of health traits in broilers (After Avendaño *et al.*, 2017.)

Trait	BW	BMY
Leg bone deformity %	0.11 to 0.29	−0.10 to 0.21
Gait score	0.23 to 0.33	−0.03 to 0.20
Tibial dyschondroplasia %	0.04 to 0.30	−0.15 to 0.05
Foot pad dermatitis %	−0.17 to −0.04	−0.02 to 0.03
Crooked toes %	0.04 to 0.18	−0.03 to 0.04
Mortality %	0.11 to 0.31	−0.02 to 0.14
Cardiovascular function %	−0.21 to −0.10	−0.11 to 0.15

Table 11.8. Correlation matrix for egg production (EP), settable eggs (ST), fertility (FT) and hatchability (HT). Standard errors for genetic parameters are given in parentheses. (Phenotypic correlations above the diagonal; heritability on the diagonal (bold); genetic correlations below the diagonal.) (After Morris, 1996.)

Trait	EP	ST	FT	HT
EP	**0.30 (0.07)**	0.30	0.08	0.11
ST	0.75 (0.29)	**0.39 (0.07)**	0.09	0.19
FT	0.07 (0.18)	0.02 (0.37)	**0.20 (0.07)**	0.26
HT	−0.06 (0.16)	−0.15 (0.33)	0.51 (0.20)	**0.11 (0.07)**

Table 11.9. Genetic (r_g) and phenotypic (r_p) correlations between juvenile body weight and growth, carcass and female traits estimated by bivariate REML. Standard errors for genetic correlations are shown in parentheses. (After Morris, 1996.)

Trait	rg	rp
Conformation	0.50 (0.01)	0.41
Feed Consumption	0.08 (0.02)	−0.01
Weight Gain	0.09 (0.02)	−0.02
Feed Conversion Ratio	−0.09 (0.03)	0.03
Breast Meat Yield	−0.04 (0.03)	0.10
Abdominal Fat	0.17 (0.02)	0.08
Hen-Day Rate Egg Production	−0.01 (0.03)	0.00
Settable Eggs	0.00 (0.04)	−0.02
Fertility	−0.13 (0.05)	0.00
Hatchability	0.26 (0.03)	−0.04

affect a trait such as percentage of fertile eggs. Using random regression models over the laying period, Wolc *et al.* (2009) showed that heritability in females ranged from 7–9% and in males from 8–11%.

Methods and results of genetic evaluation in broilers

Any broiler breeding operation must attempt to reconcile a number of apparently opposing goals: breeding for improved early growth but maintaining adult function, breeding for health and welfare as well as production traits, breeding for both 'male' and 'female' traits. One option in this scenario is to breed a number of different lines and to concentrate on improving groups of traits within each line. This is illustrated in Figs 11.7 to 11.9. Lines may concentrate on male characteristics, female characteristics, fertility, growth or FCR. Whatever strategy a broiler breeding company adopts, it must also take account of health and welfare traits within each line. The obvious way to do this is to use multi-trait selection within each line incorporating appropriate selection index weights to achieve the desired outcomes.

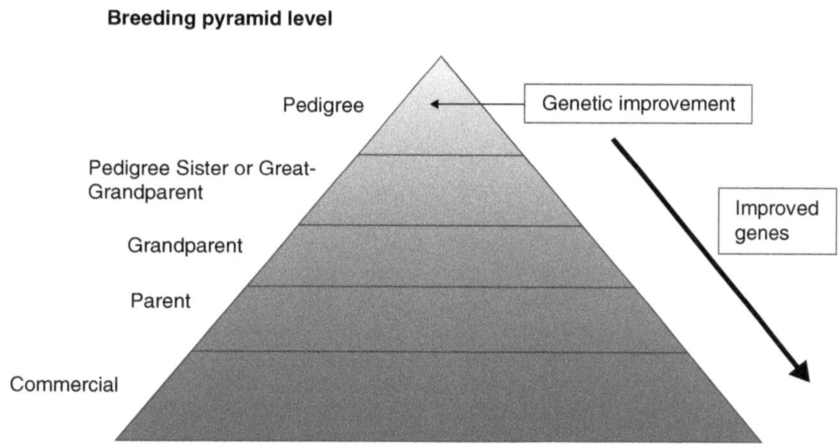

Fig. 11.7. An example breeding pyramid in the broiler sector.

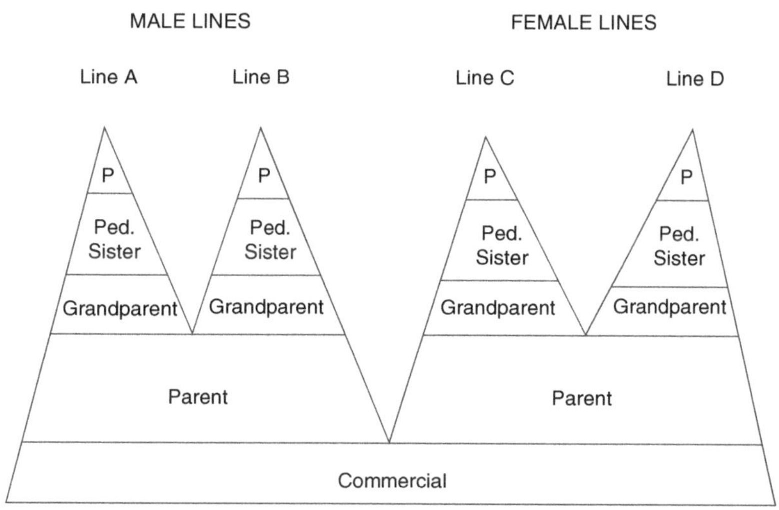

Fig. 11.8. A possible arrangement of genetic lines in a broiler breeding company showing two male lines and two female lines. P, pedigree level; Ped. Sister, pedigree sister level or great-grandparent.

Typically, a line comprises a pyramid (Fig. 11.7) with a number of strata starting with the pedigree flock at the top where all of the genetic selection occurs. This is followed by a number of multiplier layers which may comprise pedigree sister (or in some cases great-grandparent; GGP), grandparent, parent and commercial strata. Such a line may then be integrated with other lines to produce the final commercial bird, as shown in Fig. 11.8. Thus, selection for multiple traits occurs within a line and for differing sets of traits between lines. These are only brought together in the commercial birds at the base of the pyramid. There are a number of advantages to this structure. Maximal genetic progress is made within each line for a concentrated number of traits. The improved breeding stock is then multiplied up in two further strata before coming together in parent lines. This structure allows multiple objectives to be achieved and could allow integration of new lines, if these are developed independently and considered to be desirable for the overall objectives of the scheme. New traits might be incorporated in this way.

Figure 11.9 demonstrates the movement of genes on a generational basis and shows how long it takes to incorporate improved genetics at the commercial level. Typically, a structure of this type may have a generation interval of 10 months and so it may take just over 4 years to get improvements made at pedigree level to the commercial level. If one male bird is mated to 10 female birds at the pedigree level it will result in about 45 to 50 million improved birds at the commercial level. Thus, the multiplicative effect of the various strata is a very powerful tool for producing large numbers of improved birds in a relatively short time.

Use of indexes of overall economic merit in broilers

Poultry meat breeding goals have expanded enormously over the last 50 years, from being focused mainly on productivity during the 1950s to multidimensional breeding goals, including much higher emphasis given to efficiency (productive and environmental), robustness (including welfare and liveability), environmental adaptability and product quality (Fig. 11.10; Neeteson-van Nieuwenhoven *et al.*, 2013). The inclusion of welfare-related traits in chicken breeding goals is not a new feature. Antagonisms with production traits (e.g. live weight and yield) are dealt with within a multi-trait selection index framework using knowledge of the relevant genetic correlations (Kapell *et al.*, 2012a,b). One of the key features of such selection indexes is their ability to 'break' antagonistic correlations which may be contrary to the desired objectives of the breeding programme and allow progress in the desired direction in both traits. Neeteson-van Nieuwenhoven *et al.* (2013) illustrated how growth rate and leg strength can be improved simultaneously over the long term while the antagonistic genetic relationship between both traits holds within a year. This is in addition to the 'usual' benefits of index selection which are to make progress in all traits in relation to their economic importance or desired gains. Further examples of this are shown by Avendaño and Ralph (2018).

Most broiler breeding companies are multinationals and operate in a wide range of environments.

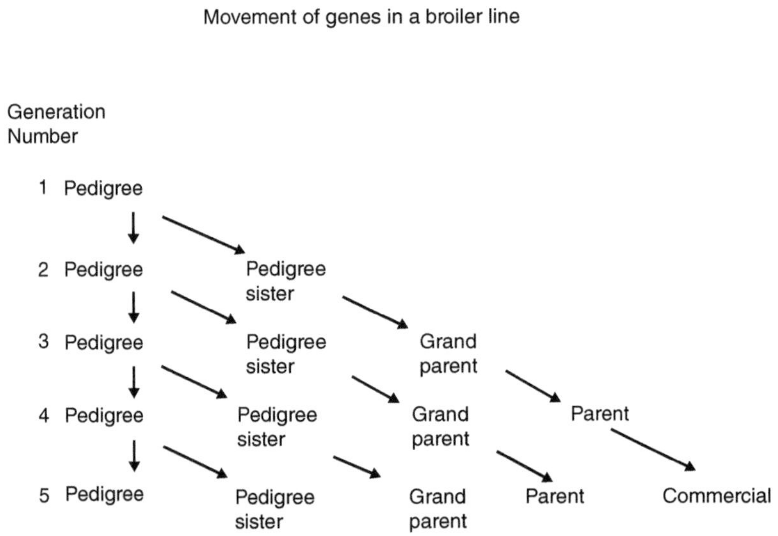

Fig. 11.9. Arrangement of lines in a possible broiler breeding programme showing the genetic lag between levels. Commercial level is four generations behind pedigree level in terms of average genetic merit. Pedigree sister level may be replaced by great-grandparent level in some situations.

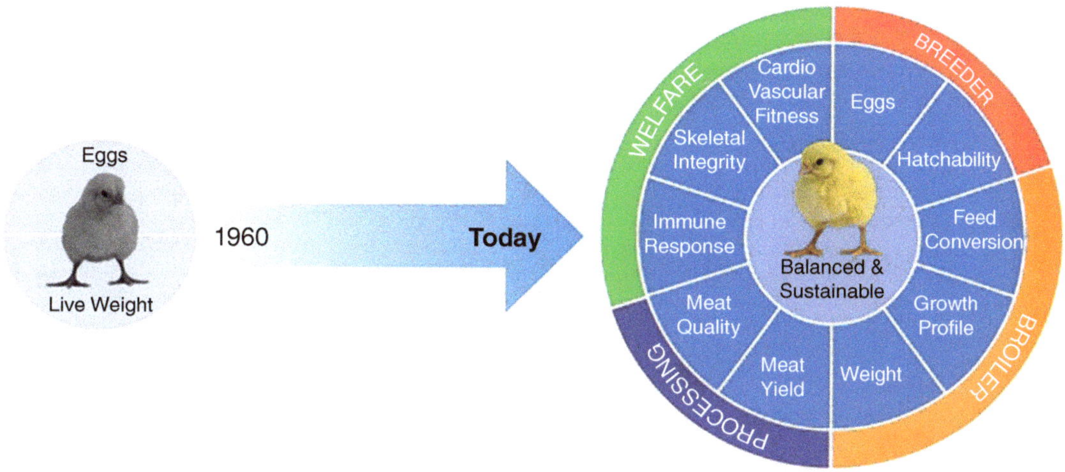

Fig. 11.10. Breeding goals in a modern broiler breeding company compared to the 1950s. (Provided by Aviagen.)

Thus genetic potential is expressed in a number of environments (production systems and geographical conditions) demonstrating that genotype-by-environment interactions (G × E) are an important consideration. Some breeding companies use a sib-testing strategy in which selection and recording takes place in highly-biosecure and high-input environments aiming to maximize expression of genetic potential. Meanwhile sibs are tested in a low-input environment with an emphasis on robustness including gut health, digestive, and immune function along with liveability, growth and uniformity (Avendaño and Ralph, 2018). These authors show two examples of G × E for broiler live weight and feed conversion rate at 35 days. The high- and low-input environments represented the top and bottom quartile of the environmental production conditions, respectively. While there was a positive correlation between breeding values across both environments of around 0.6–0.7, it was clear that the same biological trait should be handled as two different genetic traits to account for the G × E. The maximum absolute difference between both environments was about 250 g for live weight at 35 days and 70 g for feed conversion rate, which were biologically significant differences. This highlights the need to record the breeding goal traits in the relevant set of environments in which the commercial product will express its genetic potential. This inevitably adds to the cost of recording and running the breeding programme.

Future breeding goals in broiler production will become increasingly complex, using more traits and addressing multiple-trait antagonisms and multi-environmental trait expression. This extra complexity is not at odds with the sustainability of long-term genetic response. Hill (2016) concluded that continued genetic responses for production efficiency, while minimizing demand on resources without sacrificing animal health and welfare, are feasible with multi-trait selection including both fitness and production traits.

Using genomics in broiler production

In chickens, the first 3K single nucleotide polymorphism (SNP) chip was developed in 2005 with 3072 SNPs. In 2008, a 60K bead chip was developed that evenly covered the whole genome. To date, the only commercial array available is the Affymetrix 600K SNP Array. Studies of meat production quantitative trait loci have not revealed any sites with a major effect on the traits of interest and so genomic selection may be a more productive way forward. Some broiler breeders have introduced genomic selection in routine broiler breeding, with this contributing an extra 20–40% accuracy, depending on the trait. Currently, genomic selection is routinely used for breeding across broilers and layers, using single-step GBLUP (see Chapter 7). Wolc *et al.* (2016) highlight five reasons why the use of genomic selection in poultry differs markedly from, say, dairy cattle:

- **Generation intervals.** Traditional genetic improvement programmes in poultry already have short generation intervals (multiple overlapping generations per year with selection every 6 weeks in broilers, non-overlapping annual generations in layers). There is not much scope for further reducing generation intervals in broilers, as was the case for dairy cattle breeding, where bull generations can be halved in length.
- **Low value individual animals.** In poultry breeding there are very large numbers of selection candidates and high selection intensities, combined with low marginal revenues from a single selected bird. In poultry breeding programmes, tens of thousands of selection candidates are generated per line per generation, with only 1–3% of males selected for breeding. Thus, to be economically viable, genotyping has to be relatively inexpensive.
- **Inherent crossbreeding structure.** In poultry, genetic progress created in pure lines is disseminated through a comprehensive crossbreeding multiplication pyramid that has an impact on large numbers of commercial layers and broilers. Thus, a single line only contributes, say, 25% of the genes in commercial poultry compared with 100% in the purebred production systems in dairy cattle.
- **Lack of extensive AI.** In dairy cattle, large numbers of doses of semen are sold from the top bulls due to both the large volume of semen that can be produced by a bull and the ability to cryopreserve the semen for storage, shipment, and later use. In poultry, no efficient method of cryopreservation is available. Thus, highly selected males can be utilized only locally, and each cock can only inseminate a limited number of hens and for a limited time.
- **Limited pedigree recording.** In the poultry industry, there is no pedigree information on commercial descendants of the pure lines. Thus, it is difficult to track individual contributions to improved performance at the commercial level. In contrast, the dairy industry has pedigree and individual performance records on large numbers of commercial cows.

Because of limited opportunities to reduce generation intervals, the major benefit of genomic selection over pedigree-based evaluations in poultry is increasing the accuracy of estimated breeding values at puberty and for sex-limited traits. Accuracies of genomic breeding values (GEBVs) in broilers (and layers) for production, product quality, reproduction, and welfare traits have been evaluated using a range of statistical methods. In all these studies, GEBVs were more accurate than pedigree-based estimated breeding values (EBVs), but there was no clear superiority among the different genomic-based methods (as outlined in Chapter 7), i.e. no method consistently outperformed other methods across traits and populations. The use of genomic prediction is, however, particularly promising for traits that are sex limited, hard to measure, expensive to measure, or measured late in life. For traits for which phenotypes are not available on selection candidates (e.g. carcass traits), genomic predictions provide additional information and thus allow within-family selection, in contrast to traditional pedigree-based BLUP predictions (Wolc *et al.*, 2016).

Evidence of genetic change in broilers

The application of modern breeding methods in the broiler industry, described earlier and summarised by Tixier-Boichard *et al.* (2012), were responsible for rapid and consistent annual improvements in production traits, equivalent to about double the rate expected in other species such as cattle. This was helped by the much higher reproductive rate of chickens and the much shorter generation interval. As an example, Siegel (2014) quotes an improvement in FCR from 2.30 kg/kg in 1985 to 1.50 in 2010. Further evidence of large changes in broiler phenotypes from 1957 to 2001 was provided by Havenstein *et al.* (2003a,b) and are illustrated in Figs 11.11 and 11.12. In this study broilers bred in both 1957 and 2001 were compared on typical diets from both 1957 and 2001. Figure 11.11 shows how much broiler growth was changed by selection over a 25-year period. Some of this would be ascribable

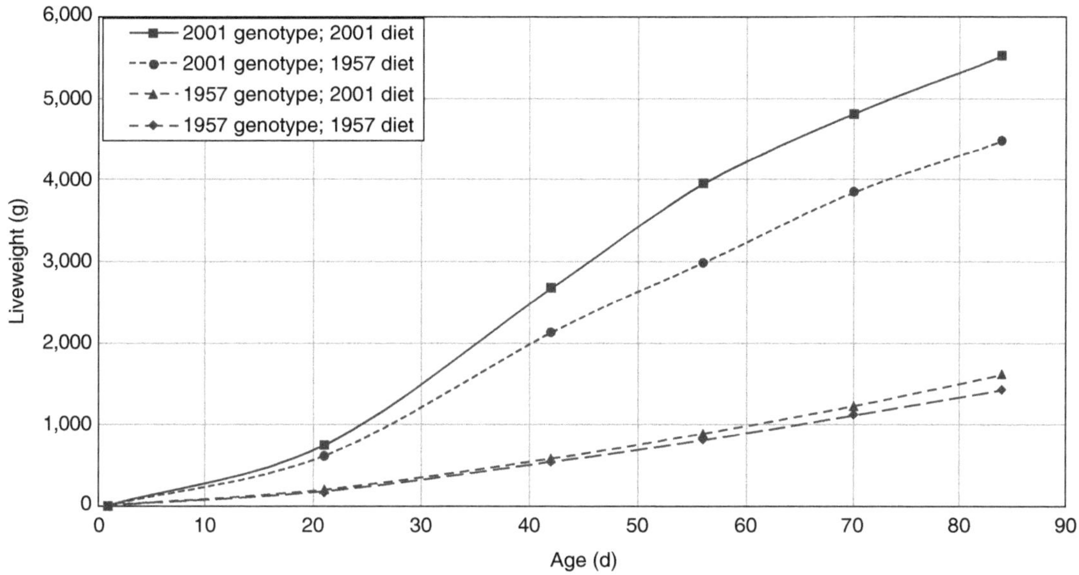

Fig. 11.11. Growth curves for broilers of two genotypes and fed on two diets, typical for 1957 and 2001. Male and female averages. (After Havenstein *et al.*, 2003a.)

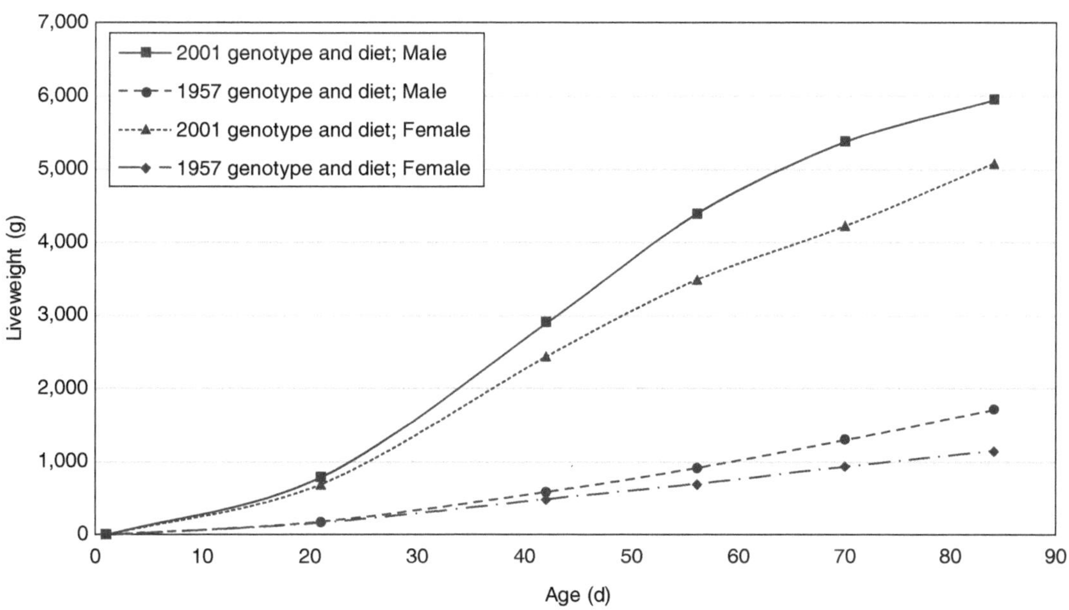

Fig. 11.12. Growth curves from male and female broilers from 1957 and 2001. (After Havenstein *et al.*, 2003a.)

to a change in feeding, but Fig. 11.11 shows this effect to be much less than the change in genetics. Havenstein *et al.* (2003a) conclude that genetics accounted for about 85–90% of the changes between 1957 and 2001 with nutrition only being responsible for 10–15%. This is another example of a genotype-by-environment interaction where the environment is the diet regime in this case.

Figure 11.12 uses the same data source to illustrate the difference between male and female broiler growth curves in both 1957 and 2001. As is commonly found in farmed species, males grow faster than females, but the effects of selection clearly affect both sexes in a similar way. Two things are of note here: females will need longer to finish than males for any given carcass weight, and females that go on to act as breeders will be very large and so will need to be managed appropriately to achieve the optimum fertility. Havenstein *et al.* (2003a) also present data for mortality and FCR on the same birds. Mortality appeared to be unchanged over the 44-year period but FCR was reduced (i.e. improved) considerably.

Carcass composition is an important trait in meat animals. Havenstein *et al.* (2003b) also described changes in carcass composition over the same 44-year period. One of the most dramatic changes was in breast meat yield at 43 days of age, which rose from about 11.5% of bodyweight to about 20% in 2001. There were similar differences over the range of ages reported. This trait is an important measure of one of the major products in broiler production. Carcass fat percentage shows a somewhat different pattern (Fig. 11.13) with 2001 genotypes always being fatter than the equivalently fed 1957 genotypes, the differences being of the order of 2% carcass fat.

Egg production

Welfare of layers

Several welfare issues are associated with layer production, including feather pecking. One of the past methods to control feather pecking has been beak trimming but recent legislation in several countries

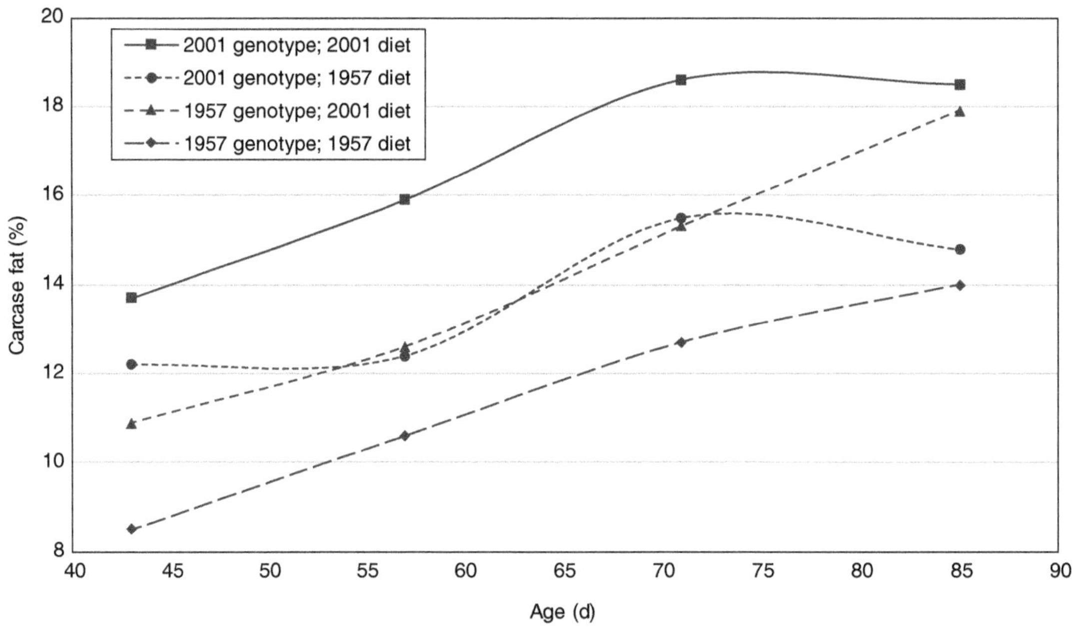

Fig. 11.13. The change in carcass fat % with age in broilers from 1957 and 2001 fed on two diets typical for these two years. (After Havenstein *et al.*, 2003b.)

has banned this practice. An alternative had to be found so both the genetics of feather pecking itself and also of beak shape have been investigated. Using new beak measuring technology, Icken *et al.* (2017) have estimated the heritability of beak shape at 45 weeks of age to be ~0.2 with some variation between lines. This suggests that some progress could be made in reducing beak length through genetic selection.

A further important welfare trait is the strength and integrity of bones in layers. Two approaches to measuring bone strength in live birds has been assessed (Andersson *et al.*, 2017). The first is a visual scoring system for keel bone deformation and the second used ultrasound of the humerus at 64 weeks of age. Both traits were shown to be heritable at about 0.2–0.3 in male lines and slightly less in female lines. Preisinger (2018) suggests that these measures of welfare show potential to be included in selection indexes.

Another important welfare issue, made more acute by the move towards cage-free layers in some countries, is the mortality and welfare impacts of cannibalism. Like several other welfare traits, it is possible to show that there is a genetic basis to this trait and so breeding to reduce it looks possible. However, additional considerations have to be made due to the social interactions involved in this trait; it is not just a trait of the aggressor but also the recipient. The genetics of cannibalism may therefore be considered in two parts; the direct effect of the bird's own survival and the social effect of the hen on its group, termed the associative effect (Ellen *et al.*, 2008). Using survival days as the trait of interest in laying hens, Ellen *et al.* (2008) found direct genetic effects to have a heritability of 0.02–0.10, but when associative effects were included this rose to 0.06–0.19. This suggests that the total genetic variability for survival was higher than the additive effects alone and that selection for reduced mortality using associative effects is a viable way forward.

Using data from the Weihenstephan Funnel Nest Box and the Electronic Pop-Hole, Icken *et al.* (2012) found similar heritabilities for egg number at the start of lay between cage and floor systems and a high genetic correlation between sibs in the two systems. The picture for egg number at peak production was somewhat different, with the correlation between the two systems being 0.18–0.44 depending on the flock of birds used.

These two new recording systems also allowed the recording of some novel traits: time spent in nest box, oviposition time and variation in the ovulation cycle. These data allowed the calculation of clutch size and the interval between consecutively laid eggs in each hen. These measurements were then used in the calculation of heritability vales for nesting behaviour traits. Icken *et al.* (2013) quote values of < 0.1 for time interval between eggs, 0.25 for clutch size, 0.23 for oviposition time and 0.27 for time spent in the nest. All traits showed usable genetic variation and could be added to selection goals.

Accuracy of recording is key for successful breeding programmes. Currently, breeding companies are mainly making use of group selection; so-called recurrent testing and reciprocal recurrent testing (selecting the pure lines on the performance of their crossbred progeny), to select modern breeds for liveability, less injurious pecking and social interaction in the field (Leenstra and Sambeek, 2014).

Layer breeding structures

The market situation outlined above is characterized by several types of housing systems, many

Table 11.10. The range of heritability estimates for layer traits estimated by REML methods using the animal model summarized from Szwaczkowski (2003).

Trait	Heritability range
Egg number (first half of laying period)	0.26–0.53
Egg number (second half of laying period)	0.16–0.40
Egg weight	0.34–0.70
Mean oviposition time	0.19–0.81
Mean within-sequence oviposition interval	0.42–0.55
Clutch number	0.11–0.22
Average clutch size	0.09–0.16
Egg density	0.34
Egg specific gravity	0.38
Eggshell colour	0.27–0.53
Eggshell thickness	0.33
Frequency of cracked eggs	0.58
Shell strength	0.27
Age at 1st egg	0.27–0.44
Fertility	0.03–0.15
Hatchability	0.05–0.24
Residual feed consumption	0.22

Table 11.11. Genetic correlations between egg production and a range of other traits in layers after Szwaczkowski (2003).

Trait 1	Trait 2	Genetic correlation
Egg number	Body weight	−0.26
	Feed cost	0.49
	Feed intake	0.28
	Residual feed consumption	−0.16/0.11
	Age at first egg	−0.41
Egg weight	Body weight	0.29/0.34
	Income feed cost	0.53
	Feed intake	0.39
	Age at first egg	0.09

countries with differing egg requirements and a range of environments being used. Since the layer breeding industry comprises a very small number of companies (< 4 at present) these companies necessarily maintain a large number of pure lines to cover all their likely selection objectives. As with broiler breeding, certain of these lines are combined in a four-way cross to produce the commercial birds producing eggs. The breeding pyramids shown in Figs 11.7 to 11.9 for broilers are basically similar to those used for layers, but with differences in the traits used as selection objectives within each line. Essentially, the heterosis generated by this crossbreeding is likely to generate an extra 10–40% productivity depending on the line and trait (Leenstra and Sambeek, 2014); the greatest effect being in the low heritability traits like survival and reproduction.

Methods and results of genetic evaluation in layers

There are many reports of genetic parameters for a wide variety of traits from layer breeds and lines by a range of different methods. For an extensive discussion of these, see the review by Szwaczkowski (2003). Key parameters from this review are summarized in Tables 11.10 and 11.11.

The heritability of various layer traits shown in Table 11.10 suggests that there is considerable usable genetic variation in many of these. As typical in many species, the heritability of the fertility traits is somewhat lower than that of production traits, but it is not zero.

The genetic correlations between egg number and weight with other layer production traits are shown in Table 11.11. These genetic correlations suggest that increasing egg number is genetically associated with lighter hens, higher feed intake and cost, little change in RFI and earlier age at first laying. Greater egg weight is genetically associated with larger hens, higher feed intake and cost, and little change in age at first lay. Note that this does not imply that breeding for one set of objectives will necessarily result in unfavourable correlated changes in other traits, as most breeding programmes use a multi-trait index approach that has the potential to 'break' unfavourable correlations and result in an overall balanced objective being met.

Use of indexes of overall economic merit in layers

A common theme in animal breeding is that selection for a single trait is rarely a useful economic route since correlated responses may negate the benefits of improving a single key trait, and profitability usually depends on multiple traits. Layer breeding is no exception to this general observation and there is plenty of evidence that breeding for egg production alone is not a viable option. Not surprisingly, therefore, breeding companies attempt to take a balanced approach to breeding by using multi-trait selection indexes in order to improve the profitability of the birds that they sell but in a manner that is sustainable in the long run. This effectively means also maintaining the health, welfare and environmental impact of the birds that they produce, and which meet the market needs of their consumers in the wide variety of markets that exist in the world. Clearly this is no mean feat and so clear objectives and good breeding structures are extremely important in this sector.

The actual selection indexes used and the economic weights (or similar) used by the major breeding companies are not in the public domain, though some of them discuss their selection objectives in a broad way (see Fig. 11.14). In addition to the use of multi-trait selection indexes with BLUP there is also the question of how much use is made of molecular genetic methods in the various companies, in particular genomic selection which has a range of advantages, not all of which may be pertinent in layer breeding programmes.

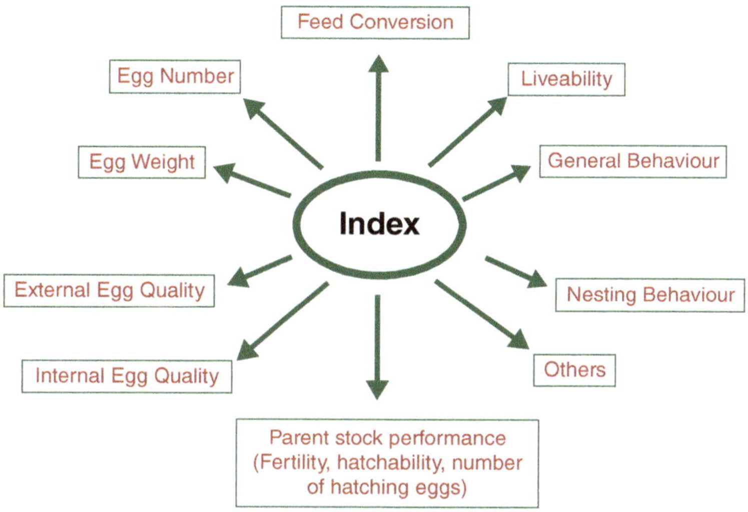

Fig. 11.14. A diagrammatic representation of selection objectives in a layer breeding company. (Provided by Professor Dr Rudi Preisinger.)

We can get some idea of the types of evaluation methods which may be relevant in layer breeding from some of the published studies in this field. Muir *et al.* (2014) discuss extensively the various options available to layer breeders for balancing direct and associated effects. Their conclusion is that kinship selection, i.e. selecting family groups rather than individuals, increases the robustness of birds. They suggest that kinship selection is easy to implement, does not require multi-trait genetic parameter estimates and so is robust to estimation errors and should improve both productivity and animal welfare but with lower levels of inbreeding. The drawback is that it needs individual animal records which may be difficult to achieve unless trap nests are available. Also, most breeding companies operate selection within lines and the effect of crossbreeding on associated effects is largely unknown.

Using genomics in layers

Using genomic selection in laying hens has the potential to supplement current schemes for a number of reasons. Traits which are important but not directly measurable on the candidate animals are one such reason. Traits like laying performance in males, crossbred performance, disease resistance and social interaction traits may be enhanced using genomic selection. Also genomic selection can be used with kinship selection to help differentiate between individuals in the group; something not possible with BLUP methods in this context (BLUP EBVs are based on parental average and so full sibs all get the same EBVs early in life). Genomic selection has another advantage in that selection can occur at a much younger age.

The study by Heidaritabar *et al.* (2014) is particularly instructive in this context. They compared genomic selection methods and BLUP using three lines of laying birds selected for seven generations. Most characteristics of the experiment were the same for all lines and methods, except that family sizes differed due to the requirements of the two estimation methods. They used a 15-trait selection index in both methods and evaluated the response to selection at the end of the trial. The GBLUP (genomic selection) methods always outperformed the BLUP methods with a 62% advantage to GBLUP in one line and an average of 39% across all lines. There was little discussion of which traits contributed to this increase between the two methods but there was an interesting comparison between the different regions found to contain altered allele frequencies between the two methods.

One of the outcomes of using genomic selection has been to highlight the need for continuing and improving the collection of phenotypes. Hence the discussion earlier in the chapter about new ways of measuring health and welfare traits in layers. Several authors have commented on how balanced selection across many traits in a multi-trait context is the key to improved poultry breeding (see, for example, Dawkins and Layton (2012) for broilers and Muir *et al.* (2014) for layers, and also Lawrence *et al.* (2004)).

Evidence of genetic improvement in layers

Some evidence of genetic trends in layer production, in the US, were suggested by Jones *et al.* (2001). Their approach was somewhat different to that of the broiler example given above, but they also used strains developed over different years and randomly bred to 'freeze' genetic progress. Three strains were used equivalent to typical birds in 1950, 1959 and 1972. They also included modern (in 1993) strains as a comparison. Birds were randomly distributed to different environmental treatments such as hatching, rearing, feeding and laying, to ensure no bias due to environmental factors. A range of layer traits were compared among the four strains of bird used, including bodyweight, onset of maturity, egg production, egg mass, egg weight, egg grades, feed intake, feed conversion ratio, mortality, feed cost and income. Not surprisingly, there were differences between the strains in all traits measured. Jones *et al.* (2001) concluded that comparing the 1950 and 1993 strains in the experiment, genetic selection had led to:

- smaller birds at the end of the laying period (–275 g);
- earlier sexual maturity (–28 days);
- greater hen-day egg production (+16%);
- greater egg mass (+15 g);
- greater egg weight (+7 g);
- higher feed consumption (+0.87 kg/bird/d);
- better feed conversion (0.107 g eggs/g feed; Note: this is the reverse measure compared to that used in broilers);
- higher feed cost (+US$0.66 /bird); and
- higher egg income (+US$5.17 /bird).

This study suggests that, as a result of genetic selection, birds are more efficient, more profitable and produce more of the eggs required by consumers. The only downside was the slightly higher mortality of the 'modern' birds. More recent studies of this sort are rare, but Hill *et al.* (2016) suggest that these trends were continuing, at least until 2009.

In Europe, Preisinger (2018) suggests that egg production has been rising by about two to three eggs per hen per year in a 13-month production cycle, body weight has been stabilized at an optimum level, and feed efficiency continues to improve. This is driven by a stable maintenance requirement and a constant daily feed intake. This is equivalent to about 0.45 kg less feed per kg of egg mass produced, which is equivalent to 57,000 t of feed or 8 million hectares of land over the last 20 years.

Practical Guidelines on Selection

In industrialized countries, most commercial poultry meat or egg producers buy replacement stock from suppliers which distribute genetic stock (either breeders or broilers) from the major breeding companies, or from rearers connected to suppliers. In the case of egg producers, most replacement stock are sourced as point-of-lay pullets. In broiler production, replacements are sourced as day-old chicks. The main opportunity for producers to influence genetic merit of their stock is via selection of the most appropriate supplier, or the most appropriate strain within supplier, for their particular circumstances (if this is not already specified by customers). This may require on-farm comparison of alternative strains.

In challenging environments in lower income settings, this matching of breed types or strains to systems is likely to be even more critical. Again, identifying suppliers, or strains within suppliers, that achieve desired levels of performance in key traits within the relevant environment will be crucial to success. While several major breeding companies supply stock bred for robustness and adaptability in low-input environments, resources such as the African Chicken Genetic Gains project may also help identify suitable breeding stock (African Chicken Gains Project, 2019).

Summary

- Poultry species have undergone dramatic changes over recent years in both the way they are kept and managed and also their genetic makeup.
- Chickens dominate the world production of both meat and eggs although a range of other species achieve importance in different regions and countries. Asia dominates the chicken production sector with countries like China and India producing large quantities of eggs and meat. The US is the largest producer of chicken meat worldwide and is ranked second for eggs.
- The demand for chicken meat is expected to rise dramatically in the future to meet the growing consumer demand for an economic source of protein. This is expected to be met by an increased industrial broiler sector worldwide.
- The majority of chicken products are produced in intensively managed systems with birds being purchased from a limited number of large, multinational breeding companies.
- Selection objectives of breeding companies include a wide range of traits covering groups of traits for weight, growth profile, feed conversion, breast meat yield, meat quality, heart/lung fitness, skeletal integrity, egg production (for breeding), hatchability and immune response.
- Egg production is also projected to rise dramatically in the near future with a demand growing by more than 1 Mt of eggs annually. This will require 50 M extra hens producing 20 kg of egg mass per hen, over a 20 to 76 weeks of age laying period.
- Consumer preferences for eggs vary considerably around the world and the legal framework for egg production varies by country. This has given rise to a variety of layer housing systems for egg production. Breeding companies need to be aware of all these factors and keep enough breeding lines to be able to satisfy each country's particular requirements.
- Layer breeding programmes contain a wide range of objectives covering egg production, egg quality, production efficiency, reproductive performance, functional traits, health, welfare and behavioural traits. New traits are required all the time as new breeding goals emerge and recent concerns over the environmental impact of layer production highlight the need to consider further improving feed conversion and digestibility.
- Despite there being over 1000 breeds of chicken in the world, modern production is based on relatively few lines produced by breeding companies. All commercial white egg chicken lines are based on the White Leghorn breed, whereas brown egg chicken lines were initially selected from Rhode Island Red and White Plymouth Rock. Broiler lines are derived from Cornish stock and the same dual-purpose breeds used for brown egg production (e.g. Barred Plymouth Rock, White Plymouth Rock, New Hampshire).
- Many of the key broiler traits are heritable and so can respond to selection (see above two points). Generally, the correlations between selection objective traits useful for broiler breeding, are favourable or neutral, and there is enough genetic variation to utilize in broiler breeding programme. Fertility is a key broiler trait and measurement and selection for both male and female fertility traits is required.
- Both layer and broiler companies use a complicated system of interlocking pyramids to arrive at the final commercial bird. Genetic improvement occurs at the top of the pyramid, the so-called pedigree level, and is multiplied up in a series of generations. Commonly four lines are used to produce a particular commercial bird. Two generations of crossing between two male lines and two female lines are required to produce the four-way cross commercial birds.
- The potential to multiply improved genetics in this structure is powerful with one male mated to 10 females in the pedigree flock resulting in over 45–50 million commercial birds in about 4 years.
- Breeding companies use multi-trait BLUP-based selection indexes within lines as the basis for identifying future breeding parents. This is often augmented with genomic selection methods, particularly for hard-to-measure-traits, and the greatest gain from using genomic selection is the greater accuracy of breeding values achieved.

- There have been dramatic changes in broiler performance over recent years due to intense selection, e.g. improvements in FCR from 2.30 kg/kg in 1985 to 1.50 in 2010, with equally dramatic changes in breast meat yield at 43 days of age, which rose from about 11.5% of bodyweight in 1976 to about 20% in 2001. Eighty-five to 90% of this change is due to genetics and only 10–15% due to improved feeding.
- Layer companies have had to introduce novel ways of measuring production in cage-free systems and to incorporate a number of new welfare and behavioural traits in their programmes.
- Layer production has also seen large increases in performance due to breeding. Over the period from 1950 to 1993 this includes smaller birds at the end of the laying period (275 g), earlier sexual maturity (28 days), greater hen-day egg production (16%), greater egg mass (15 g), greater egg weight (7 g), higher feed consumption (0.87 kg/bird/d), higher feed conversion (0.107 g eggs/g feed), higher feed cost ($0.66/bird) and egg income ($5.17/bird).
- There is no evidence that such changes in either broiler or layer production are slowing down and so they should be set to continue for many more years.

References

African Chicken Gains Project (2019) Available at: https://africacgg.net/ (accessed 21 October 2019).

Andersson, B., Icken, W., Cavero, D., Kaufmann, F. and Schmutz, M. (2017) Different methodologies to genetically improve the robustness of bones in layers. In: Bostvironnoi, C., Lessire, C. and Tixier-Boichard, M. (eds), *Proceedings of the 10th European Symposium on Poultry Genetics. St.* Malo, France, June 26-28, pp. 97. WPSA France Branch.

Avendaño, S. and Ralph, J. (2018) Economic challenges facing a global breeding company. *Proceedings of the 11th World Congress on Genetics Applied to Livestock Production* 23, 113. Available at: http://www.wcgalp.org/proceedings/2018 (accessed 16 June 2020).

Avendaño, S., Fancher B.I. and Neeteson-van Nieuwenhoven, A.M. (2017) Broiler breeding for sustainability and welfare – are there trade-offs? *Proceedings of the New Zealand Poultry Beyond 2023 Conference*, 16–20 October 2017.

Bailey, R.A., Watson, K.A., Bilgili, S.F. and Avendaño, S. (2015) The genetic basis of pectoralis major myopathies in modern broiler chicken lines. *Poultry Science* 94, 2870–2879. DOI: 10.3382/ps/pev304.

Bautista-Ortega, J., Maxwell, M.H., Robertson, G.W. and Bishop, S.C. (1999) Estimate of the heritability of, and the responses to selection for, plasma cardiac troponin T in broiler chickens. In: *Proceedings of the Poultry Genetics Symposium, 6–8 October 1999*, Mariensee, Germany, pp. 80–83.

Berthelot, F., Beaumont, C., Mompart, F., Girard-Santosuosso, O., Pardon, P. and Duchet-Suchaux, M. (1998) Estimated heritability to the resistance to cecal carrier state of *Salmonella enteritidis* in chickens. *Poultry Science* 77, 797–801. DOI: 10.1093/ps/77.6.797.

Dawkins, M.S. and Layton, R. (2012) Breeding for better welfare: genetic goals for broiler chickens and their parents. *Animal Welfare* 21, 147–155.

Ellen, E.D., Visscher, J., van Arendonk, J.A.M., and Bijma, P. (2008) Survival of laying hens: genetic parameters for direct and associative effects in three purebred layer lines. *Poultry Science* 87, 233–239. DOI: 10.3382/ps.2007-00374.

FAO (2015) *The Second Report on the State of the World's Animal Genetic Resources for Food and Agriculture*. Scherf, B.D. and Pilling, D. (eds) FAO Commission on Genetic Resources for Food and Agriculture Assessments, Rome. Available at: http://www.fao.org/3/a-i4787e.pdf (accessed 28 September 2020).

FAO (2019) FAOSTAT. Available at: http://www.fao.org/faostat/en/#data/QL/visualize (accessed 5 May 2019).

Groen, A.F. (2003) Breeding objectives and selection strategies for layer production. In: *Poultry Genetics, Breeding and Technology*. CAB International, Wallingford, UK, pp. 101–112.

Havenstein, G.B., Ferket, P.R. and Qureshi, M.A. (2003a) Growth, livability and feed conversion of 1957 versus 2001 broilers when fed representative 1957 and 2001 broiler diets. *Poultry Science* 82, 1500–1508. DOI: 10.1093/ps/82.10.1500.

Havenstein, G.B., Ferket, P.R. and Qureshi, M.A. (2003b) Carcass composition and yield of 1957 versus 2001 broilers when fed representative 1957 and 2001 broiler diets. *Poultry Science* 82, 1509–1518. DOI: 10.1093/ps/82.10.1509.

Heidaritabar, M., Vereijken, A., Muir, W.M., Meuwissen, T., Cheng, H.W. *et al.* (2014) Systematic differences in the response of genetic variation to pedigree and genome based selection methods. *Heredity* 113, 503–513. DOI: 10.1038/hdy.2014.55.

Hill, W.G. (2016) Is continued genetic improvement of livestock sustainable? *Genetics* 202, 887–881. DOI: 10.1534/genetics.115.186650.

Hill, W.G., Wolc, A., O'Sullivan, N.P. and Avendaño, S. (2016) Breeding for sustainability: maintaining and enhancing multi-trait genetic improvement. In: Burton, E., Gatcliffe, J., O'Neill, H.M. and Scholey, D. (eds), *Sustainable Poultry Production in Europe*. CAB International, Wallingford, UK.

Icken, W., Cavero, D., Schmutz, M. and Preisinger, R. (2012) New phenotypes for new breeding goals in layers. *World Poultry Science Journal* 68, 387–399. DOI: 10.1017/S0043933912000505.

Icken, W., Cavero, D. and Schmutz, M. (2017) Selection on beak shape to reduce feather pecking in laying hens. *Lohmann Information* 51, 22–27. Available at: http://www.ltz.de/en/news/lohmann-information/4-Selection-on-beak-shape-to-reduce-feather-pecking-in-laying-hens.php (accessed 9 September 2020).

Janss, L.L.G. and Bolder, N.M. (2000) Heritabilities of genetic relationships between salmonella resistance traits in broilers. *Journal of Animal Science* 78, 2287–2291. DOI: 10.2527/2000.7892287x.

Jones, D.R., Anderson, K.E. and Davis, G.S. (2001) The effects of genetic selection on production parameters of single comb White Leghorn hens. *Poultry Science* 80, 1139–1143.

Kapell, D.N.R.G., Hill, W.G., Neeteson, A-M., McAdam, J., Koerhuis, A.N.M. and Avendaño, S. (2012a) Twenty-five years of selection for improved leg health in purebred broiler lines and underlying genetic parameters. *Poultry Science* 92, 3032–3043. DOI: 10.3382/ps.2012-02578.

Kapell, D.N.R.G., Hill, W.G., Neeteson, A-M., McAdam, J., Koerhuis, A.N.M. and Avendaño, S. (2012b) Genetic parameters of foot-pad dermatitis and body weight in purebred broiler lines in 2 contrasting environments. *Poultry Science* 91, 565–574. DOI: 10.3382/ps.2011-01934.

Katanbaf, M.N. and Hardiman, J.W. (2010) Primary broiler breeding—Striking a balance between economic and well-being traits. *Poultry Science* 89, 822–824. DOI: 10.3382/ps.2009-00439.

Koch, R.M., Swiger, L.A., Chambers, D. and Gregory, K.E. (1963) Efficiency of food use in beef cattle. *Journal of Animal Science* 22, 486–494.

Kuhlers, D.L. and McDaniel, G.R. (1996) Estimates of heritabilities and genetic correlations between tibial dyschondroplasia expression and body weight at two ages in broilers. *Poultry Science* 75, 959–961. DOI: 10.3382/ps.0750959.

Laughlin, K. (2007) Poultry genetics – anticipating the industry requirements. *Lohmann Information* 42, 10.

Lawrence, A.B., Conington, J. and Simm, G. (2004) Breeding and animal welfare: practical and theoretical advantages of multi-trait selection. *Animal Welfare* 13, S191–196. Available at: https://www.ingentaconnect.com/contentone/ufaw/aw/2004/00000013/a00101s1/art00029 (accessed 28 September 2020).

Leenstra, F. and Sambeek, F. (2014) Breeding of laying hens. *Poultry Breeding. LowInputBreeds Technical Note*. Available at: www.lowinputbreeds.org. (accessed 12 July 2019).

Morris, A.J. (1996) An evaluation of genetic selection in a commercial broiler dam line. PhD Thesis, University of London, London.

Muir, W.M., Cheng, H-W. and Croney, C. (2014) Methods to address poultry robustness and welfare issues through breeding and associated ethical considerations. *Frontiers in Genetics* 5, 407. DOI: 10.3389/fgene.2014.00407.

Neeteson-van Nieuwenhoven, A-M., Knap, P. and Avendaño, S. (2013) The role of sustainable commercial pig and poultry breeding for food security. *Animal Frontiers* 3, 52–57. DOI: 10.2527/af.2013-0008.

OECD/FAO (2016) Available at: http://dx.doi.org/10.1787/agr_outlook-2016-en. (accessed 10 July 2019).

Preisinger, R. (2018) Innovative layer genetics to handle global challenges in egg production. *British Poultry Science* 59, 1–6. DOI: 10.1080/00071668.2018.1401828.

Sell-Kubiak, E., Wimmers, K., Reyer, H. and Szwaczkowski, T. (2017) Genetic aspects of feed efficiency and reduction of environmental footprint in broilers: a review. *Journal of Applied Genetics* 58, 487–498. DOI: 10.1007/s13353-017-0392-7.

Siegel, P.B. (2014) Evolution of the modern broiler and feed efficiency. *Annual Review of Animal Biosciences* 2, 375–385. DOI: 10.1146/annurev-animal-022513-114132.

Szwaczkowski, T. (2003) Use of mixed model methodology in poultry breeding: estimation of genetic parameters. In: Muir, W.M. and Aggrey, W. (eds) *Poultry Genetics, Breeding and Technology*. CAB International, Wallingford, UK, pp. 165–202.

Tixier-Boichard, M., Leenstra, F., Flock, D., Hocking, P. and Weigend, S. (2012) A century of poultry genetics. *World's Poultry Science Journal* 68, 307–321. DOI: 10.1017/S0043933912000360.

Wolc, A., White, I.M.S., Olori, V.E. and Hill, W.G. (2009) Inheritance of fertility in broiler chickens. *Genetics Selection Evolution* 41, 47. DOI: 10.1186/1297-9686-41-47.

Wolc, A. Kranis, A., Arango, J., Settar, P., Fulton, J.E. *et al.* (2016) Implementation of genomic selection in the poultry industry. *Animal Frontiers* 6, 23–31. DOI:10.2527/af.2016-0004.

Yonash, N., Leitner, G., Waiman, R., Heller, E.D. and Cahaner, A. (1996) Genetic differences and heritability of antibody response to *Escherichia coli* vaccination in young broiler chicks. *Poultry Science* 75, 683–690. DOI: 10.3382/ps.0750683.

Recommended Reading

Animal (formerly *Animal Science* and *Animal Production*; Journal of the British Society of Animal Science).

British Poultry Science.

Livestock Production Science.

Muir, W.M. and Aggrey, S.E. (2003) *Poultry Genetics, Breeding and Technology.* CAB International, Wallingford, UK.

Poultry Science.

Proceedings of the World Congresses on Genetics Applied to Livestock Production Available at: http://www.wcgalp.org/ (accessed 16 June 2020).

World's Poultry Science Journal.

12 Pig Breeding

Introduction

Pig meat, or pork, has been an important animal-source food for thousands of years. Domestic pigs first appeared in archaeological records independently in Anatolia and the Mekong valley around 9000 years ago (Frantz *et al.*, 2015; Groenen, 2016). They descended separately from the Asian and Eurasian wild boar (*Sus scrofa*) with multiple domestication centres including the Near East, Europe, China and South-East Asia, amongst other (Giuffra *et al.*, 2000; Kijas and Andersson, 2001; Larson *et al.*, 2005, 2007; Rothschild and Ruvinsky, 2011; Ottoni *et al.*, 2013; Yang et al., 2017). Multiple introgression events accompanied their domestication, including an introgression of Asian domestic pigs into European breeds during the 1700s and 1800s (Giuffra *et al.*, 2000; Kijas and Andersson, 2001).

More focused pig breeding has been undertaken since the 1960s with an acceleration of science-based breeding during the 1990s, due to higher computing power to process data and predict breeding values. Today, the modern pig breeding industry in developed countries is highly technology-based, capitalizing on the latest advances in genomic, phenomic and computing technologies. It is commonly structured as a three-tiered pyramid, with nucleus, multiplier and commercial levels, incorporating crossbreeding in the lower tiers. In fact, the wide-spread uptake of crossbreeding in the 1960s to 1990s was revolutionary in terms of increasing productivity of the pig sector (Kyriazakis and Whittemore, 2006). A number of multinational companies are key players in driving genetic gains. Pigs are also kept by smallholders, commonly in developing countries, where both the pig sector and breeding activities within it, are less structured.

In this chapter we first give some brief background to the global pig sector and pig-meat value chains. From here we discuss breeding objectives, pig breeds and lines, genetic improvement strategies for pigs (for both large-scale and smallholder systems) and use of pig reproductive technologies. The final section gives some practical guidelines for selection.

The Global Pig Sector

In 2016, the global pig population was estimated to be 982 million, with an estimated 118 million tonnes (Mt) of pig meat produced (FAO, 2019). At a continental level, the main producers of pig meat were Asia (56.1% of global pig-meat production in 2016), followed by Europe (24.5%) and North America (12.9%), see Fig. 12.1. The dominant pig-meat producing country was China, which produced an estimated 54 Mt of pig meat representing almost half (46%) of the global total and more than that for Europe and North America combined. The next ranked country for pig-meat production was the United States, which produced about one-fifth of the pig meat of China, see Fig. 12.2. The two top continents importing pig meat were Europe and Asia, which imported 3.7 and 1.5 Mt, respectively, and the two top continents exporting pig meat were Europe and North America, which exported 5.1 and 0.7 Mt, respectively. Looking toward the future (until 2030), the growth in demand for pork is expected to increase, largely in East Asia and the Pacific, and particularly China (FAO, 2011).

Pig-meat Value Chains

Pig-meat or pork value chains comprise all actors involved in pig-meat production, including the input suppliers, pig keepers/pig-meat producers, traders, processors and value adders, retailers and consumers. Value chains have competitive advantage when value is created for the consumer. This value can be created through a variety of ways, including meeting certain product specifications such as product quality or food safety, ensuring continuity of supply, and implementing measures to reduce costs, amongst others. Often this is achieved through collaborations

Genetic Improvement of Farmed Animals (G. Simm *et al.*)
DOI: 10.1079/9781789241723.0012

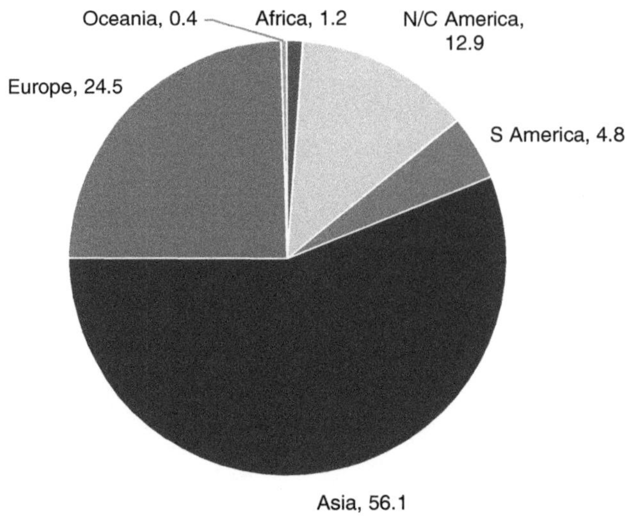

Fig. 12.1. Proportion of the world pig-meat production by continent in 2016 (%). (After FAO, 2019.)

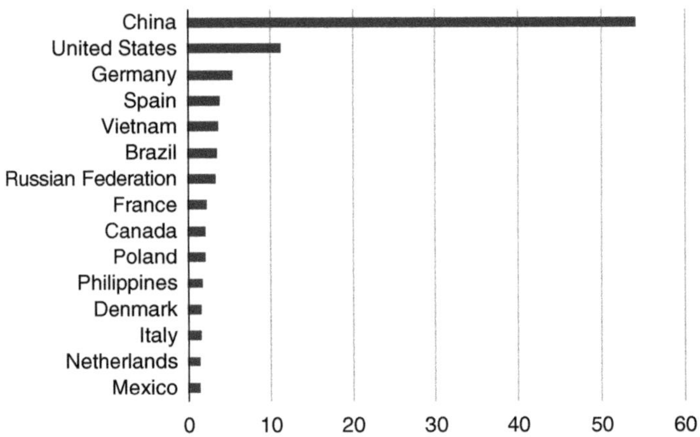

Fig. 12.2. Production of pig meat by the 15 highest-producing countries in the world in 2016 (million tonnes). (After FAO, 2019.)

or partnerships across the value chain. For the pig-meat value chains these vary in nature, from highly integrated, where one company carries out all or most of the value chain rôles, to semi-structured, such as where different actors meet and interact as part of multi-stakeholder platforms or forums, to largely informal. What is important from a genetic improvement viewpoint is that information flows across the value chains, including back from the consumers to the producer to those implementing the genetic improvement programmes, such that the producer can make an informed choice in the type of pig genetics to utilize and the breeders can ensure the improved pigs they are providing meet the various market and societal demands.

Breeding Objectives

Drivers of profitability

Pig production in commercial systems typical of developed countries is largely focused on generating economic benefits. Income is primarily generated from the sale of pigs, though there may be other sources of income, such as from the sale of manure. The main cost is that of feed: a 2016 report summarizing pig production costs in 17 countries indicated that feed accounted for 56–90% of total production costs (AHDB, 2017). Other costs include healthcare, biosecurity, breeding, replacements, labour, buildings, equipment, utilities, transport and professional fees.

There are many examples of how choice of pig genetics can influence profitability. For example, income from the enterprise depends on pig sale prices and pigs marketed per sow per year, in turn affected by sow reproductive performance, piglet growth rate, mortality rate, etc., all of which are heritable traits. Feed cost depends on several factors including feed use practices (waste reduction), feed price and feed efficiency, the latter also a heritable trait. Additionally, the choice of genetics influences the final product, for example, carcass and meat-quality attributes, and thus which markets will accept, or pay a premium for, the product.

In some societies, there is an increasing demand for pig meat to be produced from operations that have high pig welfare and health standards, and which reduce the negative environmental effects of pig-meat production while enhancing the positive. For a proportion of consumers this affects the acceptance or desirability of the product. In the most extreme examples, such requirements may be a barrier to consumer uptake and hence such standards impact on market access. In such situations, an economic value for such operations can be derived. In other circumstances there are wider societal benefits, such as reduced antibiotic use in the sector for which there is no direct economic value, but a point of difference for the marketing of pork produced in these systems.

In smallholder systems, pigs are recognized for their ability to transform low-value 'waste' (including kitchen leftovers as well as crop residues and by-products) into high-value animal-source food, either for sale or home consumption, within short time periods. Here the keeping of pigs is commonly to provide regular cash income, used to pay for household expenses such as food, clothing and school fees. Other reasons for keeping pigs in smallholder systems include the provision of manure (with the manure used as an input into crop production), insurance against emergencies (with pigs sold to pay for unexpected expenses, such as medical care), and fulfilment of cultural obligations (with pigs or their products used for particular festivals, etc.) (McOrist *et al.*, 2011; FAO, 2012; Tatwangire, 2014).

Historical and modern breeding objectives

Here we give a brief historical perspective of how breeding objectives have changed over time in commercial pig-production systems (using the example of Europe over the 1900s), discuss current breeding objectives as implemented by various breeding organizations, and finally consider how the breeding objectives may evolve in the future.

Pig breeding in Europe (Merks, 2000) was initiated in the early 1900s, by the gradual set-up of local and regional breeding programmes. Initially, the focus was largely to maintain or improve breed characteristics like type and coat colour. Attention was later placed on traits that were easy to identify and measure, such as leanness (via backfat thickness) and growth (daily gain), such that by the mid-1900s considerable genetic progress had been made in these traits. Notably though, little emphasis had been placed on reproductive performance, mainly because at the point of selection very little information was available to make such a choice. Crossbreeding was widely adopted in the 1960s through to the 1990s, resulting in specialization into sire and dam lines and breeding programmes within them. Pig-breeding companies also emerged during this time. In the later 1900s, it was recognized that selection for reproduction could be profitable, and dam lines started to be selected for litter size (Haley *et al.*, 1986) as appropriate statistical methodology became available. Farms also started to specialize into pure-breeding, multiplication and crossbreeding, and commercial enterprises, enhanced by the introduction of artificial insemination. Breeding goals began to widen, including profit-related traits like daily gain, feed efficiency and litter size, and, since about 2000, meat quality and piglet vitality, amongst others. Similar trends occurred in other developed country pig-production systems outside of Europe.

Today, breeding organizations, including both breeding companies and national breeding programmes, have sophisticated breeding objectives. These typically focus on reducing meat production costs as well as increasing meat quality, both in terms of processing and consumer acceptability. Some examples of breeding objectives for different breeding organizations are given in Table 12.1.

Table 12.1. Examples of breeding objectives from different pig-breeding organizations.

Breeding organization	Breeding objective (web reference)
Canadian Swine Improvement Program	The purpose of the Swine Improvement Strategy is to increase the competitiveness of the Canadian pork industry by maximizing genetic improvement (http://www.ccsi.ca/genetics/guide.htm)
DanBred	The DanBred breeding objective is based on the production of finishers which integrates weaner and finisher production with an emphasis on production economy (https://danbred.com/en/avlssystem-uk/breeding-objectives-of-the-future/)
Hypor	The Hypor breeding programme is focused on balanced breeding as the way to maximizing total system profitability (https://www.hypor.com/en/about-us/)
JSR genetics	Our aim is to breed pigs that perform profitably for the producer and create pork which is of exceptional eating quality for the consumer (http://www.jsrgenetics.com/about-us.php)
PIC	The PIC Genetic Improvement Programme is focused on maximizing profit potential of PIC genetics in our customers' operations (http://gb.pic.com/resources/articles_genetics/ pic_is_selecting_for_real_life_robust_performance.aspx).

The full breeding objective is typically expressed in the commercial tier, through the crossing of the sire and dam lines.

Note that the breeding objectives as presented in Table 12.1 are for the overall breeding programme, with different breeds or lines typically having their own more specific breeding objectives depending on their intended use. In general, sire breeds or lines are selected for genetic improvement in production traits, and dam lines for genetic improvement in production as well as reproduction traits. As an example of breeding objectives for the specific sire and dam lines we use that of the breeding company DanBred (https://danbred.com). Their overall breeding objective emphasizes production economy (see Table 12.1). They describe traits included in the breeding objective for their dams lines, DanBred Landrace and DanBred Yorkshire, used for sow production, as: daily growth, to shorten the time from production to slaughter and decrease the production cost; feed conversion, to increase finisher feed efficiency and reduce production costs; lean meat percentage, for good market price; conformation, to reduce risk of culling due to leg or back problems; slaughter loss, to increase carcass weight as percentage of live weight; longevity of sows, defined as the likelihood a sow will be mated after the first litter; and the number of living pigs in the litter five days after farrowing, as an indicator of sustainable reproductive output. Traits included in the breeding objective for their sire line, DanBred Duroc, used for finisher production, are described as daily growth, feed conversion, lean meat percentage, conformation and slaughter loss (for the same reasons as given above), and male fertility, as the number of living pigs in the litter.

The inclusion of pig welfare and societal traits in breeding objectives has received increasing attention over the last 10 to 15 years, in response to the demands of consumers and citizens. For example, breeding for robustness traits, such as sow longevity, farrowing and preweaning survival of piglets, is seen as being important to balance the unfavourable physiological consequences that could arise from breeding for productivity and efficiency alone (Hermesch *et al.*, 2015; Turner *et al.*, 2018). Non-castration of pigs is becoming more commonly practised by some producers, both to increase animal welfare and because entire males have better feed efficiency than castrated males. This, however, can lead to boar taint (an undesirable smell and taste in the meat from entire boars), which is now being genetically selected against. For instance, the breeding company Topigs Norsvin indicates it has included the reduction of boar taint in the breeding goals of all of its lines (Topigs Norsvin, 2018a). Breeding for social behaviour, such as less aggression, tail biting and savaging of piglets, is also being explored (Kanis *et al.*, 2005; Turner, 2011; Topigs Norsvin, 2018b; Turner *et al.*, 2018).

With increasing demand, in some societies, for pig meat to be produced from operations with high pig welfare and health standards, and which reduce the negative environmental effects of pig-meat production while enhancing the positive, it is possible that future breeding objectives may broaden from being largely focused on profitability to balancing a focus on profit, animal welfare and health, and environmental sustainability.

Breeds and Lines Used in Pig Production

A 2015 report on the state of the world's animal genetic resources for food and agriculture (FAO, 2015) identified 543 local breeds of pigs and 59 transboundary breeds of pigs currently existing. Here local breeds are defined as those found within one country only, while transboundary breeds are found within more than one country. Of these breeds, 16% were reported as being at some level of risk of extinction, 18% not at risk, and the remaining 66% of unknown risk status. An additional 107 extinct breeds were reported. As this was based on data voluntarily supplied by countries, and not all countries participated or provided full data, it is likely an underestimate of both the number of breeds currently existing and those that have become extinct.

A relatively small number of breeds dominate commercial pig production, and many others are of interest for a variety of reasons. A limited selection of these are described below, with information largely sourced from a pig-focused website called The Pig Site (www.thepigsite.com) and the Oklahoma State University Breeds of Livestock website (www.ansi.okstate.edu/breeds/swine/). For an expanded overview of the world's pig genetics, see Rothschild and Ruvinsky (2011).

The Large White breed of pig originated in Britain, the result of crossing between the white pigs from Yorkshire and other breed(s). They were first recognized in 1868 and became popular across the developed world before the end of the 1800s. Today the Large White is well established in most pig-producing countries and is the most numerous of the pig breeds globally. Large Whites are recognized for both their ability to perform under a range of environmental conditions as well as suitability for intensive and largely environmentally-controlled production systems. Large White sows are recognized for their strong maternal ability, high prolificacy, high milk production, sound legs and feet, and long productive lives. They are often crossed with Landrace to produce F_1 sows for use as a parent female in the commercial sector. Large White sires, superior for growth and lean meat percentage, are used in many terminal sire breeding programmes. Pigs of the Large White breed are large framed, with long bodies and legs. They have white or pink skin and white hair. Their faces are slightly dished and ears erect (Fig. 12.3). In the USA and Canada this breed is often referred to as the Yorkshire.

The Landrace breed of pig originated in Denmark in 1895 as a cross between the Large White and native pig breeds. The cross was then genetically improved under the control of the Danish government and helped establish Denmark as a leading bacon-exporting country. The Landrace pig was not exported from Denmark until the mid-1900s. Currently, the Landrace is well established in many pig-producing countries, used in both intensive and extensive pig-farming systems. Many different strains of Landrace exist, such as the Danish, Swedish, British, American, and so on. The Landrace breed is recognized for its prolificacy, for farrowing large pigs and for heavy milk production. They are often crossed with the Large White to produce F_1 sows for use as a parent female in the commercial sector. Pigs of the Landrace breed are long bodied. They have mostly white skin and white hair, but several strains show more or less abundant black spots. Their ears are large and droop with a forward slant.

The Duroc breed of pig originated in the United States in the early 1800s as a cross between the two red pig strains, the Duroc of New York and the Jersey Red of New Jersey. The origin of the red pig strains in the United States is not well documented,

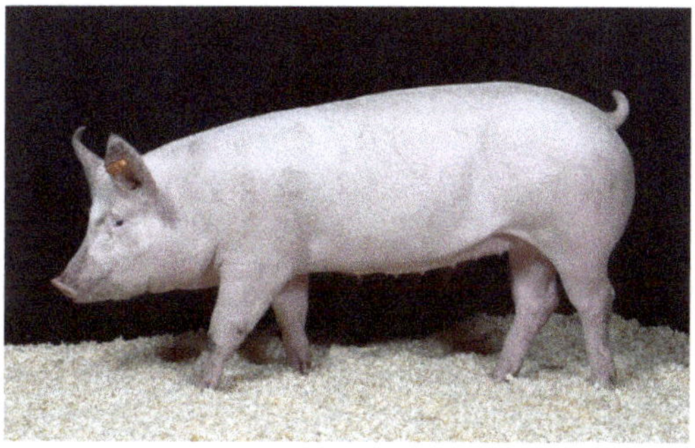

Fig. 12.3. The Large White breed of pig. (Photo credit: JSR Genetics.)

though there are some suggestions that one source was the Guinea coast of Africa. The Duroc is recognized for its ability to grow quickly and its hardiness, doing well in both warm and cold climates. Durocs are often used in crossbreeding programmes as a terminal sire. Pigs of the Duroc breed are medium to large in size and length, and also muscular. They are golden red to deep red in colour, with a thick winter coat that moults in the summer. Their faces are slightly dished and the ears are small and drooping. White Duroc are mostly crosses of Duroc with white breeds, though some animals referred to as White Duroc may contain no Duroc genes.

The Pietrain breed of pig originated as a Belgian Landrace strain in Pietrain, Belgium. Details of its origin are not known, but it become popular in the mid-1900s. The Pietrain breed is recognized for its very high yield of lean meat, and thus ability to improve the carcass produced for lean pork markets. It is most commonly used as a terminal sire, either pure or as an input into a crossbreed or synthetic. The latter is often preferred because the purebred Pietrain contains a deleterious allele variant at the halothane gene which results in animals becoming easily stressed and prone to sudden death, such as during transport. The inclusion of other breeds in the synthetic line means that the undesirable variant can be selectively bred out of the line. The breed is not commonly used in maternal lines due to its poor mothering abilities and milk production. Pigs of the Pietrain breed are medium in size, short in the legs and stocky; the loins and hams are very muscular. They are white with black spots, with rings of light pigmentation carrying white hair around the black spots (often referred to as piebald markings). Their ears are carried erect.

Taihu pigs are a group of Chinese pigs, originating from the Taihu valley of Eastern China. Meishan pigs are a sub-group of the Taihu pigs. Taihu pigs, and particularly the Meishan, have received a lot of attention due to their high prolificacy. Currently, Taihu pigs are used locally in major pig-producing areas around the Taihu valley (for example, in Jiangsu province, there are an estimated 320,000 TaiHu sows; AGTR, 2020). A small number of Taihu pigs can also be found elsewhere (e.g. Meishan conservation programmes in the United States; American Meishan Breeders Association, 2020). As mentioned, the Meishan pig is recognized for its high prolificacy, perhaps being one of the most prolific breeds in the world, with early puberty (2.5 to 3 months of age) and large litter sizes (15 to 16 piglets). The mechanisms behind their high prolificacy have been well studied (Bazer *et al.*, 1988; Haley and Lee, 1993; Li *et al.*, 2017). Meishan pigs are also extremely docile and sedentary, slow growing and able to consume large amounts of roughage. Phenotypically, they are small to medium sized with wrinkled black skin and drooping ears (Fig. 12.4). They are mentioned here as an example of a pig breed that is valued locally and of interest internationally due to specific trait characteristics. The Meishan breed has been incorporated into the dam lines of several breeding companies.

Breeding companies also develop their own sire and dam lines, which are pure breeds, or hybrids of two or more breeds selected for certain characteristics. Common breeds contributing to dam lines are the Large White and Landrace, while common breeds contributing to sire lines are Duroc and Pietrain. The exact details of the selection process used in generating these lines is usually not shared by the breeding companies, though descriptions of the lines are given and performance information in various production environments is usually available. For example, the Camborough® developed by the breeding company PIC is a dam line derived from the crossing of Landrace and Large White. It is described by PIC as having (PIC, 2020):

> prolificacy with uniform vigorous piglets, excellent mothering abilities, high birthweight-low prewean mortality; efficiency with few gilt development days, lower cost per weaned piglet from less feed usage and more lifetime pigs marketed per gilt, and weaned pigs with superior feed conversion and higher daily gain; and robustness with low sow mortality and long productive life.

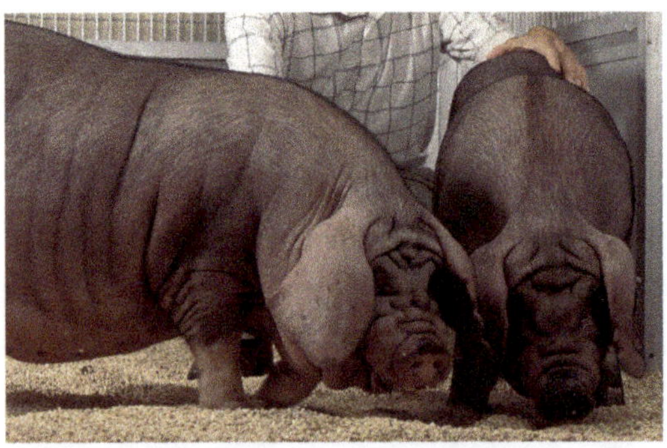

Fig. 12.4. The Meishan breed of pig. (Photo credit: USDA.)

As another example, Norsvin Duroc developed by the breeding company Topigs Norsvin is a sire line that is a purebred Duroc. It is described by Topigs Norsvin as having (Topigs Norsvin, 2020a):

> Excellent finisher performance with low feed conversion, high growth rate and high pig survival; and excellent meat quality with above average intramuscular fat levels.

Genetic Improvement Strategies within Large-scale Pig-production Systems Typical of Developed Countries

Overview

As mentioned previously, in many of the larger-scale pig-production systems typical of developed countries, pig genetic improvement currently operates as a three-tiered pyramid (Fig. 12.5). The tiers are referred to as nucleus, multiplier and commercial, with more animals in the multiplier tier compared to the nucleus, and significantly more animals in the commercial tier compared to the multiplier. Pig enterprises within the nucleus tier are responsible for generating the genetic gain, typically achieved through the breeding of separate sire and dam lines (each of which can be from one or more breeds) that have specific characteristics. Pig enterprises within the multiplier tier breed and multiply animals from the nucleus to produce large numbers of breeding animals. Crossbreeding of different lines is commonly practised as part of this multiplication stage. Commercial tier enterprises use maternal line females from the multiplier tiers, and sire line boars (most commonly semen) from either the multiplier or nucleus tiers, for piglet production. Piglets are then finished (i.e. grown to meet specific market specifications) and slaughtered. Pigs within the nucleus, multiplier and commercial tiers of the pyramid are often referred to as great grandparent (GGP), grandparents (GP) and parents (P), respectively. The genetic lag, or time delay between genetic improvements in the nucleus reaching the commercial tier, is usually 3 to 5 years (Rothschild and Ruvinsky, 2011).

The intent of the crossbreeding scheme is to create pigs that meet the needs and preferences of those in the commercial sector. Use of a three-breed (or line) terminal cross is common, where the commercial (slaughter) pigs are produced from an F_1 sow (itself produced from the cross of two breeds or dam lines) crossed to a different breed (or sire line) of boar. Note, however, that given the dam and sire lines are often hybrids of multiple breeds, the actual number of breeds contributing to the pig-breeding programme can be numerous (most commonly between 3 and 6, and up to 12).

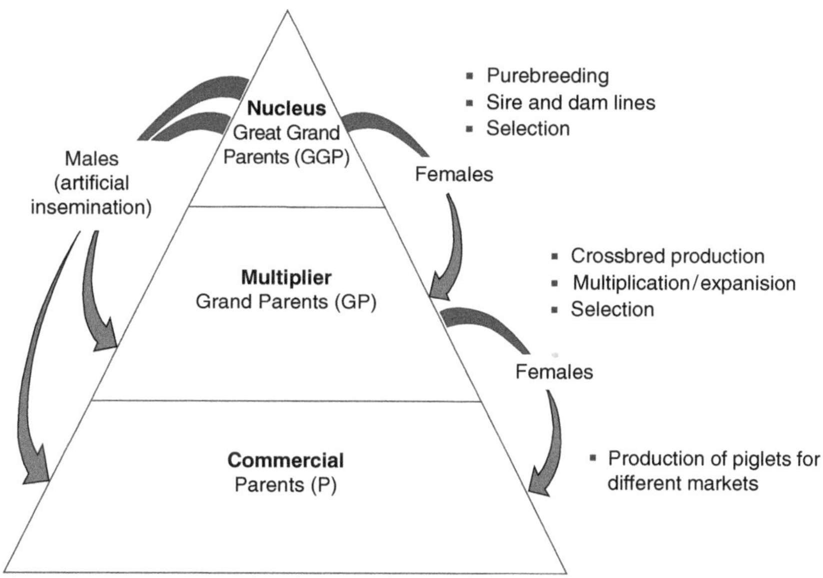

Fig. 12.5. Pig-breeding pyramid.

The crossing system takes advantage of both heterosis and breed complementarity. As a simplified example, say an F_1 sow (from a cross of dam lines A and B) improved for litter size and mothering ability is crossed with a sire (from sire line C) improved for growth and carcass quality (Fig. 12.6). Here, the crossing of these will result in a large litter as well as piglets that grow fast and have good carcass characteristics. The breed complementarity is evident, and both the slaughter piglets as well as crossbred sows also benefit from full heterosis. In reality, the breeding objectives for the maternal and terminal sire lines are more complex than this, typically including a larger number of traits (see above).

It is of note that performance information from all tiers of the pyramid, including that of the crossbred animals in the multiplier and commercial tiers, is becoming more commonly used in making breeding decisions on nucleus animals. This is because the genetic correlation between crossbred and purebred performance, while positive, is often less than one (Godinho *et al.*, 2019; Lutaaya *et al.*, 2001), meaning that the best animals for crossbred performance will differ from those for purebred performance.

The variations on the above general scheme are numerous. For example, a single enterprise may combine activities of two or more tiers, such as commercial and multiplication, or multiplication and nucleus, or a commercial enterprise may only produce piglets or finish piglets. There are also variations on the crossbreeding scheme, including: the use of different numbers of sire or dam lines as crossbred parents of the slaughter progeny (e.g. a four-breed terminal cross where crossbred boars are mated to crossbred sows; breeding programmes using up to four sire or five dam lines); and the use of different types of crossbreeding schemes such as rotational or rota-terminal (a blend of rotational and terminal) for own gilt replacement.

Systems of testing

Breeding companies

A number of companies provide much of the world's improved pig genetics, with the improved pig lines targeted for specific production systems and environments. Some major companies include: Babcock genetics (http://www.babcockgenetics.com/); Choice Genetics (http://choice-genetics.com); Danbred (https://danbred.com); Fast Genetics (http://fast-genetics.com/); Genesus Genetics (https://www.genesus.com/); Hypor (https://www.hypor.com); JSR genetics (http://www.jsrgenetics.com/); PIC (http://www.pic.com/); and Topigs Norsvin (https://topigsnorsvin.com/). These are often multinational, with pig-breeding operations and/or pig germplasm distribution in more than one country. As discussed in more detail below, they routinely use best linear unbiased prediction (BLUP), BLUP with marker or gene-assisted selection or genomic BLUP (GBLUP), including single-step, to estimate breeding values, and may also use mate allocation software to maximize rates of genetic gain while minimizing inbreeding. The number of traits measured is typically large.

The companies usually do not disclose the full details of their genetic improvement strategies, though many give an overview, often on their

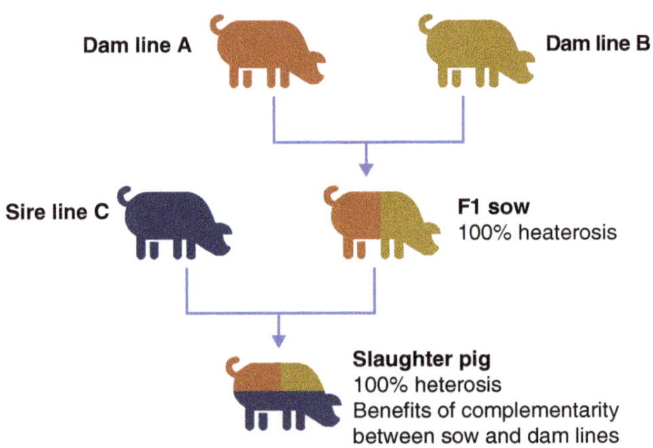

Fig. 12.6. Common three-way pig crossbreeding scheme.

websites. For example, one of the websites of PIC (https://www.picnz.co.nz/genetic-improvements) indicates 'PIC's genetic improvement programme utilizes the variation available in 17 different line populations worldwide. The performance of these lines, and the products derived from them, is measured in many different environments around the world'. Further, it says 'PIC now utilizes CBV™ (Crossbred Breeding Value) to calculate the breeding value of PIC boars. This innovative system adds additional information from the commercial level to the boar's own test performance and PICmarq® genotypes....This means that PIC now selects its pure lines and parent boars based on how their progeny are expected to perform in commercial conditions, rather than on performance of lines in the pristine GN environment' (PICmarq® genotypes refers to genetic marker information used in selection, GN refers to genetic nucleus). To support this, PIC uses a database called PICtraq™ which is described as storing 'performance information collected through the production pyramid; carcass and meat-quality performance from nucleus animals; genetic marker information acquired through PICmarq® technology; and commercial performance information from the GN Crossbred Programme'. It notes that 'information is entered into PICtraq™ 24 hours per day from nucleus and multiplier farms on every continent', and that 'PIC routinely measures 49 traits affecting pig production'.

Another major pig genetic improvement company, Topigs Norsvin, also share some information on its genetic improvement strategy on its website (https://topigsnorsvin.com/). They state that 'our ambition is to double genetic progress to 4% by working better with big data than anyone else, understanding genomics and using full-sequence information...Our next steps are using DNA patterns for precision farming and genomic management as well as new technology to faster increase and disseminate the frequency of desired functional genes within our populations' (https://topigsnorsvin.com/innovations/innovation/). They also use data from all levels of the breeding and production pyramid in calculation of their breeding values (Oldenbroek and van der Waaij, 2014).

Breeding companies are often very fast to adopt the latest breeding and associated technologies (Knap *et al*., 2001). They are highly competitive with many investing heavily in research to develop new technologies or approaches that help them maintain their competitive edge.

National genetic improvement programmes

While pig-breeding companies dominate pig genetic improvement, national genetic improvement programmes exist in a number of countries, including Austria, Canada, France, Italy and Switzerland. They essentially act as a dispersed nucleus, with animals from different breeding enterprises jointly evaluated. This requires that genetic linkages exist between animals in the different enterprises. As an example, in Canada the national swine genetic improvement programme (called the Canadian Swine Improvement Program) is coordinated by the Canadian Centre for Swine Improvement (CCSI), a national non-profit corporation (https://www.ccsi.ca/). The CCSI maintains a national database of pig performance records, with data including that generated on-farm, at testing stations, and at packing plants. It performs regular (biweekly) genetic evaluations for 18 traits including growth and feed efficiency, carcass, meat quality and sow productivity. It also calculates dam- and sire-line selection indexes, and customized indexes to suit the needs of particular clients can also be generated. Genomic selection was introduced into the programme in 2017, using a 50K single nucleotide polymorphism (SNP) chip. In 2016, more than 90,000 pigs were evaluated (CCSI, 2017).

Breed societies

Pig breed societies have historically had an important place in the maintenance of breed characteristics and herd books/pedigree, and many still exist today, either for single breeds or groups of breeds. Over time the rôle of breed societies has broadened, with functions now including breed promotion, issuing certificates of breed purity, maintenance of DNA banks, various research and capacity-building activities and, in some cases, support to genetic improvement through, for example, links to national genetic breed improvement schemes (Rothschild and Ruvinsky, 2011).

Traits recorded

The selection criteria used in different pig-breeding programmes will depend on the breeding objective as well as choice of selection criteria for each trait within the breeding objective, among other factors (Knap, 2014). Some examples of traits recorded are given below; note: due to the very high number of traits the list is not comprehensive.

Traits measured in relation to reproductive performance of the sow include litter size (number of piglets in the litter) and litter weight (weight of all piglets in the litter), as well as the number stillborn. In some cases, individual piglet birth weight is measured to allow calculation of variation in birth weight (within litters). Piglet survival to weaning is also commonly recorded, as are litter weights. Other traits include age at first farrowing, interfarrowing interval, farrowing rate, weaning to oestrus or conception interval, number of lifetime litters, days of sow life, teat number, and sow condition or weight loss during lactation. In relation to reproductivity of the boars, sperm quality (including viability) and quantity are often measured. Traits measured in relation to performance or production include growth rate and feed intake (used to calculate feed conversion ratio or feed efficiency), both usually recorded over a given live weight interval. Other traits include post-weaning mortality and various health traits, including disease resistance indicators. It should also be noted that genetic progress in feed efficiency can also be achieved through selection for reduced backfat, increased rate of lean gain, an increase in the percentage of carcass, and for insulin-like growth factor-1 (IGF-1) levels: this partially negates the need for expensive feed intake measurements. Conformation and skeletal traits can be measured, for example, osteochondrosis and various leg and pastern measures. Various genetic abnormalities such as hernias, cryptorchids (where one or both of the testicles do not descend normally), splay leg and hermaphrodites are also often recorded. Carcass measurements can include backfat depth, loin muscle depth or area, and percent lean, and killing out percentage, among others. Meat-quality traits can include meat colour, meat pH, drip loss, intramuscular fat and taste. In some cases, behavioural traits are measured, such as tail biting and skin lesions as an indicator of aggressiveness.

There are numerous publications giving genetic parameters for pig traits, and these would also be estimated on a regular basis by the pig-breeding companies using their own data, though these results are not generally published (e.g. for papers giving genetic parameters see Perez-Enciso and Gianola, 1992; Knapp *et al.*, 1997; Labroue *et al.*, 1997; Larzul *et al.*, 1997; Sonesson *et al.*, 1998; Kaufmann *et al.*, 2000; Hanenberg *et al.*, 2001; Chen *et al.*, 2002, 2003, 2010; Gilbert *et al.*, 2007; Bergsma *et al.*, 2008; Turner *et al.*, 2008, 2009; Zumbach *et al.*, 2008; D'Eath *et al.*, 2009; Bouwman *et al.*, 2010; Canario *et al.*, 2010, 2012; Windig *et al.*, 2012; Strange *et al.*, 2013; Herrero-Medrano *et al.*, 2015).

As noted in Chapter 6, genetic parameter estimates differ for the same trait for different populations. Examples are given here for Australian Large White and Landrace pigs, for reproductive, performance, carcass, and meat-quality traits (Hermesch *et al.*, 2000a,b,c). Tables 12.2 to 12.5 show examples of heritabilities and litter effects, and Tables 12.6 to 12.8 list genetic and environmental correlations. We will briefly discuss some interpretation from these tables in the following paragraphs.

Heritabilities for the reproductive traits were low to modest, with litter size (number of animals born alive per litter) the least heritable (0.08–0.09) and litter weights (the combined weight of all animals in the litter) for later parities (0.20–0.22), the most heritable of the reproductive traits. Low to modest heritabilities for reproductive traits are common across species. Litter size in first parity had a moderate positive genetic correlation with litter size in second and third parities (0.62 and

Table 12.2. Means, phenotypic standard deviations (s.d.), heritabilities, with standard errors (s.e.) in brackets, for a range of reproductive traits in Australian Large White and Landrace pigs. (Adapted from Hermesch *et al.*, 2000c.)

Trait	Mean	Phenotypic s.d.	Heritability (s.e.)
Litter size in first parity	9.61	2.43	0.08 (0.02)
Litter size in second parity	10.06	2.44	0.09 (0.02)
Litter size in third parity	10.79	2.47	0.08 (0.03)
Litter weight in first parity (kg)	12.55	2.69	0.08 (0.02)
Litter weight in second parity (kg)	13.41	2.91	0.22 (0.05)
Litter weight in third parity (kg)	14.65	3.24	0.20 (0.07)
Average piglet weight in first parity (g)	1342	352	0.15 (0.03)
Average piglet weight in second parity (g)	1390	314	0.16 (0.04)
Average piglet weight in third parity (g)	1419	282	0.15 (0.06)

Table 12.3. Means, phenotypic standard deviations (s.d.), heritabilities, litter effects, with standard errors (s.e.) in brackets, for a range of performance traits in Australian Large White and Landrace pigs. (Adapted from Hermesch *et al.*, 2000a.)

Trait	Mean	Phenotypic s.d.	Heritability (s.e.)	Litter effect (s.e.)
Average daily gain from 3 to 18 weeks (g/day)	616.0	80.1	0.27 (0.05)	0.15 (0.03)
Average daily gain from 18 to 22 weeks (g/day)	946.0	185.8	0.13 (0.04)	0.08 (0.03)
Feed intake 18 to 22 weeks (kg)	2.62	0.43	0.23 (0.04)	
Feed conversion ratio 18 to 22 weeks[a]	2.85	0.58	0.15 (0.04)	

[a]Calculated as feed intake over growth rate.

Table 12.4. Means, phenotypic standard deviations (s.d.), heritabilities, and litter effects, with standard errors (s.e.) in brackets, for a range of carcass traits in Australian Large White and Landrace pigs. (Adapted from Hermesch *et al.*, 2000a.)

Trait	Mean	Phenotypic s.d.	Heritability (s.e.)	Litter effect (s.e.)
Live animal backfat depth at P2 site (mm)	13.0	2.59	0.60 (0.05)	
Live animal backfat depth between 3rd and 4th last ribs (mm)	13.1	2.61	0.62 (0.05)	
Live animal muscle depth between 3rd and 4th last ribs (mm)	37.8	4.56	0.21 (0.04)	
Carcass backfat depth at P2 site (mm)	12.9	3.13	0.46 (0.06)	
Carcass backfat depth between 3rd and 4th last ribs (mm)	13.2	3.00	0.45 (0.07)	
Weight of whole back left leg (mm)	10.6	1.24	0.22 (0.05)	0.14 (0.03)
Weight of slash boned back left leg (kg)	5.7	0.73	0.38 (0.07)	0.13 (0.03)

Table 12.5. Means, phenotypic standard deviations (s.d.), heritabilities, with standard errors (s.e.) in brackets, for a range of meat quality traits in Australian Large White and Landrace pigs. (Adapted from Hermesch *et al.*, 2000a.)

Trait	Mean	Phenotypic s.d.	Heritability (s.e.)
Colour of the *m. longissimus dorsi*[a]	53.16	4.91	0.29 (0.06)
Colour of the *m. multifidus dorsi*[a]	45.78	4.10	0.30 (0.05)
pH recorded 45 minutes after slaughter	6.36	0.46	0.15 (0.04)
pH recorded 24 hours after slaughter	5.74	0.26	0.14 (0.04)
Drip loss percentage (%)	1.98	1.87	0.23 (0.05)
Intramuscular fat (%)	1.69	0.67	0.35 (0.06)

[a]Measured as the L value of Minolta chroma-meter: 100 = white.

Table 12.6. Genetic and environmental correlations, with standard errors (s.e.) in brackets, between pairs of reproductive traits in Australian Large White and Landrace pigs. (Adapted from Hermesch *et al.*, 2000c.)

		Correlation between traits (s.e.)	
Trait 1	Trait 2	Genetic	Environmental
Litter size in 1st parity	Litter size in 2nd parity	0.62 (0.19)	0.11
Litter size in 1st parity	Litter size in 3rd parity	0.61 (0.30)	0.09
Litter size in 2nd parity	Litter size in 3rd parity	0.95 (0.04)	0.12
Litter size in 1st parity	Litter weight in 1st parity	–0.15 (0.17)	0.42
Litter size in 1st parity	Average piglet weight in 1st parity	–0.74 (0.10)	–0.66
Litter size in 2nd parity	Average piglet weight in 2nd parity	–0.69 (0.16)	–0.67
Litter size in 3rd parity	Average piglet weight in 3rd parity	–0.56 (0.25)	–0.57

Table 12.7. Genetic and environmental correlations, with standard errors (s.e.) in brackets, between pairs of performance, carcass and meat-quality traits in Australian Large White and Landrace pigs. (Adapted from Hermesch *et al.*, 2000b.)

		Correlation between traits (s.e.)	
Trait 1	Trait 2	Genetic	Environmental
Average daily gain from 3 to 18 weeks	Average daily gain from 18 to 22 weeks	0.32 (0.23)	0.05
Average daily gain from 3 to 18 weeks	Weight of whole back left leg	0.83 (0.07)	0.74
Average daily gain from 3 to 18 weeks	pH recorded 24 hours after slaughter	0.05 (0.24)	0.06
Average daily gain from 3 to 18 weeks	Intramuscular fat	0.01 (0.18)	–0.02
Average daily gain from 18 to 22 weeks	Intramuscular fat	–0.21 (0.18)	0.10
Average daily gain from 18 to 22 weeks	Feed intake	0.82 (0.11)	0.61
Live animal backfat depth at P2 site	Carcass backfat depth at P2 site	0.93 (0.04)	0.36
Live animal backfat depth between 3rd and 4th last ribs	Live animal muscle depth between 3rd and 4th last ribs	–0.14 (0.16)	–0.07
Live animal backfat depth between 3rd and 4th last ribs	Intramuscular fat	0.27 (0.16)	0.10
Colour of the *m. longissimus dorsi*	pH recorded 24 hours after slaughter	–0.83 (0.11)	–0.47

Table 12.8. Genetic correlations, with standard errors (s.e.) in brackets, between pairs of reproductive and other traits in Australian Large White and Landrace pigs. Note that environmental correlations were not able to be estimated in this case. (Adapted from Hermesch *et al.*, 2000c.)

Trait 1	Trait 2	Genetic Correlation between traits (s.e.)
Litter size in 1st parity	Average daily gain from 3 to 18 weeks	–0.30 (0.14)
Litter weight in 1st parity	Average daily gain from 3 to 18 weeks	0.39 (0.13)
Average piglet weight in 1st parity	Average daily gain from 3 to 18 weeks	0.33 (0.12)
Litter size in 1st parity	Weight of whole back left leg	–0.45 (0.13)
Litter size in 2nd parity	Weight of whole back left leg	–0.23 (0.15)
Average piglet weight in 1st parity	Weight of whole back left leg	0.29 (0.14)
Average piglet weight in 2nd parity	Weight of whole back left leg	0.27 (0.16)
Litter size in 1st parity	Colour of the *m. multifidus dorsi*	–0.42 (0.12)

0.61, respectively), while litter size in second parity had a strong positive genetic correlation to litter size in third parity (0.95). This suggests that litter size in the first parity is genetically a different trait to litter size in later parities. The genetic, as well as environmental, correlations between litter size and average pig birth weight were negative (unfavourable), meaning that (single-trait) selection for increased litter size would lower average pig birth weight, and vice versa.

Performance, carcass and meat-quality traits had heritabilities in the range of 0.13–0.62, generally higher than the reproductive traits, as is also commonly seen across species. Additionally, the average daily gain traits, as well as the back leg weight traits, had litter effects of 0.08–0.15 (see Chapter 6 for a further discussion on litter effects). The genetic correlations between these traits varied from strong (e.g. feed intake and average daily gain from 18 to 22 weeks had a genetic correlation of 0.82, while colour of the *m. longissimus dorsi* and pH recorded 24 hours after slaughter had a genetic correlation of –0.83) to weak (e.g. average daily again from 3 to 18 weeks and pH recorded 24 hours after slaughter had a genetic correlation of 0.05, and average daily again from 3–18 weeks and intramuscular fat had a genetic correlation of 0.01).

Litter size at first parity was negatively genetically correlated with average daily gain from 3 to 18 weeks (–0.30), while first parity litter weight and average piglet weight were both positively genetically correlated to average daily gain from 3–18 weeks (0.39 and 0.33, respectively). Litter size (for both first and second parities) was negatively correlated with the weight of the whole back leg (–0.45 and –0.23, respectively), while average piglet weight (again for both first and second parities) was positively correlated with the weight of the whole back leg (0.29 and 0.27, respectively).

In general, environmental correlations were the same sign as the genetic correlations, although there were some exceptions, for example litter size and litter weight in first parity where the genetic correlation was negative (–0.15) and the environmental correlation positive (0.42).

Altogether these illustrative results reinforce the importance of using a multi-trait selection approach, as discussed in Chapter 7.

As mentioned above, the inclusion of pig welfare and societal traits in breeding objectives is becoming more common. We will discuss the genetic parameters for a few of these. One study (Turner *et al.*, 2008) monitored pigs for aggressiveness for 24 hours post-mixing and estimated heritability for several aggressiveness traits, as well as the relationships between these traits and the number of skin lesions caused by this aggressiveness. The trait duration of reciprocal aggression had a heritability of 0.47 and that of duration of delivery of non-reciprocal aggression had a heritability of 0.37. The genetic correlation between these two traits and lesion score was high at 0.79. This means that lesion score is a useful indicator trait for aggressive behaviour, which is advantageous given that lesion score is easier to measure than aggression duration traits. Another study (Breuer *et al.*, 2005) considered tail biting in Large White and Landrace pigs. Tail biting was found to be heritable in the Landrace pigs, but not the Large White pigs. In the Landrace pigs the estimated heritability was 0.05 when the trait was scored as 0–1, equivalent to a heritability of 0.27 when the trait is expressed continuously. For the Landrace, genetic correlations between tail biting and lean tissue growth rate, and between tail biting and back fat thickness, were unfavourable at 0.27 and –0.28, respectively.

Methods of Genetic Evaluation

The first use of BLUP methodology in pig breeding was in Canada in 1985 (Hudson and Kennedy, 1985). BLUP, and its successors such as GBLUP, are now commonly used in commercial pig-breeding programmes, with the software used including PEST (Groeneveld *et al.*, 1990), ASREML (Gilmour *et al.*, 2009), BLUPf90 (http://nce.ads.uga.edu/wiki/doku.php) and PIGBLUP (http://agbu.une.edu.au/pig_genetics/pigblup.html), in addition to software developed in-house by pig-breeding companies. The use of BLUP has resulted in significant increases in genetic gain in comparison to that prior to its use, particularly for traits with low heritability.

Marker-assisted selection (MAS) and gene-assisted selection have also contributed to pig genetic improvement. The first major application was initiated in the early 1990s with the use of the Hal-1843 marker test for a mutant recessive allele of the Halothane gene causing poor meat quality and malignant hyperthermia in pigs exposed to stressful conditions, also called porcine stress syndrome (OMIA 000621-9823; Fujii *et al.*, 1991; Hamilton *et al.*, 2000; Knol *et al.*, 2016a). Use of this marker test led to the elimination of the mutant allele in many lines. Other applications of MAS for single-gene traits included for the mutant dominant allele of the Rendement Napole (RN) gene causing low ultimate pH, processing yield and water-holding capacity, but reduced slice shear force in pork (OMIA 001085-9823; le Roy *et al.*, 1990; Lundström *et al.*, 1996; Hamilton *et al.*, 2000), and for the K88 receptor causing resistance to *Escherichia coli* diarrhoea (OMIA 001088-9823; Edfors-Lilja *et al.*, 1986, 1995). The use of these markers is still practised today (Knol *et al.*, 2016b). Markers of quantitative traits (traits controlled by many genes) have also played an important role in genetic improvement. The first of these explained a substantial proportion of the variance in litter size (about 12% of the phenotypic standard deviation) and targeted an oestrogen receptor gene (Rothschild *et al.*, 1996; Short *et al.*, 1997). The total number of quantitative trait loci reported for economically important traits in pigs is now in the thousands (see Ernst and Steibel, 2013, for a review).

The first porcine SNP chip was developed in 2009 (Ramos *et al.*, 2009), and a number are commercially available today. These include the Illumina PorcineSNP60 BeadChip v2 array (with ~61,000 SNPs), and the GeneSeek Genomic Profiler for Porcine LD (with ~10,000 SNPs) and HD (with ~68,000 SNPs). The availability of the SNP chip (among other factors, including decreasing genotyping cost) has led to implementation of genomic selection by some commercial pig-breeding companies and national genetic evaluation systems. For example, the breeding company PIC reported use of genomic selection in 2013 (PIC, 2016), and other companies such as Topigs Norsvin (Topigs Norsvin, 2020b) and Hypor (2020) have also reported doing so. The Canadian Swine Improvement Program incorporated genomic selection in 2016.

The advantage of genomic selection to breeding programmes is earlier selection and thus shortened generation intervals, and/or increased accuracy of breeding value estimation. In pigs, selection of boars in the nucleus herds is the most important selection step, and most production records are available at the time of selection, meaning that there is little room for earlier selection (though some reduction may be possible; Meuwissen *et al.*, 2016). The main benefit of genomic selection in pig breeding is thus from increased accuracy of breeding value estimation (Lillehammer *et al.*, 2011; Knol *et al.*, 2016a; Meuwissen *et al.*, 2016; Samorè and Fontanesi, 2016). Another potential use of genomic selection in pig breeding is to enhance the selection of purebred animals for crossbred performance. This would require additional genotypes on the crossbred animals, in comparison to the present situation where phenotypes are available on the crossbred animals, and genotypes and phenotypes on the nucleus animals. However, the effectiveness of genomic selection across breeds and cross-breeds is still to be well-demonstrated (Meuwissen *et al.*, 2016). One limitation to genomic selection in pig breeding is the fragmentation of data, which resides with multiple breeding organizations and is unlikely to be fully shared. This may result in genomic selection not achieving the very high accuracies seen in other livestock sectors where much larger reference populations can be created (Knol *et al.*, 2016a).

It was reported that up to late 2015 the most advanced genomic applications in commercial pig production was single-step evaluation (combining phenotypic, genomic and pedigree information in one model; see Chapter 7) using imputation (where high-density genotypes are imputed from low density genotypes) (Christensen *et al.*, 2012; Knol *et al.*, 2016a). The use of single-step evaluation for genomic selection has been reported to increase estimated breeding value (EBV) accuracies by half (Knol *et al.*, 2016a). The prediction for future developments was for pig breeding to benefit from an increased number of genotypes and phenotypes, as well as use results from genome-wide association studies to weight markers in the genomic breeding values, according to the trait effect they have (Knol *et al.*, 2016a). Already some breeding companies have begun to report the generation of full-sequence data on some of their animals (PIC, 2016) for use in genomic prediction.

Use of Indexes

Selection indexes, as described in Chapter 4, are commonly used in pig-breeding programmes. However, the specific details of these are not often shared by breeding companies.

Evidence of Genetic Improvement and its Value

Some pig-breeding companies, as well as national pig genetic improvement programmes, publish genetic trends as evidence of genetic improvement. Here we give two illustrative examples.

Genetic trends were estimated for Large White pigs in France by inseminating modern sows with semen of boars that were born in 1977 and 1998, about 11 selection generations apart (Sellier, 1976; Canario *et al.*, 2007a, b, 2014; Foury *et al.*, 2009a; Tribout *et al.*, 2010). The breeding goal of this pig population in the early 1980s was to increase growth rate, feed efficiency and carcass leanness. An additional breeding goal of improved meat quality was introduced in the mid-1980s, and a further additional breeding goal of increased litter size in the late 1980s. Genetic trends for growth and carcass traits are summarized in Table 12.9, with strong and favourable changes in average daily gain, feed conversion ratio (despite an increase in average daily feed intake), carcass fatness and carcass leanness (Tribout *et al.*, 2010). An analysis of farrowing characteristics (Canario *et al.*, 2007b) between the boars from 1977 and 1998 showed an increase in litter size of 1.3 ± 0.6 piglets born alive per litter, but also an increase in stillbirths of 0.7 ± 0.3 piglets per litter. Correlated responses to this selection (for lean growth rate and sow prolificacy) were also examined for a number of other traits. Here it was found that there were unfavourable changes in sow and piglet behaviour at farrowing (Canario *et al.*, 2014), lower maturity of piglets at birth (Canario *et al.*, 2007a), and changes in the functioning of the stress-response system (Foury *et al.*, 2009b). It is worth noting that these studies are quite rare in that they evaluate genetic trends via the use of gene-banked semen to produce animals that originated from different time periods. This contrasts to the more commonly used approaches that regress trait EBVs on date of birth, and thus depend on the quality of the EBV system for its power. The approach as presented in these studies may become more common in the future, due to the increase in the uptake of gene-banking. It is worth noting that similar approaches have been used in estimating poultry genetic trends, as discussed in Chapter 11.

Table 12.9. Genetic trends for French Large White pigs from 1977 to 1998, for growth and carcass traits. (Adapted from Tribout *et al.*, 2010.)

Trait (units)	Average annual genetic gain
Average daily gain (g/day)	3.7 ± 1.3
Feed conversion ratio (kg/kg)	−0.014 ± 0.005
Average daily feed intake (g)	7.6 ± 4.7
Carcass fatness - carcass average backfat thickness (mm)	−0.35 ± 0.77
Carcass leanness – loin eye area (mm^2)	0.31 ± 0.10
Carcass leanness - carcass muscle content (%)	0.41 ± 0.08

Genetic trends for the Canadian Swine Improvement Program (as described above) are provided in its annual report (CCSI, 2017). These are summarized for three breeds, the Yorkshire (Large White), Landrace and Duroc, over the time period of 2010 to 2016 (see Table 12.10). Favourable genetic changes can be observed. Of note is the higher change in lean yield and loin eye area for the Duroc in comparison to the Yorkshire and Landrace, and higher change in litter size and piglet perinatal survival for the Yorkshire and Landrace compared to the Duroc. This is in line with the Duroc being used as a sire line, and the Yorkshire and Landrace as dam lines. The genetic change from 2010 to 2016 was reported as resulting in a CAD$17.50 increase in the sire line index ($/litter) and a $19.10, $18.30 and $37.30 increase in the dam line index ($/litter) for Yorkshire, Landrace and F_1 sows, respectively.

Genetic Improvement Strategies Within the Smallholder Pig Sectors

Genetic improvement strategies within smallholder pig sectors are often less formalized or structured, and/or more heterogeneous, than that of intensive pig sectors. In some cases, smallholder pig enterprises are based on the indigenous or local pig breeds, which are well-recognized for their adaptation to the local environmental conditions. These systems often prevail in areas where the higher

Table 12.10. Genetic trends for Yorkshire (Large White), Landrace and Duroc breeds within the Canadian Swine Improvement Program from 2010 to 2016. (Source: CCSI, 2017.)

	Average annual genetic change		
Trait (units)	Yorkshire	Landrace	Duroc
Lean yield (%)	+0.02	+0.01	+0.05
Loin eye area (cm^2)	+0.06	+0.02	+0.23
Days to market weight (days)	−0.92	−0.68	−0.95
Feed conversion ratio (kg/kg)	−0.014	−0.010	−0.013
Backfat (mm)	−0.04	0.00	−0.06
Lean depth (mm)	+0.07	+0.03	+0.25
Litter size at birth (pigs/litter)	+0.16	+0.13	+0.03
Piglet perinatal survival (%)	+0.19	+0.32	+0.06
Farrowing interval (days)	+0.01	−0.02	+0.01
Functional teats (teats)	+0.06	+0.04	+0.04

inputs necessary to keep other pigs breeds (such as local by exotic cross-breeds or pure exotics) are not accessible or affordable to the smallholder, where there are strong cultural reasons to keep the local breed of pigs, or where the local breed is supplying a particular market. In other smallholder systems, particularly those that are more commercially orientated and can access a higher level of inputs (feeding, healthcare and housing), a crossbreeding system can prevail. Here it is common for the well-adapted but often poorly productive local breed(s) to be crossed with highly productive but poorly-adapted exotic breed(s). This produces crossbred animals that exhibit moderate levels of both adaptation and productivity, taking advantage of breed complementarity. As the crossbreeding system is often loosely formalized, with crossbred piglets that would be targeted for slaughter in industrial systems often retained for use as sows, and a variety of breed/crossbreed types being used in the absence of pedigree recording, the degree of heterosis retained in the final cross is highly variable. In such systems considerable genetic gain is realized through the adoption of more appropriate breed-types and crossing structures (Marshall, 2014) and thus the level of genetic improvement with a system (comprising multiple smallholder units) is highly related to the number of adopters. Smallholders may access breeding animals from a variety of sources, including neighbours, local markets, village boar keepers, government breeding farms, larger-scale pig operations, international pig companies and others (see, for example, Marshall and Huyen, 2016). The wide variation in pig genetics used, coupled with the wide variation in pig management practices across different smallholder pig farms, often results in a wide variation in pig performance with subsequent market implications. A picture of pigs kept in a smallholder system is shown in Fig. 12.7.

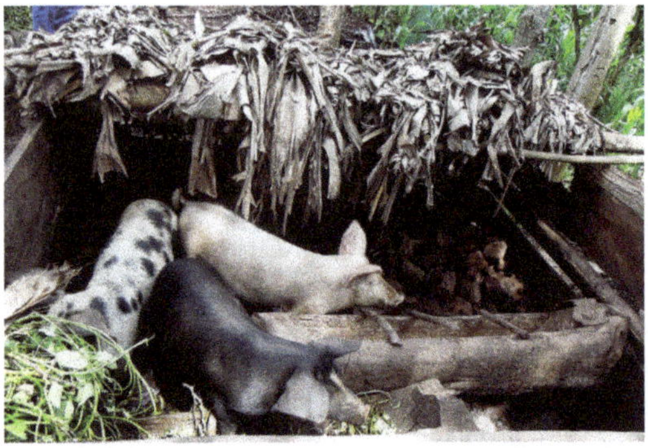

Fig. 12.7. Smallholder pig keeping in Uganda. (Photo credit: ILRI/Kristina Rösel.)

Use of reproductive technologies in dissemination of improved genetics

Use of artificial insemination, in particular, has helped in the dissemination of improved pig genetics (Knox, 2016; Rothschild and Ruvinsky, 2011). Advances in artificial insemination allow selected sires to be used widely, including across countries, in a cost effective manner. It also reduces the risk of disease transmission, which is critically important in the pig sector where high biosecurity standards are practised. A further advantage is a reduction in labour associated with pig reproduction. The use of artificial insemination (AI) with fresh semen became common in the 1990s, leading to a higher level of connectedness across herds and across-herd genetic evaluation which has been crucial for the meaningful use of BLUP (Knap *et al.*, 2001). AI using fresh semen (in extenders to increase sperm life to 3–7 days) is commonly used now, with sows typically receiving two inseminations on each day during standing oestrus (Knox, 2016). Technology advancements in AI are currently focused on lowering the number of sperm per AI dose, as well as the number of inseminations (e.g. use of a single, fixed-time AI after ovulation induction; Knox, 2016). While embryo transfer in pigs was first reported in 1951, its use has been limited due to the need for surgical procedures to collect embryos from donor sows and the difficulty in cryopreserving swine embryos (Brussow *et al.*, 2000; Martinez *et al.*, 2016; Fowler *et al.*, 2018). Research to improve embryo transfer is ongoing, and there is strong interest in using it to transfer genetics between the different tiers of the breeding pyramid.

Practical Guidelines on Selection

Breeding companies typically sell a breeding 'package', comprising both sire and dam lines, and are well placed to give good advice on what lines suit different types of producers.

Replacement breeding animals can either be purchased or generated through internal multiplication (usually for female lines). This decision largely depends on the cost:benefit of each option, in turn dependent on the scale of operation. Biosecurity considerations are also important, as the purchase of animals can risk introducing disease. Internal multiplication of breeding females can be achieved by various types of crossbreeding schemes, including terminal, rotational or rota-terminal. Depending on the crossing scheme a number of pure lines will need to be maintained, and in some cases semen from other complementary maternal lines will also be used. Tools to assist selection of replacements on-farm, based on herd records, exist (e.g. PBSELECT – AGBU, 2020).

Summary

- The dominant pig meat-producing country is China, which produces almost half of the global total.
- In developed countries, the modern pig-breeding industry is highly technology-based, capitalizing on the latest advances in genomics, phenomics, and computing technologies.
- The broad breeding objective of pig genetic improvement is typically to increase the benefit (still largely defined as profit) of the overall system. Different breeds or lines typically have their own more specific breeding objectives.
- There are numerous pig breeds/lines globally, though a limited number of these are more commonly used.
- Pig genetic improvement often operates as a three-tiered pyramid, with nucleus, multiplier and commercial tiers.
- Crossbreeding schemes are commonly used, with use of a three-breed (or line) terminal cross common. Here the commercial pig is produced from an F_1 sow crossed to a different breed (or sire line) of boar. The system takes advantage of both heterosis and breed complementarity.
- In general, sire lines are selected for production traits, and dam lines for production as well as reproduction traits.
- A relatively small number of companies provide much of the world's improved pig genetics. National genetic improvement strategies also exist.
- Artificial insemination has had a major positive impact on genetic improvement as such, as well as on the dissemination of improved pig genetics.

References

AGBU (2020) PBSELECT: The online PIGBLUP service. Available at: http://agbu.une.edu.au/pig_genetics/pdf/PBSELECT1.pdf (accessed 24 June 2020).

AGTR (2020) Taihu. Available at: http://agtr.ilri.cgiar.org/taihu (accessed 24 June 2020).

AHDB (2017) Agriculture and Horticulture Development Boars. 2017 Pig Cost of Production in Selected Countries.https://pork.ahdb.org.uk/media/274535/2016-pig-cost-of-production-in-selected-countries.pdf (accessed 24 June 2020).

American Meishan Breeders Association (2020) Available at: https://www.meishanbreeders.com/ (accessed 24 June 2020).

Bazer, F.W., Thatcher, W.W., Martinat-Botte, F. and Terqui, M. (1988) Conceptus development in large white and prolific Chinese Meishan pigs. *Journal of Reproduction and Fertility* 84, 37–42.

Bergsma, R., Kanis, E., Knol, E.F. and Bijma, P. (2008) The contribution of social effects to heritable variation in finishing traits of domestic pigs (*Sus scrofa*). *Genetics* 178, 1559–1570. DOI: 10.1534/genetics.107.084236.

Bouwman, A.C., Bergsma, R., Duijvesteijn, N. and Bijma, P. (2010) Maternal and social genetic effects on average daily gain of piglets from birth until weaning. *Journal of Animal Science* 88, 2883–2892. DOI: 10.2527/jas.2009-2494.

Breuer, K., Sutcliffe, M.E.M., Mercer, J.T., Rance, K.A., O'Connell, N.E. *et al.* (2005) Heritability of clinical tail-biting and its relation to performance traits. *Livestock Production Science* 93, 87–94. DOI: 10.1016/j.livprodsci.2004.11.009.

Brussow, K.P., Torner, H., Kanitz, W. and Ratky, J. (2000) *In vitro* technologies related to pig embryo transfer. *Reproduction Nutrition Development* 40, 469–480. DOI: 10.1051/rnd:2000111.

Canario, L., Père, M.C., Tribout, T., Thomas, F., David, C. *et al.* (2007a) Estimation of genetic trends from 1977 to 1998 of body composition and physiological state of Large White pigs at birth. *Animal* 1, 1409–1413. DOI: 10.1017/s1751731107000766.

Canario, L., Rydhmer, L., Gogué, J., Tribout, T. and Bidanel, J.P. (2007b) Estimation of genetic trends from 1977 to 1998 for farrowing characteristics in the French Large White breed using frozen semen. *Animal* 1, 929–938. DOI: 10.1017/s1751731107000511.

Canario, L., Lundeheim, N. and Bijma, P. (2010) Pig growth is affected by social genetic effects and social litter effects that depend on group size. In: *World Congress on Genetics Applied to Livestock Production*, pp. 1–4. Available at: http://www.wcgalp.org/proceedings/2010 (accessed 16 June 2020).

Canario, L., Turner, S.P., Roehe, R., Lundeheim, N., D'Eath, R.B. *et al.* (2012) Genetic associations between behavioral traits and direct-social effects of growth rate in pigs. *Journal of Animal Science* 90, 4706–4715. DOI: 10.2527/jas.2012-5392.

Canario, L., Bidanel, J.P. and Rydhmer, L. (2014) Genetic trends in maternal and neonatal behaviors and their association with perinatal survival in french large white swine. *Frontiers in Genetics* 5, 410. DOI: 10.3389/fgene.2014.00410.

CCSI (2017) *Canadian Centre for Swine Improvement 2017 Annual Report.* Available at: https://www.ccsi.ca/meetings/annual/2017AnnualReportEnglish.pdf (accessed 24 June 2020).

Chen, C.Y., Misztal, I., Tsuruta, S., Herring, W.O., Holl, J. and Culbertson, M. (2010) Influence of heritable social status on daily gain and feeding pattern in pigs. *Journal of Animal Breeding and Genetics* 127, 107–112. DOI: 10.1111/j.1439-0388.2009.00828.x.

Chen, P., Baas, T.J., Mabry, J.W., Dekkers, J.C.M. and Koehler, K.J. (2002) Genetic parameters and trends for lean growth rate and its components in U.S. Yorkshire, Duroc, Hampshire, and Landrace pigs. *Journal of Animal Science* 80, 2062–2070. DOI: 10.1093/ansci/80.8.2062.

Chen, P., Baas, T.J., Mabry, J.W., Koehler, K.J. and Dekkers, J.C.M. (2003) Genetic parameters and trends for litter traits in U.S. Yorkshire, Duroc, Hampshire, and Landrace pigs. *Journal of Animal Science* 81, 46–53.

Christensen, O.F., Madsen, P., Nielsen, B., Ostersen, T. and Su, G. (2012) Single-step methods for genomic evaluation in pigs. *Animal* 6, 1565–1571. DOI: 10.1017/s1751731112000742.

D'Eath, R.B., Roehe, R., Turner, S.P., Ison, S.H., Farish, M. *et al.* (2009) Genetics of animal temperament: Aggressive behaviour at mixing is genetically associated with the response to handling in pigs. *Animal* 3, 1544–1554. DOI: 10.1017/S1751731109990528.

Edfors-Lilja, I., Petersson, H. and Gahne, B. (1986) Performance of pigs with or without the intestinal receptor for *Escherichia coli* K88. *Animal Science* 42, 381–387. DOI: 10.1017/S000335610001816X.

Edfors-Lilja, I., Gustafsson, U., Duval-Iflah, Y., Ellergren, H., Johansson, M. *et al.* (1995) The porcine intestinal receptor for *Escherichia coli* K88ab, K88ac: regional localization on chromosome 13 and influence of IgG response to the K88 antigen. *Animal Genetics* 26, 237–242. DOI: 10.1111/j.1365-2052.1995.tb03250.x.

Ernst, C.W. and Steibel, J.P. (2013) Molecular advances in QTL discovery and application in pig breeding. *Trends in Genetics* 29, 215–224. DOI: 10.1016/j.tig.2013.02.002.

FAO (2011) Mapping Supply and Demand for Animal-Source Foods to 2030, by Robinson, T.P. and Pozzi, F. *Animal Production and Health Working Paper. No. 2.* FAO, Rome.

FAO (2012) Pig sector Kenya. *FAO Animal Production and Health Livestock Country Reviews*. No. 3. FAO, Rome.

FAO (2015) *The Second Report on the State of the World's Animal Genetic Resources for Food and Agriculture*. FAO Commission on Genetic Resources for Food and Agriculture Assessment, Rome.

FAO (2019) FAOSTAT. Available at: http://www.fao.org/faostat/en/#data/QL/visualize (accessed 10 August 2019).

Foury, A., Tribout, T., Bazin, C., Billon, Y., Bouffaud, M. *et al.* (2009a) Estimation of genetic trends from 1977 to 2000 for stress-responsive systems in French Large White and Landrace pig populations using frozen semen. *Animal* 3, 1681–1687. DOI: 10.1017/s1751731109990504.

Foury, A., Tribout, T., Bazin, C., Billon, Y., Bouffaud, M., Gogué, J.M., Bidanel, J.P. and Mormède, P. (2009b) Estimation of genetic trends from 1977 to 2000 for stress-responsive systems in French Large White and Landrace pig populations using frozen semen. *Animal* 3, 1681–1687. DOI: 10.1017/s1751731109990504.

Fowler, K.E., Mandawala, A.A., Griffin, D.K., Walling, G.A. and Harvey, S.C. (2018) The production of pig preimplantation embryos *in vitro*: Current progress and future prospects. *Reproductive Biology* 18, 203–211. DOI: 10.1016/j.repbio.2018.07.001.

Frantz, L.A.F., Schraiber, J.G., Madsen, O., Megens, H.J., Cagan, A. *et al.* (2015) Evidence of long-term gene flow and selection during domestication from analyses of Eurasian wild and domestic pig genomes. *Nature Genetics* 47, 1141–1148. DOI: 10.1038/ng.3394.

Fujii, J., Otsu, K., Zorzato, F., De Leon, S., Khanna, V.K. *et al.* (1991) Identification of a mutation in porcine ryanodine receptor associated with malignant hyperthermia. *Science* 253, 448–451. DOI: 10.1126/science.1862346.

Gilbert, H., Bidanel, J.P., Gruand, J., Caritez, J.C., Billon, Y. *et al.* (2007) Genetic parameters for residual feed intake in growing pigs, with emphasis on genetic relationships with carcass and meat quality traits. *Journal of Animal Science* 85, 3182–3188. DOI: 10.2527/jas.2006-590.

Gilmour, A.R., Gogel, B.J., Cullis, B.R., Thompson, R. and Butler, D. (2009). ASReml User Guide, release 3.0, VSN Int. Ltd, Hemel Hempstead, UK.

Giuffra, E., Kijas, J.M.H., Amarger, V., Carlborg, Ö., Jeon, J.T. and Andersson, L. (2000) The origin of the domestic pig: Independent domestication and subsequent introgression. *Genetics* 154, 1785–1791.

Godinho, R.M., Bergsma, R., Silva, F.F., Sevillano, C.A., Knol, E.F. *et al.* (2019) Genetic correlations between growth performance and carcass traits of purebred and crossbred pigs raised in tropical and temperate climates. *Journal of Animal Science* 97, 3648–3657.

Groenen, M.A.M. (2016) A decade of pig genome sequencing: A window on pig domestication and evolution. *Genetics Selection Evolution* 48, 23. DOI: 10.1186/s12711-016-0204-2.

Groeneveld, E., Kovac, M. and Wang, T. (1990) PEST, a general purpose BLUP package for multivariate prediction and estimation. In: *Proceedings of the 4th World Congress on Genetics Applied to Livestock Production*, Edinburgh (Vol. 13, pp. 488–491). Available at: http://www.wcgalp.org/ (accessed 16 June 2020).

Haley, C.S. and Lee, G.J. (1993) Genetic basis of prolificacy in Meishan pigs. *Journal of Reproduction and Fertility* 2, 247–259.

Haley, C., Avalos, E. and Smith, C. (1986) A review of selection for reproductive performance in the pig. *37th European Association of Animal Production*, Budapest.

Hamilton, D.N., Ellis, M., Miller, K.D., McKeith, F.K. and Parrett, D.F. (2000) The effect of the Halothane and Rendement Napole genes on carcass and meat quality characteristics of pigs. *Journal of Animal Science* 78, 2862–2867. DOI: 10.2527/2000.78112862x.

Hanenberg, E.H.A.T., Knol, E.F. and Merks, J.W.M. (2001) Estimates of genetic parameters for reproduction traits at different parities in Dutch Landrace pigs. *Livestock Production Science* 69, 179–186. DOI: 10.1016/S0301-6226(00)00258-X.

Hermesch, S., Luxford, B.G. and Graser, H.U. (2000a) Genetic parameters for lean meat yield, meat quality, reproduction and feed efficiency traits for Australian pigs. 1. Description of traits and heritability estimates. *Livestock Production Science* 65, 239–248. DOI: https://doi.org/10.1016/S0301-6226(00)00152-4.

Hermesch, S., Luxford, B. and Graser, H.-U. (2000b) Genetic parameters for lean meat yield, meat quality, reproduction and feed efficiency traits for Australian pigs. 2. Genetic relationships between production, carcase and meat quality traits. *Livestock Production Science* 65, 249–259. DOI: 10.1016/s0301-6226(00)00152-4.

Hermesch, S., Luxford, B.G. and Graser, H.U. (2000c) Genetic parameters for lean meat yield, meat quality, reproduction and feed efficiency traits for Australian pigs. 3. Genetic parameters for reproduction traits and genetic correlations with production, carcase and meat quality traits. *Livestock Production Science* 65, 261–270. DOI: 10.1016/S0301-6226(00)00152-4.

Hermesch, S., Li, L., Doeschl-Wilson, A.B. and Gilbert, H. (2015) Selection for productivity and robustness traits in pigs. *Animal Production Science* 55, 1437. DOI: 10.1071/an15275.

Herrero-Medrano, J.M., Mathur, P.K., Ten Napel, J., Rashidi, H., Alexandri, P. *et al.* (2015) Estimation of genetic parameters and breeding values across challenged environments to select for robust pigs. *Journal of Animal Science* 93, 1494–1502. DOI: 10.2527/jas.2014-8583.

Hudson, G.F.S. and Kennedy, B.W. (1985). Genetic evaluation of swine for growth rate and backfat thickness. *Journal of Animal Science* 61(1), 83–91.

Hypor (2020) Hypor selection. Available at: https://www.hypor.com/en/animal-breeding/selection/ (accessed 26 September 2020).

Kanis, E., De Greef, K.H., Hiemstra, A. and Van Arendonk, J.A.M. (2005) Breeding for societally important traits in pigs. *Journal of Animal Science* 83, 948–957.

Kaufmann, D., Hofer, A., Bidanel, J.P. and Künzi, N. (2000) Genetic parameters for individual birth and weaning weight and for litter size of Large White pigs. *Journal Animal Breeding and Genetics* 117, 121–128. DOI: 10.1111/j.1439-0388.2000x.00238.x.

Kijas, J.M.H. and Andersson, L. (2001) A phylogenetic study of the origin of the domestic pig estimated from the near-complete mtDNA genome. *Journal of Molecular Evolution* 52, 302–308. DOI: 10.1007/s002390010158.

Knap, P.W. (2014) Pig breeding goals in competitive markets. *Proceedings of the 10th World Congress Genetics Applied to Livestock Production*. Available at: http://www.wcgalp.org/proceedings/2014 (accessed 16 June 2020).

Knap, P.W., Van Der Steen, H.A.M. and Plastow, G.S. (2001) Developments in pig breeding and the role of research. *Livestock Production Science* 72, 43–48. DOI: 10.1016/S0301-6226(01)00265-2.

Knapp, P., Willam, A. and Sölkner, J. (1997) Genetic parameters for lean meat content and meat quality traits in different pig breeds. *Livestock Production Science* 52, 69–73. DOI: 10.1016/S0301-6226(97)00120-6.

Knol, E.F., Nielsen, B. and Knap, P.W. (2016a) Genomic selection in commercial pig breeding. *Animal Frontiers* 6, 15–22. DOI: 10.2527/af.2016-0003.

Knol, E.F., Nielsen, B. and Knap, P.W. (2016b) Genomic selection in commercial pig breeding. *Animal Frontiers* 6, 15–22. DOI: 10.2527/af.2016-0003.

Knox, R.V. (2016) Artificial insemination in pigs today. *Theriogenology* 85, 83–93. DOI: 10.1016/j.theriogenology.2015.07.009.

Kyriazakis, I. and Whittemore, C.T. (Eds) (2006) *Science and Practice of Pig Production*. Blackwell Publishing Ltd, Oxford. DOI: 10.1002/9780470995624.

Labroue, F., Guéblez, R. and Sellier, P. (1997) Genetic parameters of feeding behaviour and performance traits in group-housed Large White and French Landrace growing pigs. *Genetics Selection Evolution* 29, 451–468.

Larson, G., Dobney, K., Albarella, U., Fang, M., Matisoo-Smith, E., *et al.* (2005) Worldwide phylogeography of wild boar reveals multiple centers of pig domestication worldwide. *Science* 307, 1618–1621. DOI: 10.1126/science.1106927.

Larson, G., Albarella, U., Dobney, K., Rowley-Conwy, P., Schibler, J. *et al.* (2007) Ancient DNA , pig domestication, and the spread of the Neolithic into Europe. *Proceedings of the National Academy of Sciences* 104, 15276–15281. DOI: 10.1073/pnas.0703411104.

Larzul, C., Lefaucheur, L., Ecolan, P., Gogué, J., Talmant, A. *et al.* (1997) Phenotypic and genetic parameters for longissimus muscle fiber characteristics in relation to growth, carcass, and meat quality traits in large white pigs. *Journal of Animal Science* 75, 3126–3137. DOI: 10.2527/1997.75123126x.

le Roy, P., Naveau, J., Elsen, J.M. and Sellier, P. (1990) Evidence for a new major gene influencing meat quality in pigs. *Genetics Research* 55, 33–40. DOI: 10.1017/S0016672300025179.

Li, W.T., Zhang, M.M., Li, Q.G., Tang, H., Zhang, L.F., *et al.* (2017) Whole-genome resequencing reveals candidate mutations for pig prolificacy. *Proceedings of the Royal Society B: Biological Sciences* 284, 20172437. DOI: 10.1098/rspb.2017.2437.

Lillehammer, M., Meuwissen, T.H.E. and Sonesson, A.K. (2011) Genomic selection for maternal traits in pigs. *Journal of Animal Science* 89, 3908–3916. DOI: 10.2527/jas.2011-4044.

Lundström, K., Andersson, A. and Hansson, I. (1996) Effect of the RN gene on technological and sensory meat quality in crossbred pigs with Hampshire as terminal sire. *Meat Science* 42, 145–153. DOI: 10.1016/0309-1740(95)00034-8.

Lutaaya, E., Misztal, I., Mabry, J.W., Short, T., Timm, H.H. and Holzbauer, R. (2001) Genetic parameter estimates from joint evaluation of purebreds and crossbreds in swine using the crossbred model. *Journal of Animal Science* 79, 3002–3007.

Marshall, K. (2014) Optimizing the use of breed types in developing country livestock production systems: A neglected research area. *Journal of Animal Breeding and Genetics* 131, 329–340. DOI: 10.1111/jbg.12080.

Marshall, K. and Huyen, L.T.T. (2016) Pig breeds and breeding operations in Nghe An province, Vietnam, with a focus on the smallholder pig sector. *ILRI Research Report*, 41.

Martinez, E.A., Cuello, C., Parrilla, I., Martinez, C.A., Nohalez, A. *et al.* (2016) Recent advances toward the practical application of embryo transfer in pigs. *Theriogenology* 85, 152–161. DOI: 10.1016/j.theriogenology.2015.06.002.

McOrist, S., Khampee, K. and Guo, A. (2011) Modern pig farming in the People's Republic of China: growth and veterinary challenges. *Revue Scientifique et Technique-OIE* 30, 961–968.

Merks, J.W.M. (2000) One century of genetic changes in pigs and the future needs. *British Society of Animal Science Occasional Publication* 27, 8–19.

Meuwissen, T., Hayes, B. and Goddard, M. (2016) Genomic selection: A paradigm shift in animal breeding. *Animal Frontiers* 6, 6–14. DOI: 10.2527/af.2016-0002.

Oldenbroek, K. and van der Waaij, L. (2014) *Textbook Animal Breeding: Animal Breeding and Genetics for BSc Students*. Centre for Genetic Resources and Animal Breeding and Genomics Group, Wageningen University and Research Centre, Wageningen, The Netherlands.

Ottoni, C., Girdland Flink, L., Evin, A., Geörg, C., De Cupere, B. *et al.* (2013) Pig domestication and human-mediated dispersal in western Eurasia revealed through ancient DNA and geometric morphometrics. *Molecular Biology and Evolution* 30, 824–832. DOI: 10.1093/molbev/mss261.

Perez-Enciso, M. and Gianola, D. (1992) Estimates of genetic parameters for litter size in six strains of Iberian pigs. *Livestock Production Science* 32, 283–293. DOI: 10.1016/S0301-6226(12)80007-8.

PIC (2020) Available at: https://gb.pic.com/services/gilts/ (accessed 24 June 2020).

PIC (2016) PIC UK Newsletter August 2016. The next step-change in genetic improvement – Sequencing the PIC Genome. Available at: https://gb.pic.com/resources/pic-matters-newsletter/ (accessed 28 September 2020).

Ramos, A.M., Crooijmans, R.P.M.A., Affara, N.A., Amaral, A.J., Archibald, A.L. *et al.* (2009) Design of a high density SNP genotyping assay in the pig using SNPs identified and characterized by next generation sequencing technology. *PLoS One* 4, e6524. DOI: 10.1371/journal.pone.0006524.

Rothschild, M. and Ruvinsky, A. (2011) *The Genetics of the Pig*, 2nd edn. CAB International, Wallingford, UK. DOI: 10.1079/9781845937560.0000.

Rothschild, M., Jacobson, C., Vaske, D., Tuggle, C., Wang, L. *et al.* (1996) The estrogen receptor locus is associated with a major gene influencing litter size in pigs. *Proceedings of the National Academy of Sciences of the United States of America* 93, 201–205. DOI: 10.1073/pnas.93.1.201.

Samorè, A.B. and Fontanesi, L. (2016) Genomic selection in pigs: State of the art and perspectives. *Italian Journal of Animal Science* 15, 211–232. DOI: 10.1080/1828051X.2016.1172034.

Sellier, P. (1976) The basis of crossbreeding in pigs: A review. *Livestock Production Science* 3, 203–226. DOI: 10.1016/0301-6226(76)90016-6.

Short, T.H., Rothschild, M.F., Southwood, O.I., McLaren, D.G., De Vries, A. *et al.* (1997) Effect of the estrogen receptor locus on reproduction and production traits in four commercial pig lines. *Journal of Animal Science* 75, 3138–3142. DOI: 10.2527/1997.75123138x.

Sonesson, A.K., De Greef, K.H. and Meuwissen, T.H.E. (1998) Genetic parameters and trends of meat quality, carcass composition and performance traits in two selected lines of large white pigs. *Livestock Production Science* 57, 23–32. DOI: 10.1016/S0301-6226(98)00163-8.

Strange, T., Ask, B. and Nielsen, B. (2013) Genetic parameters of the piglet mortality traits stillborn, weak at birth, starvation, crushing, and miscellaneous in crossbred pigs. *Journal of Animal Science* 91, 1562–1569. DOI: 10.2527/jas.2012-5584.

Tatwangire, A. (2014) Uganda smallholder pigs value chain development: Past trends, current status and likely future directions. *ILRI Project Report, ILRI*, Nairobi.

Topigs Norsvin (2018a) Boar Taint Reduced by More than 50%. Available at: https://topigsnorsvin.com/news-tn1/animal-welfare/boar-taint-reduced-by-more-than-50/ (accessed 25 June 2020).

Topigs Norsvin (2018b) Breeding for Less Tail Biting. Available at: https://topigsnorsvin.com/innovation-news/breeding-for-less-tail-biting/ (accessed 25 June 2020).

Topigs Norsvin (2020a) Available at: https://norsvin.no/produkter/norsvin-duroc/ (accessed 7 November 2020).

Topigs Norsvin (2020b) Available at: https://topigsnorsvin.com/our-5-focus-areas/

Tribout, T., Caritez, J.C., Gruand, J., Bouffaud, M., Guillouet, P. *et al.* (2010) Estimation of genetic trends in French Large White pigs from 1977 to 1998 for growth and carcass traits using frozen semen. *Journal of Animal Science* 88, 2856–2867. DOI: 10.2527/jas.2009-2356.

Turner, S.P. (2011) Breeding against harmful social behaviours in pigs and chickens: State of the art and the way forward. *Applied Animal Behaviour Science* 134, 1–9.

Turner, S.P., Roehe, R., Mekkawy, W., Farnworth, M.J., Knap, P.W. and Lawrence, A.B. (2008) Bayesian analysis of genetic associations of skin lesions and behavioural traits to identify genetic components of individual aggressiveness in pigs. *Behavioural Genetics* 38, 67–75. DOI: 10.1007/s10519-007-9171-2.

Turner, S.P., Roehe, R., D'Eath, R.B., Ison, S.H., Farish, M. *et al.* (2009) Genetic validation of postmixing skin injuries in pigs as an indicator of aggressiveness and the relationship with injuries under more stable social conditions. *Journal of Animal Science* 87, 3076–3082. DOI: 10.2527/jas.2008-1558.

Turner, S.P., Camerlink, I., Baxter, E.M., D'Eath, R.B., Desire, S. and Roehe, R. (2018) Breeding for pig welfare: Opportunities and challenges. In: Spinka, M. (ed.) *Advances in Pig Welfare*. Woodland Publishing, Salt Lake City, Utah, pp. 399–414. DOI: 10.1016/B978-0-08-101012-9.00012-5.

Windig, J.J., Mulder, H.A., ten Napel, J., Knol, E.F., Mathur, P.K. and Crump, R.E. (2012) Genetic parameters for androstenone, skatole, indole, and human nose scores as measures of boar taint and their relationship with finishing traits. *Journal of Animal Science* 90, 2120–2129. DOI: 10.2527/jas.2011-4700.

Yang, B., Cui, L., Perez-Enciso, M., Traspov, A., Crooijmans, R.P.M.A. et al. (2017) Genome-wide SNP data unveils the globalization of domesticated pigs. *Genetics Selection Evolution* 49, 71. DOI: 10.1186/s12711-017-0345-y.

Zumbach, B., Misztal, I., Tsuruta, S., Sanchez, J.P., Azain, M. *et al.* (2008) Genetic components of heat stress in finishing pigs: Parameter estimation. *Journal of Animal Science* 86, 2076–2081. DOI: 10.2527/jas.2007-0282.

Recommended Reading

Knol, E.F., Nielsen, B. and Knap, P.W. (2016) Genomic selection in commercial pig breeding. *Animal Frontiers* 6, 15–22. DOI: 10.2527/af.2016-0003.

Kyriazakis, I. and Whittemore, C.T. (Eds) (2006) *Science and Practice of Pig Production*. Blackwell Publishing Ltd, Oxford. DOI: 10.1002/9780470995624.

Merks, J.W.M. (2000) One century of genetic changes in pigs and the future needs. *British Society of Animal Sciences Occasional Publication* 27, 8–19.

Proceedings of the World Congresses on Genetics Applied to Livestock Production. Available at: http://www.wcgalp.org/ (accessed 16 June 2020).

Rothschild, M. and Ruvinsky, A. (2011) *The Genetics of the Pig*. CAB International, Wallingford, UK. DOI: 10.1079/9781845937560.0000.

Turner, S.P., Camerlink, I., Baxter, E.M., D'Eath, R.B., Desire, S. and Roehe, R. (2018) Breeding for pig welfare: opportunities and challenges. In: Spinka, M. (ed.) *Advances in Pig Welfare*. Woodland Publishing, Salt Lake City, Utah, pp. 399–414. DOI: 10.1016/B978-0-08-101012-9.00012-5.

13 Aquaculture Breeding

Introduction

Aquaculture is a broad sector of farmed food production, encompassing species from highly diverse branches of the evolutionary tree. These species are also kept in a wide range of production systems and there are varying degrees of sophistication in their selective breeding programmes, with much of aquaculture production still derived from wild or near-wild broodstock animals. However, aquaculture is a rapidly growing sector, and one which is typically quick to adopt new technologies. Selective breeding and use of genetic technologies have major potential to improve production. This chapter reviews the state of play in aquaculture breeding and presents an outlook, together with opportunities and challenges, for this sector. Given the wide range of species involved, and the huge differences in the current status of their breeding programmes, we use a slightly different structure in this chapter to that in the previous five.

Aquaculture: Global Status and Trends

Fish, shellfish and crustacean production via aquaculture has a critical rôle in meeting the current and future demand for animal protein. In many of the developing and developed regions of the world, the demand for seafood has grown constantly over the past few decades. When combined with a global population expansion and urbanization, together with rising incomes in the developing world, this rise in demand will continue (Kobayashi *et al.*, 2015). Since wild-capture fishery production is widely considered to have plateaued, aquaculture has a rapidly increasing rôle in supporting global food security. Fish production via aquaculture is now approximately equal to capture fishery production for the first time in history (Fig. 13.1), and extrapolation of the production trends highlights that aquaculture will be the dominant source of aquatic food within a few decades. Global production of fish, crustaceans, molluscs and other aquatic animals reached 170.9 Mt in 2016. Of this total, capture production was 90.9 Mt, a decrease of 1.9% compared with the previous year. Aquaculture production was 80 Mt in 2016, up by 5.2% from the previous year (FAO, 2018).

Asia dominated the world's aquaculture production of fish and shellfish in 2016 (~90% by volume), followed by the Americas, Europe, Africa and Oceania. In 2016, the top ten aquaculture producers (excluding aquatic plants and non-food products) were China (49.2 Mt), India (5.7 Mt), Indonesia (4.9 Mt), Vietnam (3.6 Mt), Bangladesh (2.2 Mt), followed by Egypt (1.4 Mt), Norway (1.3 Mt), Chile and Myanmar (1 Mt each) and Thailand (0.96 Mt). It is clear that the vast majority (almost 90%) of global aquaculture production of finfish, crustaceans and shellfish occurs in Asia (Table 13.1)

The majority of food production via aquaculture is finfish, comprising 54.1 Mt (67.6%). In comparison, there are 17.1 Mt of molluscs (21.4%) produced *per annum*, 7.9 Mt of crustaceans (9.8%) and 0.9 Mt of other aquatic animal species (1.2%). The majority of aquaculture production is from inland, freshwater systems, comprising 47.5 Mt (59.3%) (note the top five finfish species in Table 13.2 are freshwater, and Atlantic salmon is included in ninth place for reference). It is noteworthy that freshwater constitutes only ~1% of the globe's surface, while the very large areas covered by sea and brackish water are comparatively underused for aquaculture production.

Aquaculture Versus Terrestrial Livestock

While production of aquatic species shares many similarities with terrestrial livestock production, there are some clear and consistent differences. Food conversion is generally more efficient in fish than in terrestrial livestock, as warm-blooded animals (homeotherms) tend to have higher energy

Genetic Improvement of Farmed Animals (G. Simm *et al.*)
DOI: 10.1079/9781789241723.0013

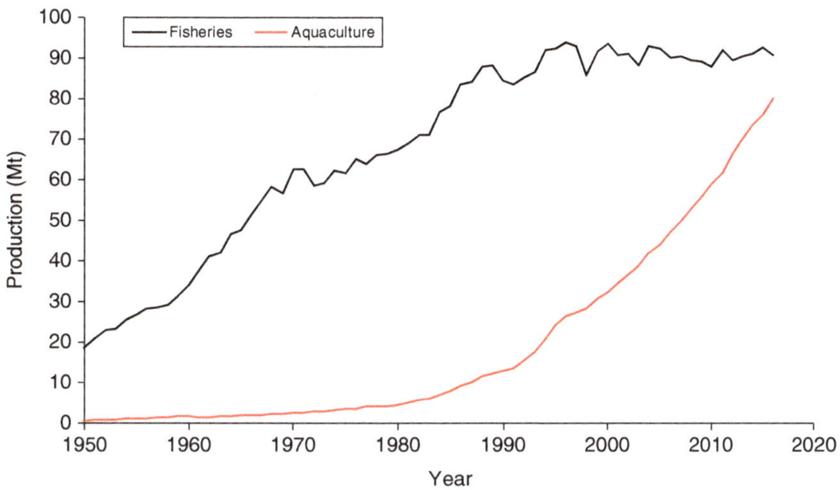

Fig. 13.1. World capture fisheries and aquaculture production 1950–2014. (Source: FAO, 2018.)

Table 13.1. Total aquaculture production (thousand tonnes, live weight) by continent in 2016. (Source: FAO, 2018.)

Category	Africa	Americas	Asia	Europe	Oceania	World
Finfish	1,972	1,978	47,722	2,332	87	54,091
Crustacea	5	795	7,055	0	7	7,862
Molluscs	6	574	15,835	613	112	17,139
Others	0	1	933	0	5	939
Total	**1,982**	**3,348**	**71,546**	**2,945**	**210**	**80,031**

requirements for maintenance and respiration compared to the cold-blooded animals (poikilotherms) used in aquaculture. It has been estimated on average that only 2% of energy consumed is converted to biomass in homeotherms, compared to an estimated average of 17 % for poikilotherms (Ytrestøyl *et al.*, 2015). Interestingly, farmed salmon derived from a selective breeding programme have been shown to exhibit 2.3- and 1.6-times higher rates of energy retention than poultry and pigs, respectively. Estimated protein retention from the diet was also higher in salmon in comparison to both poultry (1.5 times) and pigs (1.75 times) (Ytrestøyl *et al.* 2015). Further, this retention of protein has improved with selective breeding, with suggestions of a 20% improvement in Atlantic salmon after five generations of selection, mainly for higher growth rate (Thodesen *et al.*, 1999). A similar finding in coho salmon (*Oncorhynchus kisutch)* indicated that selection for growth rate over a period of 16 generations resulted in improved feed efficiency and energy allocations (Neely *et al.*, 2008).

It is also worth noting the very distinct nutritional profile of fish compared to sources of terrestrial animal protein. Fish and other seafood can be an excellent source of long-chained n-3 fatty acids. These are known to have significant benefits for human health, and are difficult to obtain by alternative means (Karr *et al.*, 2011; Abeywardena and Patten, 2012). Partly for these reasons, and partly due to their accessibility, fish are a key source of protein, micronutrients and essential fatty acids for large numbers of people in developing countries. However, while aquaculture products are routinely consumed in the diets of many Asian people, consumption is much lower in people living in sub-Saharan Africa. Per capita fish consumption in this region has grown comparatively little in recent years. This is despite potentially suitable conditions for aquaculture, and highlights that the rôle aquaculture plays in food and nutrition security is influenced by several factors including whether or not seafood is readily available from capture fisheries.

Table 13.2. Aquaculture production by groups of species in 2016. (Source: FAO, 2018). n.e.i., not elsewhere included

Species	Production ('000 t live weight)	% of total
Finfish		
Grass carp (*Ctenopharyngodon idellus*)	6,068	11
Silver carp (*Hypophthalmichthys molitrix*)	5,301	10
Common carp (*Cyprinus carpio*)	4,557	8
Nile tilapia (*Oreochromis niloticus*)	4,200	8
Bighead carp (*Hypophthalmichthys nobilis*)	3,527	7
Atlantic salmon (*Salmo salar*) (ranked ninth)	2,248	4
Other finfish	28,100	53
Finfish total	**54,091**	**100**
Crustaceans		
Whiteleg shrimp (*Penaeus vannamei*)	4,156	53
Red swamp crawfish (*Procambarus clarkii*)	920	12
Chinese mitten crab (*Eriocheir sinensis*)	812	10
Giant tiger prawn (*Panaeus monodon*)	701	9
Oriental river prawn (*Macrobrachium nipponense*)	273	4
Other crustaceans	1,000	12
Crustacean total	**7,862**	**100**
Molluscs		
Cupped oysters n.e.i. (*Crassostrea* spp.)	4,864	28
Japanese carpet shell (*Ruditapes philippinarum*)	4,229	25
Scallops n.e.i. (*Pectinidae*)	1,861	11
Marine molluscs n.e.i. (*Mollusca*)	1,154	7
Sea mussels n.e.i. (*Mytilidae*)	1,100	6
Other molluscs	3,931	23
Mollusc total	**17,139**	**100**
Other animals		
Other animals total	**939**	**100**

The Potential of Selective Breeding

Selective breeding programmes have substantial potential to help address the aforementioned requirement for increase in aquaculture production. Selective breeding can offer cumulative and permanent improvement in traits of economic, welfare and environmental relevance. Until recently, less than 10% of aquaculture production was derived from selectively bred stocks (Gjedrem *et al.*, 2012). While this is likely to have increased in recent years, it is clear that selective breeding and genetic improvement of aquaculture species generally lags significantly behind the terrestrial animal and crop breeding industries (Gjedrem *et al.*, 2012; Yáñez *et al.*, 2015; Robledo *et al.*, 2017). The consequence of this is that the majority of farmed aquatic species are either sourced directly from the wild, or are in the very early stages of a domestication process (Teletchea and Fontaine, 2014). This means that there is likely to be a huge amount of standing genetic variation for traits of relevance to production, and as such a substantial potential for genetic improvement in these traits. This is likely to have downstream benefits for global food security via greater utilization of genetically improved stocks and the positive impact of this on production traits.

The reproductive biology of aquatic species can be highly amenable to selective breeding, with potential for high selection intensity and therefore genetic gain. The reasons for this include the high fecundity that is almost universal in aquaculture species. For example, an Atlantic salmon female may produce 20,000 eggs, marine finfish such as sea bream hundreds of thousands of eggs per female, and shellfish such as oysters, millions of eggs per female. Compared to terrestrial livestock, this fecundity is orders of magnitude higher, and this presents opportunities to design breeding programmes in different ways. External fertilization is often possible, where the gametes from both sire and dam can be obtained individually (in a process known as 'stripping') and then fertilization can be performed externally. This gives great flexibility in breeding programme design. For example, it is plausible to perform effective genotype-by-environment interaction studies (discussed below) by splitting full-sib families into groups and sending each group to a different environment. Also, critically, it is possible to measure traits that are difficult or impossible to measure on the selection candidates themselves on close relatives of selection candidates, including full siblings, which facilitates accurate breeding value estimation. However, there are also related challenges to be addressed, since each species is likely to have unique reproductive biology and associated requirements to tailor a breeding programme to address these. An example of this is *mass spawning*, whereby some species will only reproduce effectively in groups, which causes downstream issues of individual tracking and avoidance of inbreeding.

History of Selective Breeding in Aquaculture

Atlantic salmon breeding programmes

The most advanced breeding programmes for any aquaculture species are those in place for Atlantic salmon. The first commercial-scale salmon farming was in Norway in the 1960s, and the first major trials of family-based breeding programmes were in the early 1970s (Gjedrem *et al.*, 2012). In these experiments, gametes from Atlantic salmon originating from ~40 Norwegian rivers were collected, and these were used to establish datasets where robust genetic parameters were obtained for important production traits. This led to the first commercial breeding programme (Gjøen and Bentsen, 1997). Similar initiatives were instigated shortly after, and included the establishment of strains such as the Mowi, the Rauma, the Jakta and the Bolaks originating from different sampling events and locations (Glover *et al.*, 2017). Today, the vast majority of global salmon aquaculture populations is derived from these original strains, including salmon farming in Chile and the UK, after a series of crossing and international export events. The exceptions are the North American-derived Atlantic salmon aquaculture strains which are predominantly farmed in the Australian (primarily Tasmanian) and Canadian industries. These strains are genetically quite distinct from the European Atlantic salmon, and even have a different chromosome number (27 pairs of chromosomes for North American versus 29 for European; Brenna-Hansen *et al.*, 2012). The continuous consolidation of breeding companies has resulted in a relatively small number of large international companies supplying eggs to most of the major salmon-producing countries. These large breeding companies, which include AquaGen (Norway), Benchmark (UK) and Hendrix Genetics (Netherlands), tend to supply eggs to the market via separate breeding programmes operating in Norway and Chile. Mowi (formerly Marine Harvest) is one of the world's largest Atlantic salmon producers and runs its own integrated breeding programme.

The initial target trait for improvement of the aforementioned family-based breeding programmes was higher growth rate. Typical heritability estimates for growth rate and other production-relevant traits in salmon are given in Table 13.3. This initial selective breeding, typically using pedigree-based best linear unbiased prediction with the focus primarily on growth rate, was exceptionally successful, with genetic gain per generation estimated at approximately 15%, which is notably superior to equivalent levels seen in most terrestrial livestock programmes (Gjedrem and Rye, 2018). Example genetic gains for this and other traits is shown in Table 13.4. The generation interval of salmon is relatively long, typically 3 to 4 years, which reduces the realized rate of genetic progress, but the rate of improvement is still impressive. Part of the reason for these levels of genetic gain is the selection intensity that is possible due to the high fecundity mentioned above. It may also relate to working with a species

Table 13.3. Example heritability estimates for production traits in salmonid fish breeding.

Trait	Example heritability estimate (s.e.)	Source
Harvest weight	0.52 (0.05)	Powell *et al.* (2008)
Fillet weight	0.53 (0.05)	Powell *et al.* (2008)
Gutted yield	0.04 (0.01)	Powell *et al.* (2008)
Fat percentage	0.18 (0.03)	Powell *et al.* (2008)
Fillet colour	0.14 (0.03)	Powell *et al.* (2008)
Feed conversion ratio	0.10 (0.05)	Kause *et al.* (2016)

Table 13.4. Genetic gain in an Atlantic salmon breeding programme after five generations. (From Thodesen *et al.* (1999), adapted from Gjedrem and Baranski (2009).)

Trait	Improvement – selected versus wild (%)
Growth rate	+113
Food consumption	+40
Protein retention	+9
Energy retention	+14
Feed conversion ratio[a]	−20

[a]kg feed per kg body weight produced.

with a very recent domestication history, which could result in high levels of genetic variability in traits of importance for farmed production. In the case of terrestrial livestock species, these have been domesticated and selected for favourable traits for farming over approximately 10,000 years (Mignon-Grasteau *et al.*, 2005), either directly or indirectly.

As the breeding programmes became more advanced and the producers' requirements changed, the breeding goals widened and began to include traits such as disease resistance, rate of sexual maturation and fillet traits (Gjedrem and Rye, 2018). As broodstock fish are usually not exposed to disease and are not harvested for consumption, incorporating these traits into the breeding goal required the use of extensive testing of close relatives to selection candidates. This was achieved by taking advantage of amenable features of salmon reproductive biology, including the external fertilization and the high levels of fecundity. The result was that a typical breeding programme structure may include a breeding nucleus of approximately 100–300 families, where each full-sib family would be split into two groups, with some full sibs remaining in the breeding nucleus while other full sibs were used for production and performance testing. This operation, known as sib testing (see Chapter 4), allows genetic progress to be made for the traits that are difficult or impossible to measure on the candidates themselves.

Salmon-breeding programmes have been early adopters of various technologies. Some of the first examples were the means to track individuals to be able to construct pedigrees. This was typically achieved by rearing individual full-sib families separately until the stage where they are large enough to be tagged. Passive integrated transponder tags can then be inserted under the skin of individuals prior to mixing of families such that the family origin can later be established during performance testing and/or selection of broodstock candidates. Parentage assignment genetic marker panels were also applied and used for a similar purpose. In addition, in the early years of the 21st century, genetic markers began to be applied to capitalize on the within-family component of genetic variation, along with the between-family genetic variation used in family-selection programmes. One of the most impactful early examples of this was the widespread application of marker-assisted selection (MAS) for favourable alleles at a major quantitative trait locus (QTL) explaining the vast majority of variation in host resistance to infectious pancreatic necrosis virus (IPNV) (Houston *et al.*, 2008, 2010; Moen *et al.*, 2009; Gheyas *et al.*, 2010). The result was a sustained decrease in the incidence of IPN outbreaks to near zero, and widespread recognition of the potential of (molecular) genetics in selective breeding to tackle infectious disease (Norris, 2017). Subsequent studies have demonstrated that most other traits of importance for salmon production are heritable but highly polygenic (for reviews, see Yáñez *et al.*, 2014b; Houston, 2017), and therefore genomic selection (GS) is the most relevant method for application of genomics to genetic improvement (discussed in more detail below).

Due to the fact that both domestication and selective breeding are relatively recent in Atlantic salmon (as with other aquaculture species), there is a close proximity between farmed and wild salmon populations. However, there are already notable genetic and phenotypic differences between farmed and wild Atlantic salmon populations. Escapees from salmon farms may have resulted in substantial introgression into wild stocks, which has the potential to impact on life history traits and associated fitness of those wild populations (e.g. Glover *et al.*, 2017). Therefore, there is a substantial body of research focused on preventing interbreeding of wild and farmed fish, including generations of triploids en masse (Benfey, 2016) – because triploids are sterile they cannot interbreed with wild stocks if they escape. There are also novel applications of genome editing to induce sterility in farmed stocks (see below). Comparisons between different populations of farmed and wild stocks are useful for detecting genetic signatures of the domestication process. Here again, salmon present an interesting model due to the passage of relatively few generations since the advent of commercial-scale farming, perhaps 12–14 generations. Analyses comparing the genomes of farmed and wild populations have revealed signals of selection that may be associated with domestication traits, and these have been linked to genes associated with growth, early sexual maturation and immune response (Gutierrez *et al.*, 2016; Liu *et al.*, 2017).

Breeding programmes for other aquaculture species

Selective breeding programmes for other aquaculture species have been established more recently than salmon and are still at a formative stage in most species. The high fecundity and low individual value of offspring resulted in early attempts to perform mass selection (see Chapter 4) for favourable traits in several finfish, shellfish and crustacean species. However, this mass selection approach was largely unsuccessful in the long term, which is to be expected given the likelihood of a large, cumulative impact of inbreeding and associated inbreeding depression (Gjedrem *et al.* 2012). Such mass selection without measures to avoid mating related animals (sharing common ancestors) is likely to be detrimental to the breeding objective in the long term. It has been well established that inbreeding causes substantial depression in economically-important traits in addition to an overall reduction in genetic variation within the breeding population (e.g. Gjerde *et al.*, 1983). Therefore, avoidance of inbreeding is particularly important in aquaculture species, where uncontrolled mating has a high likelihood of resulting in crosses between related animals. Encouragingly, alterations to mating designs and knowledge of the pedigree can very easily prevent this rapid increase in inbreeding (Sánchez *et al.*, 2003). However, even if inbreeding can be avoided, mass selection is limited to the traits that can be measured on the selection candidates and is very restrictive on the number of traits that can be included in the breeding goal. Breeding programmes for many aquaculture species have initially focused on mass selection for growth which is straightforward to measure on selection candidates, but other traits such as disease resistance and fillet traits are much more challenging to measure on the candidates themselves and typically rely solely on records from relatives, as described above.

As with Atlantic salmon, family selection is increasingly becoming standard practice for the finfish aquaculture industries for species where there is a large production volume and value. For example, the Nile tilapia (*Oreochromis niloticus*) is one of the most important aquaculture species globally and is a critical source of protein and nutrition in developing countries. As is common to many farmed fish species, an important milestone was the establishment of primarily monosex production (production of a single sex – in the case of tilapia, only using males (Shelton and Rothbard, 2006)). Monosex production for males is used to increase growth performance (because males grow faster than females) and avoids problems related to premature maturation and reproduction. Monosex technologies are discussed in more detail below. Selective breeding of tilapia is one of the highest profile success stories in aquaculture, and the development of the 'Genetically Improved Farmed Tilapia' or GIFT strain resulted in an 86% increase in growth rate in just five generations (Bentsen *et al.*, 2017). The GIFT strain broodstock were sampled from four strains of Nile tilapia reared in the Philippines (specifically, stocks derived from Israel, Singapore, Taiwan and Thailand) as well as samples from four wild populations imported from Africa (Egypt, Ghana, Kenya and Senegal; Gjedrem *et al.*, 2012). This diverse sampling was performed to ensure a high level of genetic variability in the population. GIFT and GIFT-derived strains now dominate world tilapia aquaculture production and have been the basis of new private-company breeding programmes (the major salmon breeding companies AquaGen and Benchmark have sister companies that specialize in tilapia breeding). An example of the spread of the GIFT strain is that it represents 80% of the total production of tilapia juveniles in China, 75% in Thailand, and 40% in the Philippines (Sukmanomon *et al.*, 2012; Fabrice, 2019).

The aquaculture industries for many other groups of species are in the process of establishing or consolidating breeding programmes to enhance production. These include (but are not limited to) several freshwater and marine finfish, crustacean and bivalve shellfish species. The evolutionary diversity of these species and their reproductive biology mean that tailored programmes are often required to optimize genetic improvement for a specific (group of) species. An example of the diversity of species and production environments is shown in Figs 13.2 to 13.5. In bivalve shellfish, for example, both male and female parents can produce millions of gametes each. This typically results in relatively low survival rates for fertilized embryos, and is thought to be related to the high levels of genetic diversity, high incidence of deleterious mutations and *segregation distortion* within their genomes (Plough, 2016). Nonetheless, breeding programmes that do exist have successfully improved complex traits such as growth by a similar amount per generation as has been observed in finfish (e.g. 10–15% per generation) and genomic tools have potential to allow selection for new traits such as disease resistance (Hollenbeck and Johnston, 2018).

There are other aquaculture species where, despite large production volume and value, well-managed selective breeding programmes are not

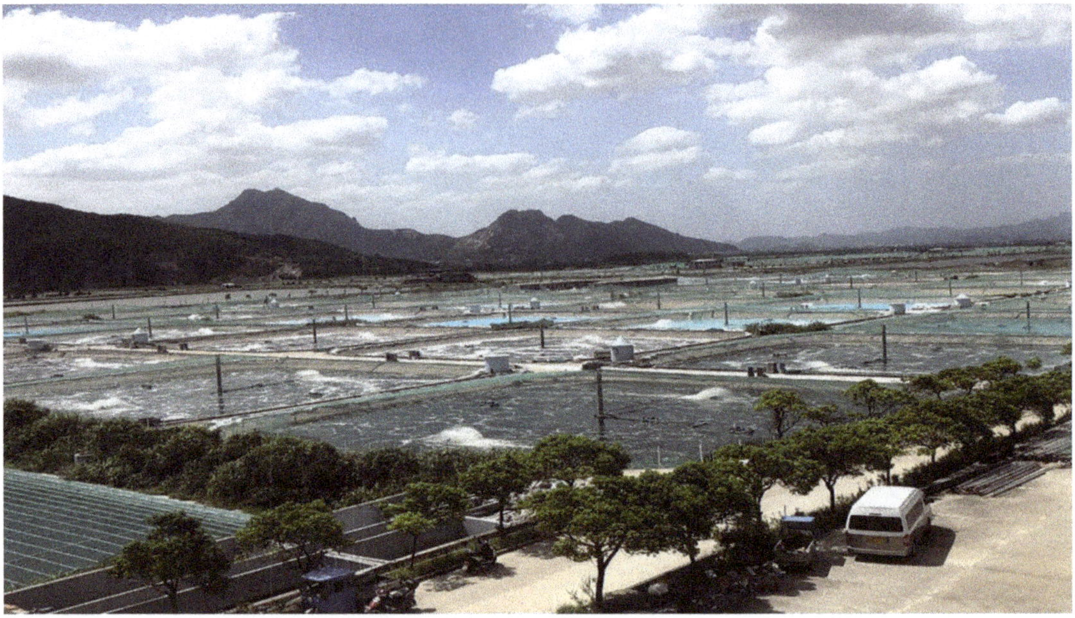

Fig. 13.2. A large Pacific white shrimp farm in China.

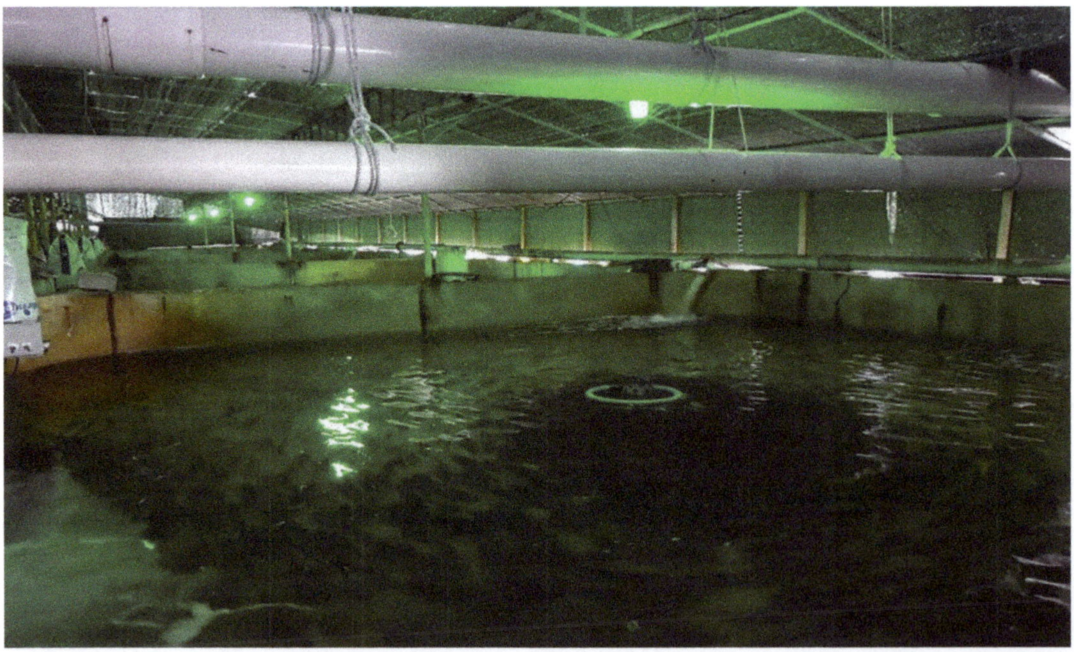

Fig. 13.3. A striped beakfish farm in South Korea.

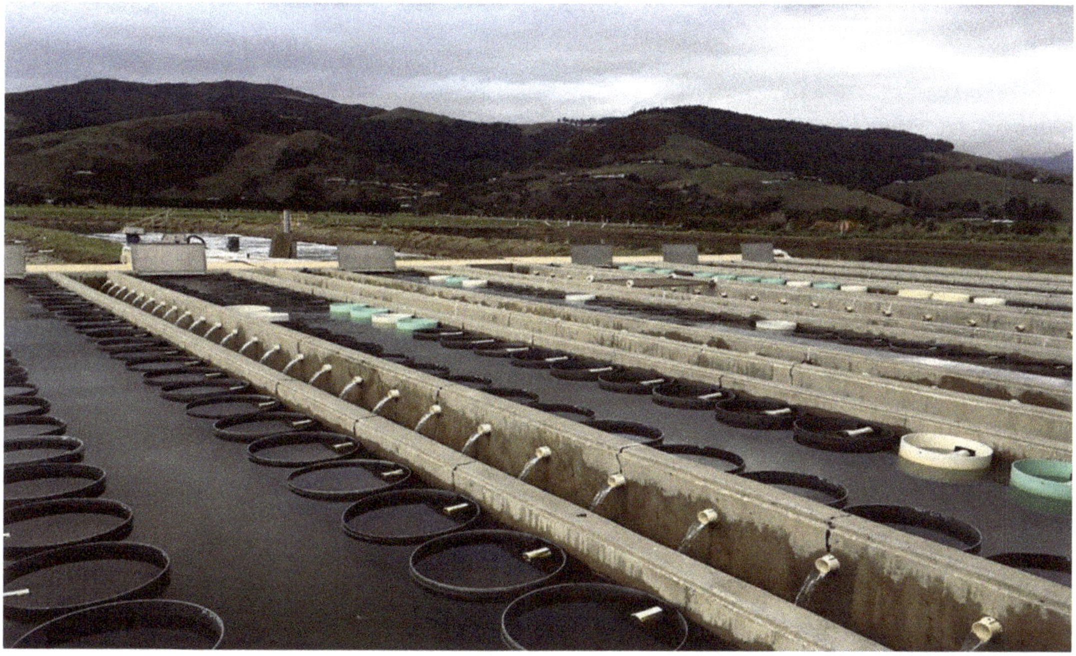

Fig. 13.4. A Pacific oyster 'grow out' facility in New Zealand.

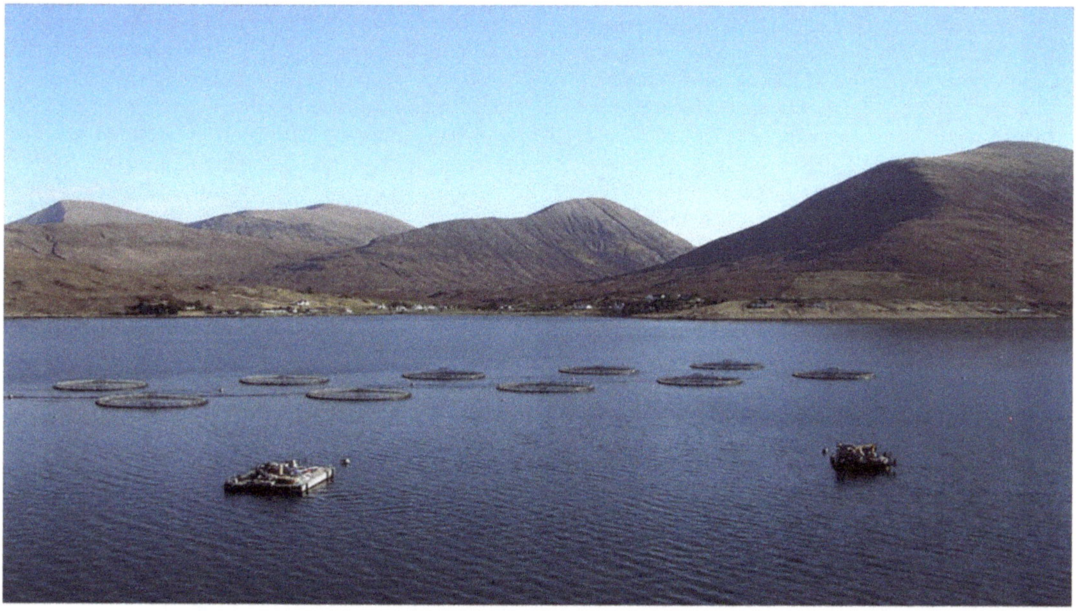

Fig. 13.5. Atlantic salmon sea cages in Scotland. (Available at: https://en.wikipedia.org/wiki/Fish_farming#/media/File:Loch_Ainort_fish_farm_-_geograph.org.uk_-_1800327.jpg; accessed 8 December 2019; Richard Dorrell / Loch Ainort fish farm / CC BY-SA 2.0.)

yet commonplace. This disparity in breeding technologies across different sectors is rather unique to aquaculture, with the salmon-breeding programmes being highly advanced, yet the majority of species being derived from wild or near-wild stocks. Crossbreeding has been utilized extensively for some species, notably carp species. A high degree of heterosis has been observed, which has been utilized by breeders and producers to improve production (e.g. Wohlfarth, 1993). However, there is movement in recent years towards family-based selective breeding programmes to enable continuous genetic gain, and the high fecundity of these species does make family selection an attractive option. Another option is continuation of cross breeding but with genetic improvement programmes within each of the founder lines, as in the pig and poultry breeding sectors, for example.

Disease resistance as a primary target trait

Infectious diseases present a major and persistent constraint to sustainable aquaculture production. Disease outbreaks can cause periodic catastrophic losses due to mortalities or the requirement to cull for biosecurity reasons. In addition, for certain endemic diseases, there are significant indirect costs associated with impaired growth during infection, and/or the substantial cost of treatments where they are available. A unique feature of aquaculture is that the farmed animals are in frequent contact with the 'wild' environment, and in particular farming marine species in the open ocean makes preventative management and biosecurity challenging (Lafferty *et al.*, 2015). It has been shown that diseases can be transmitted from farmed hosts to wild hosts in the surrounding waters and vice versa (Lafferty *et al.*, 2015). In several finfish species there are vaccines and medicines which assist with the prevention and control of infectious disease. However, they can be expensive, logistically challenging to deliver to the fish, and only partially effective. Further, obtaining regulatory approval can also be challenging (Lafferty *et al.*, 2015). To treat certain diseases, blanket treatments are applied (e.g. in feed), which can create a selective pressure for evolution of resistance in the pathogen or parasite. For example, drug-resistant strains of ectoparasitic copepod sea lice (which parasitize Atlantic salmon and other salmonid species) have emerged in Europe and Chile, due to extensive use of medicines (Aaen *et al.*, 2015). For these reasons, selective breeding for improvement of host resistance is seen as a very attractive option to help prevent or mitigate outbreaks of infectious diseases. Encouraging heritability estimates for host resistance traits have been observed in a wealth of studies (Table 13.5), suggesting that breeding for improved resistance is a feasible goal.

Disease-resistance traits are often complex and generally depend on the specific pathogen and host species in question. In the literature, disease resistance is typically used as a generic term to describe the ability of the host to limit infection, or the consequences of infection, by reducing pathogen replication (Doeschl-Wilson *et al.*, 2012). From a selective breeding standpoint, disease resistance could be considered 'the desirable trait' in this context, and the opposite to disease resistance could be considered as 'susceptibility'. However, there are several additional terms related to the broad-sense disease resistance which have been defined. The 'tolerance' of an animal can refer to its ability to reduce the impact of infection with a pathogen on performance (without necessarily impacting on the total pathogen load) (Doeschl-Wilson *et al.*, 2012). The 'infectivity' of an animal is the propensity of transmitting infection upon contact with a susceptible individual (Lipschutz-Powell *et al.*, 2012) and has also recently been suggested to be a heritable trait (Anacleto *et al.*, 2019). Disease resistance (in the general sense described above) has been a target trait for aquaculture breeders since the early 1990s as salmon-breeding programmes began to broaden their breeding goals (Gjøen and Bentsen, 1997). Typically, disease resistance is a trait that is not measured on the selection candidates, due to the biosecurity risk to the hatchery (e.g. potential carrier status of survivors and possible vertical transmission to offspring). Therefore, to perform effective breeding for disease resistance it is necessary to record accurate disease-resistance measures or correlates on relatives of the candidates (Bishop and Woolliams, 2010). In the typical sib-testing schemes of aquaculture breeding, this is plausible using experimental challenge or 'field' data from the siblings of the candidates (Bishop and Woolliams, 2014).

Highly pathogenic diseases (in particular viruses and bacteria) could be considered to be the most straightforward to tackle from a practical breeding perspective. It is possible to define resistance as survival (and/or mortality) of individuals during a natural challenge or a laboratory disease-challenge trial

Table 13.5. Heritability estimates for disease resistance in salmonid fish species. (After Yáñez *et al.*, 2014b; CC-BY 4.0.)

Salmonid species	Disease agent	$h^2 \pm$ s.e.	Reference
Atlantic salmon (*Salmo salar*)	*Neoparamoeba* spp.	0.40 ± 0.08 to 0.49 ± 0.09	Taylor *et al.* (2009)
	Renibacterium salmoninarum	0.2 ± 0.1	Gjedrem and Gjøen (1995)
	Aeromonas salmonicida	0.48 ± 0.17	Gjedrem *et al.* (1991)
	Aeromonas salmonicida	0.34 ± 0.13	Gjøen *et al.* (1997)
	Aeromonas salmonicida	0.38 ± 0.09	Ødegård *et al.* (2006)
	Aeromonas salmonicida	0.43 ± 0.02	Ødegård *et al.* (2007b)
	Aeromonas salmonicida	0.59 ± 0.06	Olesen *et al.* (2007)
	Aeromonas salmonicida	0.62	Kjøglum *et al.* (2008)
	Aeromonas salmonicida	0.47 ± 0.05	Gjerde *et al.* (2009)
	Gyrodactylus salaris	0.32 ± 0.10	Salte *et al.* (2010)
	IPNV	0.43	Guy *et al.* (2006)
	IPNV	0.5	Wetten *et al.* (2007)
	IPNV	0.55	Kjøglum *et al.* (2008)
	ISAV	0.13 ± 0.03	Gjøen *et al.* (1997)
	ISAV	0.16 ± 0.01	Ødegård *et al.* (2007a)
	ISAV	0.32 ± 0.02	Ødegård *et al.* (2007b)
	ISAV	0.24 ± 0.03	Olesen *et al.* (2007)
	ISAV	0.37	Kjøglum *et al.* (2008)
	ISAV	0.40 ± 0.04	Gjerde *et al.* (2009)
	Caligus elongatus	0.22	Mustafa and MacKinnon (1999)
	Lepeophtheirus salmonis	0.14 ± 0.02	Kolstad *et al.* (2005)
	Lepeophtheirus salmonis	0.07 ± 0.02	Glover *et al.* (2005)
	Vibrio anguillarum	0.38 ± 1.07	Gjøen *et al.* (1997)
	Vibrio salmonicida	0.13 ± 0.08	Gjedrem and Gjøen (1995)
	Caligus royercresseyi	0.10 ± 0.03	Yáñez *et al.*, (2014a)
	Caligus royercresseyi	0.12 ± 0.07 to 0.34 ± 0.07	Lhorente *et al.* (2012)
	SPDV	0.21 ± 0.005	Norris *et al.* (2008)
	Piscirickettsia salmonis	0.11 ± 0.02 to 0.41	Yáñez *et al.* (2013)
	Piscirickettsia salmonis	0.18 ± 0.03	Yáñez *et al.* (2014a)
Brook trout (*Salvelinus fontinalis*)	*Aeromonas salmonicida*	0.51 ± 0.03	Perry *et al.* (2004)
Chinook salmon (*Oncorhynchus tshawytscha*)	*Renibacterium salmoninarum*	0 ± 0.05	Beacham and Evelyn (1992)
	Aeromonas salmonicida	0.21 ± 0.14	Beacham and Evelyn (1992)
	Vibrio anguillarum	0.14 ± 0.11	Beacham and Evelyn (1992)
Coho salmon (*Oncorhynchus kisutch*)	*Renibacterium salmoninarum*	0.53 ± 0.16	Withler and Evelyn (1990)
Rainbow trout (*Oncorhynchus mykiss*)	*Yersinia ruckeri*	0.21 ± 0.05	Henryon *et al.* (2005)
	Flavobacterium psychrophilum	0.35 ± 0.09	Silverstein *et al.* (2009)
	Flavobacterium psychrophilum	0.23 ± 0.03	Leeds *et al.* (2010)
	Flavobacterium psychrophilum	0.53 ± 0.09	Vallejo *et al.* (2010)
	Flavobacterium psychrophilum	0.07 ± 0.02	Henryon *et al.* (2005)
	VHS	0.63 ± 0.26	Dorson *et al.* (1995)
	VHS	0.11 ± 0.1	Henryon *et al.* (2005)

IPNV, infectious pancreatic necrosis virus; ISAV, infectious salmon anaemia virus; SPDV, salmon pancreas disease virus; VHS, Viral haemorrhagic septicaemia.

(Ødegård *et al.*, 2011). Survival, when measured as a binary trait, has been shown typically to have a moderate heritability for a number of commercially-important diseases (e.g. Ødegård *et al.*, 2011; Yáñez *et al.*, 2014b). Therefore, disease-challenge testing has become a routine component of many advanced selective breeding programmes, particularly for finfish such as salmonids and tilapia (Yáñez *et al.*, 2014b; Elaswad and Dunham, 2018). A typical disease-challenge trial may involve infecting tagged individual juvenile fish in a standardized tank environment with a pathogen strain that is thought to be representative of those causing disease outbreaks in the production environment. Mortality (or survival) at the end of the test (when mortality returns to baseline level) is recorded, and genetic parameters for binary survival can be estimated using relatively simple linear models with adaptations to consider the trait of resistance on the underlying liability scale (Ødegård *et al.*, 2011). Binary survival can be an excellent indicator of disease resistance in the field setting, as shown by high genetic correlations between trait measures in both environments (e.g. Ødegård *et al.*, 2006). Alternative measures of disease resistance include pathogen or parasite load, for example, as measured by cell culture assays or quantitative PCR (e.g. for viral disease in shrimp) (Phuthaworn *et al.*, 2016) or biomarkers of the host immune response (e.g. Yáñez *et al.*, 2014b). For certain ectoparasites (e.g. salmon lice), the primary disease-resistance phenotype used for selection is the number of parasites attached to the fish after a standardized challenge (e.g. Tsai *et al.*, 2016).

An alternative to the artificial laboratory challenge testing described above is collection of disease data and samples from field outbreaks, which can be used opportunistically to quantify genetic resistance to infectious diseases, and also to calculate breeding values for selection candidates. It is of course necessary to first establish the genetic link between the animals in which the outbreak occurred, and those for which we wish to predict breeding values. In this scenario, typically pedigree and family assignment is performed using genetic markers. The advantage of measuring the disease in the field is that the trait is directly relevant to the production problem, and the pathogen strain is the one that is currently problematic. However, there are some drawbacks to this approach. For example, it can be challenging to discern the cause of mortality in natural outbreaks and obtaining high-quality samples from dead fish can be challenging due to both difficulty in collecting the fish, and the likelihood of degradation of tissue and DNA. In addition, certain diseases must be controlled by other means (e.g. culling of stock for notifiable viral diseases or chemotherapeutants for parasites) before the fish become sufficiently infected to obtain meaningful resistance phenotypes, and this clearly restricts the feasibility and usefulness of field trials to gather data related to genetic resistance.

While family selection has many advantages for breeding for disease resistance, mass selection approaches have also been applied in aquaculture. Mass selection can result in high selection intensity and could enable rapid genetic progress for resistance traits, albeit with a significant risk of inbreeding depression (Gjedrem and Baranski, 2009). Mass selection resulted in > 60% increase in oyster herpes virus survival compared with unselected controls after only four generations of selection of Pacific oysters (Dégremont *et al.*, 2015) and has also been successfully applied to taura syndrome virus in Panaeid shrimps (Cock *et al.*, 2009). However, as described above, mass selection is considered risky because: (i) it can result in high levels of inbreeding and associated problems; (ii) it requires breeding from broodstock, which have previously been exposed to a disease outbreak which can present a biosecurity risk to hatcheries; and (iii) it is not amenable to selection for multiple traits, which is a feature of modern breeding programmes.

Genotype × Environment Interactions

A major challenge for breeding programmes of many aquaculture species is genotype-by-environment (G × E) interaction, in which the performance of the selected animals can vary markedly across diverse production environments (e.g. in tilapia breeding; Sae-Lim *et al.*, 2016). This results in re-ranking of genotypes across environments and effectively reduces the overall response to selection within a breeding programme (Sae-Lim *et al.*, 2016). Genotype-by-environment interactions have been discussed in several earlier chapters in the book, and present a challenging issue in certain aquatic species because: (i) variation in environmental conditions can occur at distinct stages of the production cycle, for example the freshwater and marine water stages of salmon production; (ii) the 'grow out' conditions for many species occur under 'natural' conditions in ponds or seawater cages; and (iii) the large number of offspring from broodstock matings can be distributed across many different environments, and are readily shipped to a broad geographical range. All these factors suggest that G × E is an important factor to consider in aquaculture breeding programmes.

Reproductive Technologies in Aquaculture Production

As briefly highlighted earlier for Nile tilapia, the use of reproductive technology is widespread for aquaculture species. This can include generation of monosex populations and/or alterations in ploidy levels (the number of sets of chromosomes that each animal carries) in different species. These technologies are used for a variety of reasons and are often specific to the species or production system in question. There are many aquaculture species where sexual dimorphism (the difference between sexes) is challenging to detect based on visual checks alone, and/or does not occur until late in the reproductive cycle (e.g. for Atlantic salmon). Unlike most terrestrial livestock species, genetic control of sex can be polygenic (i.e. more than one sex-determining gene), which can make identification of predictive sex-linked DNA markers challenging (see Devlin and Nagahama, 2002). Sex can also be determined or heavily influenced by environment in many cultured species, and in some cases there is a genotype-by-environment interaction in sex determination. Finally, while most fish are *gonochoristic* (i.e. each animal is one sex throughout its life) some farmed fish species, such as gilthead seabream (*Sparus aurata*), are *sequential hermaphrodites* (i.e. the animals change sex at some point in their life) which adds further logistical challenges to a breeding programme.

Artificial insemination is a routine technology in most aquaculture hatchery operations and breeding programmes. External fertilization combined with high fecundity in fish makes artificial insemination or strip-spawning very efficient. A challenge related to this process is the timing of several events associated with spawning which need to be coordinated. For example, eggs can rapidly diminish in viability after ovulation/stripping, and sperm are activated almost immediately upon contact with water and has a very short period of activity. Technologies have been developed to tackle this issue, and it is now possible to extend and cryopreserve sperm of several species to increase the flexibility of the timings of reproduction.

Sterilization is used as a form of reproductive control in many aquaculture species for several reasons. Firstly, sterilization can be used to prevent the negative impacts of gonadal development on growth, flesh quality, and other traits. Secondly, it can be used as a mechanism to protect the environment and wild fish stocks, for example, to prevent interbreeding between escapees of farmed salmonids and their wild counterparts. Thirdly, sterility can be used as a form of protection for breeders by limiting the wider spread of potentially valuable genetic material derived from selective breeding programmes or potentially genetically modified organisms.

One of the primary means of inducing sterility is the artificial generation of polyploidy. Physical means of inducing polyploidy, for example by application of a pressure or temperature shock to disrupt the expulsion of the second polar body during embryo development, is widely used in aquaculture species (hybridization is not common). This physical induction of triploidy is considered the most effective means for producing sterile progeny for the majority of aquaculture sectors (Benfey, 2016). The technology has also been used in recreational fisheries to prevent breeding of non-native species (e.g. grass carp; Zajicek *et al.*, 2011) or interbreeding of stocked fish with native species (Loopstra and Hansen, 2004) and is routine in many hatcheries used for restocking salmonid species in North America.

Technologies for controlling gender are widely applied in aquaculture for maximizing production efficiency and product quality, and for restricting reproduction. For the majority of aquaculture species, one sex has an improved production performance compared to the other. Almost all aquaculture species display sexually dimorphic growth. This includes the most popular and valuable farmed fish globally, i.e. carp, salmonids, tilapia, and catfish. In addition, in most of these species, differences in growth and feed efficiency are due in part to one sex maturing earlier than the other within the production cycle. Gender control and prevention of reproduction/sterilization are often closely linked. Use of a monosex population for production has many of the benefits of sterilization, including prevention of negative effects associated with precocious maturation and the resultant overpopulation in mixed-culture pond systems. As an example, all-male populations of Nile tilapia are farmed to: (i) prevent overpopulation: (ii) prevent loss of growth and other negative side effects of reproduction: and (iii) because males grow faster than females. In contrast, for rainbow trout, all-female rainbow populations are used in production because: (i) females grow faster than males; (ii) males are more likely to display premature maturation with associated negative side effects on growth and flesh quality; and (iii) triploidy is only effective at preventing gonad development in females. It is clear that monosex and sterility technologies have many advantages for commercial aquaculture production, but that the specific reasons and methods are very particular to the species and system in question.

Use of Genomic Technology in Aquaculture Breeding

Molecular markers

While family selection is effective for aquaculture species, it only captures the between-family genetic variation in the traits of interest and cannot capture the within-family genetic variation. For highly fecund aquaculture species, the within-family genetic variation is likely to be substantial. Genomic technology, such as the development of routine genotyping for microsatellite or single nucleotide polymorphism (SNP) multiplexes (see Chapter 5), have enabled rapid and accurate family assignment (Vandeputte and Haffray, 2014) which has underpinned family selection. The routine use of molecular genetic markers may have facilitated early uptake of MAS approaches in the early 21st century, because the industry was familiar with molecular genetic technology already. Marker-assisted selection is one route for gaining information on the comparative disease resistance of selection candidates from within a full-sib family (i.e. the within-family genetic variation; Sonesson, 2007). MAS first requires detection of marker alleles linked to QTL affecting the trait of interest and selecting animals based on whether they carry favourable alleles at the QTL.

Mapping of QTL has been a major goal for aquaculture genetics and breeding research and has yielded some successful results. Aquaculture species are close to their wild ancestors from an evolutionary standpoint, and the relatively new selection and disease pressures in the farm environment raise the possibility that loci with major effects may be segregating within the populations. One of the most notable examples of this is the aforementioned case of resistance to infectious pancreatic necrosis in Atlantic salmon, where a major QTL has been demonstrated as a successful means of controlling the disease (Norris, 2017). Selected other examples of QTL affecting resistance to disease include salmonid alphavirus (Gonen *et al.*, 2015), ISAV (Moen *et al.*, 2007) and *Gyrodactylus salaris* (Gilbey *et al.*, 2006) in salmon, lymphocystis disease in Japanese flounder (Fuji *et al.*, 2006), Bonamiosis in the European Flat Oyster (Lallias *et al.*, 2009) and *Flavobacterium psychrophilum* in rainbow trout (Vallejo *et al.*, 2014). Despite this, MAS has not been routinely successful in animal breeding, which is likely to be due to the fact that the majority of economically-important traits are polygenic (Meuwissen *et al.*, 2013). While recent domestication of aquaculture species may increase the chances of an *oligogenic* genetic architecture for disease-resistance traits (i.e. controlled by several genes but including some of major effect), it is also important to consider that the effect of any given QTL may differ according to the environment and the genetic background of the population.

Genomic selection

Genomic selection is increasingly used in modern selective breeding schemes in aquaculture, particularly for Atlantic salmon, but it is at a formative stage for various other key species. In GS, genome-wide markers are used to calculate genomic breeding values, and this is done without prior knowledge of the underlying QTL affecting the trait of interest (see Chapter 7 and Meuwissen *et al.*, 2001). Genetic marker effects are estimated in a 'training' population, which must be measured for both phenotypes (e.g. disease resistance) and genotypes (e.g. a SNP chip). The training population is used to develop a model which is then used to estimate genomic breeding values on selection candidates with genotypes only. The initial idea of GS was to detect and utilize population-wide linkage disequilibrium between genome-wide markers and QTL (Meuwissen *et al.*, 2001). However, the benefits of GS also include a more accurate estimate of the genetic relationship between any two individuals than could be given by pedigree records alone, and this is especially the case within families where full sibs would otherwise be assigned identical relationships (Meuwissen *et al.*, 2013). There have been several empirical test studies of genomic selection in aquaculture species, and in all cases the use of GS has resulted in higher prediction accuracy of breeding values than the use of pedigree information alone (Ødegård *et al.*, 2014; Tsai *et al.*, 2015; Dou *et al.*, 2016; reviewed in Zenger *et al.*, 2019).

To allow GS, a platform to generate high-density SNP marker genotypes across populations of animals is required. SNP arrays have been developed for several aquaculture species, including Atlantic salmon (Houston *et al.*, 2014; Yáñez *et al.*, 2016), rainbow trout (Palti *et al.*, 2015), common carp (Xu *et al.*, 2014), Pacific oysters (Gutierrez *et al.*, 2017) and catfish (Liu *et al.*, 2014). The buy-in of the advanced aquaculture breeding companies is clear, with the major salmon companies all routinely employing GS to improve genetic gain for multiple traits (see Houston, 2017; Zenger *et al.*, 2019). However, GS is an expensive technology, primarily due to the cost of high-density SNP chip genotyping in large numbers of individuals. A further caveat is that while GS is effective when the training and test populations are closely related (e.g. within a year group of a breeding programme), the ability to predict breeding values in animals more distantly related to the training population is rather limited (Tsai *et al.*, 2016). Genotype imputation, as described in Chapter 5, is one promising avenue for reducing the costs of GS, and has been tested in several studies using both simulated (Dufflocq *et al.*, 2019), and empirical data (Tsai *et al.*, 2017; Yoshida *et al.*, 2018).

Possibilities for genome editing

Genetic engineering approaches have been applied in aquaculture species for several decades, and the first genetically modified animal to be approved for human consumption was the AquaBounty Atlantic salmon. In more recent years, genome editing technologies have allowed targeted changes to the genomic DNA at a specific location, and engineered CRISPR/Cas9 systems are now routinely applied in an experimental setting for this purpose in many species (Cong *et al.*, 2013). As described in Chapter 5, this system uses a Cas9 enzyme making a double-stranded cut in the genomic DNA at a specific target site, enabled by the design of the guide RNA. The resulting changes to the genomic DNA can be the result of non-homologous end joining (NHEJ) which will repair the DNA at the cut site in the absence of a homologous template, and will result in small insertions or deletions at the cut site that can result in loss-of-function mutations in genes of interest. Alternatively, homology-directed repair (HDR) involves the provision of a DNA template which is similar to the flanking sequence of the cut site but may contain a user-targeted change in sequence, and the cell uses the template to repair at the cut site. The successful use of CRISPR/Cas9 with NHEJ repair to generate *slc45a2* knockout salmon in the F_0 generation via microinjection into one-cell stage embryos demonstrated the efficacy of the technology in salmon (Edvardsen *et al.*, 2014), the first example in an aquaculture species. Subsequent studies have successfully applied CRISPR/Cas9 to generate sterile salmon via ablation of germ cells caused by dnd (a factor required for germ cell survival in vertebrates) knockout (Wargelius *et al.*, 2016). In addition to these successful applications *in vivo*, CRISPR/Cas9 has been successfully applied for gene knockout in a salmonid cell line (CHSE-214; Dehler *et al.*, 2016), which harnesses the possibility of using cell line models to study the biology underlying traits of interest. There are not yet published examples of the use of HDR in aquaculture species, either *in vivo* or *in vitro*, but this may be the most valuable mechanism for future applications due to the possibility of making a user-defined and precise change to the genome.

As discussed in Chapters 5 and 14, the regulatory landscape around genome editing is uncertain. Interestingly, the first approved GM farmed animal was an Atlantic salmon which was ruled as fit for human consumption by the US Food and Drug Administration and the Canadian Food Inspection Agency after a long period of regulatory limbo (Waltz, 2017). The AquAdvantage (AquaBounty Technologies) strain shows improved growth rate due to the insertion of a growth hormone (GH) gene from Chinook salmon linked to a promoter from another fish species that drives high GH expression. Ultimately, research and development relating to potential uses of gene modification and gene editing in aquaculture will continue to develop rapidly and it is important that the dialogue surrounding the regulatory framework continues in parallel.

Practical Guidelines on Selection

It is challenging to make generalized guidelines for selection across all aquaculture species, but two features they all share are high fecundity and relatively recent domestication. Since only a minority of production globally is derived from science-based breeding programmes, the main recommendation is that we need breeding programme technology to be more widely adopted, and to underpin some of the production of the world's most widely-produced species. The high fecundity can result in very large genetic gain in a short time, and with appropriate management of diversity, this can have a major positive impact on global production. At the same time, due to the recent domestication and proximity of farmed strains to wild stocks, safeguards need to be put in place to ensure that there is no negative impact on wild aquatic genetic resources. Assuming the resources and the will to introduce selective breeding programmes are there, then the high fecundity can be harnessed very effectively in sib-testing schemes. This can ensure that trait records (either experimental or field records) can be collected in very close relatives of selection candidates. This means that, even for traits that are difficult or impossible to measure on the selection candidates, rapid progress can be made and can help overcome issues with genotype-by-environment interactions. Genomic tools have many rôles to play in supporting selective breeding in aquaculture, and will be used from the very early stages of a breeding programme to inform base populations, manage genetic diversity, and potentially also for parentage assignment and marker-assisted or GS.

The companies involved in selective breeding in aquaculture tend to fall into one of three categories. The first are specialized breeding companies whose business is to sell genetically improved eggs to producers, which are most evident in Atlantic salmon (e.g. Aquagen, Benchmark), and are typically paired with equivalent companies for other sectors, including tilapia and shrimp. Such companies do not yet exist for most other aquaculture species. There are some fully-integrated companies where their breeding programme supplies only their own producers, for example, the large Atlantic salmon company Mowi. The final type of company that has a major rôle in smaller sectors is genetic services companies which manage breeding programmes on behalf of (typically) small- and medium-sized producers. Examples of this would be Akvafosk (Norway), Xelect (UK) or Center for Aquaculture Technologies (North America). There are also a number of national and international breeding programmes funded by public funds, and an example is WorldFish which is a CGIAR organization who supply genetically improved tilapia and various carp species typically to low- and middle-income countries.

Summary

- Aquaculture species cover a hugely diverse group of species from throughout the evolutionary tree, with finfish, crustacean and mollusc species all featuring in global aquaculture production.
- Aquaculture has a key future rôle in meeting global demands for seafood, as capture fisheries have little opportunity to expand. The vast majority of aquaculture production by volume and value occurs in Asia.
- There are fundamental differences in reproductive biology of aquaculture species compared to livestock species, that can represent challenges and opportunities for breeding programmes. One major advantage of most aquaculture species is that they are highly fecund and thousands to millions of offspring are possible from a single cross.
- Application of genetic improvement in aquaculture is lagging significantly behind terrestrial livestock and the level of domestication and use of objective genetic improvement is highly variable between species.
- The most advanced breeding programmes are for Atlantic salmon, where family selection, including routine genomic selection, is performed for multiple traits. The high fecundity allows for sib testing whereby traits are recorded on full sibs of selection candidates.
- Disease resistance is a key target trait for aquaculture species because infectious diseases are a major threat, and it is common that few other mitigation or control options exist.
- Genetics and breeding technology tend to transfer from Atlantic salmon to other sectors, with similar breeding programmes run for major global aquaculture species such as Nile tilapia and Pacific white shrimp.
- Avoidance of early maturation is very important in aquaculture breeding and production, and manipulation of ploidy or use of monosex production is commonplace for certain species.
- Genotype × environment interaction is a key concern for most aquaculture systems, and the high fecundity of most species allows the routine testing of close relatives in diverse environments.
- Genome editing has substantial potential to improve production and welfare traits in aquaculture, with the high fecundity potentially allowing rapid and widespread dissemination. However, a suitable regulatory and public perception environment is key to uptake of this technology.

References

Aaen, S.M., Helgesen, K.O., Bakke, M.J., Kaur, K. and Horsberg, T.E. (2015) Drug resistance in sea lice: a threat to salmonid aquaculture. *Trends in Parasitology* 31(2), 72–81. DOI: 10.1016/j.pt.2014.12.006.

Abeywardena, M.Y. and Patten, G.S. (2012) Role of ω3 longchain polyunsaturated fatty acids in reducing cardio-metabolic risk factors. *Endocrine, Metabolic & Immune Disorders - Drug Targets* 11, 232–246. DOI: 10.2174/187153011796429817.

Anacleto, O., Cabaleiro, S., Villanueva, B., Saura, M., Houston, R.D. *et al.* (2019) Genetic differences in host infectivity affect disease spread and survival in epidemics. *Scientific Reports* 9, 4929. DOI: 10.1038/s41598-019-40567-w.

Beacham, T.D. and Evelyn, T.P.T. (1992) Genetic variation in disease resistance and growth of chinook, coho, and chum salmon with respect to vibriosis, furunculosis, and bacterial kidney disease. *Transactions of the American Fisheries Society* 121, 156–489. DOI: 10.1577/1548-8659(1992)121%3C0456%3AGVIDRA%3E2.3.CO%3B2.

Benfey, T.J. (2016) Effectiveness of triploidy as a management tool for reproductive containment of farmed fish: Atlantic salmon (*Salmo salar*) as a case study. *Reviews in Aquaculture* 8, 264–282. DOI: 10.1111/raq.12092.

Bentsen, H.B., Gjerde, B., Eknath, A.E., de Vera, M.S.P., Velasco, R.R. *et al.* (2017) Genetic improvement of farmed tilapias: Response to five generations of selection for increased body weight at harvest in Oreochromis niloticus and the further impact of the project. *Aquaculture* 468, 206–217. DOI: 10.1016/j.aquaculture.2016.10.018.

Bishop, S.C. and Woolliams, J.A. (2010) On the genetic interpretation of disease data. *PloS One* 5(1), e8940. DOI: 10.1371/journal.pone.0008940.

Bishop, S.C. and Woolliams, J.A. (2014). Genomics and disease resistance studies in livestock. *Livestock Science* 166, 190–198. DOI: 10.1016/j.livsci.2014.04.034.

Brenna-Hansen, S., Li, J., Kent, M.P., Boulding, E.G., Dominik, S. *et al.* (2012) Chromosomal differences between European and North American Atlantic salmon discovered by linkage mapping and supported by fluorescence *in situ* hybridization analysis. *BMC Genomics* 13, 432. DOI: 10.1186/1471-2164-13-432.

Cock, J., Gitterle, T., Salazar, M. and Rye, M. (2009) Breeding for disease resistance of Penaeid shrimps. *Aquaculture* 286, 1–11. DOI: 10.1016/j.aquaculture.2008.09.011.

Cong, L., Ran, F.A., Cox, D., Lin, S., Barretto, R. *et al.* (2013) Multiplex genome engineering using CRISPR/Cas systems. *Science* 339, 819–823. DOI: 10.1126/science.1231143.

Dégremont, L., Nourry, M. and Maurouard, E. (2015). Mass selection for survival and resistance to OsHV-1 infection in *Crassostrea gigas* spat in field conditions: response to selection after four generations. *Aquaculture* 446, 111–121. DOI: 10.1016/j.aquaculture.2015.04.029.

Dehler, C.E., Boudinot, P., Martin, S.A.M. and Collet, B. (2016) Development of an efficient genome editing method by CRISPR/Cas9 in a fish cell line. *Marine Biotechnology* 18(4), 449–452. DOI: 10.1007/s10126-016-9708-6.

Devlin, R.H. and Nagahama, Y. (2002) Sex determination and sex differentiation in fish: An overview of genetic, physiological, and environmental influences. *Aquaculture* 208, 191–364. DOI: 10.1016/S0044-8486(02)00057-1.

Doeschl-Wilson, A.B., Bishop, S.C., Kyriazakis, I. and Villanueva, B. (2012) Novel methods for quantifying individual host response to infectious pathogens for genetic analyses. *Frontiers in Genetics* 3, 266. DOI: 10.3389/fgene.2012.00266.

Dorson, M., Quillet. E., Hollebecq, M., Torhy, C. and Chevassus, B. (1995) Selection of rainbow trout resistant to viral haemorrhagic septicaemia virus and transmission of resistance by gynogenesis. *Veterinary Research* 26 (5-6), 361–368. Available at: https://hal.archives-ouvertes.fr/hal-00902359 (accessed 10 September 2020).

Dou, J., Li, X., Fu, Q., Jiao, W., Li, Y. *et al.* (2016) Evaluation of the 2b-RAD method for genomic selection in scallop breeding. *Scientific Reports* 6, 19244. DOI: 10.1038/srep19244.

Dufflocq, P., Pérez-Enciso, M., Lhorente, J.P. and Yáñez, J.M. (2019) Accuracy of genomic predictions using different imputation error rates in aquaculture breeding programs: A simulation study. *Aquaculture* 503, 225–230. DOI: 10.1016/j.aquaculture.2018.12.061.

Edvardsen, R.B., Leininger, S., Kleppe, L., Skaftnesmo, K.O. and Wargelius, A. (2014) Targeted mutagenesis in atlantic salmon (*Salmo salar* L.) using the CRISPR/Cas9 system induces complete knockout individuals in the F0 Generation. *PLoS ONE* 9, e108622. DOI: 10.1371/journal.pone.0108622.

Elaswad, A. and Dunham, R. (2018) Disease reduction in aquaculture with genetic and genomic technology: current and future approaches. *Reviews in Aquaculture* 10, 876–898. DOI: 10.1111/raq.12205.

Fabrice, T. (2019) Fish Domestication: An Overview. In: *Animal Domestication*. IntechOpen, London. DOI: 10.5772/intechopen.79628.

FAO (2018) World Fisheries and Aquaculture. Available at: www.fao.org/publications (accessed May 2019).

Fuji, K., Kobayashi, K., Hasegawa, O., Coimbra, M.R.M., Sakamoto, T. and Okamoto, N. (2006) Identification of a single major genetic locus controlling the resistance to lymphocystis disease in Japanese flounder (*Paralichthys olivaceus*). *Aquaculture* 254(1), 203–210. DOI: 10.1016/j.aquaculture.2005.11.024.

Gheyas, A.A., Houston, R.D., Mota-Velasco, J.C., Guy, D.R., Tinch, A.E. *et al.* (2010) Segregation of infectious pancreatic necrosis resistance QTL in the early life cycle of Atlantic Salmon (*Salmo salar*). *Animal Genetics* 41, 531–536. DOI: 10.1111/j.1365-2052.2010.02032.x.

Gilbey, J., Verspoor, E., Mo, T.A., Sterud, E., Olstad, K. *et al.* (2006) Identification of genetic markers associated with *Gyrodactylus salaris* resistance in Atlantic salmon *Salmo salar*. *Dis Aquat Organ* 71(2), 119–129. DOI: 10.3354/dao071119.

Gjedrem, T. and Baranski, M. (2009) *Selective Breeding in Aquaculture: An Introduction*. Springer, New York. DOI: 10.1007/978-90-481-2773-3.

Gjedrem, T. and Gjøen, H.M. (1995) Genetic variation in susceptibility of Atlantic salmon, *Salmo salar* L., to furunculosis, BKD and cold water vibriosis. *Aquaculture Research* 26(2), 129–134. DOI: 10.1111/j.1365-2109.1995.tb00892.x.

Gjedrem, T. and Rye, M. (2018). Selection response in fish and shellfish: a review. *Reviews in Aquaculture* 10, 168–179. DOI: 10.1111/raq.12154.

Gjedrem, T., Salte, R. and Gjøen, H.M. (1991) Genetic variation in susceptibility of Atlantic salmon to furunculosis. *Aquaculture* 97(1), 1–6. DOI: 10.1016/0044-8486(91)90274-B.

Gjedrem, T., Robinson, N. and Rye, M. (2012) The importance of selective breeding in aquaculture to meet future demands for animal protein: A review. *Aquaculture* 350–353, 117–129. DOI: 10.1016/j.aquaculture.2012.04.008.

Gjerde, B., Gunnes, K. and Gjedrem, T. (1983) Effect of inbreeding on survival and growth in rainbow trout. *Aquaculture* 34, 327–332. DOI: 10.1016/0044-8486(83)90212-0.

Gjerde, B., Evensen, Ø., Bentsen, H.B. and Storset, A. (2009) Genetic (co)variation of vaccine injuries and innate resistance to furunculosis (*Aeromonas salmonicida*) and infectious salmon anaemia (ISA) in Atlantic salmon (*Salmo salar*) *Aquaculture* 287(1–2), 52–58. DOI: 10.1016/j.aquaculture.2008.10.028.

Gjøen, H.M. and Bentsen, H.B. (1997) Past, present, and future of genetic improvement in salmon aquaculture. *Ices Journal of Marine Science* 54, 1009–1014.

Gjøen, H.M., Refstie, T., Ulla, O. and Gjerde, B. (1997) Genetic correlations between survival of Atlantic salmon in challenge and field tests. *Aquaculture* 158(3–4), 277–288. DOI: 10.1016/S0044-8486(97)00203-2.

Glover, K.A., Aasmundstad, T., Nilsena, F., Storset, A. and Skaala, Ø. (2005) Variation of Atlantic salmon families (*Salmo salar* L.) in susceptibility to the sea lice *Lepeophtheirus salmonis* and *Caligus elongatus*. *Aquaculture* 245(1–4), 19–30. DOI: 10.1016/j.aquaculture.2004.11.047.

Glover, K.A., Solberg, M.F., McGinnity, P., Hindar, K., Verspoor, E. *et al.* (2017) Half a century of genetic interaction between farmed and wild Atlantic *salmon: Status* of knowledge and unanswered questions. *Fish and Fisheries* 18, 890–927. DOI: 10.1111/faf.12214.

Gonen, S., Baranski, M., Thorland, I., Norris, A., Grove, H. *et al.* (2015) Mapping and validation of a major QTL affecting resistance to pancreas disease (salmonid alphavirus) in Atlantic salmon (*Salmo salar*). *Heredity* 115(5), 405–414. DOI: 10.1038/hdy.2015.37.

Gutierrez, A.P., Yáñez, J.M. and Davidson, W.S. (2016) Evidence of recent signatures of selection during domestication in an Atlantic salmon population. *Marine Genomics* 26, 41–50. DOI: 10.1016/j.margen.2015.12.007.

Gutierrez, A.P., Turner, F., Gharbi, K., Talbot, R., Lowe, N.R. *et al.* (2017) Development of a medium density combined-species SNP array for pacific and european oysters (*Crassostrea gigas* and *Ostrea edulis*). *G3: Genes, Genomes, Genetics* 7, 2209–2218. DOI: 10.1534/g3.117.041780.

Guy, D.R., Bishop, S.C., Brotherstone, S., Hamilton, A., Roberts, R.J. *et al.* (2006) Analysis of the incidence of infectious pancreatic necrosis mortality in pedigreed Atlantic salmon, *Salmo salar* L., populations. *Journal of Fish Diseases* 29(11), 637–647. DOI: 10.1111/j.1365-2761.2006.00758.x.

Henryon, M., Berg, P., Olesen, N.J., Kjær, T.E., Slierendrecht, W.J. *et al.* (2005) Selective breeding provides an approach to increase resistance of rainbow trout (*Onchorhynchus mykiss*) to the diseases, enteric redmouth disease, rainbow trout fry syndrome, and viral haemorrhagic septicaemia. *Aquaculture* 250(3–4), 621–636. DOI: 10.1016/j.aquaculture.2004.12.022.

Hollenbeck, C.M. and Johnston, I.A. (2018) Genomic tools and selective breeding in molluscs. *Frontiers in Genetics* 9, 253. DOI: 10.3389/fgene.2018.00253.

Houston, R.D. (2017) Future directions in breeding for disease resistance in aquaculture species. *Revista Brasileira de Zootecnia* 46, 545–551. DOI: 10.1590/S1806-92902017000600010.

Houston, R.D., Haley, C.S., Hamilton, A., Guy, D.R., Tinch, A.E. *et al.* (2008) Major quantitative trait loci affect resistance to infectious pancreatic necrosis in Atlantic salmon (*Salmo salar*). *Genetics* 178, 1109–1115. DOI: 10.1534/genetics.107.082974.

Houston, R.D., Haley, C.S., Hamilton, A., Guy, D.R., Mota-Velasco, J.C. *et al.* (2010) The susceptibility of Atlantic salmon fry to freshwater infectious pancreatic necrosis is largely explained by a major QTL. *Heredity* 105, 318–327. DOI: 10.1038/hdy.2009.171.

Houston, R.D., Taggart, J.B., Cézard, T., Bekaert, M., Lowe, N.R. *et al.* (2014) Development and validation of a high density SNP genotyping array for Atlantic salmon (*Salmo salar*). *BMC Genomics* 15(1), 90. DOI: 10.1186/1471-2164-15-90.

Karr, J.E., Alexander, J.E. and Winningham, R.G. (2011) Omega-3 polyunsaturated fatty acids and cognition throughout the lifespan: A review. *Nutritional Neuroscience* 14, 216–225. DOI: 10.1179/1476830511y.0000000012.

Kause, A., Kiessling, A., Martin, S.A.M., Houlihan, D. and Ruohonen, K. (2016) Genetic improvement of feed conversion ratio via indirect selection against lipid deposition in farmed rainbow trout (*Oncorhynchus mykiss* Walbaum). *The British Journal of Nutrition* 116, 1656–1665. DOI: 10.1017/S0007114516003603.

Kjøglum, S., Henryon, M., Aasmundstad, T. and Korsgaard, I. (2008) Selective breeding can increase resistance of Atlantic salmon to furunculosis, infectious salmon anaemia and infectious pancreatic necrosis. *Aquaculture Research* 39(5), 498–505. DOI: 10.1111/j.1365-2109.2008.01904.x.

Kobayashi, M., Msangi, S., Batka, M., Vannuccini, S., Dey, M.M. and Anderson, J.L. (2015). Fish to 2030: The role and opportunity for aquaculture. *Aquaculture Economics and Management* 19, 282–300. DOI: 10.1080/13657305.2015.994240.

Kolstad, K., Heuch, P.A., Gjerde, B., Gjedrem, T. and Salte, R. (2005) Genetic variation in resistance of Atlantic salmon (*Salmo salar*) to the salmon louse *Lepeophtheirus salmonis*. *Aquaculture* 247, 145–151. DOI: 10.1016/j.aquaculture.2005.02.009.

Lafferty, K.D., Harvell, C.D., Conrad, J.M., Friedman, C.S., Kent, M.L. *et al.* (2015) Infectious diseases affect marine fisheries and aquaculture economics. *Annual Review of Marine Science* 7, 471–496. DOI: 10.1146/annurev-marine-010814-015646.

Lallias, D., Gomez-Raya, L., Haley, C.S., Arzul, I., Heurtebise, S. *et al.* (2009) Combining two-stage testing and interval mapping strategies to detect QTL for resistance to Bonamiosis in the european flat oyster *Ostrea edulis*. *Marine Biotechnology* 11, 570. DOI: 10.1007/s10126-008-9173-y.

Leeds, T.D., Silverstein, J.T., Weber, G.M., Vallejo, R.L., Palti, Y. *et al.* (2010) Response to selection for bacterial cold water disease resistance in rainbow trout. *Journal of Animal Science* 88(6), 1936–1946. DOI: 10.2527/jas.2009-2538.

Lhorente, J.P., Gallardo. J.A., Villanueva, B., Araya, A.M., Torrealba, A.B. *et al.* (2012) Quantitative genetic basis for resistance to *Caligus rogercresseyi* sea lice in a breeding population of Atlantic salmon (*Salmo salar*). *Aquaculture* 324–325, 55–59. DOI: 10.1016/j.aquaculture.2011.10.046.

Lipschutz-Powell, D., Woolliams, J.A., Bijma, P. and Doeschl-Wilson, A.B. (2012) Indirect genetic effects and the spread of infectious disease: are we capturing the full heritable variation underlying disease prevalence? *PloS One* 7(6), e39551. DOI: 10.1371/journal.pone.0039551.

Liu, L., Ang, K.P., Elliott, J.A.K., Kent, M.P., Lien, S. *et al.* (2017) A genome scan for selection signatures comparing farmed Atlantic salmon with two wild populations: Testing colocalization among outlier markers, candidate genes, and quantitative trait loci for production traits. *Evolutionary Applications* 10, 276–296. DOI: 10.1111/eva.12450.

Liu, S., Sun, L., Li, Y., Sun, F., Jiang, Y. *et al.* (2014) Development of the catfish 250K SNP array for genome-wide association studies. *BMC Research Notes* 7, 135. DOI: 10.1186/1756-0500-7-135.

Loopstra, D.P. and Hansen, P.A. (2004) *Fishery Data Series No. 08-22: Induction of Triploidy in Rainbow Trout* (Oncorhynchus mykiss) *using Hydrostatic Pressure*. Alaska Department of Fish and Game, Divisions of Sport Fish and Commercial Fisheries, USA.

Meuwissen, T.H.E., Hayes, B.J. and Goddard, M.E. (2001) Prediction of total genetic value using genome-wide dense marker maps. *Genetics* 157(4), 1819–1829. Available at: http://www.genetics.org/content/157/4/1819.short (accessed 14 September 2020).

Meuwissen, T., Hayes, B. and Goddard, M. (2013). Accelerating improvement of livestock with genomic selection. *Annual Review of Animal Biosciences* 1(1), 221–237. DOI: 10.1146/annurev-animal-031412-103705.

Mignon-Grasteau, S., Boissy, A., Bouix, J., Faure, J.M., Fisher, A.D. *et al.* (2005) Genetics of adaptation and domestication in livestock. *Livestock Production Science* 93, 3–14. DOI: 10.1016/j.livprodsci.2004.11.001.

Moen, T., Sonesson, A.K., Hayes, B., Lien, S., Munck, H. and Meuwissen, T.H. (2007) Mapping of a quantitative trait locus for resistance against infectious salmon anaemia in Atlantic salmon (*Salmo salar*): comparing survival analysis with analysis on affected/resistant data. *BMC Genetics* 8, 53. DOI: 10.1186/1471-2156-8-53.

Moen, T., Baranski, M., Sonesson, A.K. and Kjoglum, S. (2009) Confirmation and fine-mapping of a major QTL for resistance to infectious pancreatic necrosis in Atlantic salmon (*Salmo salar*): population-level associations between markers and trait. *BMC Genomics* 10, 368. DOI: 10.1186/1471-2164-10-368.

Mustafa, A. and MacKinnon, B.M. (1999) Genetic variation in susceptibility of Atlantic salmon to the sea louse *Caligus elongatus* Nordmann, 1832. *Canadian Journal of Zoology* 77(8), 1332–1335. DOI: 10.1139/z99-096.

Neely, K.G., Myers, J.M., Hard, J.J. and Shearer, K.D. (2008) Comparison of growth, feed intake, and nutrient efficiency in a selected strain of coho salmon (*Oncorhynchus kisutch*) and its source stock. *Aquaculture* 283, 134–140. DOI: 10.1016/j.aquaculture.2008.06.038.

Norris, A. (2017) Application of genomics in salmon aquaculture breeding programs by Ashie Norris: Who knows where the genomic revolution will lead us? *Marine Genomics* 13, 13–15. DOI: 10.1016/j.margen.2017.11.013.

Norris, A., Foyle, L. and Ratcliff, J. (2008) Heritability of mortality in response to a natural pancreas disease (SPDV) challenge in Atlantic salmon, *Salmo salar* L., post-smolts on a West of Ireland sea site. *Journal of Fish Diseases* 31(12), 913–920. DOI: 10.1111/j.1365-2761.2008.00982.x.

Ødegård J., Olesen I., Gjerde B. and Klemetsdal G. (2006) Evaluation of statistical models for genetic analysis of challenge test data on furunculosis resistance in Atlantic salmon (*Salmo salar*): prediction of field survival. *Aquaculture* 259, 116–123 DOI: 10.1016/j.aquaculture.2006.05.034

Ødegård, J., Olesen, I., Gjerde, B. and Klemetsdal, G. (2007a) Evaluation of statistical models for genetic analysis of challenge-test data on ISA resistance in Atlantic salmon (*Salmo salar*): Prediction of progeny survival. *Aquaculture* 266(1–4), 70–76. DOI: 10.1016/j.aquaculture.2007.02.012.

Ødegård, J., Olesen, I., Gjerde, B. and Klemetsdal, G. (2007b) Positive genetic correlation between resistance to bacterial (furunculosis) and viral (infectious salmon anaemia) diseases in farmed Atlantic salmon (*Salmo salar*). *Aquaculture* 271(1–4), 173–177. DOI: 10.1016/j.aquaculture.2007.06.006.

Ødegård, J., Baranski, M., Gjerde, B. and Gjedrem, T. (2011) Methodology for genetic evaluation of disease resistance in aquaculture species: challenges and future prospects. *Aquaculture Research* 42(s1), 103–114. DOI: 10.1111/j.1365-2109.2010.02669.x.

Ødegård, J., Moen, T., Santi, N., Korsvoll, S.A., Kjøglum, S. and Meuwissen, T.H.E. (2014) Genomic prediction in an admixed population of Atlantic salmon (*Salmo salar*). *Frontiers in Genetics* 5, 402. DOI: 10.3389/fgene.2014.00402.

Olesen, I., Hung, D. and Ødegård, J. (2007) Genetic analysis of survival in challenge tests of furunculosis and ISA in Atlantic salmon. Genetic parameter estimates and model comparisons. *Aquaculture* 272, S297–S298. DOI: 10.1016/j.aquaculture.2007.07.155.

Palti, Y., Gao, G., Liu, S., Kent, M.P., Lien, S. *et al.* (2015) The development and characterization of a 57K single nucleotide polymorphism array for rainbow trout. *Molecular Ecology Resources* 15(3), 662–672. DOI: 10.1111/1755-0998.12337.

Perry, G.M.L., Tarte, P., Croisetière., S., Belhumeur, P. and Bernatchez, L. (2004) Genetic variance and covariance for 0+ brook charr (*Salvelinus fontinalis*) weight and survival time of furunculosis (*Aeromonas salmonicida*) exposure. *Aquaculture* 235(1–4), 263–271. DOI: 10.1016/j.aquaculture.2004.03.002.

Phuthaworn, C., Nguyen, N.H., Quinn, J. and Knibb, W. (2016) Moderate heritability of hepatopancreatic parvovirus titre suggests a new option for selection against viral diseases in banana shrimp (*Fenneropenaeus merguiensis*) and other aquaculture species. *Genetics Selection Evolution* 48, 64. DOI: 10.1186/s12711-016-0243-8.

Plough, L.V. (2016) Genetic load in marine animals: A review. *Current Zoology* 62, 567–579. DOI: 10.1093/cz/zow096.

Powell, J., White, I., Guy, D. and Brotherstone, S. (2008) Genetic parameters of production traits in Atlantic salmon (*Salmo salar*). *Aquaculture* 274, 225–231. DOI: 10.1016/j.aquaculture.2007.11.036.

Robledo, D., Palaiokostas, C., Bargelloni, L., Martínez, P. and Houston, R. (2017) Applications of genotyping by sequencing in aquaculture breeding and genetics. *Reviews in Aquaculture* 10, 670–682. DOI: 10.1111/raq.12193.

Sae-Lim, P., Gjerde, B., Nielsen, H.M., Mulder, H. and Kause, A. (2016) A review of genotype-by-environment interaction and micro-environmental sensitivity in aquaculture species. *Reviews in Aquaculture* 8, 369–393. DOI: 10.1111/raq.12098.

Salte, R., Bentsen, H.B., Moen, T., Tripathy, S., Bakke, T.A. *et al.* (2010) Prospects for a genetic management strategy to control *Gyrodactylus salaris* infection in wild Atlantic salmon (*Salmo salar*) stocks. *Canadian Journal of Fisheries and Aquatic Sciences* 67(1), 121–129. DOI: 10.1139/F09-168.

Sánchez, L., Bijma, P. and Woolliams, J.A. (2003) Minimizing inbreeding by managing genetic contributions across generations. *Genetics* 164, 1589–1595.

Shelton, W.L. and Rothbard, S. (2006) Exotic species in global aquaculture: a review. *The Israeli Journal of Aquaculture-Bamidgeh* 58, 3–28.

Silverstein, J.T., Vallejo, R.L., Palti, Y., Leeds, T.D., Rexroad III, C.E. *et al.* (2009) Rainbow trout resistance to bacterial cold-water disease is moderately heritable and is not adversely correlated with growth. *Journal of Animal Science* 87(3), 860–867. DOI: 10.2527/jas.2008-1157.

Sonesson, A.K. (2007) Within-family marker-assisted selection for aquaculture species. *Genetics Selection Evolution* 39(3), 301–317. DOI: 10.1051/Gse:2007005.

Sukmanomon, S., Kamonrat, W., Poompuang, S., Nguyen, T.T.T., Bartley, D.M. *et al.* (2012) Genetic changes, intra- and inter-specific introgression in farmed Nile tilapia (*Oreochromis niloticus*) in Thailand. *Aquaculture* 324–325, 44–54. DOI: 10.1016/j.aquaculture.2011.10.025.

Taylor, R.S., Kube, P.D., Muller, W.J. and Elliot, N.G. (2009) Genetic variation of gross gill pathology and survival of Atlantic salmon (*Salmo salar* L.) during natural amoebic gill disease challenge. *Aquaculture* 294(3–4), 172–179. DOI: 10.1016/j.aquaculture.2009.06.007.

Teletchea, F. and Fontaine, P. (2014) Levels of domestication in fish: implications for the sustainable future of aquaculture. *Fish and Fisheries* 15, 181–195. DOI: https://doi.org/10.1111/faf.12006

Thodesen, J., Grisdale-Helland, B., Helland, S.J. and Gjerde, B. (1999) Feed intake, growth and feed utilization of offspring from wild and selected Atlantic salmon (*Salmo salar*). *Aquaculture* 180, 237–246. DOI: 10.1016/S0044-8486(99)00204-5.

Tsai, H.Y., Hamilton, A., Tinch, A.E., Guy, D.R., Gharbi, K. *et al.* (2015) Genome wide association and genomic prediction for growth traits in juvenile farmed Atlantic salmon using a high density SNP array. *BMC Genomics* 16, 969. DOI: 10.1186/s12864-015-2117-9.

Tsai, H.-Y., Hamilton, A., Tinch, A.E., Guy, D.R., Bron, J.E. *et al.* (2016) Genomic prediction of host resistance to sea lice in farmed Atlantic salmon populations. *Genetics Selection Evolution* 48(1), 47. DOI: 10.1186/s12711-016-0226-9.

Tsai, H.-Y., Matika, O., Edwards, S.M., Antolín-Sánchez, R., Hamilton, A. *et al.* (2017) Genotype imputation to improve the cost-efficiency of genomic selection in farmed Atlantic salmon. *G3: Genes, Genomes, Genetics* 7(4) 1377–1383. DOI: 10.1534/g3.117.040717.

Vallejo, R.L., Wiens, G.D., Rexroad III, C.E., Welch, T.J., Evenhuis, J.P. *et al.* (2010) Evidence of major genes affecting resistance to bacterial cold water disease in rainbow trout using Bayesian methods of segregation analysis. *Journal of Animal Science* 88(12), 3814–3832. DOI: 10.2527/jas.2010-2951.

Vallejo, R.L., Palti, Y., Liu, S., Evenhuis, J.P., Gao, G. *et al.* (2014) Detection of QTL in rainbow trout affecting survival when challenged with *Flavobacterium psychrophilum*. *Marine Biotechnology* 16(3), 349–360. DOI: 10.1007/s10126-013-9553-9.

Vandeputte, M. and Haffray, P. (2014). Parentage assignment with genomic markers: a major advance for understanding and exploiting genetic variation of quantitative traits in farmed aquatic animals. *Frontiers in Genetics* 5, 432. DOI: 10.3389/fgene.2014.00432.

Waltz, E. (2017) First genetically engineered salmon sold in Canada. *Nature* 548, 148. DOI: 10.1038/nature.2017.22116.

Wargelius, A., Leininger, S., Skaftnesmo, K.O., Kleppe, L., Andersson, E. *et al.* (2016) *Dnd* knockout ablates germ cells and demonstrates germ cell independent sex differentiation in Atlantic salmon. *Scientific Reports* 6, 21284. DOI: 10.1038/srep21284.

Wetten, M., Aasmundstad, T., Kjøglum, S., Storset, A. *et al.* (2007) Genetic analysis of resistance to infectious pancreatic necrosis in Atlantic salmon (*Salmo salar* L.). *Aquaculture* 272(1–4), 111–117. DOI: 10.1016/j.aquaculture.2007.08.046.

Withler, R. and Evelyn, T. E.-T. (1990) Genetic variation in resistance to bacterial kidney disease within and between two strains of coho salmon from British Columbia. *Transactions of the American Fisheries Society* 119, 1003–1009. DOI: 10.1577/1548-8659(1990)119%3C1003:GVIRTB%3E2.3.CO;2.

Wohlfarth, G.W. (1993). Heterosis for growth rate in common carp. *Aquaculture* 113, 31–46. DOI: https://doi.org/10.1016/0044-8486(93)90338-Y.

Xu, J., Zhao, Z., Zhang, X., Zheng, X., Li, J. *et al.* (2014) Development and evaluation of the first high-throughput SNP array for common carp (*Cyprinus carpio*). *BMC Genomics* 15, 307. DOI: 10.1186/1471-2164-15-307.

Yáñez, J.M., Bangera, R., Lhorente, J.P., Oyarzún, M. and Neiraac, R. (2013) Quantitative genetic variation of resistance against *Piscirickettsia salmonis* in Atlantic salmon (*Salmo salar*). *Aquaculture* 414–415, 155–159. DOI: 10.1016/j.aquaculture.2013.08.009.

Yáñez, J.M., Lhorente, J.P., Bassinib, L.N., Oyarzún, M., Neira, R. and Newman, S. (2014a) Genetic co-variation between resistance against both *Caligus rogercresseyi* and *Piscirickettsia salmonis*, and body weight in Atlantic salmon (*Salmo salar*). *Aquaculture* 433, 295–298. DOI: 10.1016/J.AQUACULTURE.2014.06.026.

Yáñez, J.M., Houston, R.D. and Newman, S. (2014b) Genetics and genomics of disease resistance in salmonid species. *Frontiers in Genetics* 5, 415. DOI: 10.3389/fgene.2014.00415.

Yáñez, J.M., Newman, S. and Houston, R.D. (2015). Genomics in aquaculture to better understand species biology and accelerate genetic progress. *Frontiers in Genetics* 6(April), 1–3. DOI: 10.3389/fgene.2015.00128.

Yáñez, J.M., Naswa, S., López, M.E., Bassini, L., Correa, K. *et al.* (2016) Genome-wide single nucleotide polymorphism (SNP) discovery in Atlantic salmon (*Salmo salar*): validation in wild and farmed American and European populations. *Molecular Ecology Resources* 16, 1002–1011. DOI: 10.1111/1755-0998.12503.

Yoshida, G.M., Carvalheiro, R., Lhorente, J.P., Correa, K., Figueroa, R. *et al.* (2018) Accuracy of genotype imputation and genomic predictions in a two-generation farmed Atlantic salmon population using high-density and low-density SNP panels. *Aquaculture* 491, 147–154. DOI: 10.1016/j.aquaculture.2018.03.004.

Ytrestøyl, T., Aas, T.S. and Åsgård, T. (2015) Utilisation of feed resources in production of Atlantic salmon (*Salmo salar*) in Norway. *Aquaculture* 448, 365–374. DOI: 10.1016/j.aquaculture.2015.06.023.

Zajicek, P., Goodwin, A.E. and Weier, T. (2011) Triploid grass carp: triploid induction, sterility, reversion, and certification. *North American Journal of Fisheries Management* 31, 614–618. DOI: 10.1080/02755947.2011.608616.

Zenger, K.R., Khatkar, M.S., Jones, D.B., Khalilisamani, N., Jerry, D.R. and Raadsma, H.W. (2019). Genomic selection in aquaculture: Application, limitations and opportunities with special reference to marine shrimp and pearl oysters. *Frontiers in Genetics* 9, 693. DOI:. 10.3389/fgene.2018.00693.

Recommended Reading

Gjedrem, T. and Baranski, M. (2009) *Selective Breeding in Aquaculture: An Introduction*. Springer, New York. DOI: 10.1007/978-90-481-2773-3.

Gjedrem, T. and Rye, M. (2018) Selection response in fish and shellfish: a review. *Reviews in Aquaculture* 10, 168–179. DOI: 10.1111/raq.12154.

Gjedrem, T., Robinson, N. and Rye, M. (2012) The importance of selective breeding in aquaculture to meet future demands for animal protein: A review. *Aquaculture 350–353*(null), 117–129. DOI: 10.1016/j.aquaculture.2012.04.008.

Proceedings of the World Congresses on Genetics Applied to Livestock Production. Available at: http://www.wcgalp.org/ (accessed 16 June 2020).

Robledo, D., Palaiokostas, C., Bargelloni, L., Martínez, P. and Houston, R. (2017) Applications of genotyping by sequencing in aquaculture breeding and genetics. *Reviews in Aquaculture* 10, 670–682. DOI: 10.1111/raq.12193.

Sae-Lim, P., Gjerde, B., Nielsen, H.M., Mulder, H. and Kause, A. (2016) A review of genotype-by-environment interaction and micro-environmental sensitivity in aquaculture species. *Reviews in Aquaculture* 8, 369–393. DOI: 10.1111/raq.12098.

Vandeputte, M. and Haffray, P. (2014) Parentage assignment with genomic markers: a major advance for understanding and exploiting genetic variation of quantitative traits in farmed aquatic animals. *Frontiers in Genetics* 5, 432. DOI: 10.3389/fgene.2014.00432.

Yáñez, J.M, Houston, R.D. and Newman, S. (2014) Genetics and genomics of disease resistance in salmonid species. *Frontiers in Genetics* 5, 415. DOI: 10.3389/fgene.2014.00415.

Zenger, K.R., Khatkar, M.S., Jones, D.B., Khalilisamani, N., Jerry, D.R. and Raadsma, H.W. (2019) Genomic selection in aquaculture: Application, limitations and opportunities with special reference to marine shrimp and pearl oysters. *Frontiers in Genetics* 9, 693. DOI: 10.3389/fgene.2018.00693.

14 Future Directions

Introduction

In the previous chapters we have discussed the history of farm animal breeding and genetics, the methods currently employed in the major farmed species, and the technologies likely to have an impact in the future. We can expect continuing innovation in the tools available for genetic improvement from advances in molecular, quantitative and statistical genetics, from reproductive biology, and from precision agriculture and the new opportunities for data collection and new phenotypes that this brings. The purpose of this final chapter is to explore some of the key challenges facing farm animal production in general, and animal breeding and genetics in particular, and to discuss how livestock breeders might respond to ensure wide societal and animal benefits.

There are many global drivers that will shape future food and agricultural systems, and the rôle of livestock breeding within these. The world population is expected to approach 11 billion by the end of this century (UN, 2019b). Currently, around a third of the global population is affected by one or more forms of malnutrition – be that hunger, obesity or micronutrient deficiency (WHO, 2017; FAO, IFAD, UNICEF, WFP and WHO, 2019). Globally, we already use much of the land capable of supporting agriculture, although potential marine aquaculture sites are comparatively underexploited. Many current agricultural practices have adverse environmental consequences, and competition for resources (e.g. water, energy, fuel) is a major issue. Achieving sustainable, healthy diets underpins many of the United Nations' Sustainable Development Goals – especially those concerned with hunger, poverty, health, gender equality, land use, responsible consumption and production, and climate action (FAO, 2018; UN, 2019a). Feeding the world's growing population well, while protecting the natural systems on which we all depend, is one of the greatest challenges we face as a society. The rôle that livestock should play in our future food systems is strongly contested, ranging from those who expect an increasing rôle to those who see no rôle at all (see e.g. Garnett *et al.*, 2017).

In many parts of the world, genetic improvement of farmed livestock has been a highly effective strategy for altering the performance of farmed animals. While some methods of genetic improvement, for example within-breed selection, produce less immediate changes than some other methods, such as improved feeding, its benefits are permanent and cumulative, and in most cases it is highly cost effective. Hence, it has contributed to increasing the availability and affordability of highly nutritious food, and so to food security, and it has improved resource-use efficiency per unit of product. However, livestock-derived food requires more land and other resources than plant-based food, per unit of protein or energy produced. Also, the availability of relatively cheap livestock products is a major driver of the so-called 'livestock revolution' – the rapid growth in global demand for livestock products, which exacerbates the environmental impact of our food systems. So, how do we achieve more sustainable livestock production?

The concept of sustainability became popular following the publication of the 'Brundtland Report' in 1987 (World Commission on Environment and Development, 1987). The core tenet of that report is that sustainable development 'meets the needs of the present without compromising the ability of future generations to meet their own needs'. Over the last few decades there have been many developments intended to improve the sustainability of animal breeding, as we have discussed in previous chapters. These include:

- selection for improved resource-use efficiency and reduced waste;
- improving knowledge and practice of conservation and sustainable use of farm animal genetic resources;

Genetic Improvement of Farmed Animals (G. Simm *et al.*)
DOI: 10.1079/9781789241723.0014

- incorporation of, and increasing emphasis on, animal health and welfare-related traits in breeding programmes;
- investigation, and in a few cases adoption in breeding programmes, of traits intended to directly reduce environmental impact; and
- regulation or guidance on the use of certain technologies in animal breeding deemed to have detrimental effects on animal welfare.

It is often helpful to think of economic, environmental and societal dimensions of sustainability, which overlap. In the following sections we briefly consider the challenges in each of these areas, and the contributions that future breeding programmes could make.

Towards Sustainable Livestock Production

Economic dimension

The livestock sector makes an important economic contribution in many countries, accounting for around 40% of the value of global agricultural output (FAO, 2019a). Over the last few decades, genetic improvement programmes operating in many parts of the world have helped to increase the value of livestock products, by improving alignment with consumer demand (e.g. by improving carcass leanness) and reducing costs of production (e.g. by improving feed conversion efficiency). In previous chapters we have given examples of impressive rates of return on investment in genetic improvement, at farm and national levels. Similar or higher rates of return can be expected in the future, depending on the level of uptake of the existing and new technologies described in earlier chapters. In particular, the aquaculture sector may be poised for a large and rapid uptake of selective breeding, as there are large components of this sector which rely on wild or near-wild strains (Gjedrem *et al.*, 2012).

Livestock production also makes a related but broader contribution to livelihoods. For example, livestock have a crucial economic rôle in around 60% of rural households in developing countries – including smallholder farmers, agro-pastoralists and pastoralists. They contribute to the livelihoods of about 1.7 billion poor people, 70% of whom are women (FAO, 2019b). In many cultures, livestock have important rôles as a source of economic and social capital, fibre, hides, fertilizer, draught power or transport, as well as an important source of food. While the priorities may be different, the livestock sector also contributes substantially to the economy in the Global North (e.g. contributing around €168 billion annually to the European economy, 45% of the total agricultural activity; Animal Task Force, 2019).

While primary agricultural production is of lower direct economic importance in most industrialized nations in comparison to lower income countries, it often underpins major food processing sectors with a significant share of employment. For example, food and drink manufacturing is the largest manufacturing sector in the UK; the food supply chain employs around 4 million people and generates over £121 billion of added value *per annum* (Food and Drink Federation, 2019).

Over the last few decades, the global production and consumption of livestock products has grown dramatically – the livestock revolution referenced earlier. The growth has been especially dramatic in Asia, and especially in the poultry and pig sectors (see Figs 14.1 and 14.2). Consumption of aquaculture species is also growing globally, with farmed fish now accounting for around half of all consumption, again with Asia being the primary driver of this growth. This growth has arisen partly because of the growing human population, but also because of growing wealth, which tends to lead to an increase in the consumption of livestock-sourced foods in many cultures (Fig. 14.3). Innovation in livestock production, including modern livestock genetic improvement programmes, has contributed by making livestock products more affordable. On one level, this is an economic success story. However, there are hidden costs or 'externalities' which we discuss below.

Environmental dimension

Livestock production has many problematic environmental impacts and some positive ones. It is a major user of land – both directly for livestock production, and indirectly for livestock feed production. Increasingly, land use for livestock production is competing with other interests, including the provision of other ecosystem services apart from provisioning (regulating, supporting and cultural services), production of crops for direct human consumption, the production of biofuels, land uses

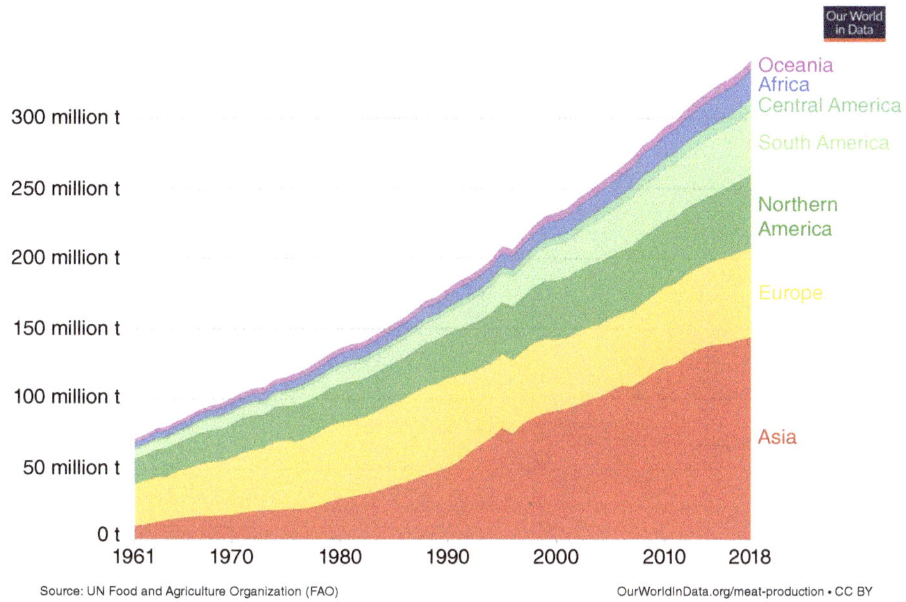

Fig. 14.1. Global meat production by region. (Our World in Data, 2020, CC-BY, based on data from FAO, 2020.)

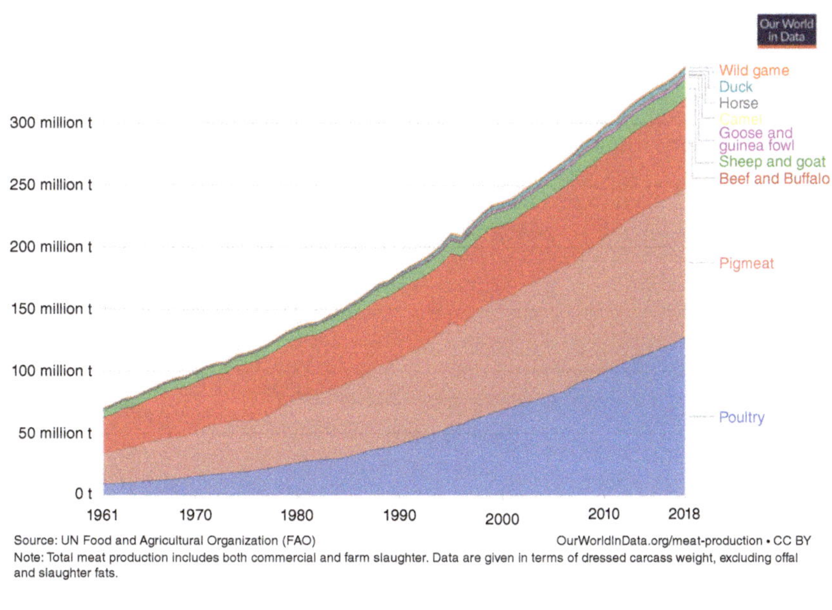

Fig. 14.2. Global meat production by livestock type. (Our World in Data, 2020, CC-BY, based on data from FAO, 2020.)

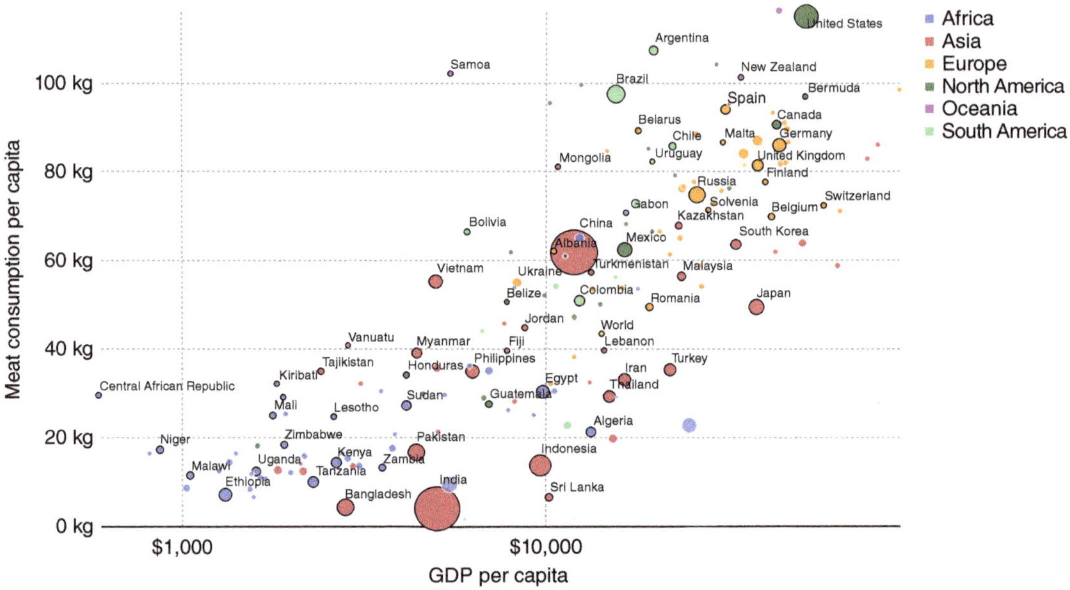

Fig. 14.3. Share of calories from animal protein vs GDP per capita. (Our World in Data, 2019, CC-BY, based on data from FAO, 2017.)

intended to increase carbon sequestration (e.g. planting trees or restoring peatlands) or restoration of lost biodiversity, and the spread of cities. Livestock production is also a major user of water globally.

Agriculture is essentially all about harnessing solar energy to grow plants to feed humans directly, or to feed to livestock, whose products in turn feed humans. The processes of capturing solar energy by plants, and of using plants to grow livestock, are both inherently inefficient. However, as livestock production involves both steps, the inefficiencies are compounded. Where ruminants are involved, there is an additional step – plants are feeding rumen microbes that in turn, to a large extent, feed the host animal. Hence, livestock production, especially with ruminants, requires a greater land area and more inputs to produce a unit of energy or protein than producing crops for direct consumption. For example, Fig. 14.4, based on the results of Poore and Nemecek (2018), shows results of a metanalysis of land area required to produce a unit of protein from different food types. As expected, this shows a much greater requirement for land to produce beef and lamb than for other livestock products or food crops. The advantage to pigs and poultry has been accentuated by several decades of selection for production and feed conversion efficiency, as well as naturally higher reproductive rates. (Poore and Nemecek (2018) also highlight the wide range in environmental performance within species between systems – a clear target for further genetic improvement.) The trends towards increasing consumption of products from the more efficient species is helpful in terms of resources required per unit of product, but the growth in consumption *per capita* is challenging. Also, the disadvantage to ruminants in terms of land use or feed conversion can be exaggerated in this sort of comparison as, in many parts of the world, ruminants use land that is unsuitable for crop production because of its altitude, topography, soil type, low or high rainfall, etc. – so while the land area needed is greater, much of it cannot be switched readily to other agricultural uses. (Though some of it may be suitable for other land uses with biodiversity or carbon sequestration benefits.)

Frequently, livestock are fed co-products from other agri-food systems or crops of a quality unsuitable for processing, so direct competition with crops for direct consumption is lower than it first appears (see, for example, the study of Mottet *et al.*, 2017). Recent modelling studies show that land use for human food production is not minimized by

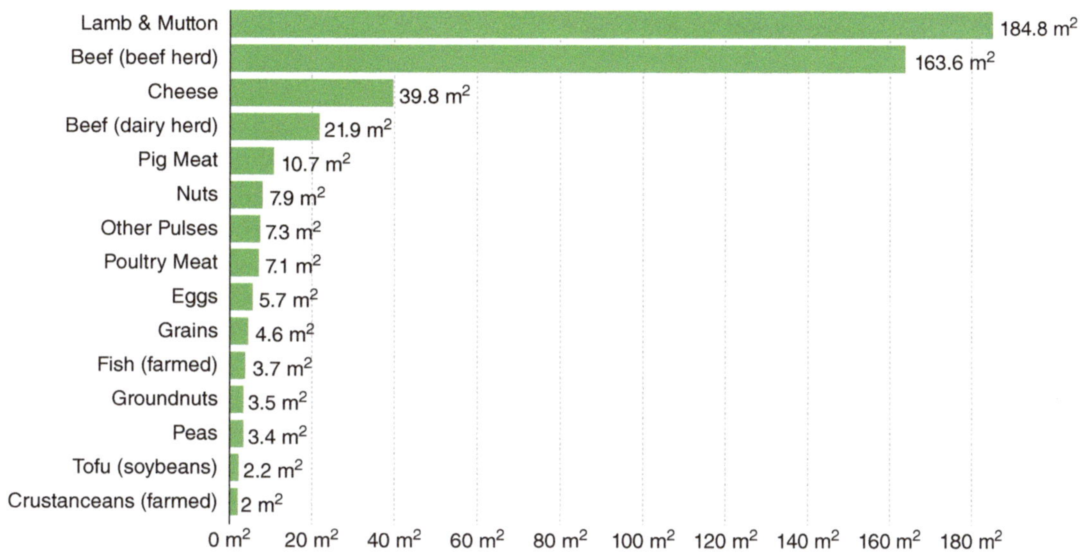

Fig. 14.4. Land area required to produce a unit of protein from different food types. (Our World in Data, 2019, CC-BY, based on data from Poore and Nemecek, 2018.)

removing livestock-sourced food from the diet altogether, as some assume. It is lowest when part of our daily protein needs (9–23 g of the ~50–60 g *per capita* needed) is derived from livestock raised in systems that prioritize the use of feed sources that are not directly useful for human consumption, such as food waste and grassland. This reduces competition for land for food production for direct human consumption (see review by Van Zanten *et al.*, 2018). In these studies, the optimal use of livestock-derived food by humans depends on the quality and quantity of waste/co-products available and the area of grassland available with a low opportunity cost for livestock grazing (i.e. less suitable for other cropping, biodiversity or carbon sequestration uses). Paradoxically, while many of our pig and poultry breeds were developed to be efficient converters of waste products to high-value, human-edible products, and our ruminant livestock breeds to be efficient converters of grass and forage, breeding programmes for most species in industrialized countries today usually prioritize efficiency of conversion of grain-based livestock diets. Hence, if there is a switch to a greater dependence on lower quality feeds in many parts of the world, this should prompt investigations into whether or not genotype × environment interactions exist, and if these are present, a reformulation of breeding goals and/or testing regimes. While the use of livestock in a circular bioeconomy minimizes their land use, systems including ruminants are likely to result in higher methane emissions than those without ruminants, or with ruminants fed higher quality diets. However, breeding or other technological approaches to reduce methane emissions may reduce such trade-offs (see e.g. Dijkstra *et al.*, 2018; Huws *et al.*, 2018; Breider *et al.*, 2019).

The FAO report *Livestock's Long Shadow* (FAO, 2006) was one of the first reports to draw attention to the environmental impacts of livestock production, reporting that livestock production was responsible for around 18% of global greenhouse gas (GHG) emissions as a result of land use and land use change, feed production, animal production, manure management and processing and international transport, as well as a major contributor to water use and pollution and loss of biodiversity. (More recent estimates suggest that the proportion of GHG emissions attributable to livestock production are slightly lower (e.g. 14.5 %; Gerber *et al.*, 2013), largely due to increases in other sectors between the first and second publications.) The findings of the report have been broadly accepted and ignited an important debate on the future of livestock production globally.

Agricultural systems produce methane as a result of enteric fermentation (fermentation in the digestive tract) by ruminants and manure management; nitrous oxide as a result of excretion by livestock and application of manure and fertilizer to land; and carbon dioxide as a result of feed production, land use change and machinery use. Methane emissions from ruminants are especially important, accounting for around 80% of all livestock emissions, with cattle responsible for the majority of these (Gerber *et al.*, 2013).

Improvements in breeding, feeding and managing ruminants have reduced emissions per unit product (emissions intensity) over the last few decades. For example, Capper *et al.* (2009) estimated that compared to US dairy systems in 1944, those in 2007 required 21% of the animals, 23% of the feedstuffs, 35% of the water and only 10% of the land per billion kg of milk. Similarly, 2007 dairy systems producing 24% of the manure, 43% of methane and 56% of the nitrous oxide per billion kg of milk compared with 1944 systems. Genetic improvement is a major contributor to these changes.

A number of possible responses have been advocated to further reduce emissions: (i) reducing the numbers of livestock globally; (ii) breeding more efficient/lower-emitting animals, as mentioned in earlier chapters; (iii) improving the health, feeding and management of livestock to reduce system-level losses; and (iv) direct interventions to reduce methane emissions, including the use of dietary additives to suppress emissions.

In some circumstances, depending on soil and vegetation type, age of grassland, rainfall, stocking rate and a range of other factors, grazing systems can contribute to carbon sequestration, though not usually sufficiently to fully offset methane emissions of the grazing animals themselves (Garnett *et al.*, 2017). Improving previously poorly managed grasslands is one of the most effective measures (Smith, 2014; Conant *et al.*, 2017).

As well as being a major source of GHG emissions globally, livestock can be an important source of pollution locally. This can arise through the production of ammonia from intensive livestock houses, effluent or run-off from manure, slurry or silage stores, run-off from fertilized land with nitrogen and phosphorus entering water courses or groundwater, and the environmental impact of veterinary medicines and treatments. Animal pathogens in the environment can also be a direct risk to human health (in addition to the risks posed from direct contact or via livestock products). The high use of antibiotics in livestock production in many parts of the world increases the prevalence of antimicrobial resistance, which is a risk to human and animal health. Most of these risks are best mitigated by system-level regulation (see e.g. European Commission, 2019b), though breeding for livestock disease resistance or resilience can reduce the use of medicines and the environmental impact of these.

While the area of land needed to grow food of different types is of significant concern in its own right, it is the conversion of native forest, grasslands or bush to cropping, especially to grow livestock feed, that has rightly caused most concern. For instance, deforestation in Brazil is often attributed to growing global demand for soya beans for use in livestock feed. It is clear that dramatic measures are needed to halt the loss of biodiversity and habitats, and the threat to ecosystems posed by the expansion of livestock production globally. While it is less often discussed, livestock breeds and strains are themselves part of biodiversity and worthy of conservation for this, as well as utilitarian reasons.

Overgrazing is a cause of serious biodiversity loss, land and soil degradation. Conversely, well-managed livestock farming systems, especially grazing or mixed farming systems with intermediate stocking rates, contribute to biodiversity, e.g. by maintaining habitats suitable for particular plant species, and providing feed sources for particular insects, and in turn, bird species (FAO, 2016b; HNV, 2019).

While technological solutions can make an important contribution to addressing the environmental impacts of growing livestock production and to waste reduction, it is hard to see how these alone will deal rapidly enough with this problem today, let alone with the impact of the global growth in demand for livestock products. The annual growth in consumption of livestock products, and hence their total environmental footprint, is growing about threefold to sixfold faster than the improvements in resource-use efficiency mentioned above in the US dairy sector, and these are unlikely to be replicated globally. Hence, interest in some countries with higher consumption on measures to limit demand, such as via taxation (Wirsenius *et al.*, 2011; Chatham House, 2015; see also the Food Ethics Council (2019), which analyses some of the pros and cons of this approach) or promotion of alternatives to meat and milk (Ritchie *et al.*, 2018).

The impacts of aquaculture production have many similarities to those of terrestrial livestock, but also some unique features. Aquaculture is considered to be the fastest growing food production sector in percentage terms, predicted to grow by 31% in the next 10 years (OECD/FAO, 2018). There is less competition for space, in particular in the marine environment. Further, aquaculture production is considered very efficient in terms of food conversion and protein retention compared to most terrestrial livestock (Fry *et al.*, 2018). However, there are serious concerns over the impact on marine or fresh-water environments, and sustainable growth will need to consider methods to minimize this. For example, a rather unique feature of aquaculture is the proximity of farmed species to their wild counterparts, and the high probability of interaction and interbreeding between the two groups. Technology targeting production of sterile animals holds promise in this area, including the ploidy manipulation and genome editing solutions described in Chapter 13.

Societal dimension

Livestock products form an important part of the human diet in many cultures. Nutritionally, they are a particularly valuable source of protein, energy and highly bioavailable micronutrients, such as calcium, iron and vitamin B12. Small amounts of livestock-derived foods can make a significant contribution to the wellbeing of pregnant and lactating mothers, and the physical and cognitive development of their children in the first 1000 days of life (Grace *et al.*, 2018). A recent FAO-sponsored report highlighted the importance of livestock in future food systems (HLPE, 2016). Further, farmed seafood provides a major source of long chain fatty acids considered essential for human development and health.

As well as making a direct economic contribution, livestock farming, and its support services, often make a disproportionate contribution to socially and economically fragile regions globally. Livestock have a particularly important rôle in supporting nomadic communities, and those living in areas of protracted conflict (FAO, 2016a)

Livestock farming is a longstanding activity in many rural areas, and a strong part of their history, heritage and culture. Many livestock breeds have strong regional roots and have played an important rôle in the development of regional economies. Some have played an important rôle in the economic and social development of whole nations (see e.g. Defra, 2006; FAO 2015).

Livestock farming has often had an important rôle in shaping landscapes. For instance, grazing has influenced many landscapes in the hills and uplands of Europe. The presence of livestock themselves, and their regional diversity, is often highly valued by those who live in, work in, or visit the countryside (Defra, 2006).

There are also widespread societal concerns over aspects of livestock breeding and production – especially relating to their environmental impacts, as discussed above, and to the ethical and welfare implications of some breeding practices and technologies. As the latter are so central to the subject of this book, we discuss them at greater length in the next section.

Ethical implications of livestock breeding

Many fields of human endeavour lead to ethical dilemmas, and agriculture is certainly no exception. While there are ethical dilemmas in many areas of agriculture, the application of new technologies, particularly in animal production, is perhaps the area where there is most public concern. Views on the use of animals by humans range from those who regard any use of animals as immoral, to those who feel any use of animals in the interest of humans is justified. However, the majority of people in most countries accept the use of animals for a range of purposes including food production, providing that the animals are treated humanely.

It is still difficult to decide whether particular treatments of animals are humane, and some form of ethical analysis is often used to help reach rational decisions. There are two main schools of thought in ethical analysis (Mepham, 1996). The first is consequentialism – that the ethics of certain actions can be judged solely by the consequences, or that 'the ends justify the means'. Applied to animal production, this approach would allow any treatment of animals to be justified, providing that the benefits for humans were high enough. The second is deontology, which states that rights and duties are of overriding importance, irrespective of consequences. Applied to animal production, this approach would rule out certain procedures, regardless of the benefits. In practice, it is difficult to solve ethical dilemmas using only one of these approaches (Mepham, 1996).

Although it was produced several decades ago, the report of the Banner Committee provides one of the most relevant, and balanced, assessments of ethical issues in animal breeding, and it has influenced much later thinking on the topic. The Banner Committee was formed by the UK government 'to consider the ethical implications of emerging technologies in the breeding of farm animals; to advise on the adequacy of the existing legal and other safeguards in those areas; and to make recommendations' (MAFF, 1995). The committee used both approaches outlined above to produce a framework for ethical discrimination among new breeding technologies in farm animals.

The crux of their report is that the humane use of animals respects three principles (MAFF, 1995):

> (a) Harms of a certain degree and kind ought under no circumstances to be inflicted on an animal.
> (b) Any harm to an animal, even if not absolutely impermissible, nonetheless requires justification and must be outweighed by the good which is realistically sought in so treating it.
> (c) Any harm which is justified by the second principle ought, however, to be minimized as far as is reasonably possible.

In other words, there are some procedures that should simply never be used on animals, no matter what the potential benefits. There are others that could be used, even if there is potential harm to the animal. If there is any harm, this needs to be justified by the benefits expected, and steps need to be taken to make sure that the harm is minimized. These principles recognize that a cost:benefit analysis alone is not sufficient to justify the use of harmful procedures. The report also emphasizes that harm does not just mean physical harm, but also includes treatment of animals which might be considered degrading, or disrespectful of the nature of the animal. The committee applied the three principles to each of the breeding technologies mentioned above, to help discriminate them on ethical grounds. They recognized that some individuals and groups disagree with any use of animals for food production, but applied the principles from the majority view that the humane use of animals for this purpose is acceptable.

The first principle would exclude the use of technologies which are regarded as intrinsically objectionable. Many of the organizations consulted during the production of the report had objections to the use of new breeding technologies. These included the views that use of these technologies treated animals as 'raw materials', disrespected the 'integrity of nature', or allowed practitioners to 'play God'. However, the committee felt that the uses of the new technologies were not *automatically* objectionable on these grounds since many of them simply accelerate the selection process possible by natural means. Even those which directly modify the genetic makeup by gene transfer can still respect the essential nature and wellbeing of the animal. As an example they cited three hypothetical uses of gene transfer. The first aimed at increasing the protein content of cows' milk, the second aimed at producing only female chicks from an egg-laying line of poultry, and the third aimed at improving feed efficiency in pigs by reducing their sentience and responsiveness. The committee reasoned that neither of the first two of these aims was intrinsically objectionable, since they did not affect the animals' 'defining characteristics, nor threaten the achievement of its natural ends or good'. However, they argued that the third use would be intrinsically objectionable since it was designed specifically to modify the normal behaviour of pigs.

The committee felt that the use of DNA from different species to create transgenic animals could be considered in the same framework, since in most cases this was aimed at the addition of a trait without significantly modifying the animal's natural characteristics, rather than creating a new type of animal. For example, some of the earliest transgenic sheep produced had an additional human protein secreted in their milk, but in all other respects they were normal sheep. However, the use of DNA across species does create problems for people with dietary restrictions for religious or other reasons. Other committees have considered this issue and suggested appropriate labelling of foods from modified animals to ensure freedom of choice for consumers.

The report emphasizes that while there may be no intrinsic objections about the 'ends' or aims of a particular technology, there would be objections if the 'means' to that end seriously compromise animal welfare (see MAFF, 1995 or Simm, 1998 for more details).

Techniques requiring the use of non-therapeutic surgery were considered unacceptable for routine use by the Banner Committee, as they have been by other groups in the veterinary profession in the UK and several other countries. While this is a reasonable prior choice of boundary, it appears that laparoscopy itself may compromise welfare no more than some routine handling operations on sheep, in so far as this can be measured by blood hormones which act as indicators of stress (Haresign *et al.*, 1995). However, the procedure causes pain in humans for some days afterwards, and it is probable that it is painful for sheep too, hence a recommendation that analgesia be used. Although a great deal of research effort has gone into finding alternative methods of artificial insemination (AI) in sheep, as yet there are no alternatives which produce consistently high conception rates with frozen semen. Also, there are concerns about the welfare implications of some of the alternative non-surgical methods of AI.

The committee also had a welfare concern over the use of AI in poultry. The concern here was not with the technique itself, but due to the fact that in some strains of turkey its use is necessary because heavily muscled birds are incapable of natural mating. This was considered intrinsically objectionable. These strains have been created in the past by conventional selection, which highlights the fact that ethical concerns are not restricted to the use of new breeding technologies. Many people regard as intrinsically objectionable the high incidence of caesarean sections in homozygous double-muscled cattle, or the congenital defects common in some dog breeds due to selection for particular breed characteristics.

The committee reached similar conclusions on the use of superovulation, embryo transfer and other embryo technologies to those reached for AI. Where non-surgical procedures can be used for embryo recovery or transfer, they were not regarded as inherently bad for welfare. Where surgical procedures are required, such as in sheep and pigs, the committee recommended similar restrictions to those for laparoscopic AI in sheep. There were concerns that although several of the techniques did not inherently compromise welfare, some associated procedures could do so. For instance, some embryo culture procedures are thought to be implicated in the birth of abnormally large calves from *in vitro*-produced embryos. Similarly, the use of recipients of an inappropriate breed-type or degree of maturity may increase the incidence of difficult calvings following embryo transfer, and so compromise welfare. Hence the recommendations include consideration of these wider risks to welfare, as well as risks from the technologies themselves.

In a similar vein, a welfare checklist has been proposed to help deliberations on the use of new technologies in cattle breeding (Webster, 1994). This includes assessing: (i) pain and fear associated with the technique itself, or its immediate consequences; (ii) periparturient problems associated with the technique (e.g. oversize calves associated with some *in vitro*-produced embryos, or calving difficulties associated with twinning); (iii) physical or psychological problems demonstrable in all or most of the genetically modified offspring (such as those seen in the modified pigs mentioned earlier); and (iv) increased incidence of disease or disability only demonstrable by observation of relatively large populations over several generations (e.g. increased incidence of mastitis or lameness). A two-stage review process was proposed so that problems of types (i) to (iii) would need to be solved before a technique was approved for wider use, but a second stage of controlled use on a wider scale would be needed to detect problems of the sort outlined in (iv).

The Banner Committee did not regard genetic modification in its own right as a threat to animal welfare, although there may be consequences which affect welfare, such as the high incidence of lameness and arthritis in the earliest examples of modified pigs and sheep. Both the creation of genetically modified organisms, and breeding from them, are controlled procedures already in many countries. Before a licence is granted in the UK, the likely 'adverse effects' on the animal have to be weighed against the likely benefits of the modification. Hence, possible threats to welfare should be considered already, and the committee supported the existing controls. However, they recommended that if consideration of 'adverse effects' does not already encompass intrinsic objections, such as damage to the natural integrity of the animal, it should be broadened to do so. Additionally, the committee recommended greater uniformity across species in the legislation governing some of the technologies and made suggestions on training of operators to safeguard animal welfare.

In many countries there are stringent regulatory processes before genetically modified plants or animals can be approved for use in food production (see review by Van Eenennaam and Young, 2018). Often these apply the so-called precautionary principle, that new techniques should not be permitted unless potential harm can be ruled out. In the US, intentional nucleotide insertions, substitutions or deletions in animals are treated as new drugs. Current EU legislation regulates the release of genetically modified organisms into the environment. (Other EU legislation is relevant too – see Hoppe (2018) for a fuller discussion of this, and wider legal governance of animal biotechnologies, and European Commission (2019a)). In practice, at the time of writing, only one genetically modified animal product – AquAdvantage® salmon – has been approved for food purposes, several decades after being produced. This is in contrast to the situation in crops, where many genetically modified strains have been approved for food use in many countries. Van Eenennaam and Young (2018) and Lanzerath (2018) highlight inconsistencies in several countries or regions in the regulation of genetically modified animals and plants, and in the treatment of older (e.g. radiation-induced mutagenesis in plants; traditional selective breeding resulting in extreme phenotypes) versus newer techniques for effecting genetic change. These inconsistencies have become widely debated with the advent of the gene editing techniques discussed in Chapter 5. These produce far more precise changes in the genome, do not involve introduction of 'foreign' DNA, and appear to have fewer of the unintended welfare consequences seen in early livestock genetic modification experiments. However, those with intrinsic objections to directly altering the genome of animals are likely to continue to have concerns. The Nuffield Council on Bioethics (2019) is currently investigating the ethical implications of genome editing in farmed livestock.

Van Eenennaam and Young (2018) argue for regulation in this area to be more proportional and based on the risks of new technologies. Likewise, there is much current interest in 'responsible innovation' and in moving towards regulation which supports innovation (Tait, 2017). While future regulatory processes may accelerate the approval of genetically modified animal products, it remains unclear how consumers in many countries would respond. For instance, research shows that consumers are generally opposed to genetic engineering of animals to increase food animal productivity, though they may be more supportive of applications intended to improve welfare (Van Eenennaam and Young, 2018).

There has been much debate on the issue of patenting genetically modified animals, and the techniques involved in producing them. Those in favour often argue that the protection offered by patents is essential to encourage biotechnology companies to invest in research and development. Those against often argue that it is immoral to patent modified animals or associated techniques, since this encourages the view that animals are simply industrial commodities. The issue was considered by the Banner Committee, which concluded that patents were not objectionable in principle, but that consideration of patent applications should include moral criteria as well as technical ones. They also suggested that the threat to small producers from very widely drawn claims to patent protection be monitored.

While the report of the Banner Committee is particularly relevant to the discussion in this chapter, other approaches have been proposed elsewhere. For instance, an ethical matrix has been proposed to help evaluate the impact of new biotechnologies from the perspective of the animals, producers, consumers and the 'biota' or wider environment (Mepham, 1996). In each case three ethical principles are considered: respect for wellbeing, autonomy and justice. Applying these principles to animals, wellbeing equates to welfare, animal autonomy includes freedom to express normal behaviour, and justice equates to respect for the integrity and nature of the animal. In the case of consumers, wellbeing would encompass any health risks posed by food produced by new biotechnological processes, autonomy would encompass consumer choice, and justice would encompass product price, which affects the ability of different groups to benefit from the product. While this approach is interesting, there is a risk that it leads to such wide thinking that the practical problems remain unsolved. (See also de Boer *et al.*, 1995.) Lanzerath (2018) argues for greater dialogue on the type of food production system we wish to see as a society, and whether or not we are ready to move to a more technologically-led system.

The majority of this book has concentrated on the technical aspects of farm animal breeding. However, it is entirely appropriate that analyses of the technical aspects of a breeding scheme be accompanied by an analysis of the ethical implications. Many of the breeding techniques and selection goals described throughout the book are likely to be neutral with respect to animal welfare. But, based on experience in many species, the sustained pursuit of some breeding goals, such as higher output alone, may have unfavourable consequences for animal welfare. For example, selection for milk yield in dairy cattle is associated with a higher incidence of mastitis.

However, with a better understanding of the genetics of the production traits and diseases involved it is possible to turn this situation around and develop breeding goals which limit the deterioration in resistance to disease, and ideally improve it. It is important not to forget that many of the new breeding technologies provide opportunities for great good in this respect, as well as the possibility of harm. For instance, the use of acceptable reproductive technologies could allow more rapid progress in selection for disease resistance or calving ease. Similarly, gene editing may allow rapid genetic changes in some traits conferring benefits to animals as well as humans.

By their very nature, ethical problems are difficult to solve. The frameworks mentioned above are not easy to apply in all circumstances. However, they provide an important foundation for a more open dialogue in what is clearly an area of great public concern. In the longer term, this must help to increase public confidence in livestock farming and science, while allowing maximum benefit to be derived from those technologies which are considered acceptable.

Tailpiece

Our food and farming systems in general, and the livestock sector in particular, are facing unprecedented challenges in feeding the growing global human population well, while protecting the natural systems on which we all depend. The expansion of livestock production globally is a major contributor to the challenge. Livestock breeding has made a significant contribution to human wellbeing for several centuries, by improving the availability, cost and environmental impact of animal-sourced foods. The responsible use of the approaches and technologies we have outlined in this book promise even greater gains, for the benefit of humans, animals and this environment. We hope that this book will help to equip and inspire future generations of students, researchers and practitioners to rise to these massive challenges, and develop even more sustainable livestock breeding practices in future.

Summary

- Livestock production has a range of economic, social and environmental costs and benefits. The dramatic growth in global consumption of livestock products is having significant environmental consequences. Hence, the rôle that livestock should play in our future food systems is strongly contested.
- Future breeding programmes should aim to reduce the economic, social and environmental costs of livestock production and increase the benefits.
- Both traditional methods and new breeding technologies can give rise to ethical concerns. Ethical appraisal and wider public dialogue will be important in ensuring public confidence in livestock breeding and production, while allowing maximum benefit to be derived from those technologies which are considered acceptable.

References

Animal Task Force (2019) Why We Promote a Sustainable Livestock Sector. Available at: http://animaltaskforce.eu/Our-work/Why-we-promote-a-sustainable-livestock-sector (accessed 6 March 2019).

Breider, I.S., Wall, E. and Garnsworthy, P.C. (2019) Heritability of methane production and genetic correlations with milk yield and body weight in Holstein-Friesian dairy cows. *Journal of Dairy Science* 102, 7277–7281. DOI: 10.3168/jds.2018-15909.

Capper, J.L., Cady, R.A. and Bauman, D.E. (2009) The environmental impact of dairy production: 1944 compared with 2007. *Journal of Animal Science* 87, 2160–2167. DOI: 10.2527/jas.2009-1781.

Chatham House (2015) Changing Climate, Changing Diets: Pathways to Lower Meat Consumption. Available at: https://www.chathamhouse.org/publication/changing-climate-changing-diets (accessed 30 June 2019).

Conant, R.T., Cerri, C.E.P., Osborne, B.B. and Paustian, K. (2017) Grassland management impacts on soil carbon stocks: a new synthesis. *Ecological Applications* 27, 662–668. DOI: 10.1002/eap.1473.

de Boer, I.J.M., Brom, F.W.A. and Vorstenbosch, J.M.G. (1995) An ethical evaluation of animal biotechnology: the case of using clones in dairy cattle breeding. *Animal Science* 61, 453–463. DOI: 10.1017/S1357729800014028.

Defra (2006) UK National Action Plan on Farm Animal Genetic Resources. Available at: https://assets.publishing.service.gov.uk/government/uploads/system/uploads/attachment_data/file/69397/pb12190-fangr-actionplan.pdf (accessed 30 June 2019).

Dijkstra, J., Bannink, A., France, J., Kebreab, E. and van Gastelen, S. (2018) Antimethanogenic effects of 3-nitrooxypropanol depend on supplementation dose, dietary fiber content, and cattle type. *Journal of Dairy Science* 101, 9041–9047. DOI: 10.3168/jds.2018-14456.

European Commission (2019a) Genetically Modified Organisms. Available at: https://ec.europa.eu/food/plant/gmo_en (accessed 28 June 2019).

European Commission (2019b) The Nitrates Directive. Available at: http://ec.europa.eu/environment/water/water-nitrates/index_en.html (accessed 30 June 2019).

FAO (2006) Livestock's Long Shadow. Environmental Issues and Options. Available at: http://www.fao.org/3/a-a0701e.pdf (accessed 30 June 2019).

FAO (2015) The Second Report on the State of the World's Animal Genetic Resources for Food and Agriculture. Commission on Genetic Resources for Food and Agriculture, Food and Agriculture Organization of the United Nations, Rome. Available at: http://www.fao.org/3/a-i4787e.pdf (accessed 14 May 2019).

FAO (2016a) Livestock in Protracted Crises. Guidance Note. Available at: http://www.fao.org/3/a-i6637e.pdf (accessed 17 June 2019).

FAO (2016b) Principles for the Assessment of Livestock Impacts on Biodiversity. Available at: http://www.fao.org/3/a-i6492e.pdf (accessed 17 June 2019).

FAO (2017) FAOSTAT. Available at: http://www.fao.org/faostat/en/?#data/ (accessed 20 November 2019).

FAO (2018) The Future of Food and Agriculture. Alternative Pathways to 2050. Available at: http://www.fao.org/3/I8429EN/i8429en.pdf (accessed 17 June 2019).

FAO (2019a) Animal Production. Available at: http://www.fao.org/animal-production/en/ (accessed 6 March 2019).

FAO (2019b) Decent Rural Employment. Available at: http://www.fao.org/rural-employment/agricultural-sub-sectors/livestock/en/ (accessed 6 March 2019).

FAO, IFAD, UNICEF, WFP and WHO (2019) The State of Food Security and Nutrition in the World 2019. Safeguarding against economic slowdowns and downturns. FAO, Rome. Available at: http://www.fao.org/3/ca5162en/ca5162en.pdf (accessed 18 November 2019).

Food and Drink Federation (2019) Our Industry at a Glance. Available at: https://www.fdf.org.uk/public-general/our-industry-at-a-glance-2019.pdf (accessed 6 March 2019).

Food Ethics Council (2019) Food Policy on Trial. Available at: https://www.foodethicscouncil.org/app/uploads/2019/05/Food-Policy-On-Trial-Meat-tax-Jury-verdict-final.pdf (accessed 17 June 2019).

Fry, J.P., Mailloux, N.A., Love, D.C., Milli, M.C. and Cao, L. (2018) Feed conversion efficiency in aquaculture: do we measure it correctly? *Environmental Research Letters* 13, 024017. DOI: 10.1088/1748-9326/aaa273.

Garnett, T., Godde, C., Muller, A., Röös, E., Smith, P. *et al.* (2017) Grazed and Confused? FCRN, University of Oxford. Available at: https://www.fcrn.org.uk/sites/default/files/project-files/fcrn_gnc_report.pdf (accessed 17 June 2019).

Gerber, P.J., Steinfeld, H., Henderson, B., Mottet, A., Opio, C. *et al.* (2013) Tackling Climate Change Through Livestock – A global assessment of emissions and mitigation opportunities. Food and Agriculture Organization of the United Nations (FAO), Rome. Available at: http://www.fao.org/3/a-i3437e.pdf (accessed 30 June 2019).

Gjedrem, T., Robinson, N. and Rye, M. (2012) The importance of selective breeding in aquaculture to meet future demands for animal protein: A review. *Aquaculture* 350–353, 117–129. DOI: 10.1016/j.aquaculture.2012.04.008.

Grace, D., Dominguez-Salas, P., Alonso, S., Lannerstad, M., Muunda, E. *et al.* (2018) The influence of livestock-derived foods on nutrition during the first 1,000 days of life. *ILRI Research Report 44*. International Livestock Research Institute, Nairobi. Available at: https://cgspace.cgiar.org/handle/10568/92907 (accessed 18 June 2019).

Haresign, W., Williams, R.J., Khalid, M. and Rodway, R. (1995) Heart rate responses and plasma cortisol and β-endorphin concentrations in ewes subjected to laparoscopy and its associated handling procedures. *Animal Science* 61, 77–83. DOI: 10.1017/S1357729800013540.

HLPE (2016) Sustainable Agricultural Development for Food Security and Nutrition. A report by The High Level Panel of Experts on Food Security and Nutrition. Available at: http://www.fao.org/fileadmin/user_upload/hlpe/hlpe_documents/HLPE_Reports/HLPE-Report-10_EN.pdf (accessed 30 June 2019).

HNV (2019) High Nature Value Farming. Available at: http://www.high-nature-value-farming.eu/ (accessed 17 June 2019).

Hoppe, N. (2018) The Legal Governance of Animal Biotechnologies. In: Niemann, H. and Wrenzycki, C. (eds) *Animal Biotechnology 2. Emerging Breeding Technologies.* Springer, Springer International Publishing, New York, pp. 235–250.

Huws, S.A., Creevey, C.J., Oyama, L.B., Mizrahi, I., Denman, S. *et al.* (2018) Addressing global ruminant agricultural challenges through understanding the rumen microbiome: Past, present and future. *Frontiers in Microbiology* 9, 2161. DOI: 10.3389/fmicb.2018.02161.

Lanzerath, D. (2018) Ethical aspects of animal biotechnology. In: Niemann, H. and Wrenzycki, C. (eds), *Animal Biotechnology 2. Emerging Breeding Technologies.* Springer, Springer International Publishing, New York. pp. 251–273. DOI: 10.1007/978-3-319-92348-2.

MAFF (1995). *Report of the Committee to Consider the Ethical Implications of Emerging Technologies in the Breeding of Farm Animals.* HMSO, London.

Mepham, T.B. (1996) Ethical impacts of biotechnology in dairying. In: Phillips, C.J.C. (ed.) *Progress in Dairy*

Science. CAB International, Wallingford, UK, pp. 375–395.
Mottet, A., de Haan, C., Falcucci, A., Tempio, G., Opio, C. and Gerber, P. (2017) Livestock: On our plates or eating at our table? A new analysis of the feed/food debate. *Global Food Security* 14, 1–8. DOI: 10.1016/j.gfs.2017.01.001.
Nuffield Council on Bioethics (2019) Genome Editing and Farmed Animals. Available at: http://nuffieldbioethics.org/current-work (accessed 30 June 2019).
OECD/FAO (2018) *OECD-FAO Agricultural Outlook 2018-2027*. OECD Publishing, Paris/Food and Agriculture Organization of the United Nations, Rome. Available at: https://doi.org/10.1787/agr_outlook-2018-en (accessed !8 November 2019).
Poore, J. and Nemecek, T. (2018) Reducing food's environmental impacts through producers and consumers. *Science* 360, 987–992.
Ritchie, H., Reay, D.S. and Higgins, P. (2018) Potential of meat substitutes for climate change mitigation and improved human health in high-income markets. *Frontiers in Sustainable Food Systems* 2, 16. DOI: 10.3389/fsufs.2018.00016
Simm, G. (1998) *Genetic Improvement of Cattle and Sheep*. CAB International, Wallingford, UK.
Smith, P. (2014) Do grasslands act as a perpetual sink for carbon? *Global Change Biology* 20, 2708–2711. DOI: 10.1111/gcb.12561.
Tait, J. (2017) From responsible research to responsible innovation: challenges in implementation. *Engineering Biology* 1, 1–5. DOI: 10.1049/enb.2017.0010.
UN (2019a) United Nations Sustainable Development Goals. Available at: https://sustainabledevelopment.un.org/sdgs (accessed 17 June 2019).
UN (2019b) United Nations World Population Prospects 2019. Available at: https://population.un.org/wpp/ (accessed 18 June 2019).
Van Eenennaam, A.L. and Young, A.E. (2018). Gene editing in livestock: promise, prospects and policy. *CAB Reviews,* 13, No. 027.
Van Zanten, H.H.E., Herrero, M., Van Hal, O., Röös, E., Muller, A. *et al.* (2018) Defining a land boundary for sustainable livestock consumption. *Global Change Biology* 24, 4185–4194. DOI: 10.1111/gcb.14321.
Webster, J. (1994) New breeding technologies: ethical and animal welfare issues. *British Cattle Breeders Club Digest* 49, 41–44.
Wirsenius, S., Hedenus, F. and Mohlin, K. (2011) Greenhouse gas taxes on animal food products: rationale, tax scheme and climate mitigation effects. *Climatic Change* 108, 159–184. DOI: 10.1007/s10584-010-9971-x.
World Commission on Environment and Development (1987) Our Common Future. Available at: https://sustainabledevelopment.un.org/content/documents/5987our-common-future.pdf (accessed 17 June 2019).
World Health Organization (WHO) (2017) The Double Durden of Malnutrition. Policy brief. Available at: https://apps.who.int/iris/bitstream/handle/10665/255413/WHO-NMH-NHD-17.3-eng.pdf?ua=1 (accessed 18 November 2019).

Recommended Reading

Garnett, T., Godde, C., Muller, A., Röös, E., Smith, P. *et al.* (2017) Grazed and Confused? FCRN, University of Oxford. Available at: https://www.fcrn.org.uk/sites/default/files/project-files/fcrn_gnc_report.pdf (accessed 17 June 2019).
ILRI (2019) Options for the livestock sector in developing and emerging economies to 2030 and beyond. *Meat: The Future Series*. World Economic Forum, Geneva, Switzerland.
IPCC (2019) Climate Change and Land: an IPCC special report on climate change, desertification, land degradation, sustainable land management, food security, and greenhouse gas fluxes in terrestrial ecosystems. Available at: https://www.ipcc.ch/report/srccl/ (accessed 18 November 2019).
Van Zanten, H.H.E., Herrero, M., Van Hal, O., Röös, E., Muller, A. *et al.* (2018) Defining a land boundary for sustainable livestock consumption. *Global Change Biology* 24, 4185–4194. DOI: 10.1111/gcb.14321.

Appendix

Table A.1. Values of selection intensity for different proportions of animals selected.[a] (After: Becker, W.A. (1984) *Manual of Quantitative Genetics*, 4th edn. Academic Enterprises, Pullman, Washington, USA.)

	No. in population						
No. selected	5	10	15	20	25	30	35
1	1.163	1.539	1.736	1.867	1.965	2.043	2.107
2	0.829	1.270	1.492	1.638	1.745	1.829	1.898
3	0.553	1.065	1.311	1.469	1.584	1.674	1.748
4	0.291	0.893	1.162	1.332	1.455	1.550	1.628
5		0.739	1.032	1.214	1.345	1.446	1.527
6		0.595	0.916	1.110	1.248	1.354	1.439
7		0.457	0.809	1.016	1.161	1.271	1.360
8		0.318	0.708	0.928	1.081	1.196	1.288
9		0.171	0.611	0.846	1.006	1.126	1.222
10			0.516	0.767	0.936	1.061	1.160
11			0.422	0.692	0.869	1.999	1.102
12			0.328	0.619	0.805	0.941	1.047
13			0.230	0.547	0.743	0.884	0.994
14			0.124	0.476	0.683	0.830	0.944
15				0.405	0.624	0.777	0.895
16				0.333	0.566	0.726	0.848
17				0.259	0.508	0.676	0.803
18				0.182	0.451	0.627	0.758
19				0.098	0.394	0.579	0.714
20					0.336	0.530	0.672
21					0.277	0.483	0.629
22					0.216	0.435	0.588
23					0.152	0.387	0.546
24					0.082	0.338	0.505
25						0.289	0.464
26						0.239	0.423
27						0.186	0.382
28						0.131	0.340
29						0.070	0.298
30							0.255
31							0.210
32							0.164
33							0.115
34							0.062

[a]Estimates of the selection intensity for numbers between the rows or columns of this table may be obtained by a linear approximation.

Genetic Improvement of Farmed Animals (G. Simm *et al.*)

	No. in population						
No. selected	40	45	50	75	100	150	200
1	2.161	2.208	2.249	2.403	2.508	2.649	2.746
2	1.957	2.008	2.052	2.217	2.328	2.478	2.580
3	1.810	1.864	1.911	2.084	2.201	2.357	2.463
4	1.694	1.750	1.799	1.980	2.101	2.263	2.372
5	1.596	1.654	1.705	1.893	2.018	2.185	2.297
6	1.510	1.571	1.624	1.818	1.947	2.118	2.233
7	1.434	1.497	1.552	1.752	1.884	2.060	2.177
8	1.365	1.430	1.487	1.693	1.828	2.007	2.127
9	1.301	1.369	1.427	1.638	1.777	1.960	2.082
10	1.242	1.312	1.372	1.588	1.730	1.916	2.040
11	1.187	1.258	1.320	1.542	1.686	1.876	2.002
12	1.134	1.208	1.271	1.498	1.645	1.838	1.966
13	1.084	1.160	1.225	1.457	1.607	1.803	1.932
14	1.037	1.114	1.181	1.418	1.571	1.770	1.901
15	0.991	1.071	1.139	1.381	1.536	1.738	1.871
16	0.947	1.029	1.099	1.346	1.504	1.708	1.843
17	0.904	0.988	1.060	1.312	1.472	1.680	1.816
18	0.862	0.949	1.022	1.279	1.442	1.652	1.790
19	0.822	0.911	0.986	1.248	1.413	1.626	1.766
20	0.782	0.873	0.951	1.217	1.386	1.601	1.742
21	0.744	0.837	0.916	1.188	1.359	1.577	1.720
22	0.706	0.802	0.882	1.160	1.333	1.554	1.698
23	0.668	0.767	0.849	1.132	1.308	1.531	1.677
24	0.631	0.733	0.817	1.105	1.283	1.509	1.656
25	0.595	0.699	0.786	1.079	1.259	1.488	1.636
26	0.558	0.665	0.754	1.053	1.236	1.467	1.617
27	0.522	0.633	0.724	1.028	1.214	1.447	1.598
28	0.486	0.600	0.693	1.003	1.192	1.428	1.580
29	0.450	0.568	0.663	0.979	1.170	1.409	1.563
30	0.414	0.535	0.634	0.956	1.149	1.390	1.545
31	0.378	0.503	0.604	0.932	1.128	1.372	1.529
32	0.341	0.471	0.575	0.910	1.108	1.354	1.512
33	0.304	0.439	0.546	0.887	1.088	1.337	1.496
34	0.267	0.407	0.517	0.865	1.069	1.320	1.480
35	0.228	0.375	0.488	0.843	1.050	1.304	1.465
36	0.188	0.342	0.459	0.821	1.031	1.287	1.450
37	0.147	0.309	0.430	0.800	1.012	1.271	1.435
38	0.103	0.276	0.401	0.779	0.994	1.255	1.421
39	0.055	0.242	0.372	0.758	0.976	1.240	1.407
40		0.207	0.343	0.738	0.958	1.225	1.393
41		0.171	0.313	0.717	0.941	1.210	1.379
42		0.133	0.283	0.697	0.923	1.195	1.366
43		0.093	0.253	0.677	0.906	1.181	1.352
44		0.050	0.221	0.657	0.889	1.166	1.339
45			0.189	0.637	0.873	1.152	1.327
46			0.156	0.617	0.856	1.138	1.314
47			0.122	0.598	0.840	1.125	1.301
48			0.085	0.578	0.824	1.111	1.289
49			0.046	0.559	0.808	1.098	1.277
50				0.539	0.792	1.085	1.265

	No. in population			
No. selected	75	100	150	200
51	0.520	0.776	1.072	1.253
52	0.501	0.760	1.059	1.242
53	0.481	0.745	1.046	1.230
54	0.462	0.729	1.034	1.219
55	0.443	0.714	1.021	1.208
56	0.423	0.699	1.009	1.197
57	0.404	0.684	0.997	1.186
58	0.384	0.669	0.985	1.175
59	0.365	0.654	0.973	1.165
60	0.345	0.639	0.961	1.154
61	0.325	0.624	0.949	1.144
62	0.305	0.609	0.937	1.133
63	0.285	0.594	0.926	1.123
64	0.265	0.580	0.914	1.113
65	0.244	0.565	0.903	1.103
66	0.223	0.551	0.892	1.093
67	0.202	0.536	0.881	1.083
68	0.180	0.521	0.869	1.073
69	0.158	0.507	0.858	1.064
70	0.135	0.492	0.847	1.054
71	0.112	0.478	0.837	1.044
72	0.087	0.463	0.826	1.035
73	0.061	0.449	0.815	1.026
74	0.032	0.434	0.804	1.016
75		0.420	0.794	1.007
76		0.405	0.783	0.998
77		0.391	0.773	0.989
78		0.376	0.762	0.980
79		0.361	0.752	0.971
80		0.346	0.742	0.962
81		0.332	0.731	0.953
82		0.317	0.721	0.944
83		0.302	0.711	0.936
84		0.286	0.701	0.927
85		0.271	0.691	0.918
86		0.256	0.680	0.910
87		0.240	0.670	0.901
88		0.224	0.660	0.893
89		0.208	0.650	0.884
90		0.192	0.640	0.876
91		0.176	0.631	0.868
92		0.159	0.621	0.860
93		0.142	0.611	0.851
94		0.124	0.601	0.843
95		0.106	0.591	0.835
96		0.088	0.581	0.827
97		0.068	0.572	0.819
98		0.048	0.562	0.811
99		0.025	0.552	0.803
100			0.542	0.795

	No. in population			No. in population
No. selected	150	200	No. selected	200
101	0.533	0.787	151	0.414
102	0.523	0.779	152	0.407
103	0.513	0.771	153	0.400
104	0.504	0.763	154	0.392
105	0.494	0.755	155	0.385
106	0.484	0.748	156	0.378
107	0.474	0.740	157	0.370
108	0.465	0.732	158	0.363
109	0.455	0.724	159	0.356
110	0.445	0.717	160	0.348
111	0.436	0.709	161	0.341
112	0.426	0.702	162	0.333
113	0.416	0.694	163	0.326
114	0.406	0.686	164	0.318
115	0.397	0.679	165	0.311
116	0.387	0.671	166	0.303
117	0.377	0.664	167	0.296
118	0.367	0.656	168	0.288
119	0.357	0.649	169	0.280
120	0.348	0.641	170	0.273
121	0.338	0.634	171	0.265
122	0.328	0.626	172	0.257
123	0.318	0.619	173	0.249
124	0.308	0.612	174	0.242
125	0.298	0.604	175	0.234
126	0.287	0.597	176	0.226
127	0.277	0.590	177	0.218
128	0.267	0.582	178	0.210
129	0.257	0.575	179	0.202
130	0.246	0.567	180	0.194
131	0.236	0.560	181	0.185
132	0.225	0.553	182	0.177
133	0.215	0.546	183	0.169
134	0.204	0.538	184	0.160
135	0.193	0.531	185	0.152
136	0.182	0.524	186	0.143
137	0.171	0.516	187	0.134
138	0.160	0.509	188	0.125
139	0.148	0.502	189	0.116
140	0.137	0.495	190	0.107
141	0.125	0.487	191	0.098
142	0.113	0.480	192	0.089
143	0.101	0.473	193	0.079
144	0.088	0.465	194	0.069
145	0.075	0.458	195	0.059
146	0.062	0.451	196	0.048
147	0.048	0.444	197	0.038
148	0.033	0.436	198	0.026
149	0.018	0.429	199	0.014
150		0.422		

Glossary of Technical Terms

Glossary words are italicized on first use in the book; the singular form of the word is listed in the glossary.

accuracy of predicted breeding values (or transmitting abilities) – The correlation between predicted and true breeding values or predicted and true transmitting abilities.

accuracy of selection – The correlation between the selection criterion (e.g. an index) and the breeding goal.

additive - Type of gene action where the value of a heterozygote is midway between both homozygoytes.

additive correction factors – Amounts that are added to, or subtracted from, the performance records of animals which belong to particular classes (e.g. singles or twins) to adjust for non-genetic effects when predicting genetic merit.

additive genetic relationship (A) – The proportion of the genome that any two animals have in common, e.g. 0.5 for sire and offspring.

additive genetic relationship matrix (A matrix) – A table showing the expected proportion of the genome in common for all animals in the pedigree file (i.e. the additive genetic relationships between them).

additive genetic standard deviation – Square root of the additive genetic variance.

additive genetic variance (or variation) – Variance (or variation) in a trait due to the combined effects of genes with additive action.

AI-REML - Average information restricted maximum likelihood – A method for calculating variance components used to estimate genetic parameters.

allele – A particular sequence of bases at a given locus or site on a chromosome. There may be many alternative sequences possible at a particular locus in the breed as a whole, but individual animals either carry copies of two different alleles (one on each member of the pair of chromosomes concerned – these animals are heterozygotes), or two copies of the same allele (these animals are homozygotes). The alternative sequences of bases at a particular site are termed alleles or genes interchangeably.

analysis of variance (ANOVA) – A ubiquitous set of statistical models used to analyse differences between animals (or any other set of measurements) for traits of interest and the factors that affect these traits. Basic methods are found in many statistical textbooks and software packages.

artificial insemination (AI) – Deposition of semen into the reproductive tract of a female animal, either via the vagina or directly into the uterus using a laparoscope. The semen is often extended to allow wider use, and frozen to allow long-term storage.

artificial selection – Selection of animals by humans, rather than, or in addition to, natural selection. Like natural selection, artificial selection acts on the many differences between individual animals, but the choice is based on characteristics of perceived benefit to the breeder, rather than on fitness for a particular natural habitat, environment, and so on.

associative effect - The genetic part of a social interaction effect.

assortative mating – A mating plan where like is mated to like, e.g. better males for growth may be mated to the better females for the same trait. It is the opposite of random mating.

autosomal – Relating to chromosomes other than the sex chromosomes. *See* autosomes

autosomes – All chromosomes apart from the sex chromosomes. Genes on these chromosomes are said to be autosomal.

autozygous – Alleles that are identical because they were inherited from a common ancestor.

backcross – Animal resulting from backcrossing.

backcrossing – Mating of a crossbred animal back to one of the parent breeds.

base (chemical) – The chemical substances which, when paired, make up the 'rungs' of a DNA 'ladder'. There are four different bases in DNA: adenine (A), thymine (T), guanine (G) and cytosine (C).

base population – The oldest group of animals with unknown parents in the pedigree used for genetic evaluation. Usually their breeding values sum to zero and the breeding values of animals in subsequent generations are expressed relative to those of the base animals. However, the breeding values of all animals may also be expressed relative to the mean of animals born in a particular year (see genetic base for full details).

best linear unbiased prediction (BLUP) – A statistical procedure for predicting animal breeding values. Can be applied under several sets of assumptions or models which account for different relationships between animals. BLUP estimates environmental effects and predicts breeding values simultaneously, and so disentangles genetics from management, feeding, etc. more effectively, and produces better predictions of breeding value than other methods.

between-breed selection – Substitution of one breed by another; comparison of two or more breeds followed by selection of the most appropriate.

bioinformatics – The science of collecting and analysing molecular genetic data, such as large volumes of nucleic acid sequence data. Includes analysing data from the 'omic' sciences. Covers many topics and software routines, including statistics.

bloodlines – A general term relating to a group of closely related animals of similar characteristics within a breed, herd or flock.

Bonferroni correction – When the same analysis is carried out many times using one set of data but with many different categories to work with this is said to be 'multiple testing'. Under multiple testing there is a greater tendency to find statistically significant differences within the categories. The Bonferroni correction adjusts the probability test value to account for this tendency.

breed – A recognized group of interbreeding animals within a domestic species. Often animals of a breed are of fairly uniform appearance, but in some cases animals are considered to belong to a breed purely by virtue of their geographical location.

breed society – An organization formed to promote a particular breed, and to record details of ancestry (and sometimes performance data also) of animals of the breed, registered by members.

breed substitution – A method of genetic improvement involving replacing one breed by another. Often this is achieved more gradually by continually crossing to the new breed. *See* grading up.

breeding goal (or selection objective) – The characteristic(s) which selection is intended to improve, e.g. carcass lean content, margin between milk production and feed costs.

breeding value – The additive genetic merit of an animal. Double the expected progeny performance compared to the population mean. An animal's true breeding value cannot be measured directly but it can be predicted from various sources of information. These include the animal's own performance, that of its relatives and genomic information.

broodstock – A group of sexually mature individuals used in aquaculture for breeding purposes.

candidate gene – A gene which potentially contributes to variation in a trait of interest. A gene with a known or suspected link to the trait of interest which may be chosen as a marker (e.g. a gene coding for a hormone known to affect milk yield or growth rate).

carrier – A term used in Mendelian genetics to indicate that an animal is heterozygous and contains a recessive version of a gene/SNP such that its effect is not seen in the phenotype.

causal component of variance – Variance due to a particular biological effect e.g. additive genes, dominance etc. See Table 6.2 for a more extensive list of such components.

centimorgan – *See* morgan.

centromere – Part of a chromosome which is located near the middle of the chromosome, or at one end. During the initial phases of duplication of chromosomes, the two copies remain joined at the centromere.

chromatid – A chromatid is one of the two identical copies of a replicated chromosome in a cell.

chromatin – A complex of DNA and proteins that forms chromosomes within the nucleus of eukaryotic cells (eukaryotes are organisms with cell nuclei enclosed within membranes).

chromosomes – Structures found in the nuclei of all cells, which are made up of DNA, and on which genes are sited. Chromosomes occur in pairs in the nuclei of body cells, and singly in gametes (sperm and eggs).

cloning (of embryos) – The production of groups of identical embryos either by physically splitting embryos or by transferring cultured cells into eggs from which the nucleus has been removed (nuclear transfer).

co-dominance – Type of gene action in which heterozygotes show characteristics of each of the homozygous types (e.g. as with roan coat colour in Shorthorn cattle).

coding – The process whereby genes provide the basis for the production of proteins.

coding sequence (CDS) – The portion of a gene's DNA that codes for proteins.

codon – A sequence of three bases in mRNA which codes for the production of a particular amino acid (the building blocks which proteins are made from).

coefficient of variation – The ratio of the standard deviation to the mean.

collateral relatives – Relatives from the same generation as the animal of interest, e.g. sibs, cousins.

combining ability – The ability of particular breeds to produce high-performing offspring, as a result of high heterosis, when they are crossed.

complementarity – An outcome of some crossbreeding schemes, in which the overall efficiency of a production system is improved by crossing breeds which have high genetic merit in different traits, e.g. use of large, lean terminal sire breeds on dam breeds of intermediate size and good maternal performance.

complete dominance – The type of gene action in which the presence of one allele completely masks the effect of another allele at the same locus in a heterozygote (e.g. the black coat colour gene in cattle).

complex trait – *See* quantitative characteristics.

composite – A new (synthetic) breed formed by crossing two or more breeds, then selecting within the new population.

contemporary animals/contemporary groups – Animals that have been treated in a similar way, e.g. born over a relatively short period of time, on the same farm, and fed and managed similarly.

contemporary comparison – An early method of breeding value estimation measuring animals against those kept on the same farm, at the same time usually in the same physical group.

contigs – A set of overlapping DNA segments that together indicate the sequence in a particular region.

core selective sweep – Selective sweep regions with consecutive signals within 1 Mb of each other.

correlated response (to selection) – The change in the phenotypic or genetic mean of other traits when directional selection has occurred, in a population, for a specific trait or set of traits.

correlation coefficient – A value between –1 and +1 which measures the direction and strength of the association between two characteristics, or between the same characteristic at different times. Positive values indicate that as one trait increases, the other generally increases too (e.g. live weight and fatness). Negative values indicate that as one trait increases, the other generally decreases (e.g. milk yield and milk protein %). There are several types of correlations but two of the most widely used in animal breeding are the phenotypic correlation, or correlation between measurements on animals, and the additive genetic correlation, or correlation between breeding values.

covariance – A measure of the association between traits, used in its own right, and in calculating correlation coefficients. Covariances between two traits are calculated in a similar way to calculating the variance of a single trait.

crossbred (animal) – Animal with parents of different breeds or strains.

crossbreeding – Mating parents of two or more different breeds, strains or species together.

crossing over – *See* recombination.

cryopreservation – Storing semen, ova or embryos by freezing them to a very low temperature ready for later use.

culled – An animal removed from a herd or flock, e.g. because it has a poor predicted breeding value.

***de novo* sequencing** – The construction of a genetic sequence using overlapping contigs to order the results.

deoxyribonucleic acid (DNA) – The chemical substance that chromosomes are made of. DNA has a ladder-like structure with pairs of four different bases (adenine, thymine, guanine and cytosine) making up the 'rungs'. This structure, together with the fact that these bases always pair in the same way, provides a very reliable mechanism for copying DNA during cell division. Genes or alleles are simply sequences of bases on one side of a DNA molecule. Different genes or alleles at a particular locus are sequences which differ slightly, often only in one base pair. Also found in mitochondria.

deregressed predicted breeding values – A method for calculating genetic merit by reversing the 'shrinking' that goes on to account for accuracy in calculating PBVs in order to get back to average daughter performance corrected for environmental effects.

DFREML – Derivative-free restricted maximum likelihood – A method for calculating variance components from pedigree and performance data using sire or animal models.

diploid – The state in which the chromosomes occur in pairs. This is the case for all body cells in terrestrial livestock, except the gametes. For example, cattle have 30 pairs of chromosomes in body cells. Certain aquaculture species have more than two pairs of chromosomes per cell which is known as polyploidy.

direct breeding value – The genetic merit of an animal for its direct (as opposed to maternal) genetic influence on a trait (e.g. its influence on weaning weight via genes for growth as opposed to genes for uterine capacity and milk production).

direct genomic breeding value (DGV) – The genetic merit of an animal that is estimated using only the SNP genotype information on that animal and SNP solutions. It is calculated as the product of the genotypic information on that animal and the SNP solutions.

DNA probe – A single-stranded molecule of DNA used to detect the presence of a complementary DNA strand in samples of DNA or in intact chromosomes. Probes can be 'labelled' by making them either radioactive or fluorescent.

dominance – *See* complete dominance.

double muscling – The result of a genetic change in the myostatin gene which produces animals with more muscle fibres. Examples have been found in most farmed species.

draft animals – Animals chosen to be removed from a flock/herd, sometimes for further breeding (e.g. hill ewes moving to less harsh farm environments).

economic selection index – Selection index with the weighting on different breeding goal traits based on their relative economic values.

economic value (of a trait) – The marginal profit resulting from a genetic change of one unit in that trait, e.g. the increase or decrease in profit resulting from a change of 1 kg in live weight compared to the current average value, with no change in other traits in the breeding goal. Used to apportion emphasis to different traits in selection indexes.

electrophoresis – Application of an electric current to a film of gel on which DNA samples have been placed, to separate fragments of DNA of different size and charge.

elite or nucleus breeders/herds/flocks – Breeders/herds/flocks at the top of the improvement pyramid supplying breeding stock to other breeders/units in tiers below.

embryo transfer – A process used to transfer embryos from a (donor) female into (recipient) female(s). May be used after multiple ovulation and *in vivo* fertilization, or after collection and *in vitro* fertilization of ova.

environmental correlation – A measure of the extent to which environmental conditions that are favourable for one character are favourable or unfavourable for a second character (range from –1 to +1).

environmental effect – Any non-genetic influence on an animal.

environmental variation – Variance (or variation) in a trait due to non-genetic effects, including differences in feeding and management, etc. not removed by adjusting records of performance.

epigenetics – The study of phenotypic changes that do not involve alterations in the DNA sequence but are due to differential gene expression.

epistasis – Occurs when the presence of an allele at one locus masks or enhances the effect of an allele at another locus (i.e. there is an interaction between alleles at different loci). Visible examples include interactions between alleles at different coat colour loci in several species.

error variance – *See* residual variance.

estimated breeding value (EBV) – *See* predicted breeding value.

estimated transmitting ability (ETA) – *See* predicted transmitting ability.

exon – The protein-coding DNA sequence of a gene and the RNA it produces.

expected progeny differences (EPD) – *See* predicted transmitting ability.

extended haplotype homozygosity – A long run of homozygosity which can be detected when positive selection causes a rapid increase in the frequency of a favourable allele in a short time period, giving rise to an unusually long haplotype.

family selection – A type of selection where whole families are chosen as the parents of the next generation, based on their family average performance.

fixation or fixed – When all the animals in a population have only one version of a sequence of bases/alleles/genes or haplotype at a particular locus.

fixed base – The group of animals (e.g. those born in a particular year) from which deviations in breeding value are expressed. The group usually remains fixed for several evaluations. *See* genetic base.

fixed effect – A term in a statistical model that has a specific number of levels, e.g. when animals in a population are male, female or castrates the term for differences between the sexes in the model has three levels.

functional annotation – Collecting together all known biological information about a DNA feature such as a gene, usually in a database.

gametes – A sex cell, i.e. a sperm in the male, and an unfertilized egg (ovum) in the female.

gene – A sequence of bases on one side of a DNA molecule. Commonly refers to a DNA feature which codes for the production of proteins. Also can be used to refer to any DNA feature on a genome. The alternative forms of the sequence of bases at a particular site are termed genes or alleles interchangeably. The word gene is also used to describe the site on a chromosome where a particular gene occurs. More properly, this is termed a locus.

gene editing – A group of technologies such as CRISPR/Cas9 that allow targeted alterations to genomic DNA at a specific position in the genome of an individual.

gene frequency – The proportion or percentage of genes (alleles) of each type at a particular locus, in a herd, flock or other group of animals. Must add up to 1 or 100% for all alleles at this locus.

gene mapping – *See* genome mapping.

gene pool – A general term used to indicate the genetic material available for a selection programme.

gene transfer – Insertion of DNA from one animal into the genome of another. This transfer may be between individuals of the same or different breeds, species or even classes of organism.

generation interval – The weighted average age of parents when their offspring are born.

genetic base – The group of animals born in a particular year and whose mean predicted breeding value is set to equal zero. Other animals' PBVs are expressed as deviations from this base. It is called a fixed base if the definition of base animals remains unchanged for a few years. Alternatively it is called a rolling base if PBVs are expressed relative to the merit of the current population and so they change with each new evaluation.

genetic correlation – A measure of the direction and strength of the association between breeding values for two characters measured on the same (or related) animals in a population, e.g. live weight and fat depth (range from –1 to +1).

genetic distance – Genetic distance is a measure of the genetic divergence between species or between populations within a species, whether the distance measures time from common ancestor or degree of differentiation. Populations with many similar alleles have small genetic distances.

genetic drift – The change in gene frequencies over generations due to chance.

genetic evaluation – The prediction of breeding values.

genetic groups – Groups of animals of different average merit e.g. from different countries. In genetic evaluations base animals are assigned to different genetic groups to avoid bias in predicting breeding values.

genetic links – Links between contemporary groups provided by related animals. These links are necessary in order for BLUP to estimate environmental effects and predict breeding values simultaneously, and to enable comparison of PBVs across groups, herds, flocks or years.

genetic merit – A general term to mean the sum of the total effects of genes on a trait of interest in a particular animal, or group.

genetic parameters – A collective term used to include some or all of the heritability, repeatability, genetic and phenotypic correlations, variances and covariances for a set of traits in a population.

genetic trend – The change in mean predicted breeding value in a population of animals over time.

genochoristic – A species where the individual animals belong to one of at least two distinct sexes throughout their life (typical of mammals and birds, but not all aquaculture species).

genome – The entire genetic code of an animal contained in the full set of chromosomes and mitochondria.

genome annotation – The process of identifying the locations of genes, coding regions, and regulatory regions in a genome and assigning their function.

genome browser – A graphical interface for the display of information from a biological database of genomic data.

genome maps/mapping – A description of the location of functional genes, or other sequences of DNA, on the chromosomes of the species concerned. Genome maps include linkage or genetic maps, and physical maps.

genome-wide association study (GWAS) – A statistical method using SNPs or SNVs to investigate the link between individual sections of the genome and the phenotype of the animal in order to locate genes which affect a particular trait.

genome sequencing – The process of finding the order of DNA along the chromosomes of a living organism.

genomic breeding values – Estimated breeding values obtained using a genomic prediction model, via the use of genome-wide genetic markers.

genomic heritability – A method that uses all the SNPs in a particular study and attempts to combine all their effects on a trait to compute the heritability of that trait.

genomic imprinting – Type of gene action in which the expression of a gene in offspring depends on which sex of parent contributed it (e.g. the *callipyge* gene affecting muscularity in sheep).

genomic prediction – A statistical method which uses SNPs or SNVs to predict the breeding value of a population of animals.

genomic relationship matrix (G matrix) – A matrix containing the estimation of the proportion of total genomic DNA shared by any two individuals based on genome-wide genetic marker data.

genomic selection – The selection of breeding individuals for genetic improvement of a trait of interest based on the use of genome-wide genetic markers to estimate genomic breeding values. The relationships among genetic marker genotypes and animal phenotypes are first measured in a reference population, in order to predict breeding values of selection candidates that have genotypes only.

genotype – The particular combination of genes or alleles which an animal inherits.

genotype × environment (G × E) interaction – Occurs when genotypes do not rank the same in different environments, or when the advantage to a particular genotype in one environment is smaller or greater in another.

genotype frequency – The proportion or percentage of animals of each genotype in a herd, flock or other group. Must add up to 1, or 100%, over all possible genotypes. May apply at any level: animal, gene, SNP or base position.

grading up – Repeated mating of females, and subsequently their female offspring, to males of a new breed. *See* breed substitution.

gross margin – A financial indicator of success in a business. Calculated as gross income minus variable costs of production.

group breeding scheme – Co-operative breeding scheme with a nucleus of elite animals screened from members, flocks or herds. Recording and selection are concentrated in the nucleus, which then produces breeding stock for members.

H matrix – A matrix of genetic relationships among animals that is constructed by combining information from pedigrees of non-genotyped animals and SNP information from genotyped animals.

haploid – The state in which chromosomes occur singly, rather than in pairs. This is the case in gametes, e.g. the sperm or eggs of cattle carry 30 chromosomes.

haplotype – A group of alleles at polymorphic loci within an organism that are inherited together.

hapmap project – A coordinated programme to develop a database of whole genome sequences or SNP panels for individual animals in a breed.

Hardy–Weinberg equilibrium (or law) – If there is no selection for or against particular alleles at a locus, no mutation and no movement of animals into or out of a large, random-mating population of animals, then the gene and genotype frequencies in that population tend to stay the same from one generation to the next. This is described mathematically as: $p^2 + 2pq + q^2 = 1$ where p and q are the allele frequencies of two alleles at a locus and the three terms in the model relate to the genotype frequencies of a homozygous, heterozygous and the alternate homozygous genotype respectively.

heritability (h^2) – The proportion of superiority of parents in a trait (i.e. the proportion of the selection differential) which, on average, is passed on to offspring. Or, the additive genetic variation in a trait (the variation in breeding values), expressed as a proportion of the total phenotypic variation in that trait.

heterosis – The difference in performance of crossbred animals compared to the mid-parent mean.

heterozygote/heterozygous – Animals which carry copies of two different alleles at a particular locus (e.g. RW).

homology (of DNA sequence) – The high degree of similarity between parts of the genome of different mammalian species.

homology directed repair (HDR) – A laboratory procedure that involves the provision of a DNA template which is similar to the flanking sequence of a cut site (but may contain a user-targeted change in sequence); the cell uses the template to repair the genomic DNA at the cut site.

homozygote/homozygous – Animals which carry two copies of the same allele at a particular locus (e.g. RR).

hybrid vigour – *See* heterosis

ICAR (International Committee on Animal Recording) – An international non-governmental organization set up to coordinate and set standards for livestock recording across countries.

identical by descent (IBD) – When the two alleles at a specific locus of an individual are the same because they are derived from a known common ancestor.

identical by state (IBS) – When the two alleles at a specific locus of an individual are the same but are not derived from a known common ancestor.

improvement lag – The difference in genetic merit between tiers (e.g. nucleus, multiplier, commercial) of a livestock industry.

imputation – A bioinformatic method to use SNP or SNV data from a group of animals with high-density genotyping to infer the haplotypes of animals with low-density genotyping usually within the same breed.

inbreeding – The practice of mating related animals. This may be done deliberately, as in line-breeding. It is also an inevitable consequence of long-term selection in a closed population.

inbreeding coefficient (F) – A measure of the amount of inbreeding, defined as the probability that two alleles at any locus are 'identical by descent'.

inbreeding depression – The decline in performance (especially in traits associated with fitness, such as reproductive rate and disease resistance) which is a consequence of inbreeding.

incomplete penetrance – Occurs when a character appears to be entirely controlled by a single gene, but not all animals of a given genotype show the expected phenotype (e.g. malignant hyperthermia in pigs). (This may be a result of epigenetic or environmental influences, or different mutations within the same gene.)

independent culling levels – A method of selection for more than one trait. Involves setting minimum qualifying standards, or thresholds, in each trait of interest. To qualify for selection, animals must then surpass the qualifying standard in each trait.

index coefficients (or weights) – The weighting factors applied to the phenotypic measurements of one or more traits on an animal, or its relatives, to derive a single index score on which to base selection.

index measurements – The set of measurements of performance on candidates for selection, to which index coefficients are applied to calculate an index score. May be the same as traits in the breeding goal if these can all be measured in both sexes, and on the live animal, or they may be different from the goal traits e.g. if these are only available on one sex, or are measured after slaughter.

index selection – Selection on an overall score (or index) of genetic merit which combines information on several traits of importance, or from different classes of relatives.

individual heterosis – Heterosis as a result of the individual animal (rather than its sire or dam) being crossbred.

individual selection – *See* mass selection.

inherited – A term used to indicate genes or characteristics passing from one generation to the next, as a result of genes of the parents passing to offspring.

interbred – An animal derived from a cross or – interbreeding – the act of crossing two different breeds.

international conversions – In the early stages of international trade in dairy cattle semen, and prior to the introduction of MACE, international conversions provided the means by which PBVs from one country could be expressed on the scale of another.

international predicted genetic merit (PGM) – Values used to convert an animal's performance in one country into the equivalent scale in a second country. *See* MACE.

introgression – Introduction of a single gene for a favourable characteristic to an existing breed by crossing to a new breed carrying the gene, and then backcrossing to the original breed for several generations. This is followed by mating of males and females from the final backcross generation to produce animals which are homozygous for the introgressed gene.

intron – A non-protein coding sequence in a gene.

***in vitro* production of embryos** – Laboratory production of embryos, following collection of unfertilized eggs from the ovary of a slaughtered female or from a live donor via ovum pick up. These eggs are first matured, then fertilized and cultured further before transfer.

karyotype – A picture of the full set of an animal's chromosomes obtained after staining and viewing with a microscope.

linebreeding – The practice of deliberately mating closely related animals. This was widely used by early improvers of farm livestock. It is far less common in large animal breeding today because of the risks of producing non-viable lines as a result of inbreeding depression.

linkage – Occurs when two loci are close together on the same chromosome. Because segments of the chromosome are involved in crossing over, genes which are closer together on the same chromosome will tend to cross over together more often than genes which are far apart on the same chromosome. This can lead to associations between characters.

linkage disequilibrium (LD) – Linkage disequilibrium is the non-random association of alleles at different loci in a given population.

linkage equilibrium (LE) – Occurs when the haplotype frequencies in a population have the same value that they would have if the genes at each locus were combined at random.

linkage map – A map that shows the recombinational or genetic distance between pairs of markers on the same chromosome. This is achieved by measuring the frequency with which the markers separate from one generation to the next, as a result of recombination.

locus – The site ('address') of a gene on a chromosome.

major gene – A single gene with a large effect, such as those affecting coat colour, polledness and double muscling.

marker – Any variable or measurable characteristic of an animal which can potentially be used as a predictor of performance or can be used to create a linkage map (e.g. genotype at a molecular marker locus, blood group, milk protein type).

marker-assisted introgression (MAI) – The use of markers to speed up the introduction of a gene of interest from one breed to another by: (i) identifying backcrosses carrying the particular favoured allele from the new breed, and possibly (ii) amongst animals with one or two copies of this allele, identifying those with least of their genome from the new breed.

marker-assisted selection (MAS) – The use of markers to accelerate selection by identifying animals likely to have a favourable genotype for the trait of interest. The gene of interest, to which the marker is linked, may be a single gene with a large effect, or it may be one of many genes affecting a quantitative trait (a QTL).

mass selection – The mating of those animals with the highest phenotypic values for the trait or traits of interest.

mass spawning – Reproduction of aquaculture species in groups with release of high numbers of eggs and sperm into the water, where fertilization occurs externally.

maternal breeding value – The genetic merit of an animal for its maternal (as opposed to direct) genetic influence on a trait (e.g. its influence on weaning weight via genes for uterine capacity and milk production rather than via genes for growth).

maternal heterosis – Heterosis in reproduction and other maternal traits as a result of the breeding female being crossbred.

meiosis – The type of cell division which occurs during production of the gametes (sperm and eggs). During meiosis, the cells which become sperm or eggs receive only a single (haploid) set of chromosomes (although in tetraploid fish, gametes contain two pairs of chromosomes). Also, recombination leads to a mixing of segments of the maternally-derived and paternally-derived chromosomes.

Mendelian genetics – A branch of genetics dealing with traits controlled by a single gene, named after Gregor Mendel who initiated such studies. Depending on the mode of inheritance, it may be possible to infer the genotype directly from the phenotype.

Mendelian sampling – On average, the predicted breeding values of offspring are expected to equal the average of their parents' breeding values. This follows from the fact that offspring get exactly half of their genes from each parent. However, there is variation in which particular sample of genes the offspring inherit from each parent. Some may get a particularly 'good' sample for the trait of interest, and others a 'bad' sample. This becomes apparent when the offspring get records of performance of their own, or from their progeny, or when genomic breeding values are available. This chance effect is termed Mendelian sampling and it may be included as a term in a model explaining the deviation from parental average breeding value.

Mendelian segregation ratios – The ratio of expected offspring genotypes from matings between specific parental genotypes in Mendelian genetics.

messenger RNA (mRNA) – RNA is a substance very similar to DNA. Messenger RNA is a type of RNA which transfers the code for the production of a protein from the DNA in the nucleus of a cell, to the ribosomes ('protein factories') in the cytoplasm of the cell.

metric trait – *See* quantitative trait.

microarray – A laboratory tool used to detect the expression of a very large number of genes at the same time.

microsatellite – A region in the genome where the same sequence of base pairs is repeated several times, end to end. The repeated sequences are two to six or more base pairs long. The number of times a given sequence of bases is repeated varies greatly between alleles but is typically five to 50 times. Because of this variation, microsatellites can be used as markers in genome mapping and for marker-assisted selection.

mitochondria – Small structures in cells responsible for generating energy to 'fuel' the activities of the cell – the cell's 'power stations'. They also contain DNA which is passed down through the maternal line in a separate manner from nuclear DNA.

mitochondrial (cytoplasmic) inheritance – Transmission of small amounts of genetic information from mothers to daughters via mitochondrial DNA.

mitosis – The type of cell division which occurs during normal growth and development. Each of the 'daughter' cells produced receives a copy of the complete original (diploid for most animals) set of chromosomes.

mixed-animal model – A statistical method commonly used in animal genetics to estimate the breeding values of animals or the genetic parameters for a set of traits, or both. It comprises both fixed and random effects. The fixed effects remove variation often due to environmental or management variables with a fixed number of levels, while the random effects account for genetic variation as well as a residual (sometimes called the error term) to account for unexplainable variation.

model – A model is an equation that describes a particular relationship in mathematical terms. In the context of animal breeding it often outlines the possible fixed effects that we are aware of that influence the performance of animals for the trait of interest, and also the random effects. It also sets out the assumptions used in predicting breeding values (or estimating genetic parameters); these differ in sophistication. The name of the model indicates the relationships used and the animals for which breeding values are predicted, e.g. sire model BLUP predicts BVs for sires from their progeny records; an animal model BLUP predicts BVs for all animals included in the evaluation, using all relationships amongst them.

molecular genetic marker – Any identifiable segment of DNA in the genome. Markers may be all or part of a 'functional' gene, or they may be a part of the rest of the genome which does not code directly for the production of a protein. SNPs are commonly used molecular markers in livestock genome mapping and analysis and prediction of genomic breeding values.

Morgan or centimorgan (cM) – An historic unit measuring the distance between two positions on a chromosome. A centimorgan is the distance between two 'genes' which are likely to have an average number of crossovers between them of 1% per generation.

multiple ovulation and embryo transfer (MOET) – A series of reproductive techniques including superovulation of a donor female, mating, recovery of the resulting embryos, and transfer of fresh or frozen embryos to recipient females.

multiplicative correction factors – Values which are used to adjust performance records of animals which belong to particular classes (e.g. singles or twins) for non-genetic effects when predicting genetic merit.

multiplier (breeders/herds/flocks/tiers) – Breeders/herds/flocks/tiers in the middle of the improvement pyramid buying breeding stock from elite breeders above, and supplying pure or crossbred breeding stock to commercial producers below.

multi-trait across-country evaluation (MACE) – A method for predicting breeding values of animals using information from different countries. Based on multi-trait BLUP evaluation, but rather than evaluating many different traits at once, MACE treats records on the same trait from different countries as if they were different traits. This allows for differences amongst countries in the heritability of the trait of interest and allows for different genetic correlations between this trait recorded in different countries.

multi-trait animal model – A mixed model used to analyse several traits at once.

multi-trait (BLUP) evaluation – Prediction of breeding values for several traits simultaneously commonly using the multi-trait mixed-animal model. This improves the accuracy of the evaluation, if the traits are correlated, provided that accurate estimates of these correlations are used in the evaluation.

multi-trait selection – Selection to alter several traits simultaneously, e.g. by using a selection index.

mutation – Chromosomal mutations involve changes in the number or structure of chromosomes. Gene or point mutations occur when mistakes are made in copying DNA, and these are not corrected by repair enzymes. If gene mutations occur in the reproductive organs, they lead to a change in the genetic code of offspring. Gene mutations are an important source of genetic variation.

natural selection – The process by which animals, and other forms of life, which are best suited to their particular environment or niche, stand a higher chance of surviving and reproducing than those that do not ('survival of the fittest'). Natural selection acts on the many (and at least partly inherited) differences between individual animals.

next-generation sequencing (NGS) – The sequencing of millions of small fragments of DNA from an individual animal at the same time resulting in rapid sequencing of genomes or genomic regions at low cost.

nick – When two breeds or lines combine well when crossed. *See* combining ability.

non-additive genetic variance (or variation) – Variance (or variation) in a trait due to the combined effects of genes with non-additive action, e.g. dominance.

non-homologous end joining (NHEJ) – A laboratory method to repair the DNA at a cut site in the absence of a homologous template which will result in small insertions or deletions at the cut site.

normally-distributed trait – A trait which has measured values evenly distributed about the mean with a 'bell-shaped' pattern, and the peak being at the mean.

nuclear transfer – Transfer of cells from an embryo, or from cell culture, into an unfertilized egg from which the nucleus has been removed. A method of producing clones.

nucleus (cell) – The part of a cell containing the chromosomes.

nucleus (herd, flock or population) – A group of highly selected animals; animals of high genetic merit.

nucleus breeding scheme – A breeding scheme in which recording and selection are concentrated on an elite (nucleus) group of animals. These may be in a central herd or flock or dispersed over several herds or flocks.

numerator relationship matrix – *See* additive genetic relationship matrix.

observational component of variance – Variance due to the genetic relationship among the groups in a genetic analysis. For instance, an ANOVA for half sib data has sires, and dams nested within sires, as sources of variance. The sire and dam variances estimated from the expected mean squares are referred to as the observational components of variance.

oligogenic – A trait controlled by multiple genes but typically including one or more gene(s) of major effect.

'omics' – A general term used to indicate a group of disciplines based around molecular genetics; incudes genomics, transcriptomics, proteomics, metabolomics, and so on.

overdominance – Type of gene action in which the performance of heterozygous animals exceeds that of both homozygous types (e.g. the Inverdale fertility gene in sheep).

ovum pick up (OPU) – Collection of eggs from donors through an ultrasonically guided needle inserted into the ovary.

partial dominance – The type of gene action in which the performance of heterozygotes is closest to that of animals homozygous for one of the alleles concerned (e.g. the Booroola gene with respect to litter size).

paternal heterosis – Heterosis in reproductive performance as a result of sires being crossbred.

pedigree – A record of the ancestry of an animal.

pedigree (registered) animal – An animal whose ancestry is known, or more usually, whose ancestry is recorded by a breed society or similar organization.

pedigree (stud) breeder – A breeder of purebred animals who usually registers details of these, especially ancestry, with a breed society or similar organization.

pedigree index – An index combining information on ancestors' performance/breeding values.

pedigree selection – Selection based on ancestors' information.

performance test – A comparison of (and subsequently selection amongst) animals based on their own performance, commonly from groups of animals kept together.

permanent environmental effects – Non-genetic effects which influence an animal's performance throughout its life.

phenotype – Outward appearance (e.g. coat colour), or performance of animals measured in some way (e.g. milk yield). In some cases the phenotype is determined solely by the genotype (e.g. coat colour). In many other cases it is the result of both genetic and non-genetic (environmental) factors and many genes.

phenotypic correlation – A measure of the direction and strength of the association between observed performance, or phenotype, in two characters, e.g. live weight and fat depth measured on the same animals (range from –1 to +1).

physical map (mapping) – A map showing the physical location of genes or markers on individual chromosomes.

plasticity – When some genotypes may perform differently in different environments.

pleiotropy – Occurs when an allele at a single locus influences more than one characteristic of the animal (e.g. the double muscling gene in cattle affects both muscularity and fertility).

polygenic traits – Traits under the control of many loci, each typically of small effect.

polymerase chain reaction (PCR) – A method of rapidly multiplying sequences of DNA 'in a test tube' rather than in living cells.

polymorphism – Different versions of a gene or base.

polyploidy – When a cell or an organism has more than two sets of chromosomes.

predicted breeding value (PBV) – Prediction of the additive genetic merit of an animal. May be based on various sources of information including the animal's own performance, and that of its relatives, and on genomic information. Double the expected deviation in progeny performance compared to the population mean.

predicted transmitting ability (PTA) – Prediction of the additive genetic merit of an animal. May be based on various sources of information including the animal's own performance, and that of its relatives, and on genomic information. The expected deviation in progeny performance compared to the population mean (i.e. half of the predicted breeding value).

primer – A short, single-stranded DNA sequence used in the polymerase chain reaction.

primordial germ cells – Highly specialized cells that form the gametes; after meiosis they become sperm or ova.

probe – *See* DNA probe.

progeny test or testing – A comparison of animals (and subsequently selection amongst them) based on the performance of their progeny.

Punnett square – A pictorial representation (named after its inventor) used in Mendelian genetics to show all possible offspring genotypes from matings between parents of two specific genotypes. Used to calculate genotypic (segregation) ratios from specific matings.

purebred (straightbred) – Animal with both parents of the same breed.

purebreeding – The practice of mating animals belonging to the same breed.

qualitative characteristics – Characteristics like coat colour and polledness, where the animals can be divided into discrete types with no intermediates. These traits are often entirely controlled by genes and are unaffected by non-genetic influences. Also used to describe a trait which is based on judgement rather than measurement.

quantitative characteristics – Characteristics that are either expressed in units which can be counted (e.g. numbers of lambs born or weaned, number of services per conception) or, more often, measured on a continuous scale (e.g. kg of live weight, litres of milk, mm of fat) rather than falling into discrete categories. Most of these quantitative traits are affected by many genes, rather than single genes. Additionally, most of these traits are affected, to a greater or lesser extent, by non-genetic influences. Also known as metric, polygenic or complex traits.

quantitative trait locus (QTL) – A locus affecting a quantitative trait such as milk yield and quality, growth rate or wool production.

random effect – A term used in a statistical model comprising a sample of the possible large number of levels, e.g. animals in a population.

random regression – A statistical method used to account for variation between repeated measurements on a particular trait for individual animals. It is used for traits which vary across, for example, time or age periods. For instance test day milk yield throughout lactation or body weight at several ages.

reaction norm – A measure of plasticity describing how the performance of a genotype varies across a range of environments. Often analysed using random regression.

recessive – A type of gene action where the effect of the gene is only seen in the phenotype of individuals homozygous for that gene/allele.

recombination (crossing over) – The crossing over of segments of the maternally-derived and paternally-derived members of a pair of chromosomes during meiosis.

recombination loss – The loss of heterosis as a result of the breakdown of favourable 'epistatic blocks' of alleles from parental breeds, where these blocks have been established by many generations of selection.

reference genome – A digital nucleic acid sequence database, assembled by scientists as a representative example of a species' genetic makeup, commonly derived from a single animal.

reference population – Population of animals used in genome mapping or to detect useful associations between markers and traits of economic importance.

reference population (for genomic selection) – In genomic selection, the population of animals which have both genotypes and phenotypes, where the genetic marker effects are estimated, and the data are then used to predict breeding values for selection candidates.

regression coefficient – A statistic which measures the direction and strength of association between two characters, or between the same character at different times, or between the same character on related animals. Regression coefficients measure the rate of change in one character per unit change in another character, in the units of measurement.

relationship matrix – *See* additive genetic relationship matrix.

reliability of predicted breeding values (or transmitting abilities) – The squared accuracy of PBVs, i.e. the squared correlation between predicted and true breeding values (or transmitting abilities).

repeatability – The correlation between repeated records from the same animal – a measure of the value of repeated records in selection.

residual (or error) variance – A term fitted in most statistical models to account for unattributable variation between animals.

response (to selection) – The change in the mean performance in a population of animals as a result of selection. Usually measured per annum or per generation using EBVs.

restricted maximum likelihood (REML) – A statistical method to estimate variance components taking environmental factors into account.

restriction enzymes – Enzymes produced by bacteria, which are capable of 'cutting up' sequences of DNA. Different restriction enzymes 'recognize' different sequences, usually of four to eight base pairs long in DNA.

restriction fragment length polymorphism (RFLP) – Variation between animals in the number and position of sites at which a given restriction enzyme will cut the DNA. RFLP can be used to detect variation in the DNA sequence of different animals, and hence they were used as markers in genome mapping – a task more commonly carried out with SNP markers now.

Ribonucleic acid (RNA) – Molecules similar to DNA which carry out many functions in the cell, such as the coding, decoding, regulation and expression of genes. Commonly derived from a DNA template, these molecules can exist in the cell as a single strand (unlike DNA).

ribosomes – Small structures in the cytoplasm of cells responsible for assembling amino acids to produce proteins, using instructions from genes carried by messenger RNA. Ribosomes are the cell's 'protein factories'.

rolling base – The group of animals (e.g. the most recent age group included in an evaluation) from which deviations in breeding value are expressed. This group usually changes at each evaluation.

rotational crossing – This involves the use of the same two or three (or more) breeds in successive generations in a crossbreeding programme.

runs of homozygosity (ROH) – Lengths of the genome which contain identical haplotypes on both chromosomes.

Sanger sequencing – The process of determining the order of nucleotides in DNA developed by Frederick Sanger. It is based on the selective incorporation of chain-terminating dideoxynucleotides by DNA polymerase during *in vitro* DNA replication. It can only sequence a single DNA fragment at a time.

seedstock/stud breeder/herd/flock – *See* elite breeder/herd/flock.

segregation – The separation and chance sampling of paternally- and maternally-derived genes during meiosis in the production of a sperm or egg.

segregation distortion – A phenomenon where the observed genotype frequencies at a locus fall outside the expected Mendelian segregation ratio.

segregation ratios – The ratios of different offspring genotypes expected from matings between particular parental genotypes.

selection between breeds or strains – *See* between-breed selection.

selection criterion (criteria) – The measurement(s) on which selection is based (e.g. live weight at a certain age, egg weight, fleece weight). May contain several traits, particularly when index selection is used.

selection differential – The difference between the mean performance of selected animals (i.e. those identified to become parents of the next generation) and the overall mean of the group of animals from which they were selected.

selection index – An overall score of genetic merit which combines information on several measured traits, and/or from different classes of relatives. The emphasis on each trait in the index usually depends on the strength of its association with traits in the breeding goal, and the relative economic values of breeding goal traits.

selection intensity (i) – The superiority of animals selected (the selection differential) expressed in standard deviation units.

selection limit or plateau – The point at which no further response to selection can be achieved, as a result of exhaustion of genetic variation in the trait under selection. A state not commonly reached in livestock breeding.

selection objective – *See* breeding goal.

selection within breeds or strains – *See* within-breed selection.

selective sweeps – Stretches of the chromosome which contain identical runs of homozygosity in all animals within a breed/population. Often indicative of a breed characteristic being located on that stretch of DNA.

semen (or embryo) sexing – Sorting of semen (or embryos) by a variety of methods according to whether they are carrying X or Y chromosomes.

sequence – In genomics, the order of DNA bases on a segment of a chromosome or the whole genome.

sequential hermaphrodites – Where an individual in a species is born as one sex but can later change into the opposite sex.

sex-influenced gene action – When expression of a gene is influenced by the sex of the animal, without the gene being sex-linked or the trait sex-limited, e.g. presence of horns in some sheep breeds.

sex-limited gene action – When expression of a gene is influenced by the sex of the animal, as the trait is only measurable in one sex, e.g. milk yield.

sex-linked gene – A gene located on one of the sex chromosomes.

shotgun sequencing – A laboratory method for the analysis of DNA sequences longer than 1,000 base pairs, up to and including entire chromosomes. This requires the target DNA to be broken into random fragments. After sequencing individual fragments, the sequences can be reassembled on the basis of their overlapping regions but the assembly is complex, particularly with sequence repeats often causing gaps in the genome assembly.

sibs (siblings) – Animals with one or both parents in common, i.e. brothers or sisters. Full sibs have both parents in common, half sibs have only one parent in common.

sib test (sib selection) – A comparison of animals (and subsequently selection amongst them) based on the performance of siblings.

signatures of selection – Regions of the genome which are conserved over many generations due to the fact that they confer enhanced fitness or productive ability to individuals in the population. Such conserved regions are thus preferentially kept in the population, with the frequency of favorable alleles, and of particular haplotypes in the region, driven towards fixation.

single nucleotide polymorphism (SNP; pronounced 'snip') – Variation in DNA sequence in the genome occurring when the single nucleotide (adenine, thymine, cytosine or guanine) present at a specific base position differs between individuals. *See* single nucleotide variant.

single nucleotide variant (SNV) – A base position derived from NGS data where there is a different base in some individuals compared to the reference genome. *See* single nucleotide polymorphism.

single-step method – A statistical method to estimate genomic breeding values which combines all available pedigree and performance data with genotypes from a subset of animals.

single-trait BLUP – A BLUP model used to estimate breeding values for one trait.

sire-maternal grandsire model – A method of genetic evaluation using only sires and maternal grandsires in the pedigree.

sire model – A genetic analysis using the sires of measured animals as the main genetic group.

Previously used quite commonly but largely superseded by the animal model now.

SNP key – When estimating genomic breeding values we calculate a set of equations that relate SNP information for the reference set of sires with their offspring average performance. Solving this set of equations provides the solutions for the SNPs which we call the SNP key.

SNP marker – A SNP used to indicate where a change in base affects a trait of interest.

social interaction model – Animals have the phenotypic ability to compete for resources, which is termed the social interaction effect. It has a genetic component and an environmental component. This model is used in genetic evaluations for these sorts of traits using BLUP equations such that PBV effects due to the direct effects of the genes of the individual and those due to the associative effect are estimated simultaneously.

standard deviation – A statistical measure of a population describing the spread of measured values about their mean (average). The square root of the variance.

standard deviation of true breeding values – Another name for the additive genetic standard deviation.

structural annotation – A process identifying the position of genomic elements on the genome (e.g. genes).

suckler cows – Cows rearing their own young in beef production.

surrogate-sire technology – A laboratory method used in the creation of males that lack their own germline cells. Instead, they possess transplanted spermatogonial stem cells from other donor males. The recipient males have their germline ablated, e.g. via genome-editing-targeted knockout of the genes essential for germ cell development.

tandem selection – A method of selection for more than one trait. Involves selection for one trait for one or more generations, followed by selection for a second trait for one or more generations, possibly followed by selection on more traits, eventually returning to selection on the first, and so on. Largely superseded by index selection.

temporary environmental effects – Non-genetic effects which have a relatively short impact on animal performance, e.g. affecting only one lactation, or one weight record.

terminal sire – Sire, strain or breed selected for specialized meat production characteristics.

test day records – Milk records obtained on sampling days (usually at monthly intervals) which are usually then used to predict full lactation yields of milk, fat and protein in milk-recording schemes.

threshold model – A statistical method used to analyse a polygenic trait with two or more states which has an underlying normally-distributed liability, e.g. disease susceptibility measured as susceptible or not susceptible.

transcription – The first step in gene expression involving the copying of a gene's DNA sequence to make an RNA molecule using enzymes called RNA polymerases.

transfer RNA – A type of RNA involved in transporting free amino acids in the cell to ribosomes for assembling proteins.

transformation (mathematical) – An arithmetic method to convert data with a skewed distribution to being normally distributed. Common methods include taking the log, square root, etc.

transgene – A gene from another organism inserted into the genome of an animal.

transgenic (animal) – A genetically modified animal whose genome contains 'foreign' DNA, e.g. from another animal of a different breed or species.

translation – The second stage of gene expression, after transcription, when the ribosomes in the cytoplasm synthesize proteins from the RNA in the cell's nucleus.

triplet – A sequence of three bases in DNA which codes for the production of a particular amino acid (the building blocks which proteins are made from), or signals where a gene stops or starts.

two-stage selection – Selection amongst animals initially on one trait (or set of traits) and then, amongst the remaining animals, on a second trait (or set). Two-stage selection is usually practised when a second trait (or set of traits) becomes available later in life, or when it is too expensive or difficult to measure on all animals.

two-step procedure – A statistical procedure to calculate GEBVs. Firstly, conventional BLUP is carried out for all animals in the population with performance records and pedigree records. Secondly, the DGVs of the younger animals from

GBLUP or SNP-BLUP are combined with the parent averages from the conventional BLUP evaluations using their reliabilities as weights.

validation animals (or population or set) – The group of animals used to verify the accuracy of genomic prediction after computing SNP solutions in the reference population. In the validation animals, genomic breeding values are computed based only on their genotypes and this is correlated with their de-regressed breeding values or yield deviations to estimate accuracy.

variable expressivity – Type of gene action in which animals show the expected phenotype, but to varying degrees (e.g. mulefoot in cattle and pigs).

variance – A statistical measure of a population describing the spread of measured values about their mean (average). The standard deviation squared.

variance components – Measures of variation associated with random variables in livestock populations. See Table 6.2 for an extensive list of different variance components relevant to livestock data.

variant – A change in sequence at a particular base position (or positions) compared to the reference genome.

whole genome sequence (WGS) – The order of bases along the genome of an animal from the beginning of Chromosome 1 to the end of the last chromosome.

wild type – The phenotype or genotype of an animal as it naturally occurs in the wild.

within-breed selection – The process of genetic improvement by selecting animals of the best genetic merit within a particular breed as parents of the next generation.

within-family selection – A method of organizing a selection programme to minimize inbreeding. It starts by dividing the population into 'families' in a notional circle, and then keep female replacements in the family in which they were born, but move replacement males from the family in which they were born, to the next family in the circle.

Index

Page numbers in **bold** type refer to figures and tables.

www.ingramcontent.com/pod-product-compliance
Lightning Source LLC
LaVergne TN
LVHW070845210926
848482LV00016B/871